Osteoporosis Rehabilitation

Christina V. Oleson

Osteoporosis Rehabilitation

A Practical Approach

Springer

Christina V. Oleson, MD
Department of Rehabilitation Medicine
Thomas Jefferson University
Philadelphia, PA, USA

ISBN 978-3-319-45082-7 ISBN 978-3-319-45084-1 (eBook)
DOI 10.1007/978-3-319-45084-1

Library of Congress Control Number: 2016958117

Printed on acid-free paper

This Springer imprint is published by Springer Nature
The registered company is Springer International Publishing AG
The registered company address is: Gewerbestrasse 11, 6330 Cham, Switzerland

To my mother, Alexandra,

without whom

neither I nor this book

would be possible.

Thank you for teaching me

how to write and how to live.

Foreword

Osteoporosis is a major public health problem in America. Twenty-four million people, 80 % of whom are women, are afflicted with the disease: 10 million already suffer from osteoporosis, and 14 million experience low bone mass and other risk factors that can lead to this condition. It is also a worldwide health problem with 200 million people affected. Initial fracture is the major risk factor for the next fracture that may occur. Therefore, it behooves not only orthopedic surgeons but physiatrists and internists to be well aware of all aspects of the condition. Dr. Oleson has brilliantly outlined multiple aspects of the disease across 20 chapters of her single-authored book, which is well written, comprehensive, and easy to read, from the etiology, physiology, epidemiology, and pathophysiology to diagnosis, prevention, interventions, and treatments. Particularly interesting and unique to me are the descriptions of osteoporosis in men, the effects of neurologic disease on osteoporosis, and the treatment after spinal injury as well as the impact of rheumatologic disease, gastrointestinal disease, and bariatric surgery on osteoporosis.

This is clearly a seminal work and something that practitioners of every variety need to have on their shelf and turn to in treating patients with this incredibly important disease. The economies of the free world cannot afford to be unaware of such a significant public health issue. Dr. Oleson's book will help us with the awareness, treatment, and prevention of osteoporosis. I look forward to having the book on my shelf and sharing it with my residents and colleagues at our hospital who treat rheumatologic and metabolic bone disease.

Sincerely,

Todd J. Albert, MD
Surgeon in Chief and Medical Director
Hospital for Special Surgery
New York, NY, USA

Preface and Acknowledgments

When I first began to write about osteoporosis, it was meant to be a chapter in a rehabilitation textbook. But I found that I had much more to say. My initial ideas have now taken shape as a book unto itself with a clearly defined purpose: to assess the current state of our knowledge about osteoporosis and to make these findings available to the broad community of professionals who serve those afflicted with the disease. The central focus of this undertaking is the transition from the diagnosis of osteoporosis to early treatment, extended rehabilitation, and comprehensive management options.

This volume offers an expansive perspective, beginning with causes and consequences of the disease as such and extending to its manifestations within the context of related disorders as well as its wider professional, social, and economic ramifications. The concentric circles of osteoporosis, given in Fig. 1. of the opening chapter, delineate this construct. Several crosscutting themes, based on research and practice conducted in recent decades, emerge from this analysis. Some are based on new scientific findings such as the growing prominence of the concept of "bone quality" to supplement "bone density" as a measure of skeletal health. Others center on technological advances that have led to more effective tools for diagnosing and measuring the progress of osteoporosis, thereby promoting earlier assessments of the disease and improving quality of life. In addition, innovative, interdisciplinary approaches have enabled physicians, nurses, nutritionists, physical and occupational therapists, and pharmacists to bring their varying expertise to bear on the individual needs of patients. New medications directed at both prevention and treatment are continually emerging, with promising results. Medical and public awareness of the scope of osteoporosis, particularly its occurrence in men, and of the need to improve adherence to both nonpharmacologic and pharmacologic therapies is increasing, but still needs to improve. It is hoped that this book will advance understanding of these issues on a general level and provide a guide for those seeking to learn more in detail about the different manifestations of the disease.

In this undertaking, I have benefited from the insight, guidance, and hard work of a number of people. In the first instance, I want to express my appreciation to colleagues who have contributed to several chapters related to their specialized interests: Amanda Morina, PT, DPT; Tracy Ransom, PsyD; Mendel Kupfer, MD; and Akinpelumi Beckley, MD.

To readers who reviewed and critiqued individual chapters, I am indebted to Alec Beekley, MD; Robert Downie, MD; and Edward Filippone, MD.

Matthew DeLuca, BA; Devarshi Desai, BS; Sylvester Douglas, DO; Brittany Hayes, MS; Pengcheng Lu, MD, PhD; Maheen Rana, BS; Jacquelyn White, BA; and Rosalind West, PT, DPT, provided invaluable assistance in article identification, manuscript preparation, and technical production.

Special thanks are due to my colleagues in the Department of Rehabilitation and the Spinal Cord Injury Center at Thomas Jefferson University for their support, particularly my immediate working partners, Ralph J. Marino, MD, and Kristopher J. Feeko, DO. Finally, I am enormously grateful to the patients I serve whose medical needs and experiences influenced my writing.

It was a pleasure to collaborate with all of these individuals, and I am beholden to them for their dedication to this effort.

Philadelphia, PA, USA Christina V. Oleson, MD

Contents

About the Author

Christina V. Oleson MD is an Associate Professor of Rehabilitation Medicine at Thomas Jefferson University, Philadelphia PA. She is board-certified in both Physical Medicine/Rehabilitation and in Spinal Cord Injury Medicine. She earned her BA from Harvard University and her MD at the University of Massachusetts Worcester. Following completion of residency in Physical Medicine and Rehabilitation at Thomas Jefferson University, Dr. Oleson pursued a Spinal Cord Injury Medicine fellowship at the Rehabilitation Institute of Chicago of Northwestern University. Her current research focuses on immobilization osteoporosis in those with traumatic spinal cord injury. She serves as the principal investigator in a NIDLRR-funded investigational study examining the benefit of an agent to prevent osteoporosis in newly-injured spinal cord patients. Dr. Oleson has published numerous scientific articles and chapters, covering aspects of spinal cord injury, osteoporosis, and vitamin D deficiency.

Contributors

Akinpelumi A. Beckley, MD Department of Rehabilitation and Regenerative Medicine, Columbia University Medical Center, New York, NY, USA. (Dr. Beckley served as a contributing author for Chapter 7)

Mendel Kupfer, MD Department of Rehabilitation Medicine, Thomas Jefferson University/Magee Rehabilitation Hospital, Philadelphia, PA, USA. (Dr. Kupfer served as the primary author for Chapter 11)

Amanda B. Morina, PT, DPT, ATP, NCS Department of Physical Therapy, Thomas Jefferson University/Magee Rehabilitation Hospital, Philadelphia, PA, USA. (Ms. Morina served as the secondary author of Chapters 2, 4, 5, and 15)

Tracy E. Ransom, PsyD Department of Rehabilitation Medicine, Thomas Jefferson University/Magee Rehabilitation Hospital, Philadelphia, PA, USA. (Dr. Ransom served as the secondary author of Chapters 7 and 19)

Chapter 1
Introduction to Osteoporosis

Christina V. Oleson

Osteoporosis is a skeletal condition involving progressive bone loss and microarchitectural deterioration, leading to increased bone fragility and susceptibility to fractures. It is the most prevalent metabolic bone disease among adults worldwide. The magnitude of the disease is immense. A 2014 study of Americans aged 50 and older estimated that 10.2 million US adults have osteoporosis at the femoral neck and lumbar spine and another 43.4 million have low bone mass, meaning that over one-half of the total US adult population is affected [1]. Approximately 8.2 million women and 2.0 million men had osteoporosis and another 27.3 million women and 16.1 million men had low bone mass. As the number of older Americans continues to increase, these numbers are likely to increase markedly.

Osteoporosis has become one of the leading health problems of the elderly and those with medical conditions adversely affecting bone. In 2015, the first study to examine the *global* burden of fracture probability [2] projected that by 2040, approximately 319 million people will be at risk of fracture compared to 158 million in 2010. In the United States, over two million fragility fractures occur annually at an estimated cost of $19 million in direct medical care for prevention and treatment [3]. Singer et al. have estimated that osteoporotic fractures among postmenopausal women resulted in more than a half-million hospitalizations, 800,000 emergency room visits, and 180,000 nursing home admissions [4]. Moreover, they indicated that fracture incidence in these women is greater than that of heart attack, stroke, and breast cancer combined.

On a practical level, physicians encounter a number of different circumstances in dealing with osteoporosis. Often patients arrive for treatment only after encountering an acute consequence of the disease such as a hip fracture. Many do not realize that they may have had osteoporosis for years. In these cases, therapy must be aggressive but comprehensive planning for future care is also essential. In other instances, patients with adverse medical conditions such as acute stroke present for rehabilitation, yet they too may already have subclinical osteoporosis requiring

C.V. Oleson, *Osteoporosis Rehabilitation*, DOI 10.1007/978-3-319-45084-1_1

early management and future prevention. Not only are they at increased risk of falls as a result of recent medical events, but given their weak bones, they will continue to be at high risk for fractures. Some patients may have experienced a traumatic event including a head or spinal cord injury. Even if they are relatively young and their bones are healthy, they face months, perhaps even years, of immobilization which is detrimental to bone health. Little information is available to help clinicians distinguish among specific individual needs. A key objective of this volume is to help fill that void.

This book presents an overview of our current understanding of osteoporosis together with a discussion of existing and promising treatment options in the form of nutrition, medication, surgery, physical therapy, and lifestyle changes. Whereas much of the current literature on osteoporosis focuses on physiology and epidemiology, this analysis is directed at the critical association among causal factors, diagnosis, early treatment, and subsequent rehabilitation—an approach that has received only limited attention. It discusses the range of circumstances surrounding osteoporosis, emphasizing the need to consider the ramifications of this "silent disease" in the context of other disorders that both admittedly and ostensibly demand greater attention.

This text is organized into four divisions (Fig. 1). *Part I (chapters 2–6)* deals with the defining characteristics of osteoporosis, encompassing causes and risk factors; diagnostic tools and tests; and preventative measures including dietary supplements, exercise, and nonpharmacologic, pharmacologic, and surgical interventions to treat osteoporosis. A special chapter is devoted to osteoporosis in men, recognizing that men account for one-third of hip fractures worldwide and face higher mortality rates compared with women [5].

Part II (chapters 7–11) considers adult osteoporosis in the context of its neurological comorbidities, including disorders of the brain, spinal cord, and peripheral neuropathies.

Part III (chapters 12–16) examines medical comorbidities, ranging from rheumatologic disorders to cardiopulmonary, liver and kidney diseases, and cancer. A brief description of the coexistent disease precedes a more detailed analysis of the nature, severity, and treatment of osteoporosis as it occurs in each case. Although different diseases present different challenges, several commonalities should be noted. Age is, of course, a prevailing factor. Since osteoporosis is most closely associated with the aging process, patients are likely to have experienced or are in the midst of experiencing other diseases and disorders that will affect osteoporosis diagnosis and treatment. Too often, physicians and specialists tend to focus on the "primary disease," leaving osteoporosis, if present, to stand by silently. Drugs and other therapies for many of these diseases also may have a detrimental effect on bone health. Advances in treating illnesses that once resulted in death at a much earlier age have now expanded life spans, increasing the prospect of developing osteoporosis. To deal with concomitant disorders, a multidisciplinary approach is now a priority.

Part IV (chapters 17–19) centers on the onset of osteoporosis in childhood and adolescence and its progression into adulthood. In such cases, a common challenge

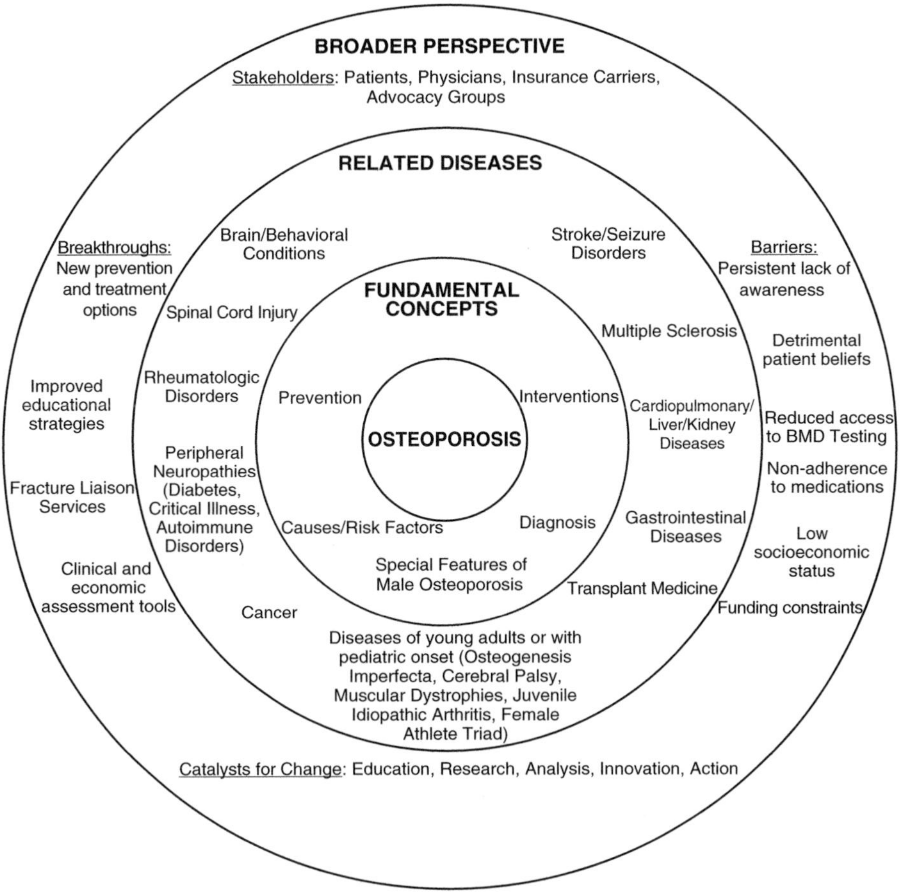

Fig. 1 The concentric circles of osteoporosis: Fundamental concepts, related diseases, and broader dimensions of osteoporosis

is posed by the transition to adult care, when a family-centered, supportive approach gives way to a more detached, impersonal environment demanding greater responsibility on the part of the patient. Planning for a smooth transition requires a multipronged approach rooted in close collaboration between pediatric and adult providers. This organization is illustrated in Fig. 1.

The final chapter considers the broader dimensions of osteoporosis—from the impact on its immediate stakeholders to its long-term economic and social consequences. The burden of osteoporosis reaches far beyond the individual patient to nations across the world, with Asia and Latin American recently emerging as areas of great concern. Osteoporosis is not inevitable. Advanced diagnostic technologies and improved therapies ensure that it is both preventable and treatable. What is needed is greater awareness of its consequences as well as determined action to advance adherence to treatment options, patient and physician education, and promising research.

References

1. Wright NC, Looker AC, Saag KG, Curtis JR, Deizell ES, Randall S, et al. The recent prevalence of osteoporosis and low bone mass in the United States based on bone mineral density at the femoral neck and lumbar spine. J Bone Miner Res. 2014;29(11):2520–6.
2. Oden A, McCloskey EV, Kanis JA, Harvey NC, Johansson H. Burden of high fracture probability worldwide: secular increases 2010–2040. Osteoporos Int. 2015;26:2243–8. doi:10.1007/s00198-015-3154-6.
3. Ajayi A, Powell M, Obremskey WT, Jahangir A, Sethi MK. Osteoporosis: the orthopaedic health policy perspective. AAOS Now. 2012:1–4. http://www.aaos.org/AAOSNow/2012/Jan/advocacy/advocacy6/?ssopc=1.
4. Singer A, Exuzides A, Spangler L, O'Malley C, Colby C, Johnston K, et al. Burden of illness for osteoporotic fractures compared with other serious diseases among postmenopausal women in the United States. Mayo Clin Proc. 2015;90 9(1):53–62.
5. Eberling P. Osteoporosis in men, why change needs to happen. International Osteoporosis Foundation. 2014. http://share.iofbonehealth.org/WOD/2014/thematic-report/WOD14-Report.pdf. Accessed 3 Sep 2015.

Chapter 2
Causes and Risk Factors of Osteoporosis

Christina V. Oleson and Amanda B. Morina

Bone is a complex matrix of organic collagen upon which inorganic hydroxyapatite, composed of calcium and phosphate, is layered. The internal collagen, often referred to as the scaffolding of bone, has a triple helical, lamellar arrangement that is further cross-linked by a compound of collagen fibers termed pyridinolines. Bone undergoes periodic remodeling—the dual processes of bone formation and resorption—through the action of multicellular units comprised of two types of bone cells—osteoblasts and osteoclasts. Osteoblast cells initially build and continually replace bone throughout the life span; osteoclast cells remove weakened sections of bone. Remodeling leads to thicker and stronger bones until approximately the age of 25; subsequently bone is essentially maintained or slowly lost until age 50 when effects of aging and hormonal changes occur (Fig. 1) [1, 2].

Pathophysiology

Osteoporosis is caused by the excessive breakdown of bone structure, inadequate bone formation, or an imbalance in the activity between the bone cells responsible for bone remodeling. It results from the increased number or activity of osteoclasts, the cells of bone resorption; the decreased number or activity of osteoblasts, the cells of bone formation; or areas of bone that demonstrate both of these abnormal bone cell characteristics [3]. Osteoporosis is evaluated by a bone mineral density (BMD) test which measures the amount of mineral per square centimeter and can be performed by a number of radiological densitometry procedures, most often dual energy x-ray absorptiometry (DXA) [4]. The most common areas evaluated are the lumbar spine or proximal hip and distal radius. With osteoporosis, bone mineral density is decreased due to the breakdown of bone without compensatory, subsequent remodeling [5].

C.V. Oleson, *Osteoporosis Rehabilitation*, DOI 10.1007/978-3-319-45084-1_2

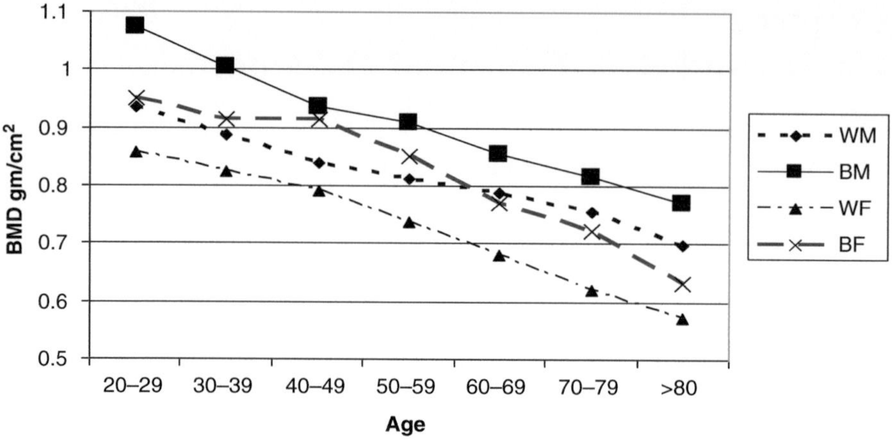

Fig. 1 Mean BMD at the femoral neck by age in the United States, *WM* white males, *WF* white females, *BM* black males, *BF* black females (*Source*: Data from Looker AC)

Compromised bone density results in decreased ability to withstand trauma. Bone loss can accelerate rapidly in certain conditions of high bone turnover such as menopause when estrogen levels fall sharply, neoplasia, metabolic abnormalities, or sudden immobility such as spinal cord injury (SCI) [6]. Bone fractures may occur with minimal external trauma forces such as a mechanical fall or internal trauma resulting from the force of a cough or sneeze. Due to weakened microarchitecture of bone and normal forces of gravity and routine, daily activities can result in spontaneous fractures, particularly in vulnerable populations.

The anatomical characteristics of bone in certain regions of the body can cause increased susceptibility to damage from osteoporosis. Although 80 % of the total skeleton is comprised of densely packed cortical bone, this type of bone is principally found in outer layers of long bones of the appendicular skeleton and is designed for structural support. Cortical bone has low bone turnover rates and is thus less likely to fracture than trabecular bone [7]. Characterized by increased porosity and reduced tensile strength, trabecular bone is heavily concentrated in the axial skeleton of the spine and is constantly being shaped and remodeled. Both the appendicular and axial skeleton are at risk of a fracture after a fall or other sustained trauma [7].

Epidemiology

Osteoporosis has generally been divided into two categories: primary and secondary osteoporosis. Primary osteoporosis is age related, affects 95 % of women and about 80 % of men, and is related to estrogen loss in women and a testosterone deficiency in men; other factors include low calcium and vitamin D intake as well as hyperparathyroidism. In contrast, secondary osteoporosis stems from other conditions including hormonal imbalances, diseases, and medications that predispose to bone

Table 1 Risk factors in the development of osteoporosis

Controllable	Uncontrollable
Inadequate dietary calcium or vitamin D	Age >75 years
Inadequate fruit and vegetable consumption	Female
Excessive protein, sodium, or phosphorous intake	Postmenopausal
Sedentary lifestyle	Family history
Ethyl alcohol (EtOH)	Low body weight/thin build
Smoking	Genetics
Weight loss	Hormonal levels (may be controlled with medications if diagnosed)
Medications	Environment with low sunlight

loss. It may arise at any age and affects both men and women [8]. The risk of osteoporosis and its severity is influenced by a variety of controllable and uncontrollable factors. Controllable factors include dietary deficiencies in vitamin D and calcium and in certain fruits and vegetables that enhance calcium absorption by limiting urinary excretion of calcium; in contrast, diets high in animal protein or sodium favor calciuria or bodily elimination of calcium through urine. Vitamin D is essential for calcium absorption which, if impaired, leads to an increase in parathyroid hormone (PTH) produced by the parathyroid glands. If calcium levels are low, these glands, the most important regulators of calcium levels in the blood, respond by secreting more PTH, resulting in increased calcium levels which, in turn, trigger bone resorption [9]. Other controllable factors range from high caffeine intake and an inactive lifestyle to smoking, alcohol consumption, and intentional weight loss beyond one's ideal body weight or implemented at the expense of overall nutritional status [1, 6]. Uncontrollable risk factors include age greater than 75 years old, female gender, postmenopausal status, family history of osteoporosis, and low body weight, thin build, or sudden unintentional weight loss from illness [1, 6].

Gender differences can affect the prevalence and severity of osteoporosis. Beginning at age 40, both sexes lose axial bone mass at relatively slow rates, but women lose bone mass more rapidly because of the onset of menopause in the late 40s or early 50s, contributing to increased risk of fracture to the axial skeleton. For men, who do not experience the sudden loss of gonadal sex steroid secretion, the reduction of reproductive hormones is more gradual, and bone loss occurs at a slower rate [10] (Table 1).

Medications Leading to Osteoporosis

Several medications have been shown to contribute to the development of osteoporosis. Glucocorticoids (aka corticosteroids), the leading secondary cause of osteoporosis, decrease bone formation by downregulating osteoblasts and prolonging their life span [11]. In addition, an inhibitory effect on sex hormones influences bone formation. When used chronically in high doses, glucocorticoids restrict intestinal vitamin D-dependent calcium absorption, increase calcium excretion, and can cause osteomalacia, a softening of bone generally caused by vitamin D deficiency.

Thiazolidinediones given to persons with diabetes mellitus can lead to osteoporosis by their direct action on bone cell differentiation. A Diabetes Outcome Progression Trial (ADOPT) found that patients randomized to rosiglitazone have a higher risk of fractures than those receiving metformin or glyburide [12, 13].

Unfractionated heparin given for greater than one year has been associated with decreased bone formation and increased resorption, but the effects are notably less with low molecular weight heparin [14]. Proton pump inhibitors moderately impede the calcium resorption essential to bone formation; some studies show that H2 blockers have a smaller adverse effect, yet others report a neutral effect [11]. Significant doses of thyroxine suppress thyroid-stimulating hormone (TSH) causing bone loss. Vitamin A (greater than10,000 units/day) and vitamin D (greater than 2,000 units/day) have a similar effect.

Immune modulating drugs can also lead to decreases in BMD. Methotrexate decreases osteoblast activity and bone resorption in a dose-dependent manner. Calmodulin–calcineurin phosphatase inhibitors, used for immunosuppression post organ transplants, have been implicated in osteoporosis because they increase bone turnover; however the exact mechanism is unknown. Their effect is further complicated because they are often used concurrently with glucocorticoids [15, 16]. Long-term use of the antiepileptic drugs (AEDs) carbamazepine, phenobarbital, phenytoin, and valproic acid have been associated with decreased BMD due to elevated vitamin D catabolism, elevated parathyroid hormone, or increased osteoclastic activity [17, 18]. Increasing evidence points to a negative association between antidepressant drugs, particularly selective serotonin reuptake inhibitors (SSRIs), and low bone density coupled with fracture risk. A study of 5,008 adults over the age of 50, conducted by the Canadian Multicentre Osteoporosis Research Group, found that patients taking SSRIs on a daily basis experienced an increased risk of fragility fracture, increased chance of falling, and lower BMD at the hip and spine than those not taking the drugs [19].

Fractures

Statistics show that approximately 50 % of women and 25 % of men will break a bone due to osteoporosis [20]. Worldwide, it is estimated that there are 8.9 million fractures annually, resulting in an osteoporotic fracture every three seconds [21]. A prior fracture is associated with an 86 % increased risk of any future fracture [22]. A 10 % loss of bone mass in the vertebrae can double the risk of vertebral fractures; similarly, a 10 % loss of bone mass in the hip can result in a 2.5 times greater risk of hip fracture [23].

By 2050, the worldwide incidence of hip fracture is projected to increase 310 % in men and 240 % in women, as a result of longer life spans in the developed and developing world [20]. The number of patients hospitalized due to an osteoporotic complication is comparable to the number hospitalized for hypertensive-related heart disease, and the disease causes greater disability than that caused by cancer.

Vertebral Compression Fractures

Vertical compression fractures occur when trauma causes the vertebra in the spine to compress and eventually collapse. Unlike most spine fractures of a traumatic nature, individuals with vertebral compression fractures may present without complaints of pain; indeed, approximately two-thirds of vertebral compression fractures are painless [24]. Regardless of pain intensity, if a vertebral fracture goes unrecognized, it can result in cumulative damage including further breakdown of bone structure, producing loss of vertebral height, increased curving of the spine leading to a "hunchback" deformity (spinal thoracic kyphosis, Fig. 2), and spinal cord compression. Vertebral fractures most often occur in the lower thoracic and upper lumbar portions of the spine because of the higher proportion of trabecular bone to cortical bone [25].

Clinical consequences of an osteoporotic compression fracture range from mild to severe. Significant kyphoscoliosis, a combination of outward curvature (kyphosis) and lateral curvature (scoliosis) of the spine, can lead to decreased pulmonary function from reduced lung surface area [26] or altered sitting or standing posture, resulting in compromised thoracic expansion. Larger fractures in the spine can progress to spinal instability through angulation of the vertebral column. If such changes compromise the spinal canal, cord compression can be observed, creating an urgent need for surgical decompression to avert devastating neurological consequences, including motor or sensory loss [26].

Hip Fractures

Hip fractures account for increased morbidity and mortality in people with osteoporosis. One in four adults who lived independently before their hip fracture is forced to reside in a nursing home for at least a year after injury. Approximately one in five hip fracture patients dies within a year of injury, and only 60 % of patients with a hip fracture return to their pre-fracture functional level [27].

The hip is a ball-and-socket joint linking two bones, the thighbone or femur and the pelvis; the ball is the head of the femur while the socket is a curved section of the pelvic bone. There are three types of high fractures. *Intracapsular fractures* occur near the neck and head of the femur, generally within the capsule, the soft tissue envelope that contains the lubricating and nourishing fluid of the high joint. By pressing on blood vessels, it may cut off blood circulation to the ball of the hip. *Intertrochanteric fractures* occur about 3–4 inches away from the joint, between the neck of the femur and a lower projection of bone called the lesser trochanter, an "attachment point" for one of the major muscles of the hip (Fig. 3). This type of fracture does not restrict blood flow to the femur. *Subtrochanteric fractures* occur even further down the bone, below the lower trochanter (Fig. 4) [28].

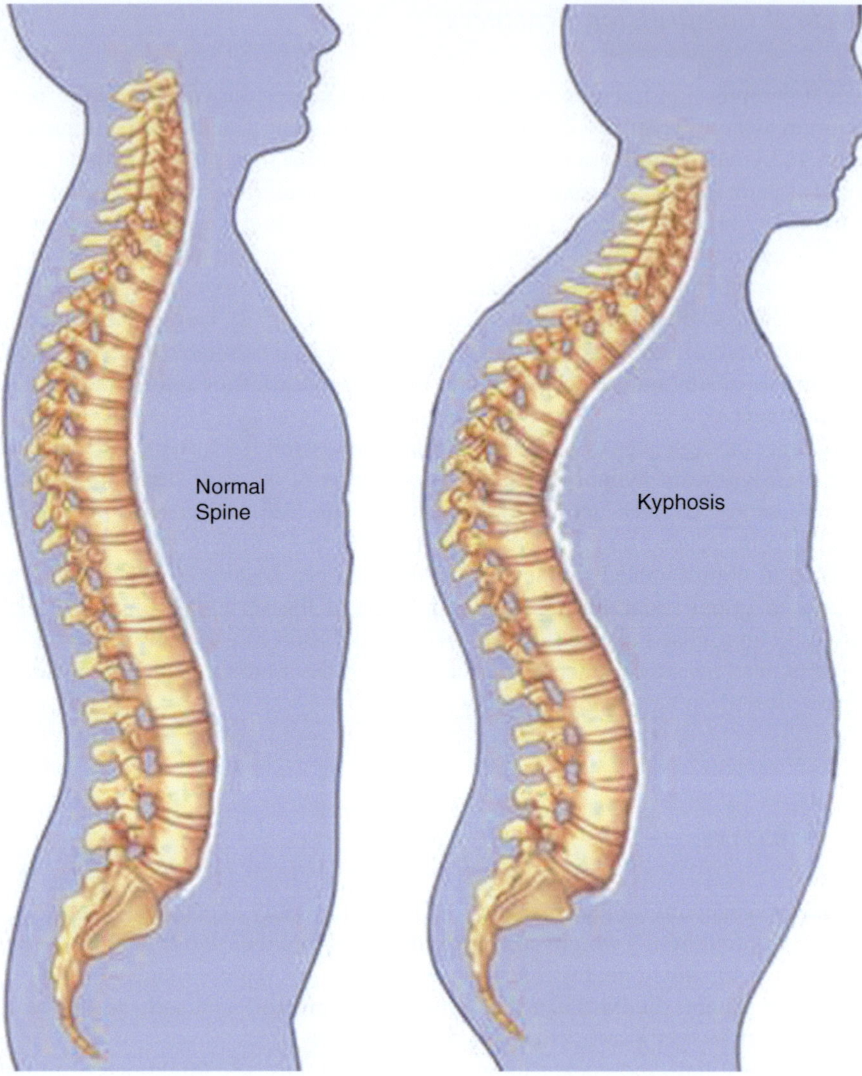

Fig. 2 Image showing a normal and kyphotic spine (*Source*: Used with permission from Mayo Clinic Foundation for Education and Research)

Anatomic Changes

Pain due to osteoporosis can be acute, progressive, or chronic [29]. As bones become increasingly osteoporotic, kyphoscoliosis develops secondary to stress and strain on the posterior ligamentous structures of the spine. With this weakening, eventual collapse of the vertebral body and the formation of an osteoporotic compression fracture occur. This type of fracture can happen even with low-amplitude, low-force

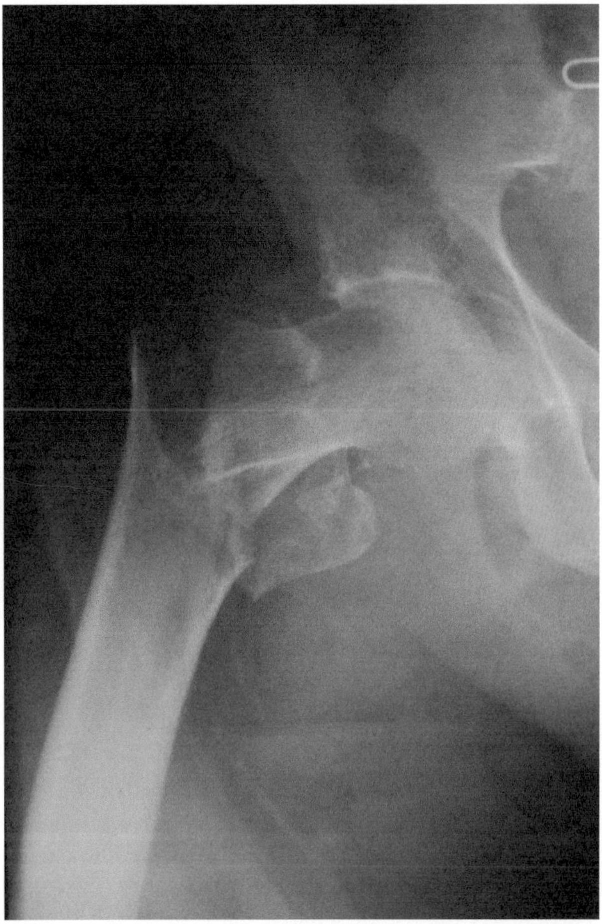

Fig. 3 Radiographic image showing an intertrochanteric fracture (*Source*: Wikipedia public domain [WPD] 1.0)

motions. Coughing, bending over to pick up an object, and other activities of daily living (ADL) can lead to fracture.

Kyphotic posture kinematically places the spine at a disadvantage for proper recruitment of back extensors, resulting in decreased extensor strength and an imbalance in the core musculature [30]. Other pertinent consequences of excessive kyphosis are altered balance and instability of posture in sitting or stance. Balance has been defined as the ability to maintain the body's center of mass over its base of support. Studies have shown that kyphotic subjects have less anteroposterior displacement of the center of mass, resulting in greater mediolateral displacement. This imbalance between center of mass and the base of support (i.e., the greater the displacement, the greater the imbalance) increases an individual's fall risk to one side or the other.

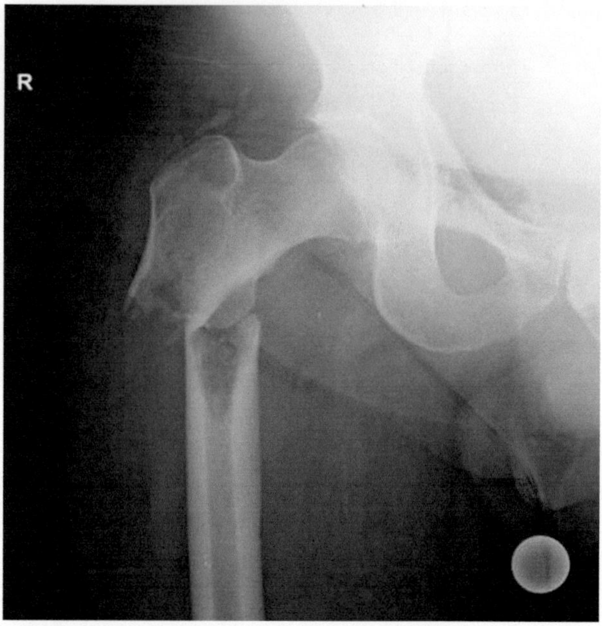

Fig. 4 Radiographic image showing a subtrochanteric fracture (Courtesy of Thomas Jefferson University, Philadelphia, PA)

Falls

As Nevitt et al. point out, the direction of the fall determines the type of fracture. It is likely that women who suffer wrist fractures have fallen to the side or straight down, whereas women who experience hip fractures have fallen, landing on an outstretched hand [31]. Intrinsic age-related changes in vision, strength, cognition, lack of coordination, dizziness posture, and polypharmacy (the use of four or more medications), particularly the use of sedatives, are among the factors contributing to postural instability and increased risk of falls. Regardless of having a diagnosis of osteoporosis, aging patients may exhibit impaired peripheral sensory input, resulting in altered proprioception or decreased muscle strength. Studies reveal that osteoporotic patients with a recent history of falls carry greater risk for fractures than osteoporotic or non-osteoporotic individuals without such history [32–34]. Other than vertebral fractures which can be traumatic or spontaneous, fractures at other body sites are usually the result of a fall [35]. Computerized dynamic posturography has linked thoracic kyphosis to falls [30, 36]. Increased energy expenditure is observed during standing activities in osteoporotic patients with kyphosis, compared to those without kyphosis [37]. Elderly patients may experience fatigue from standing and ambulation for other medical reasons, compounding the risk of falls.

Extrinsic risk factors include safety hazards in the home and community: slippery and uneven surfaces; poor lighting; loose rugs; clutter on floors, walks, and yards; and inappropriate footwear and poorly designed walking aid. Intrinsic factors are most likely the cause of falls in persons age 80 and over because loss of consciousness (indicating a medical factor) is more common in this population. In persons under 75, falls are most often caused by extrinsic factors [38].

References

1. International Osteoporosis Foundation. Boning up on osteoporosis: a guide to prevention and treatment. Washington, DC: National Osteoporosis Foundation; 2008.
2. Looker AC, Wahner HW, Dunn WL, Calvos MS, Harris TB, Heyse SR, et al. Updated data on proximal femur bone mineral levels of U.S. adults. Osteoporos Int. 1998;8:468–89.
3. Reid IR. Overview of pathogenesis. In: Rosen CJ, editor. Primer on the metabolic bone diseases and disorders of mineral metabolism. Washington, DC: Wiley-Blackwell; 2013. p. 357–60.
4. Blake G, Adams JE, Bishop N. DXA in adults and children. In: Rosen CJ, editor. Primer on the metabolic bone diseases and disorders of mineral metabolism. Washington, DC: Wiley-Blackwell; 2013. p. 251–63.
5. Harvey N, Dennison E, Cooper C. The epidemiology of osteoporotic fractures. In: Rosen CJ, editor. Primer on the metabolic bone diseases and disorders of mineral metabolism. Washington, DC: Wiley- Blackwell; 2013. p. 348–56.
6. National Osteoporosis Foundation. Clinician's guide to prevention and treatment of osteoporosis. Washington, DC: National Osteoporosis Foundation; 2013. p. 12–3.
7. Eriksen EF, Axelrod DW, Melson F. Bone histomorphometry. New York: Raven Press; 1994.
8. Merck and Company. Osteoporosis. The Merck manual, professional edition. www.merckmanual.com/professional/musculosketalandconnectivetissuedisorders/osteoporosis. Merck & Co. 2012. Accessed 2 Apr 2015.
9. University of Maryland Medical Center. Osteoporosis. 2013. http://umm.edu/health/medical/reports/articles/osteoporosis. Accessed 20 Mar 2015.
10. Clarke B, Khosla S. Physiology of bone loss. Radiol Clin North Am. 2010;48:483–95.
11. Pitts CJ, Kearns AE. Update on medications with adverse skeletal effects. Mayo Clin Proc. 2011;86:338–43.
12. Kahn SE, Haffner SM, Heise MA, Herman WH, Holman RR, Jones NP, et al. Glycemic durability of rosiglitazone, metformin, or glyburide monotherapy. N Engl J Med. 2006;355:2427–43.
13. Kahn SE. Glycemic durability on monotherapy for diabetes. N Engl J Med. 2007;356:1378–80.
14. Le Templier G, Rodger MA. Heparin-induced osteoporosis and pregnancy. Curr Opin Pulm Med. 2008;14:403–7.
15. Hruska KA, Teitelbaum SL. Renal osteodystrophy. N Engl J Med. 1995;333:166–74.
16. Goffin E, Devogelaer JP, Lalaoui A, Depressenx G, De Naeyer P, Squifflet JP, et al. Tacrolimus and low-dose steroid immunosuppression preserves bone mass after renal transplantation. Transpl Int. 2002;15:73–80.
17. Lee RH, Lyles KW, Colon-Emeric C. A review of the effect of anticonvulsant medications on bone mineral density and fracture risk. Am J Geriatr Pharmacother. 2010;8:34–46.
18. Verrotti A, Coppola G, Parisi P, Mohn A, Chiarelli F. Bone and calcium metabolism and antiepileptic drugs. Clin Neurol Neurosurg. 2010;112:1–10.
19. Richards JB, Papaioannou A, Adachi JD, Joseph L, Whitson HE, Prior JC, et al. Effect of selective serotonin reuptake inhibitors on the risk of fracture. Arch Intern Med. 2007;167:188–94.
20. Gullberg B, Johnell O, Kanis JA. World-wide projections for hip fracture. Osteoporos Int. 1997;7:407–13.
21. Johnell O, Kanis JA. An estimate of the worldwide prevalence and disability associated with osteoporotic fractures. Osteoporos Int. 2006;17:1726–33.
22. Kanis JA, Johnell O, De Laet C, Johansson H, Oden A, Delmas P, et al. A meta-analysis of previous fracture and subsequent fracture risk. Bone. 2004;35:375–82.

23. Klotzbuecher CM, Ross PD, Landsman PB, Abbott TA, Berger M. Patients with prior fractures have an increased risk of future fractures: a summary of the literature and statistical synthesis. J Bone Miner Res. 2000;15:721–39.
24. Longo UG, Loppini M, Denaro L, Maffuli N, Denaro V. Conservative management of patients with an osteoporotic vertebral fracture: a review of the literature. J Bone Joint Surg. 2012;94:152–7.
25. Griffith JF, Adams JE, Genant HK. Diagnosis and classification of vertebral compression fractures. In: Rosen CJ, editor. Primer on the metabolic bone diseases and disorders of mineral metabolism. Washington, DC: Wiley Blackwell; 2013. p. 317–35.
26. Schlaich C, Minne HW, Bruckner T, Wagner G, Gebest HJ, Grunze M, et al. Reduced pulmonary function in patients with spinal osteoporotic fractures. Osteoporos Int. 1998;8:261–7.
27. National Osteoporosis Foundation. America's bone health: the state of osteoporosis and low bone mass in our nation. Washington, DC: National Osteoporosis Foundation; 2002. http://www.nof.org/advocacy/prevalence. Accessed 30 Mar 2013.
28. Hip fractures. American Academy of Orthopaedic Surgeons. Orthoinfo. http://orthoinfo.AAOS.org/topic/cfn?topic=A00392. Accessed 25 Mar 2015.
29. Sinaki M. Critical appraisal of physical rehabilitation measures after osteoporotic vertebral fracture. Osteoporos Int. 2003;14:773–9.
30. Sinaki M, Brey RH, Hughes CA, Larson DR, Kaufman KR. Significant reduction in risk of falls and back pain in osteoporotic-kyphotic women through a Spinal Proprioceptive Extension Exercise Dynamic (SPEED) program. Mayo Clin Proc. 2005;80:849–55.
31. Nevitt MD, Cummings SR. Type of fall and risk of hip and wrist fractures: the study of osteoporotic fractures. The Study of the Osteoporotic Fractures Research Group. J Am Geriatr Soc. 1993;41:1226–34.
32. Geusens P, Autier P, Boonen S, Vanhoof J, Declerk K, Raus J. The relationship among history of falls, osteoporosis, and fractures in postmenopausal women. Arch Phys Med Rehabil. 2002;83:903–6.
33. McClung M, Geusen P, Miller P, Zippel H, Bensen WG, Roux C, et al. Effect of risedronate on the risk of hip fracture in elderly women. N Engl J Med. 2001;344:333–40.
34. Cummings SR, Black DM, Thompson DE, et al. Effect of alendronate on risk of fracture in women with low bone density but without vertebral fractures: results from the fracture intervention trial. JAMA. 1998;280:2077–82.
35. Sinaki M. Fall, fractures, and hip pads. Curr Osteoporos Rep. 2004;2:131–7.
36. Sinaki M, Brey RH, Hughes CA, Larson DR, et al. Balance disorder and increased risk of falls in osteoporosis and kyphosis: significance of kyphotic posture and muscle strength. Osteoporos Int. 2005;16:1004–10.
37. Lombardi Jr I, Oliveira LM, Monteiro CR, Confesssor YQ, Barros TL, Natour J, et al. Evaluation of physical capacity and quality of life in osteoporotic women. Osteoporos Int. 2004;15:80–5.
38. Todd C, Skelton D. What are the main risk factors for falls among older people and what are the most effective interventions to prevent these falls? WHO Regional Office for Europe (Health Evidence Network report). 2004. Copenhagen. http://www.euro.who.int/document/E82552.pdf. Accessed 10 Mar 2015.

Chapter 3
Diagnosis of Osteoporosis

Christina V. Oleson

Screening for osteoporosis is the initial step in making a diagnosis. Primary care physicians are becoming increasingly attuned to populations at risk for this condition which affects significant numbers of women and older men in the United States and abroad. This chapter will focus on the key components of diagnosis: relevant family and personal history that might contribute to risks for osteoporosis, physical examination findings, imaging, and laboratory studies. All four components are important in the diagnosis and initial care of a patient at risk for osteoporosis as well as a patient in the early phases of established osteoporosis.

Assessment Tools

Medical History and Physical Examination

The National Osteoporosis Foundation (NOF) recommends that all postmenopausal women and men 50 and older should be evaluated for risk of osteoporosis, beginning with a medical history and physical evaluation to determine whether bone mineral density (BMD) testing and/or vertebral imaging are warranted. The history should take into account the following: age, gender, personal history of fractures as an adult and family history of broken bones and osteoporosis, smoking or drinking habits, diet, medications, physical activity, eating disorders, menstrual patterns in women and testosterone levels in men, genetic diseases such as cystic fibrosis and rheumatologic and autoimmune diseases, neurological and musculoskeletal risk factors, and endocrine, gastrointestinal, and hematologic diseases.

The physical examination should include a height and spine check [1]. The results of these screenings are critical in determining whether to move forward with BMD testing.

C.V. Oleson, *Osteoporosis Rehabilitation*, DOI 10.1007/978-3-319-45084-1_3

Radiographic Studies

Bone Mineral Density (BMD) Testing

As a general guideline, the US Preventive Services Task Force (USPSTF) advises that BMD testing be performed on women age 65 and older and on younger women whose fracture risk is equal to or greater than that of white women, with no additional risk factors [2]. As of 2011, the USPSTF indicates that current evidence is insufficient to weigh the costs/benefits of testing in men [2]. However, the NOF 2014 report advises that men age 50–69 with clinical risk factors for fracture should be tested [1].

Only a bone density test can diagnose osteoporosis before a broken bone actually happens. Measurements of BMD are obtained by dual-energy x-ray absorptiometry (DXA). The DXA machine calculates bone mineral content in grams by summing pixels in a given region viewed by the scanner and dividing that number by the bone area examined in cm^2. A patient's results can be interpreted as a standard deviation from the mean of sex-matched peak bone mass (*T*-score) [3].

The World Health Organization defines osteoporosis as a *T*-score at or below 2.5 standard deviations from the mean BMD of a young normal adult of the same gender under age 30. It is designed for those who have already reached peak bone mass [1]. Another measure known as the *Z*-score employs standard deviations from the mean of age- and sex-matched bone mass. The *Z*-score is often used for patients below age 30 in which peak bone mass has not been achieved, but it is a useful measure for all premenopausal women and men <50 years [4]. A given patient is assigned a *T*- or *Z*-score for a given location (in this case the lumbar spine) based on established norms as illustrated in Fig. 1 [5]. The *T*-score determines whether a patient has normal bone, osteopenia, or osteoporosis as summarized in Table 1 [6].

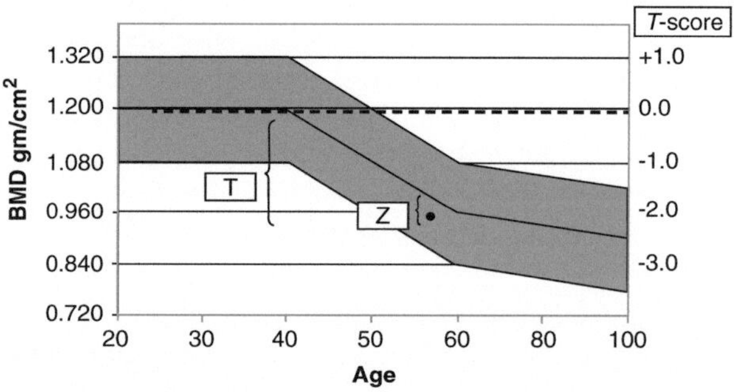

Fig. 1 Normal, osteopenic, and osteoporotic bone by *T* and *Z*-scores (*Source*: National Osteoporosis Foundation [5]. Reproduced with permission)

Table 1 Definitions of normal bone, osteopenia, and osteoporosis by DXA values as established by International Society for Clinical Densitometry (ISCD)

Classification	BMD for young-adult reference population (healthy adult < age 30)	T-score
Normal bone	Within 1 SD of the mean level	−1.0 and above
Osteopenia	Between 1.0 and 2.5 SD below that of the mean level	Between −1.0 and −2.5
Osteoporosis	2.5 SD or more below that of the mean level	At or below −2.5
Severe osteoporosis	2.5 SD or more below that of the mean level	At or below −2.5 with one or more fractures

Source: Mayo Clinic. Tests and Procedures [6]

The *Z*-score is also used to identify high-risk patients, who may not be osteoporotic, but are below expected bone density for their age and should be followed more closely [4]. While there is no specific *T*-score that correlates with fracture threshold, the more negative the *T*-score, the greater the risk [6]. In able-bodied postmenopausal females, several prospective studies indicate that half of patients with incident fractures had baseline BMD assessed by DXA above the diagnostic threshold of osteoporosis [7–9].

Vertebral Imaging

Quite apart from a patient's BMD, the presence of a vertebral fracture is considered by most clinicians to be sufficient for a diagnosis of osteoporosis as well as an important factor in predicting subsequent fractures. Because these fractures tend to be asymptomatic and may be undiagnosed for years, the NOF has established guidelines for the implementation of vertebral imaging tests encompassing women age 65 and older and men age 70 and older if their *T*-score is ≤ -1.5 or below and for women age 70 and men age 80 and older, if their *T*-score at the spine, total hip, and femoral neck is ≤ -1.0 [1].

In patients whose clinical evaluations suggest osteoporosis, radiologists use a lateral thoracic and lumbar spine x-ray or a lateral vertebral fracture assessment; the latter is available on DXA machines and can be performed at the same time as the BMD test [1]. It should be noted, however, that clinicians and radiologists may fail to detect a fracture. Lenchik et al. refer to several studies that demonstrate this failure [10]. For example, a study of 934 hospitalized women aged 60 and over identified moderate to severe vertebral fractures in 14 % of the population; only 50 % of contemporaneous radiology reports note these fractures [11]. Factors contributing to these failed diagnoses include lack of standardization in the interpretation of radiologic results, inaccurate readings by radiologists, and ambiguous terminology used in the reports [10].

Fracture Risk Assessment Tool (FRAX)

Because osteoporosis may initially present asymptomatically, screenings for osteoporosis in high-risk populations are advisable. While it is optimal that such screening be done as a standard of care, many individuals experience osteoporotic fractures in advance of ever receiving a DXA scan in the community. In fact, initial recognition that individuals are experiencing the effects of osteoporosis often comes when they present in an acute care hospital with a fracture.

To improve screening for fractures, the World Health Organization (WHO) created the Fracture Risk Assessment Tool (FRAX) which calculates the 10-year probability of hip fracture and of a major osteoporotic fracture based on US fracture and mortality rates [10]. The development of FRAX was motivated by the recognition that clinical risk factors are vital in understanding fracture risk. The risk factors used in the FRAX are given in Table 2 [12].

Here, the distinction between diagnosing osteoporosis and assessing fracture risk is important. Whereas FRAX is an assessment tool, BMD measurement remains the most clinically recognized and validated method used to diagnose osteoporosis and predict fractures [13]. However, studies show that 50 % of fractures would not be detected if only a BMD measurement were used. The

Table 2 FRAX risk factors

Age
Sex
Weight in kg
Height in cm
Previous fracture: denotes more accurately a previous fracture in adult life occurring spontaneously or a fracture arising from trauma which, in a healthy individual, would not have resulted in a fracture
Parent with fractured hip: a history of hip fracture in the patient's mother or father
Current smoking
Glucocorticoids: exposed to oral glucocorticoids or has been exposed to oral glucocorticoids for more than three months at a dose of prednisolone of 5 mg daily or more (or equivalent doses of other glucocorticoids)
Rheumatoid arthritis: a confirmed diagnosis of rheumatoid arthritis or no such diagnosis
Secondary osteoporosis: a disorder strongly associated with osteoporosis, including type I (insulin-dependent) diabetes, osteogenesis imperfecta in adults, untreated long-standing hyperthyroidism, hypogonadism or premature menopause (<45 years), chronic malnutrition, or malabsorption and chronic liver disease
Alcohol: three or more units of alcohol daily. A unit of alcohol varies slightly in different countries from 8 to 10 g of alcohol. This is equivalent to a standard glass of beer (285 ml), a single measure of spirits (30 ml), a medium-sized glass of wine (120 ml), or on measure of an aperitif (60 ml)
Bone mineral density (BMD): the manufacturer of DXA scanning equipment used and the actual femoral neck BMD (in g/cm2). Alternatively, the *T*-score based on the NHANES III female reference data can be used

Source: World Health Organization [12]

combination of BMD testing with FRAX provides the most effective means of determining the next steps in managing patients at risk and of providing essential anticipatory guidance [13].

Laboratory Studies

In situations where a patient's *Z*-score (age-matched BMD) is below expected levels, laboratory tests can assist the practitioner in identifying secondary causes of osteoporosis. Suggested studies include complete blood count, serum calcium, vitamin D, thyroid-stimulating hormone (TSH), and liver enzymes. Urine calcium or spot urine calcium/creatinine ratio may detect hypercalciuria, the excessive urinary calcium excretion that is the primary cause of kidney stones [14]. Estrogen plays a central role in osteoblast maturation and production of growth factors to form procollagen as essential building blocks of mature bone [15, 16]. Low estrogen levels are widely known to cause osteoporosis after menopause, but estrogen-deficient states can also be seen in women with premature menopause following total abdominal hysterectomy, with salpingo-oophorectomy (removal of the fallopian tube and ovary) [17, 18] or even among teens and young adults with anorexia nervosa or athletic amenorrhea [19]. In the latter special cases, laboratory investigation should be undertaken even before BMD testing, since early correction of hormonal abnormalities will reduce or even eliminate development of secondary osteoporosis [20, 21]. In men, low testosterone levels can indicate hypogonadism [22].

The best laboratory indicator of vitamin D adequacy is the serum 25-hydroxyvitamin D (D25OH) concentration. There is no consensus on the optimal D25OH concentration for skeletal or extraskeletal health. The Institute of Medicine (IOM) suggests that a level of 20 ng/mL (50 nmol/L) is adequate [23], while Heaney et al. [24] maintain that a minimum level of 32 ng/ml is needed to prevent upregulation of parathyroid hormone and impaired calcium resorption. All patients presenting to an acute hospital with any concern for osteoporotic related disease should at least have a screening involving serum vitamin D 25-OH, serum calcium, and intact parathyroid hormone. These studies are easily obtained in any inpatient facility. Table 3 summarizes initial laboratory workup which should be performed for those with *Z*-scores indicating advanced osteopenia or osteoporosis [14]. These studies will alert clinicians to primary metabolic, endocrine, or renal disorders that predispose patients to osteoporosis.

More advanced laboratory studies are advisable in patients with clinical concern for osteoporosis or in whom screening studies and lab values described above indicate additional workup is needed. If a DXA scan indicates a patient has osteopenia or osteoporosis, the question arises as to whether manifestation of the disease is due to inadequate bone formation, excessive bone loss, or a combination of both. Biochemical bone markers may be used to assess the rate of bone formation and bone resorption. Values for serum N-terminal propeptide (s-CTX) and procollagen type I N-terminal propeptide (P1NP) are not included in the FRAX

Table 3 Initial laboratory workup performed for those with *Z*-scores indicating advanced osteopenia or osteoporosis

Laboratory test	Reason
Complete blood count (CBC)	Marker of general nutrition. Evaluates anemia as source of weakness
Serum total calcium OR	To calculate albumin adjusted calcium. Not universal but may be useful to correct total calcium measurements skewed by abnormal albumin levels
Ionized calcium	More accurate measure of calcium homeostasis
Phosphorus	Detect conditions associated with hypercalcemia, i.e., primary hyperparathyroidism or hypocalcaemia and subsequent secondary hyperparathyroidism causing bone loss
Magnesium	Monitoring needed in relation to calcium and phosphorous
Renal function	To detect renal failure which can affect bone health
Serum creatinine	
Glomerular filtration rate (GFR)	
Liver function tests	Abnormal levels may impair processing of vitamin D
Serum alkaline phosphatase (ALP)	Useful to detect Paget's disease, osteomalacia, fracture healing, metastatic bone disease. May not be sensitive enough to detect changes in bone remodeling in most cases of uncomplicated osteoporosis
25(OH)D	Reflects one measure of overall bone health
Parathyroid hormone (PTH)	To help investigate calcium level abnormality; significantly elevated in setting of severe vitamin D deficiency
Thyroid-stimulating hormone (TSH) +/− free T4	TSH is a direct inhibitor of osteoclasts. Low levels in setting of hyperthyroidism indicate probable bone resorption. Elevated T4 levels are confirmatory for hyperthyroid states which involve increased osteoclastic activity
Blood and erythrocyte sedimentation rate (ESR)	For general health and for inflammatory diseases which often cause bone loss
Consider in selected patients	
Serum protein electrophoresis (SPEP), serum immunofixation, serum-free light chains	To exclude multiple myeloma which causes major bone loss
Total testosterone and gonadotropin in younger men	To exclude multiple myeloma which causes major bone loss
Tissue transglutaminase antibodies (IgA and IgG)	Screening for thyrotoxicosis and hypogonadism
Tryptase	To detect celiac disease
Urinary histamine	To detect celiac disease
Urinary free cortisol level	To detect celiac disease
	To detect Cushing's syndrome
Bone turnover markers	
Serum C-telopeptide (s-CTX) or urine N-telopeptide (u-NTX)	Indicates upregulation of osteoclastic activity which indicates bone resorption
s-P1NP	A measure of osteoblastic activity, representing bone building metabolic activity

Source: Lee and Vasikaran [14]. Adapted with permission.

because the results have been inconsistent due to the use of different markers and different methodologies and leading to calls for greater standardization in these measurements [14].

Bone formation markers include bone-specific alkaline phosphatase (BALP) and P1NP; the latter has the greatest specificity for bone, but all markers have limitations in clinical interpretation [25, 26]. Markers of bone resorption include urine and serum carboxy-terminal cross-linking telopeptide of type I collagen. Both bone formation and resorption markers guide clinicians to types of treatment that are most appropriate for osteoporosis and provide indicators of relative success of pharmacologic interventions, such as bisphosphonate therapy [25, 26]. The above studies may be carried out in either the inpatient or outpatient setting but generally require specialty labs for processing, outside of the immediate clinical setting of the patient. The results are best followed by a practitioner well versed in the literature and intervention strategies since findings may alter treatment choices. Clinicians ordering these tests should become familiar with pretesting requirements since food or medications can interfere with result interpretation.

Early detection is a critical first step in treating osteoporosis. However, further research is needed to provide direct evidence that screening reduces fracture-related morbidity and mortality and to determine the long term outcomes of screened versus non-screened populations. In addition, studies are lacking on the occurrence of fractures in nonwhite and ethnic groups [2].

References

1. National Osteoporosis Foundation. Clinician's guide to prevention and treatment of osteoporosis. Washington, DC: National Osteoporosis Foundation; 2013. p. 14–23.
2. U.S. Preventive Services Task Force. Final recommendation statement: osteoporosis: screening. 2011. http://uspreventiveservicestaskforce.org/Page/Document/RecommendationStatement. Accessed 5 Dec 2013.
3. Adams J, Bishop N. DXA in adults and children. In: Rosen CJ, editor. Primer on the metabolic bone diseases and disorders of mineral metabolism. Washington, DC: Wiley- Blackwell; 2008. p. 152–8.
4. International Society for Clinical Densitometry. Official positions. International Society for Clinical Densitometry. http://www.iscd.org. Accessed 12 Apr 2013.
5. National Osteoporosis Foundation. ISCD bone densitometry clinician course, lecture 5. 2008. http://www.nof.org. Accessed 5 Dec 2013.
6. Mayo Clinic. Bone density test. http://www.mayoclinic.org/tests-procedures/bone-density-test/basics/definition/PRC-20020254
7. Schuit SC, van der Klift M, Weel AE, DeLaet CE, Burgher H, Seeman E, et al. Fracture incidence and association with bone mineral density in elderly men and women: the Rotterdam study. Bone. 2004;34(1):195–202.
8. Miller PD, Siris ES, Barrett-Connor E, Faulkner KG, Wehren LE, Abbott TA, et al. Prediction of fracture risk in postmenopausal white women with peripheral bone densitometry: evidence from the National Osteoporosis Risk Assessment. J Bone Miner Res. 2002;17(12):2222–30.
9. Stone KL, Seeley DG, Lui LY, Cauley JA, Ensrud K, Browner WS, et al. BMD at multiple sites and risk of fracture of multiple types: long-term results from the study of osteoporotic fractures. J Bone Miner Res. 2003;18(11):1947–54.

10. Lenchik L, Rogers LF, Delmas PD. Diagnosis of osteoporotic vertebral fractures: importance of recognition and description by radiologists. Am J Roentgenol. 2004;183(4):949–58.
11. Gehlbach SH, Bigelow C, Heimisdottir M, May S, Walker M, Kirkwood JR. Recognition of vertebral fracture in a clinical setting. Osteoporos Int. 2000;11(7):577–82.
12. World Health Organization. FRAX assessment tool. FRAX WHO fracture risk assessment tool. 2008. http://www.shef.ac.uk/FRAX/tool.jsp?country=9. Accessed 18 Oct 2013.
13. Chandran A. Is BMD measurement still useful with the advent of the FRAX fracture risk assessment tool? Medicographia. 2010. http://www.medicographia.com/2010/07/is-bmd-measurement-still-useful-with-the-advent-of-the-frax%C2%AE-fracture-risk-assessment-tool/. Accessed 19 Oct 2013.
14. Lee J, Vasikaran S. Current recommendations for laboratory testing and use of bone turnover markers in management of osteoporosis. Ann Lab Med. 2012;32(2):105–12.
15. Chow J, Tobias JH, Colston KW, Chambers TJ. Estrogen maintains trabecular bone volume in rats not only by suppression of bone resorption but also by the stimulation of bone formation. J Clin Invest. 1992;89(1):74–8.
16. Qu Q, Perala-Heape M, Kapanen A, Dahllund S, Salo J, Vaananen HK, et al. Estrogen enhances differentiation of osteoblasts in mouse bone marrow culture. Bone. 1998;22(3):201–9.
17. Aitken JM, Hart DM, Anderson JB, Lindsay R, Smith DA, Speirs CF. Osteoporosis after oophorectomy for non-malignant disease in premenopausal women. BMJ. 1973;2(5862):325–8.
18. Simões RD, Baracat EC, Szjenfeld VL, de Lima GR, Gonçalves WJ, Bortoletto CD. Effects of simple hysterectomy on bone loss. Sao Paulo Med J. 1995;113(6):1210–6.
19. Cohen A, Shane E. Premenopausal osteoporosis. In: Rosen CJ, editor. Primer on the metabolic bone diseases and disorders of mineral metabolism. Washington, DC: Wiley- Blackwell; 2013. p. 514–9.
20. Legroux-Gérot I, Vignau J, D'Herbomez M, Collier F, Marchandise X, Duguesnoy B, et al. Evaluation of bone loss and its mechanisms in anorexia nervosa. Calcif Tissue Int. 2007;81(3):174–82.
21. Mehler PS, Cleary BS, Gaudiani JL. Osteoporosis in anorexia nervosa. Eat Disord. 2011;19(2):194–202.
22. Barzel US. Recommended testing in patients with low bone density. J Clin Endocrinol Metab. 2003;88(3):1404–5.
23. Ross AC, Taylor CL, Yaktine AL, Del Valle HB. Dietary reference intakes for calcium and vitamin D. Washington, DC: National Academies Press; 2010.
24. Heaney RP, Dowell MS, Hale CA, Bendich A. Calcium absorption varies within the reference range for serum 25-hydroxyvitamin D. J Am Co Nutr. 2003;22(2):142–6.
25. Vasikaran S, Cooper C, Eastell R, Griesmacher A, Morris HA, Trenti T, et al. International Osteoporosis Foundation and International Federation of Chemistry and Laboratory Medicine position on marker standards in osteoporosis. Clin Chem Lab Med. 2011;49(8):1271–4.
26. Schafer AL, Vittinghoff E, Ramachandran R, Mahmoudi N, Bauer DC. Laboratory reproducibility of biochemical markers of bone turnover in clinical practice. Osteoporos Int. 2010;21(3):439–45.

Chapter 4
Prevention of Osteoporosis

Christina V. Oleson and Amanda B. Morina

Prevention of osteoporosis should be a lifelong concern for both women and men, particularly those who exhibit controllable risk factors. Although the disease is generally associated with middle-aged and older women, there is growing evidence that, as has been said, "Osteoporosis is a pediatric disease with geriatric consequences" [1]. Maximizing bone mineral density (BMD) is the essential prerequisite for assuring good bone health. As children grow into adulthood, their bone density increases until it reaches peak bone mass—the largest amount of bone tissue that can be achieved in life [2]. The National Institute of Arthritis and Musculoskeletal and Skin Diseases states that up to 90 % of peak bone mass in women occurs by age 18 and in men by age 20 [3]. Although bone mass is determined largely by genetic factors, other influences including vitamins, diet, exercise, and lifestyle can significantly influence bone health. This chapter will provide an overview of the principal preventive measures and then focus specifically on the needs of children and adolescents—an increasingly important age group for osteoporosis prevention.

Nutrition and Vitamin Supplements

Together, vitamin D and calcium are the essential building blocks of bone tissue. Individuals with adequate intake of these two nutrients have better bone health because they achieve peak bone mass earlier in life and experience less bone loss as they age. Moreover, controlled trails have demonstrated that vitamin D in combination with calcium reduces the risk of falls in older individuals in stable health by as much as 20 % [4–6].

A 2010 Institute of Medicine (IOM) panel calls for 600 IU of vitamin D for all ages up to age 70 and 800 IU after age 71 [7]. For adults 71 years and older, 800 IU is the recommended daily allowance (RDA). In cases of fracture, higher amounts should be prescribed during and subsequent to the healing process [8]. A population-based survey of the ambulatory US population 60 years of age and older

C.V. Oleson, *Osteoporosis Rehabilitation*, DOI 10.1007/978-3-319-45084-1_4

Table 1 Calcium and vitamin D recommendations

Children and adolescents	**Calcium (daily)**	**Vitamin D (daily)**
1 through 3 years	500 mg	200 IU[a]
4 through 8 years	800 mg	200 IU[a]
9 through 18 years	1300 mg	200 IU[a]
Adult women and men	**Calcium (daily)**	**Vitamin D_3 (daily)**[b]
19 through 49 years	1000 mg	400–800 IU
50 years and over	1200 mg	800–1000 IU
Pregnant and breastfeeding women	**Calcium (daily)**	**Vitamin D_3 (daily)**[b]
18 years and under	1300 mg	400–800 IU
19 years and over	1000 mg	400–800 IU

Source: Adapted from National Osteoporosis Foundation [10]
Vitamin D_3 is also known as cholecalciferol; vitamin D_2 is also known as ergocalciferol
[a]The National Osteoporosis Foundation does not have specific vitamin D recommendations for these groups. These suggestions are from the Institutes of Medicine of the National Academies and National Institutes of Health, Office of Dietary Supplements
[b]When available, a supplement of vitamin D_3 is recommended over vitamin D_2

showed that increased 25-hydroxyvitamin D concentrations were associated with improved lower extremity function (Table 1) [9, 10].

The IOM RDA for calcium varies according to age group [7]. Children under the age of nine should be consuming at least 700–1000 mg/day. For adolescents 9–18, levels as high as 1300 mg/day are advocated because this is a crucial time for bone remodeling, impacting bone structure throughout adulthood. Based upon IOM guidelines, adults under the age of 50 should consume 1000 mg/day. Males age 50–70 should aim for 1200 mg/day with 2000 mg/day age 71 and over. Females require 1200 mg/day from age 50–70. These numbers have been questioned by several experts in the field who maintain that the vitamin D RDA is too low, whereas the calcium RDA may be too high; the IOM itself indicates that more data is needed regarding the interaction of vitamin D and calcium on bone health [11].

Vitamin D

Vitamin D plays a crucial role in calcium homeostasis, bone metabolism, and balance and risk of falling. Low vitamin D levels are linked to impaired calcium absorption and an increase in parathyroid hormone (PTH) which can result in excessive bone resorption. Without sufficient vitamin D, calcium absorption fails to satisfy the body's requirements, even when calcium intake is adequate.

Serum 25(OH)D levels, reflecting vitamin D levels produced cutaneously as well as those obtained from food, are the most effective measure of vitamin D. The principal sources of vitamin D are sunlight, food, and supplements. The skin synthesizes vitamin D from the ultraviolet rays (UVB) of the sun which vary depending on time of day, season, skin pigmentation, and other factors; in some areas, vitamin D production may not occur at all in winter. In addition, the use of sunscreen can

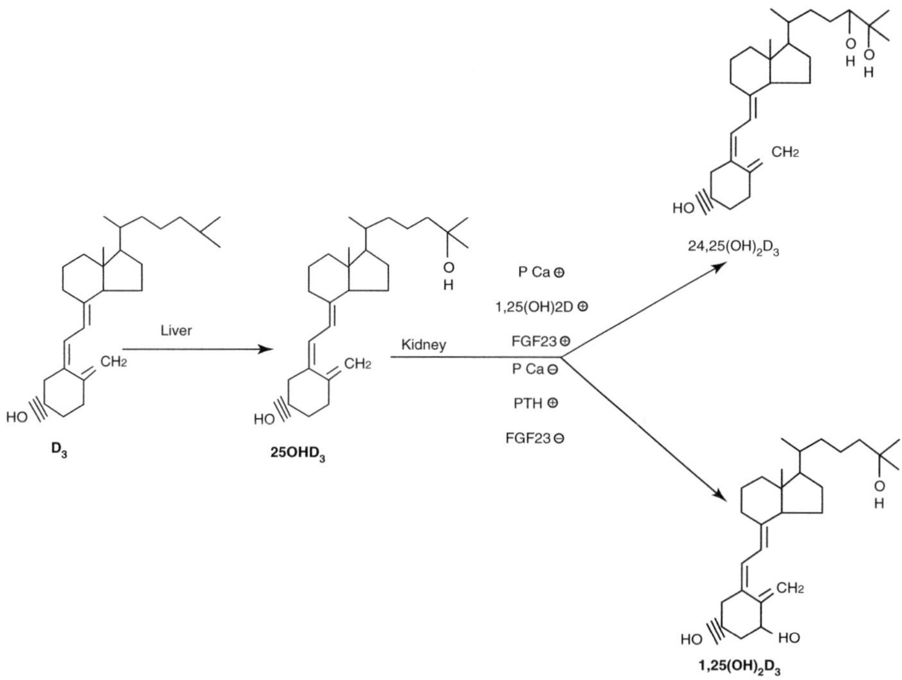

Fig. 1 The photolysis of ergosterol and 7-dehydrocholesterol to vitamin D_2 (ergocalciferol) and vitamin D_3 (cholecalciferol). An intermediate is formed after photolysis, which then undergoes a thermally activated isomerization to create the final form of vitamin D. The rotation of the A-ring positions the 3β-hydroxyl group into a different orientation with respect to the plane of the A-ring during production of vitamin D. (*Source*: Bikle et al. [59]. Used with permission)

severely limit the skin's ability to make vitamin D [12]. The pathway of absorption of vitamin D from sunlight and dietary sources is illustrated in Figs. 1 and 2. Sources of vitamin D in naturally occurring foods are extremely limited and are primarily restricted to fatty fish (salmon, swordfish, tuna), fish liver oil, and egg yolks. Most of the vitamin D in American diets comes from fortified foods such as fluid milk (400 IU per quart), ready-to-eat breakfast cereals, yogurt, cheese, and juices [13]. Since it is difficult to obtain the recommended level of vitamin D from sunlight and food, supplements in the form of vitamin D2 (ergocalciferol) and vitamin D3 (cholecalciferol) may be recommended. Whereas the two forms were once regarded as equivalent, recent studies indicate that vitamin D3 is more effective at raising serum 25(OH)D concentrations than is vitamin D2 [14]. Manufacturers appear to be producing more vitamin D3 than vitamin D2 as well as increasing the levels in multivitamin supplements from the former 400 IU per daily dose to as much as 1000–1500 IU/day. Adequate oral intake of vitamin D is also a factor in preventing falls because it addresses several components of the fall-fracture construct including strength, balance, bone density, lower extremity function, and risk of hip and non-vertebral fractures [5, 6]. Table 2 summarizes the vitamin D content in common food group [15].

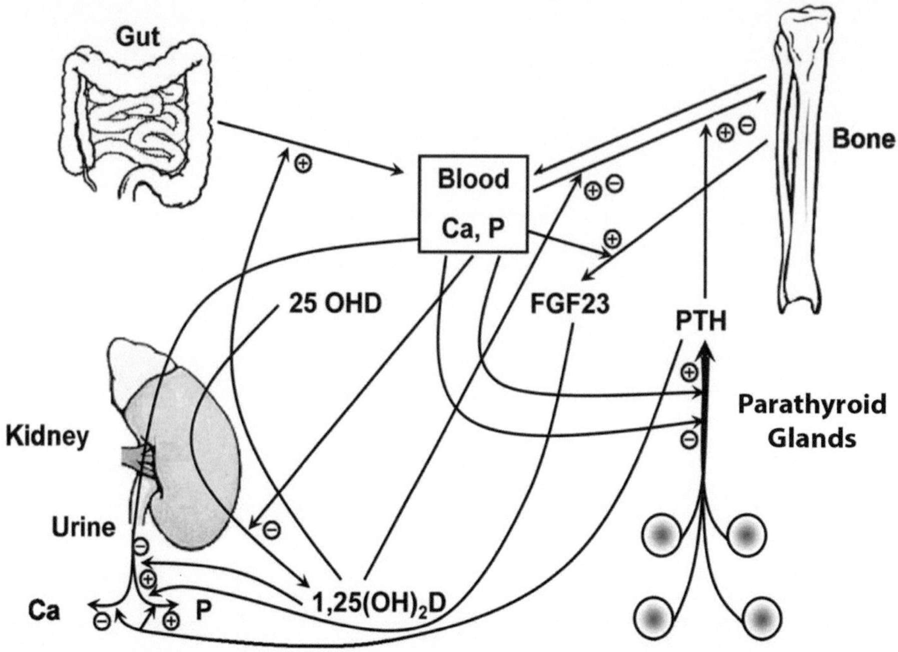

Fig. 2 Interaction of vitamin D with other hormones. 1,25(OH)$_2$D interacts with other hormones, in particular FGF23 and PTH, to regulate calcium and phosphate homeostasis. FGF23 inhibits whereas PTH stimulates, 1,25(OH)$_2$D production by the kidney. In turn, 1,25(OH)$_2$D inhibits PTH production but stimulates that of FGF23. (*Source*: Bikle et al. [59]. Used with permission)

Calcium

Calcium is the most abundant mineral in the body, and 99 % of it is stored in bones and teeth. A number of nutrients play a role in bone health, but calcium is accorded special attention not only because it is essential in bone composition but also because the average American's intake of calcium is far below the amount recommended for optimal bone health, in part because food preferences such as soda have led to reduced consumption of dairy products [16]. Only 30 % of calcium intake is absorbed by the body; factors influencing calcium absorption include vitamin D intake, age, and, to an extent, the amount of phytic acid and oxalic acid in food. Some absorbed calcium is eliminated in the form of urine, feces, and sweat [17]. When calcium intake is insufficient, bone tissue is resorbed, bone mass is reduced, and bone strength is diminished. Bone resorption is controlled by PTH in response to extracellular fluid calcium ion homeostasis rather than to a structural need for bone mass. PTH is also implicated as a cause of bone fragility through its stimulation of bone resorption [18]. "Optimal" calcium intake is defined as the level of calcium consumption required

Table 2 Vitamin D content of foods

Food item	Serving size	Estimated vitamin D content in international units (IUs)
Dairy		
Whole, nonfat, reduced fat (fortified with vitamin D)	8 oz. (1 cup)	115–124
Yogurt (fortified with 20 % of the DV for vitamin D)	6 oz.	80
Margarine (fortified)	1 tbsp.	60
Egg (vitamin D in yolk)	1 large	41
Cheese, Swiss	1 oz.	6
Meat		
Liver oil, cod	3 oz.	1360
Swordfish (cooked)	3 oz	566
Salmon, sockeye (cooked)	3 oz.	447
Tuna (canned in water and drained)	3 oz.	154
Sardines (canned in oil and drained)	2 sardines	46
Liver, beef (cooked)	3 oz.	42
Cereal and fruit juice		
Orange juice (fortified with vitamin D)	8 oz. (1 cup)	137
Cereal (fortified with 10 % of the DV for vitamin D)	8 oz. (1 cup)	40

Source: Adapted from National Institutes of Health [15]
DV percent daily value

to maximize peak adult bone mass, to maintain that mass, and to minimize bone loss later in life. In this sense, calcium serves as a "threshold" nutrient meaning that below a critical level, the effect of calcium on bone mass is limited by the amount of available calcium, whereas above that level, increased calcium intake provides no added benefit [19].

Calcium-rich foods include dairy products such as low-fat and nonfat milk, cheese, and yogurt; vegetables including kale and broccoli; fish such as sardines and salmon; and calcium fortified foods, particularly fruit juices, cereal, bread, and bottled water. Table 3 gives the calcium content of several of the most common foods [10]. To ensure bone health, the dairy group is most important, providing 20–75 % of recommended calcium, protein, phosphorus, magnesium, and potassium. As Weaver and Heaney point out, the rising consumption of soft drinks and the growing recognition of lactose intolerance have occurred concurrently with a significant decline in milk intake in the United States; alternative foods containing milk's nutrients are not consumed in sufficient amounts to replace what milk can provide [18]. Recommended calcium levels for healthy individuals vary according to age group, as discussed above. If calcium intake through food is insufficient, two common forms of supplements may be advised. Calcium carbonate is inexpensive, available in several over-the-counter antacids, and absorbed most effectively when taken with

Table 3 Calcium content of foods

Food item	Serving size	Estimated calcium content in milligrams (mg)
Milk		
Whole	8 oz. (1 cup)	275
Low-fat	8 oz. (1 cup)	290
Skim	8 oz. (1 cup)	305
Yogurt		
Plain yogurt, fat-free or low-fat	8 oz. (1 cup)	415
Fruit yogurt, low-fat	8 oz. (1 cup)	245–385
Frozen yogurt, vanilla, soft-serve	8 oz. (1 cup)	205
Ice cream, low-fat or high-fat	8 oz. (1 cup)	70–90
Cheese		
American	1 oz.	175
Cheddar, shredded	1 oz.	205
Cottage cheese, 1 % milk fat	1 cup	140
Mozzarella, part skim	1 oz.	145–205
Parmesan, grated	1 tbsp.	70
Ricotta, part skim	4 oz. (½ cup)	335
Swiss	1 oz.	220–270
Fish and shellfish (canned)		
Sardines, in oil with bones	3 oz.	325
Salmon, pink with bones	3 oz.	180
Shrimp	3 oz.	50
Vegetables		
Bok choy (Chinese cabbage), raw	8 oz. (1 cup)	75
Broccoli, cooked and drained	8 oz. (1 cup)	60
Kale, cooked	8 oz. (1 cup)	95
Soybeans, mature, cooked, and drained	8 oz. (1 cup)	175
Turnip greens, fresh, cooked, and drained	8 oz. (1 cup)	200
Fruits		
Oranges	1 whole	50
Dried figs	2 figs	55
Fortified foods		
Fruit juice with added calcium	6 oz.	200–260
Cereal with added calcium (without milk)	1 cup	100–1000
Tofu prepared with calcium	4 oz. (½ cup)	205
Soy milk with added calcium	8 oz. (1 cup)	80–500

The calcium content listed for most foods is estimated and may vary due to multiple factors such as fortification and fat content

Source: Adapted from National Osteoporosis Foundation [10]

food. Calcium citrate is easier to absorb, can be taken with or without food, and causes less constipation than the carbonate form [17]. Whether calcium is obtained from foods or from supplements, it is best absorbed in amounts of 500–600 mg or less. People with osteoporosis or those at risk are often referred to a registered dietician for nutrition counseling.

Other Dietary and Lifestyle Factors

Sodium Intake

On average, Americans consume about 3400 mg of sodium per day as opposed to the recommended 2300 mg [20]. Over the past quarter century, studies have shown a correlation between sodium intake and urinary calcium excretion, some of which comes directly from bones. Researchers led by R. Todd Alexander at the University of Alberta have demonstrated a molecular link between sodium and calcium loss, observing that the epithelial sodium/proton exchanger, NHE3, which is responsible for sodium absorption also regulates calcium loss. The greater the intake of sodium, the greater the loss of calcium through the urine [21]. In another study, Nordin et al. have shown that with sodium as the determining factor, 100 mmol of sodium removes approximately 1 mmol of calcium in the urine, which is the equivalent of 1 % extra bone loss each year. Moreover, sodium-dependent calcium loss can continue indefinitely [22]. Adhering to the recommended guidelines of 2300 mg/day, with 1500 mg over age 50 is critical to good bone health.

Alcohol Consumption

Avoidance of excessive alcohol intake, particularly during adolescence and young adulthood, also prevents general bone deterioration and risk of falls. Hormones, vitamins, and growth factors act together to regulate the distribution of calcium between bone and blood. Chronic heavy drinking disrupts that interaction by affecting the substances that regulate calcium metabolism, including PTH, calcitonin, and vitamin D. In addition, alcohol causes men to generate less testosterone, a hormone linked to the production of osteoblasts that promote bone formation. Similarly alcohol leads to irregular menstrual cycles in women, reducing estrogen production and leading to osteoporosis [23]. The effect of alcohol on balance and gait leads to an increased number of falls and particularly hip fractures.

Current dietary guidelines for Americans define heavy drinking as seven drinks or more per week for women and 14 drinks or more per week for men. Moderate drinking is defined as one drink per day for women and two drinks per day for men

[20]. A few recent studies have indicated that moderate drinking may be linked with decreased fracture risk in postmenopausal women, most notably, a study of 14,000 subjects by Naves Diaz et al. found that women age 65 and over who drank alcohol on more than five days per week had a reduced risk vertebral deformity compared with those who consumed alcohol less than once a week [23]. Other studies show no beneficial results. Further research is needed to clarify these findings.

Tobacco

Many studies have shown a link between tobacco use and deteriorating bone health, citing the effect of heavy smoking in terms of lower bone density, a higher risk of bone fracture, and a decrease in the mineralization of hip, hand, forearm, and heel bones; in bone formation, and in bone healing. Other studies have failed to confirm these findings. What is known is that factors associated with smoking do have a deleterious effect. They include lower body weight among smokers, decreased physical activity, a tendency to drink more alcohol, poor diet, and earlier onset of menopause. Given the detrimental effect of smoking on overall health, the avoidance of tobacco altogether or participation in smoking cessation programs is strongly advocated [24].

Caffeine and Carbonated Drinks

One of the principal issues in drinking too much coffee or soda is that they become a substitute for milk or fortified juices. Caffeine in high amounts can contribute to bone loss by interfering with calcium absorption; however, the effect is primarily in postmenopausal women with low calcium intake [25]. Sufficient intake of calcium through food or supplements can help to obviate the negative effect of caffeine. Evidence shows that there is an association between low bone mineral density and high intake of cola but no other carbonated beverages. The phosphorus in cola can increase PTH, leading to bone breakdown [26]. The recommended amount of caffeine per day is up to 400 mg which is the equivalent of four cups of brewed coffee or ten cans of cola [27].

Exercise

Multiple clinical trials and organizations dedicated to the prevention of osteoporosis recommend weight-bearing and strength training exercises to avoid BMD loss [28, 29]. These exercises affect the remodeling of bone consistent with Wolff's law, a theory which states that bone in a healthy individual will adapt to the loads under which it is placed [30]. The internal architecture of the trabeculae undergoes adaptive changes with subsequent alteration of the external cortical portion of bone. The inverse is true as well: if the loading on a bone decreases, the bone will become weaker due to turnover. Moreover, no stimulus for continued remodeling is required to maintain bone mass [31]. During growth, mechanical loading is critical for developing weight-bearing bones, but after full skeletal development has been achieved, bones lose their ability to increase in circumference and exercise shifts from building bone to maintaining bone strength and preventing bone loss [32].

A body of research demonstrates an increase in BMD with weight-bearing exercise and a subsequent decrease in BMD when weight-bearing activity is replaced with non-weight-bearing exercise [33]. With weight-bearing exercise, bone adapts to the impact of weight and pull of muscle by building more bone cells, resulting in increased bone density. In one study, a significant increase in density occurred in the lumbar spine, hip, and femoral neck of those participating in a weight-bearing exercise program, while these values decreased in the group without exercise [34, 35]. Exercises for strengthening the hip girdle and core musculature are proposed as preventive measures to decrease the risk of hip fracture. Common exercise options include walking, running, and team sports. Although swimming and cycling do not entail weight-bearing, benefits from resistance with these activities can contribute to bone remodeling [28, 29, 36]. Based on individual goals of the patients and baseline BMD, some forms of exercise are safer and more appropriate for individual patients. Table 4 gives a summary of four classes of exercise intensity with activities divided according to level [10].

At the same time, several studies indicate only a modest increase in bone mass attributable to exercise. Rubin et al. [37] point to research demonstrating that high-resistance strength training in young women increased muscle strength but had no effect on bone mass. Bone mass is also less responsive to mechanical stimuli in the aging body. Further studies on how mechanical signals, generated by exercise, act on bone are needed to fully understand their role in achieving and maintaining bone strength. The process of how mechanical signals are transformed into anabolic agents for bone development is called "mechanotransduction" and serves as the basis for a new way of treating osteoporosis [37].

Physical/Occupational Therapies and Education

Physical and occupational therapy can be used in patients with osteoporosis for either a preventive approach or post osteoporosis-related fracture. Preventive physical and occupational therapies include fall reduction programs, education in proper body mechanics to decrease compressive forces on the spine, and exercise programs [38]. Because falls that involve direct impact on the hip are correlated with a 30-fold increased rate of fracture [39–42], a fall prevention and technique simulation program can be instituted. To help limit falls or, in cases where falls are inevitable, to illustrate how to descend to the ground safely, therapists instruct patients to direct forces away

Table 4 Levels of exercise intensity

Group 1:	
Weight-bearing high-impact/resistance activities	
Aerobic dancing	Basketball
Dancing	Field hockey
Gymnastics	Hiking
Jogging or running	Jumping rope
Lacrosse	Racquet sports
Soccer	Stair climbing
Tennis	Volleyball
Weight lifting	Resistance
Group 2:	
Weight-bearing low-impact activities	
Cross-country ski machines (avoid if you have balance problems and are at risk of falls)	
Downhill and cross-country skiing (avoid if you have balance problems and are at risk of falls)	
Elliptical training machines	
Low-impact aerobics	
Stair-step machines	
Treadmill walking	
Walking	
Group 3:	
Nonimpact/balance/functional exercises	
Balance training exercises	
Functional exercises	
Pilates (avoid forward-bending exercises)	
Posture exercises	
Tai Chi	
Yoga (avoid forward-bending exercises)	
Group 4:	
Non-weight-bearing nonimpact activities	
Bicycling and indoor cycling	
Deep-water walking	
Stretching and flexibility exercises (avoid forward-bending exercises)	
Swimming	
Water aerobics	

Source: Adapted from National Osteoporosis Foundation [10]
The activities in Group 1 are the most effective for building bone. If you have low bone mass and osteoporosis or are frail, choose safer options from Groups 2, 3, and 4

from the hip and on to the buttock. A monitored strength training program will decrease osteoporotic bone remodeling by exerting forces on the bones through weight-bearing and applying muscle tension with resistance directly to the bone.

Other multifactorial interventions include Tai Chi and other exercise programs, individual risk assessment taking into account any vision difficulties or complications from medications, home and community assessment with attention to poor lighting, slippery and uneven surfaces, loose rugs, clutter on floors, and other common hazards. Dual-tasking strategies have also proved effective, particularly for the elderly. A recent study demonstrated that gait variability in an older population engaged in dual tasking (as examined in the landmark "stops walking when talking" test) and multitasking could be reduced through a music-based physical exercise program; the results showed that gait and balance were improved and that the fall risk decreased 54 % as compared to a fall reduction rate of 37 % for Tai Chi interventions [43].

Gait aids and protective pads are nonpharmacological options for the prevention of osteoporotic fractures. However studies on the use of padded hip protectors indicate only marginally decreased rates of hip fracture in institutionalized and community settings [44–46]. Noncompliance is also one of the principal limiting factors in the effectiveness of hip protectors, particularly with regard to long-term adherence [40, 47–51].

While techniques of fall prevention as well as specific exercises can be implemented in the inpatient rehabilitation setting, reviewing and reinforcing these techniques once the patient is home may not be feasible or realistic, even if therapy is ordered in the home setting upon hospital discharge.

Dietary Intake and Other Preventive Strategies Specific to Childhood and Adolescence

Increasing attention is being focused on prevention of osteoporosis from the very beginning of life. Recent evidence points to the fact that attaining peak bone mass may begin in utero. Not only is low birth weight linked to lower BMD but vitamin D deficiency, lack of exercise, and maternal smoking may adversely affect bone mineral acquisition in the development of the fetus. Vitamin D monitoring in pregnant women should be considered [52]. For calcium intake, the IOM recommends 200 mg/day for infants age birth to six months, 260 mg/day for ages 7–12 months, 700 mg/day for ages 1–3, increasing to 1000 mg/day for ages 4–8. Recommended vitamin D intake ranges from 400 IU/day for 0–12 months to 600 IU/day from age 1 through adolescence and indeed until age 70 [53]. Because very few foods contain vitamin D, the American Academy of Orthopedic Surgeons recommends that children from infancy through adolescence take vitamin D supplements to reach an intake of 1000 IU/day [54].

Research on the impact of exercise on bone health in young children is limited. Among the most significant is the Iowa Bone Development Study involving more than 300 children and focusing on objectively measured moderate and vigorous physical activity and BMD age 5. Using accelerometry-based monitors, Janz et al. [55] found evidence of a sustained benefit for bone mineral content associated with exercise at the whole body, spine, and hip, implying that unless children are physically active at an early age, they may be unable to reach the highest peak bone mass possible later in life. The 5-year-old boys in the study were 28 % more active than the girls, resulting in more mechanical loading of bone and potentially greater benefits [55]. Adolescence is the key period for the development of peak bone mass. Girls generally begin puberty between the ages of 10–14 and boys between the ages of 12–16. Both sexes age 10–20 require at least 1300 mg of calcium per day combined with 600 IU/day of vitamin D; if intake is insufficient, calcium and vitamin D supplements are required. Given the relative lack of sunlight in winter, the administration of a single dose of 150,000 IU of vitamin D in early winter can help maintain desirable serum 25(OH)D levels [56]. Weight-bearing exercises including walking, running, and such sports as soccer, basketball, volleyball, and gymnastics are essential to maximize bone strength during the teen years. However, young women who exercise excessively can experience the consequences of the female athlete triad: eating disorders, menstrual dysfunction, and low BMD, leading to osteoporosis (Chap. 19).

Several programs designed to educate adolescents about the dangers of osteoporosis have recently been instituted with positive results. Using lectures, slides, and posters, Hightower [1] developed an inexpensive classroom presentation dealing with the need for calcium and vitamin D, effects of diet, smoking, and alcohol on bone, and the importance of appropriate exercise. Teens suffering from the effects of bone loss often agreed to participate in these sessions, giving the audience an opportunity to question them about their experience. Surveys of the participants conducted before and after the presentations indicated an 80 % increase in knowledge about the risk factors for osteoporosis [1]. "Jump Start Your Bones©," a highly interactive school-based osteoporosis prevention program developed at Rutgers University, is aimed at seventh to eighth grade students, encompassing minority groups as well as children with African-American, Asian, and Hispanic backgrounds. Based on extensive research, it focuses on calcium nutrition and physical activity, emphasizing both their immediate and long-term benefits [57].

The internet is also becoming an important source of information for educating students and, in many cases, is more effective in altering health practices than is print material. For example, TWEEDS—The Tailored Web-Education System Tool and Site Development—produces a website for viewing educational materials interactively. Designed primarily for grades 9–12 when children have become accustomed to using computers, the question-and-answer format enables users to receive personalized messages reflecting their specific concerns and to evaluate the site's effectiveness. The response to a pilot study of the site indicates that students advanced their understanding of osteoporosis, changed their perceptions of the seriousness of the disease, and expressed intent to adopt osteoporosis prevention practices. To further evaluate the potential of tailored web-based education, participants will need to be further evaluated to determine how much information they retain and whether they actually implement a new diet and exercise regime and continue to follow it over time [58]. Studies of osteoporosis, once focused almost solely on postmenopausal women, are now providing valuable information about action that can be taken much earlier in life to help alleviate the physical and mental burdens of the disease.

References

1. Hightower L. Osteoporosis: pediatric disease with geriatric consequences. Orthop Nurs. 2000;19(5):59–62.
2. National Osteoorosis Foundation. Facts about bone health in children and adolescents. Arlington: National Osteoporosis Foundation; 2015. http://nof.org/articles/bone-health-children-adolescents. Accessed 14 Mar 2015.
3. National Institute of Arthritis and Musculoskeletal and Skin Diseases. Osteoporosis: peak bone mass in women. Bethesda, MD: 2015. http://www.niams.nih.gov/Health_Info/Bone/Osteoporosis/bone_mass.asp. Accessed 24 Mar 2015.
4. Murad MH, Elamin KB, Nisrin O, Elmour A, Elamin MB, Alkaatib AA, et al. Clinical review: the effect of vitamin D on falls: a systematic review and meta-analysis. J Clin Endocrinol Metab. 2011;96(10):2997–3006. doi:10.1210/jc.2011-1193.
5. Bischoff-Ferrari HA, Dawson-Hughes B, Staehelin HB, Orav JE, Stuck AE, Retal T, et al. Fall prevention with supplemental and active forms of vitamin D: a meta-analysis of randomised controlled trials. BMJ. 2009;339:b3692. doi:10.1136/bmj.b3692.
6. Bischoff-Ferrari HA, Willett WC, Wong JB, Giovannucci E, Dietrich T, Dawson-Hughes B. Fracture prevention with vitamin D supplementation: a meta-analysis of randomised control trials. JAMA. 2005;293(18):2257–64.
7. Institute of Medicine. Dietary reference intakes for calcium and vitamin D: report brief. Washington, DC: Institute of Medicine; 2010. http://iom.nationalacademies.org/Reports/2010/Dietary-Reference-Intakes-for-Calcium-and-Vitamin-D.aspx. Accessed 2015.
8. Dawson-Hughes B, Mithal A, Bonjour JP, Boonan S, Burckhardt P, Fleishman GE, et al. IOF position statement: vitamin D recommendations for older adults. Osteoporos Int. 2010;21(7):1151–4. doi:10.1007/s00198-010-1285-3.
9. Bischoff-Ferrari HA, Dietrich T, Orav EJ, Hu FB, Zheng Y, Carlson EW, et al. Higher 25-hydroxyvitamin D concentrations are associated with better lower extremity function in both active and inactive persons aged > or =60 y. Am J Clin Nutr. 2004;80(3):752–8.
10. National Osteoporosis Foundation. Boning up on osteoporosis: a guide to prevention and treatment. Washington, DC: National Osteoporosis Foundation; 2008.
11. Scoff-Ferrari HA, Willett WC. Comment on the IOM vitamin D and calcium recommendations. In: Harvard school of public health nutrition source. 2015. http://www.hsph.harvard.edu/nutritionsource/vitamin-d-fracture-prevention. Accessed 31 Mar 2015.
12. National Osteoporosis Foundation. Calcium and vitamin D: what you need to know. Arlington: National Osteoporosis Foundation; 2015. http://www.nof.org/calcium. Accessed 24 Mar 2015.
13. Ross AC, Taylor CL, Yaktine AL, Del Valle H, editors. Institute of Medicine Committee to Review Intakes for Vitamin D and Calcium. Dietary reference intakes for calcium and vitamin D. Washington, DC: National Academies Press; 2013. http://www.nebi.nlm.nih.gov/books/NBK56061/. Accessed 27 Mar 2015.
14. Tripkovic L, Lambert H, Hart K, Smith CP, Bucca G, Penson S, et al. Comparison of vitamin D2 and vitamin D3 supplementation in raising serum 25-hydroxyvitamin D status: a systematic review and meta-analysis. Am J Clin Nutr. 2012;95(6):1357–64. doi:10.3945/ajcn.111.031070.
15. National Institutes of Health. Fact sheet for health professionals: vitamin D. 2014. https://ods.od.nih.gov/factsheets/VitaminD-HealthProfessional/. Accessed 22 Dec 2015.
16. U.S. Department of Health and Human Services. Bone health and osteoporosis: a report of the surgeon general. Rockville: Office of the Surgeon General; 2004. p. 115–7.
17. National Institutes of Health, Office of Dietary Supplements. Calcium: dietary supplement. 2013. http://ods.od.nih.gov/factsheets/Calcium-HealthProfessional. Accessed 26 Mar 2015.
18. Weaver CN, Heaney RP. Nutrition and osteoporosis. In: Rosen CJ, editor. Primer on the metabolic bone diseases and disorders of mineral metabolism. Ames: Wiley-Blackwell; 2013. p. 361–6.

19. National Dairy Council. Calcium. http://www.ndc.ie/Why_Dairy/Calcium.asp. Accessed 16 Mar 2015.
20. Dietary Guidelines Advisory Committee. Scientific report of the 2015 dietary guidelines advisory committee: dietary guidelines for Americans. 2015. http://www.healthy.gov/dietaryguidelines.2015.asp. Accessed 16 Mar 2015.
21. Pan W, Borovac J, Spicer Z, Hoenderop JG, Bindels RJ, Shull GE, et al. The epithelial sodium/proton exchanger, NHE3, is necessary for renal and intestinal calcium (re)absorption. Am J Physiol Renal Physiol. 2012;302(8):F943–56. doi:10.1152/ajprenal.00504.2010.
22. Nordin BE, Need AG, Morris HA, Horowitz M. The nature and significance of the relationship between urinary sodium and urinary calcium in women. J Nutr. 1993;123(9):1615–22.
23. Naves Diaz M, O'Neill TW, Silman AJ. The influence of alcohol consumption on the risk of vertebral deformity. Osteoporos Int. 1997;7(1):65–71.
24. NIH Osteoporosis and Related Bone Diseases National Resource Center. Smoking and bone health. Washington, DC: National Institutes of Health; 2016. http://www.niams.nih.gov/health_info/bone/Osteoporosis/conditions_Behaviors/bone_smoking.asp. Accessed 30 May 2016.
25. Cooper C, Atkinson EJ, Wahner HW, O'Fallon WM, Riggs BL, Judd HL, et al. Is caffeine consumption a risk factor for osteoporosis? J Bone Miner Res. 1992;7(4):465–71.
26. Tucker KL, Morita K, Qiano N, Hannab MT, Cupples LA, Kiel DP. Colas, but not other carbonated beverages, are associated with low bone mineral density in older women: the Framingham Osteoporosis Study. Am J Clin Nutr. 2006;84(4):936–42.
27. Mayo Clinic Staff. Caffeine: how much is too much? Rochester: Mayo Clinic; 2015. http://www.mayoclinic.org/healthy-lifestyle/nutrition-and-healthy-eating/in-depth/caffeine/art-20045678. Accessed 24 Mar 2015.
28. Ryan AS, Treuth MS, Hunter GR, Elahi D. Resistive training maintains bone mineral density in postmenopausal women. Calcif Tissue Int. 1998;62(4):295–9.
29. Malmros B, Mortensen L, Jensen MB, Charles P. Positive effects of physiotherapy on chronic pain and performance in osteoporosis. Osteoporos Int. 1998;8(3):215–21.
30. Frost HM. Wolff's Law and bone's structural adaptations to mechanical usage: an overview for clinicians. Angle Orthod. 1994;64(3):175–88.
31. Wolff J. The law of bone remodeling. 1st ed. New York: Springer; 1986 (translation of the German 1892 edition).
32. Turner CH. Biochemical aspects of bone formation. In: Bronner F, Farach-Carson MC, editors. Bone formation. New York: Springer; 2004. p. 86.
33. Iwamoto J, Takeda T, Ichimura S. Effect of exercise training and detraining on bone mineral density in postmenopausal women with osteoporosis. J Orthop Sci. 2001;6(2):128–32.
34. Lin JT, Lane JM. Nonpharmacologic management of osteoporosis to minimize fracture risk. Nat Clin Pract Rheumatol. 2008;4(1):20–5. doi:10.1038/ncprheum0702.
35. Sinaki M. Nonpharmacologic interventions: exercise, fall prevention, and role of physical medicine. Clin Geriatr Med. 2003;19(2):337–59.
36. Kemmler W, Engelke K, Weineck J, Hensen J. The Erlangen fitness osteoporosis prevention study: a controlled exercise trial in early postmenopausal women with low bone density-first-year results. Arch Phys Med Rehabil. 2003;84(5):673–82.
37. Rubin CT, Rubin UJ, Judex S. Exercise and the prevention of osteoporosis. In: Rosen CJ, editor. Primer on the metabolic bone diseases and disorders of mineral metabolism. Ames: Wiley-Blackwell; 2013. p. 396–402.
38. Pfeifer M, Sinaki M, Geusens P, Boonen S, Preisinger E, Minne HW. Musculoskeletal rehabilitation in osteoporosis: a review. J Bone Miner Res. 2004;19(8):1208–14.
39. Sinaki M, Brey RH, Hughes CA, Larson DR, Kaufman KR. Significant reduction in risk of falls and back pain in osteoporotic-kyphotic women through a Spinal Proprioceptive Extension Exercise Dynamic (SPEED) program. Mayo Clin Proc. 2005;80(7):849–55.
40. Sinaki M. Falls, fractures, and hip pads. Curr Osteoporos Rep. 2004;2(4):131–7.
41. Sinaki M, Brey RH, Hughes CA, Larson DR, Kaufman KR. Balance disorder and increased risk of falls in osteoporosis and kyphosis: significance of kyphotic posture and muscle strength. Osteoporos Int. 2005;16(8):1004–10.

42. Kessenich C. Nonpharmacological prevention of osteoporotic fractures. Clin Interv Aging. 2007;2(2):263–6.
43. Trombetti A, Hars M, Hermann FR, Kressig RW, Ferrari S, Rizzoli R. Effect of music-based multi-tasked training on gait, balance and fall risk in elderly people. Arch Intern Med. 2011;171(6):525–33.
44. Parker MJ, Gillespie WJ, Gillespie LD. Effectiveness of hip protectors for preventing hip fractures in elderly people: systemic review. BMJ. 2006;332(7541):571–4.
45. Fleurence RL. Cost-effectiveness of fracture prevention treatments in the elderly. Int J Technol Assess Health Care. 2004;20(2):184–91.
46. Singh S, Sun H, Anis AH. Cost-effectiveness of hip protectors in the prevention of osteoporosis related hip fracture in elderly nursing home residents. J Rheumatol. 2004;31(8):1607–13.
47. van Schoor NM, Smit JH, Twisk JW, Bouter LM, Lips P. Prevention of hip fractures by external hip protectors: a randomized controlled trial. JAMA. 2003;289(15):1957–62.
48. van Schoor NM, Deville WL, Bouter LM, Lips P. Acceptance and compliance with external hip protectors: a systematic review of the literature. Osteoporos Int. 2002;13(12):917–24.
49. Kannus P, Parkkari J. Prevention of hip fracture with hip protectors. Age Ageing. 2006;35(2):ii51–4.
50. Patel S, Ogunremi L, Chinappen U. Acceptability and compliance with hip protectors in community-dwelling women at high risk of hip fracture. Rheumatology (Oxford). 2003;42(6):769–72.
51. Cameron ID, Quine S. External hip protectors: likely non-compliance among high risk elderly people living in the community. Arch Gerontol Geriatr. 1994;19(3):273–81.
52. Grossman JM. Osteoporosis prevention. Curr Opin Rheumatol. 2011;23(2):203–10.
53. National Institutes of Medicine. New recommended daily amounts of calcium and vitamin D. NIH medline plus, the magazine. Washington, DC: National Institutes of Health and Friends of the National Library of Medicine. 2011;5(4):10–15.
54. American Academy of Orthopaedic Surgeons. Healthy bones at every age. Orthoinfo. http://orthoinfo.aaos.org/topic.cfm?topic=a00127. Accessed 31 Mar 2015.
55. Janz KF, Letuchy EM, Eichenberger-Gilmore JM, Burns TL, Turner JC, Willing MC, Levy SM. Early physical activity provides sustained bone health benefits later in childhood. Med Sci Sports Exerc. 2010;42(6):1072–8.
56. Docio S, Riancho JA, Perez A, Olmos JM, Amado JA, Gonzalez-Macias J. Season deficiency of vitamin D in children: a potential target for osteoporosis-preventing strategies? J Bone Min Res. 1998;13(4):544–8.
57. Klotzbach-Shimomura K, Keenan DP. Jump start your bones©: a school-based osteoporosis prevention program. Raleigh: The Forum for Family and Consumer Issues (FFCI); 2001. http://ncsu.edu/ffci/publications/2001/v6-n3-2001-fall/jump-start.php. Accessed 24 Mar 2015.
58. Randi Schoenfeld E, Ng P, Henderson K, Wu SY. Using the internet to educate adolescents about osteoporosis: application of a tailored web-education system. Health Promot Pract. 2010;11(1):104–11. doi:10.1177/1524839908321730.
59. Bikle D, Adams JS, Christakos S. Vitamin D: production, metabolism, mechanism of action, and clinical requirements. In: Rosen CJ, editor. Primer on the metabolic bone diseases and disorders of mineral metabolism. Ames, Iowa: Wiley; 2013.

Chapter 5
Interventions and Management of Complications of Osteoporosis

Christina V. Oleson and Amanda B. Morina

The treatment and management of osteoporosis has undergone a major transformation in recent decades. Increasing knowledge about the underlying molecular mechanisms of osteoporosis has led to significant advances in surgical techniques as well as in pharmacologic and nonpharmacologic approaches aimed at improving bone density, reducing fracture risk, alleviating pain, and improving quality of life. New surgical techniques; more effective medications including bisphosphonates and the monoclonal antibody, denosumab; enhanced bracing mechanisms; exercise regimens, and fall prevention programs are all described in this chapter. However, it should be noted that their availability coexists with the need for greater physician awareness of these options as well as greater patient adherence to prescribed treatment and rehabilitation programs.

Surgical Interventions

Hip Fractures

Unlike spine fractures which are known to occur as a result of osteoporosis [1], hip fractures are primarily caused by falls. In a study examining the epidemiology of fractures among 169 community dwellers over the age of 50, only 1.2 % of fractures occurred spontaneously, with just two patients noting pain in the hip immediately prior to the fall. The remaining 167 patients (98.8 %) experienced fractures as a result of falls, with 33 % of falls due to tripping or slipping on objects, 21 % caused by weakness in legs or balance problems from neurological conditions, and the others suspected to occur from syncope and dizziness related to cardiovascular conditions [2]. Although rehabilitation strategies are generally the same for osteoporosis patients sustaining hip fracture as they are for those without osteoporosis, a number of factors unique to patients with osteoporosis should be considered by the surgeon

C.V. Oleson, *Osteoporosis Rehabilitation*, DOI 10.1007/978-3-319-45084-1_5

and physiatrist. Elderly patients with osteoporosis are particularly susceptible to hip fractures, and, in this subgroup, recovery is significantly more complex. For the surgeon, the primary challenge is to select a management strategy that relieves pain through stable fixation but also facilitates early mobilization and minimizes morbidity.

Older adults are at increased risk of experiencing the malignant effects of immobilization, including pressure ulcers [3] from extended bed rest, as well as deep vein thrombosis, urinary retention, urinary tract infections, and physical deconditioning [4]. Delays in fracture treatment of more than 24 hours are known to increase mortality in the elderly [4, 5] or compromise quality of life [6]. Every effort should be made to perform surgery within the first 24–48 hours of the fracture, recognizing that such intervention may be impossible in patients who require reversal of anticoagulation from chronic warfarin use or those requiring preoperative cardiac clearance and associated testing [4].

Hip fractures can be classified by location and degree of displacement or instability (Fig. 1). Intertrochanteric and subtrochanteric fractures are considered as extracapsular, whereas fractures in the femoral neck are classified as intracapsular. The incidence above age 50 is estimated at 49 % intertrochanteric, 37 % femoral neck, and 14 % subtrochanteric [2]. The incidence of intertrochanteric and femoral neck fracture is similar in patients aged 65–99 [7]. Surgical intervention varies depending on fracture type and degree of displacement.

Greater trochanteric fractures may be caused by direct injury or may occur following forceful activity of the gluteus medius or minimus muscles, as in certain jumping sports. If found in isolation and displacement is less than 1 cm, without risk of further separation, these fractures can be treated nonoperatively with protected weight-bearing for 6–8 weeks [8]. However, greater trochanteric fractures are commonly found in conjunction with intertrochanteric fractures, which occur in the proximal femur but distal to the femoral neck (Fig. 2). In this case operative intervention for the combined injury would be recommended. Options include sliding screw plate devices that allow for increased osseous healing by bridging bony fragments together, while imparting less stress on the device. A second common intervention used for intertrochanteric fractures is the dynamic hip screw. This may be accompanied by cerclage wires in the case of high-velocity falls (motor vehicle accidents or sports injuries) or when combined with a greater trochanteric injury (Fig. 3).

Alternatively, intertrochanteric fractures at low velocity are often seen in those with established osteoporosis. Postoperatively, the patient is made partially weight-bearing (10 %) for 4–6 weeks, depending on the degree of stability. When adequate intertrochanteric healing is evident, progressive weight-bearing is permitted [9]. Subtrochanteric fractures constitute a subgroup of intertrochanteric fractures in which the fracture extends beyond the intertrochanteric line. As with intertrochanteric fractures, the majority of patients are managed with open reduction and internal fixation rather than with an endoprosthesis [2].

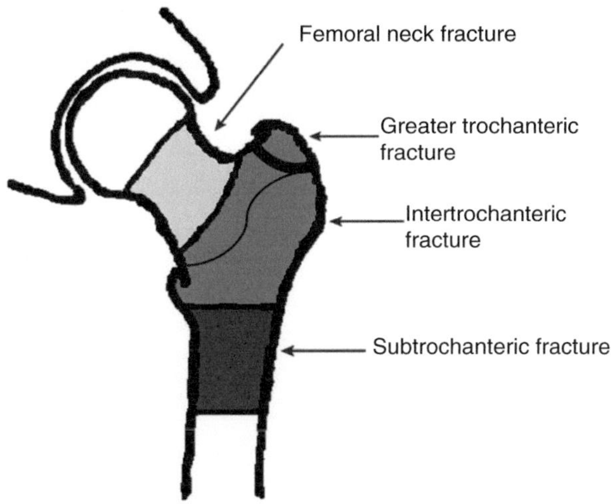

Fig. 1 Types of hip fractures (*Source*: Adapted from Wikipedia Public Domain [WPD]. Accessed 15 April 2016)

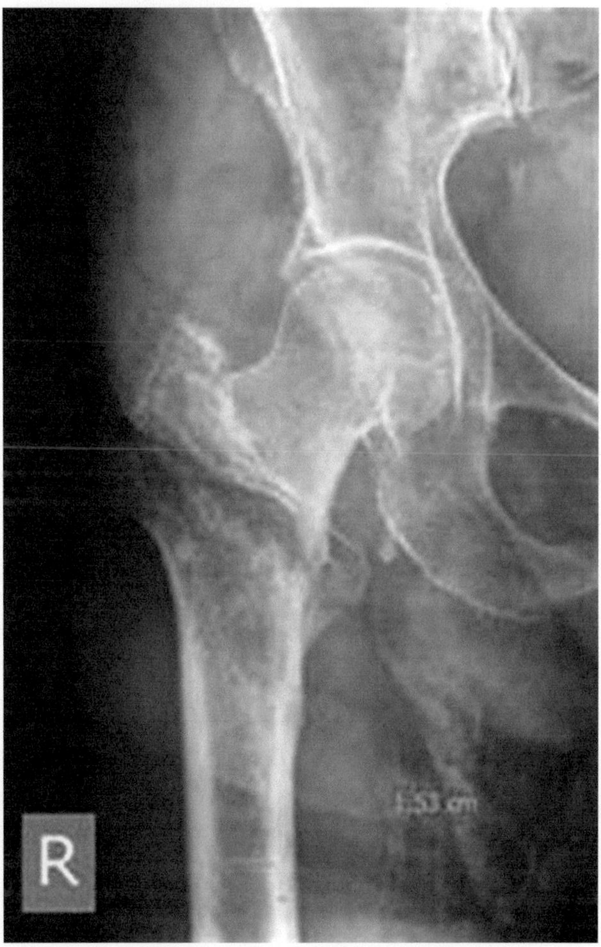

Fig. 2 Greater trochanter and intertrochanteric fracture in a single patient. This patient experienced a high velocity fall during a sporting activity. The intertrochanteric fracture is nondisplaced and the greater trochanter is minimally displaced. (*Source*: Courtesy of Thomas Jefferson University Hospital, Philadelphia, PA)

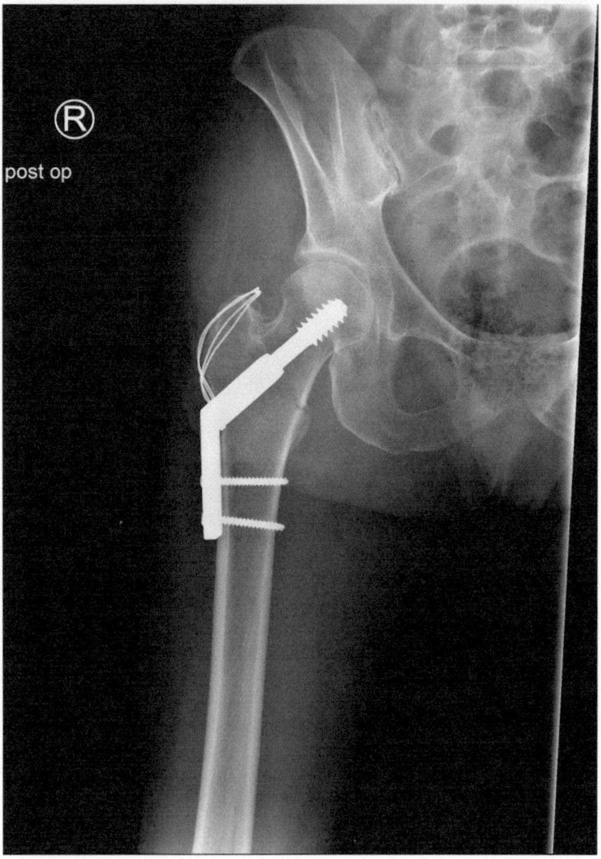

Fig. 3 Dynamic hip screw with cerclage wires used in intertrochanteric fracture repair (*Source*: Courtesy of Thomas Jefferson University Hospital, Philadelphia, PA)

Femoral Neck Fractures

Occurring proximal to the greater trochanter, femoral neck fractures (Figs. 4 and 5) carry the added risk of avascular necrosis due to the proximity of the arteries supplying the region of fracture. The Garden classification system I–IV, based on the degree of displacement, is the most commonly used method to characterize femoral neck fractures. Garden I fractures are minimally displaced and incomplete; Garden II fractures are non-displaced and complete; Garden III fractures are partially displaced and complete; and Garden IV fractures are completely displaced. Elderly patients with Garden I or II fractures can be treated with screw fixation.

Patients with displaced fractures require arthroplasty—the surgical reconstruction or replacement of a joint [10]. The advantages of arthroplasty include lower rates of reoperation, earlier recovery, and possible reduction in the risk of avascular necrosis. Disadvantages are an increase in blood loss and risk of deep wound infection [11]. Patients who are nonambulatory or who have significant medical comorbidities may

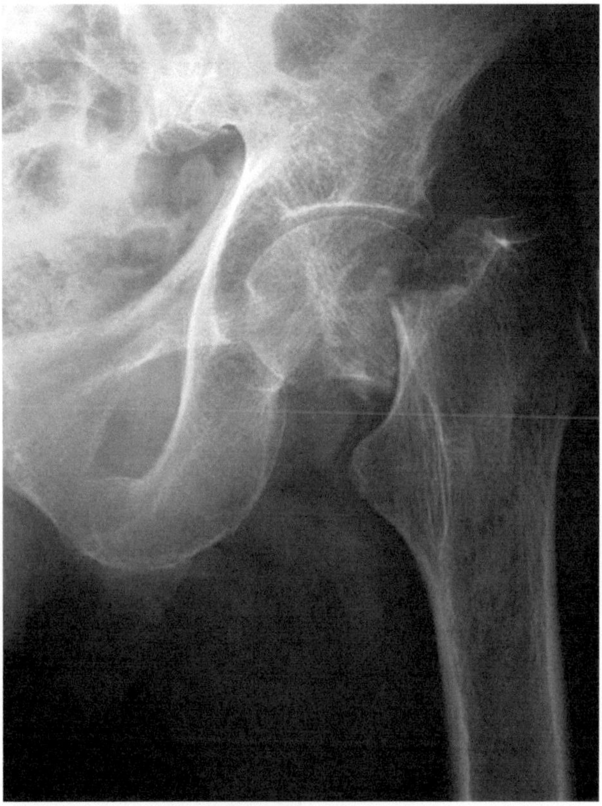

Fig. 4 Femoral neck fracture, moderately displaced, left hip (*Source*: WPD. Accessed 5 Nov 2015)

be treated nonoperatively. However, opting to forego surgery when it is recommended carries an extremely high mortality rate. One study found a 56 % mortality at 12 months post fracture for patients who declined surgery for exclusively economic reasons [12].

One of the benefits of hip arthroplasty is earlier weight-bearing on the surgical limb. For patients with osteoporosis who have undergone arthroplasty for hip fracture, only 22.4 % of those were permitted weight-bearing as tolerated as opposed to 77.7 % of those without osteoporosis [13]. Moreover, the Siebens study [13] found that patients with weight-bearing restrictions were less likely to be discharged home. Ariza-Vega et al. found non-weight-bearing status following hip fracture surgery was associated with diminished functional outcomes after one year [14].

Femoral Shaft and Distal Femur Fractures

For femoral shaft and more distal femur fractures (Fig. 6), pin and screw fixations can be difficult in weakened or osteoporotic bone. The fixation is more robust with the use of a locking compression plate which can provide three times the stability of

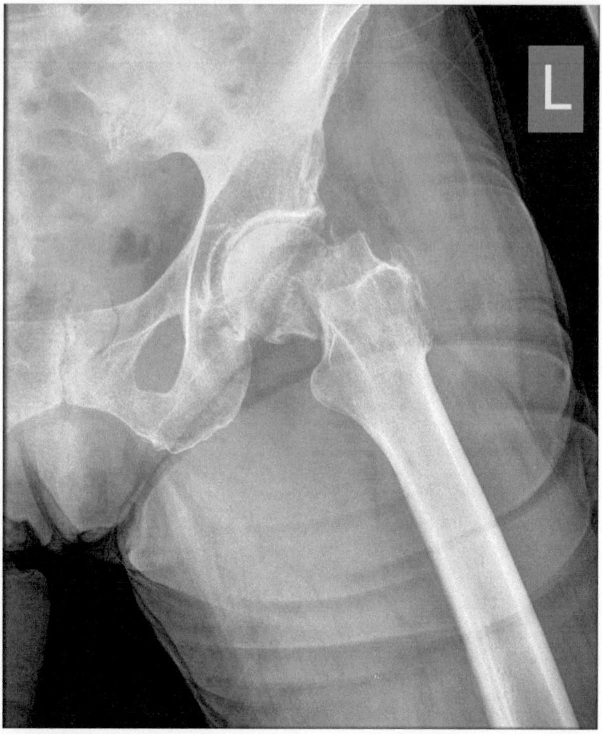

Fig. 5 Acute, displaced, comminuted and transverse fracture of the left subcapital femoral neck. This fracture was sustained in a fall from several steps in an elderly female with established osteopenia. (*Source*: Department of Radiology, Thomas Jefferson University)

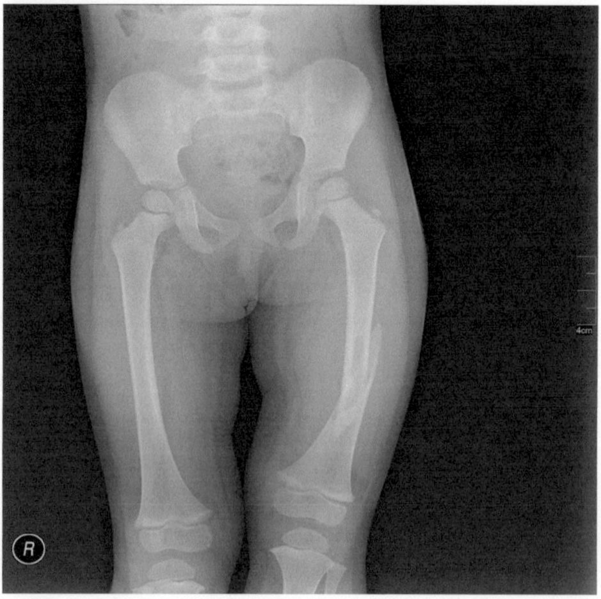

Fig. 6 *Left* distal femur fracture (*Source*: Adapted from WPD. Accessed 5 Nov 2015)

the standard lateral condylar buttress plates and 2.5 times the strength of the condylar plate in axial loading [15]. However, locking compression plates cannot be placed in cases of periprosthetic fractures, which instead require plates using wires for fixation around the femoral shaft. Periprosthetic fractures can also occur in the supracondylar region but primarily in those patients who have undergone total knee arthroplasty rather than hip arthroplasty [16]. One of the major risk factors for supracondylar periprosthetic fractures after knee surgery comes from a loss of bone mineral density of 19–44 % in the first year postoperatively [17].

From a rehabilitation standpoint, every effort should be made to prevent a periprosthetic fracture following primary or revision hip arthroplasty, given the fact that fixation in this type of injury is so challenging. For this reason and to prevent additional second fractures from falls after an initial injury, large sections of this chapter and those of a number of orthopedic textbooks for training are devoted to prevention of second fractures and healing of initial injuries through nutrition, medication, and physical intervention efforts. If a periprosthetic fracture does occur, the additional surgery necessarily predisposes the patient to further delays in weight-bearing and potentially in restricted weight-bearing for more time than had been the case from surgery for their original hip fracture.

Spinal Fractures

The most common type of spinal fracture in patients with osteoporosis is the anterior wedge compression fracture (Figs. 7 and 8) [18, 19]. As discussed in previous sections, these fractures are most frequently nontraumatic or due to minimal trauma that would not otherwise lead to fracture in a non-osteoporotic patient. Because these injuries typically occur in the thoracic or lumbar spine and involve only the anterior spinal column, the majority of compression fractures are stable and can be managed solely with a thoracolumbosacral orthosis (TLSO brace) [19]. However, patients with severe osteoporosis can experience significant and progressive loss of vertebral body height that can result in increased pain, pulmonary compromise, altered sitting posture, and reduced mobility. In the above situations, surgical options should be strongly considered. In cases where anterior wedging becomes more pronounced and involves 50 % or greater vertebral body height loss, disruption of the posterior longitudinal ligament, and related posterior spinal elements can be assumed. These fractures would then be considered unstable and warrant surgical intervention [20].

Measures of mechanical instability are best seen on a computerized tomography (CT) scan and include a widened interspinous and interlaminar distance, greater than 2 mm of translation in an anterior–posterior direction, kyphosis of more than 20°, dislocation, height loss of greater than 50 %, and the presence of articular process fractures [21]. If a patient with osteoporosis is being managed with just a TLSO brace and experiences either continued severe mid to low back pain with therapy or a sudden increase in back pain, additional imaging by either CT or a combination of anterior–posterior radiographs with a lateral radiograph should be performed [20].

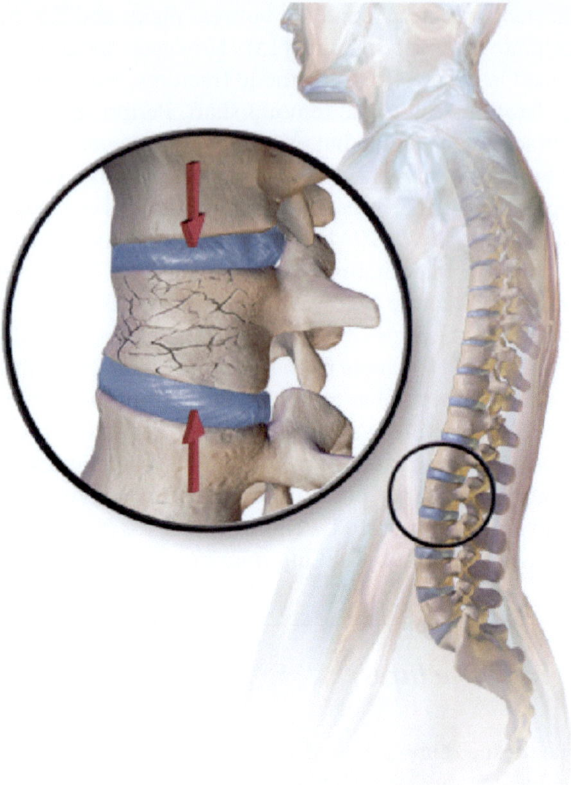

Fig. 7 Diagram showing the microscopic fracture lines within the vertebrae, contributing to a developing compression fracture (*Source*: WPD. Accessed 23 Nov 2015)

Practitioners need to ensure that a fracture has not progressed to the point of involving posterior ligamentous structures or undergone further vertebral collapse. If the posterior vertebral angle calculated on lateral radiographs exceeds 100° angulation, then a more unstable burst fracture is suspected [22]. In many cases, the lateral view and other assessment tools using a combination of plain radiographs are insufficient to ensure stability, thus making CT imperative [21]. For any patient with suspected spinal fracture instability, therapy should be suspended and flat bed rest reinstated until a confirmatory CT of the thoracolumbar spine can be performed. If any change in the sensory examination accompanies increased pain, an MRI is also required to rule out spinal cord compression or edema [20].

Surgical approaches vary according to the fracture site, the extent of collapsed vertebra, and the degree of osteoporosis, but all practitioners attempt to avoid ending a fusion at the level of greatest mobility such as the thoracolumbar junction. Instead the construct usually extends beyond this junction by one or two levels to avoid termination at the apex of kyphosis [18]. For osteoporotic compression fractures at the thoracolumbar level, the posterior surgical approach provides a relatively safe and direct means of reconstructing damage to posterior spinal elements. Short-segment fusion with two-rod distraction constructs provides correction of kyphotic posture, but this type of surgery carries a high failure rate unless multiple segments both above and below the fracture site are also fused [23]. The

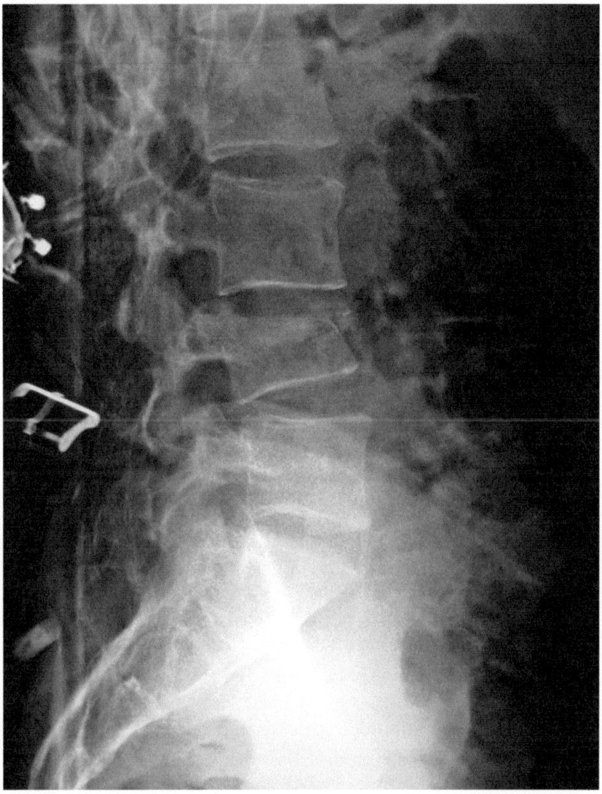

Fig. 8 X-ray of an L4 vertebral body compression fracture (*Source*: WPD. Accessed 23 Nov 2015)

additional segments fused will almost certainly compromise spinal mobility postoperatively and create additional challenges in rehabilitation, particularly for activities such as sit-to-stand transfers and reaching. Alternatively, additional placement of an anterior interbody device may decrease risk of posterior construct failure and simultaneously reduce the need for such an extensive posterior fusion [18]. The drawback of a combined anterior and posterior approach is more pain, an additional surgery, and greater risk to a patient with cardiopulmonary disease undergoing anesthesia.

For patients who cannot undergo surgery and who have intractable pain despite opiates, bracing, and rehabilitation strategies, a new hope exists in the form of percutaneous fracture stabilization with polymethyl methacrylate (PMMA). Vertebroplasty involves direct injection of PMMA into a collapsed vertebral body but does not restore vertebral height reduction. In contrast, kyphoplasty uses a balloon tamp to create a void in the bone and expand the vertebra, thereby correcting height loss [24, 25]. While these procedures offer significant pain relief [24, 26], both techniques carry the risk of cement extravasation, although this complication is less frequent with kyphoplasty due to the use of viscous form of PMMA [24, 25].

Another concern with procedures involving PMMA is weakening of adjacent spinal segments. There are inherent risks of incorporating a hard material in close proximity to fragile osteoporotic bone at neighboring vertebral segments. In verte-

Table 1 Adverse effects of medications for osteoporosis treatment

Drug	Adverse reactions	Contraindications
Alendronate	Nausea, abdominal pain, musculoskeletal pain, acid regurgitation, flatulence, dyspepsia, constipation, diarrhea	Delayed esophageal emptying, hypocalcemia, inability to be upright for >30 minutes, increased aspiration risk
Ibandronate	Influenza, nasopharyngitis, abdominal pain, dyspepsia, constipation, arthralgia, back pain, extremity pain, myalgia, headache, diarrhea, UTI	Hypocalcemia, delayed esophageal emptying, inability to be upright for >60 minutes
Zoledronic acid	Pain, chills, dizziness, N/V, osteoarthritis, fatigue, dyspnea, headache, HTN, influenza-like illness, myalgia, arthralgia, pyrexia	Hypocalcemia, CrCl <35 mL/min, acute renal impairment
Denosumab	Back pain, anemia, vertigo, upper abdominal pain, peripheral edema, cystitis, URTI, pneumonia, hypercholesterolemia, extremity pain, musculoskeletal pain, bone pain, sciatica, arthralgia, nasopharyngitis	Hypocalcemia, pregnancy
Raloxifene	DVT, PE, hot flashes, leg cramps, infection, flu, headache, N/V, diarrhea, peripheral edema, arthralgia, vaginal bleeding, pharyngitis, sinusitis, cough	VTE history, pregnancy, nursing, women who may become pregnant
Calcitonin	Rhinitis, nasal symptoms, back pain, anthralgia, epistaxis, headache	No absolute contraindications
Teriparatide	Nausea, dizziness, headache, leg cramps, acute dyspnea, allergic reactions, edema, hypercalcemia, injection-site reactions, urticaria, muscle spasm	Hypercalcemia, hyperparathyroidism, CrCl <30 mL/min

broplasty patients, long-term follow-up demonstrates a small but significant rise in adjacent segment fracture, relative to segments without PMMA [27]. In one investigation examining kyphoplasty outcomes, a decreased rate of adjacent segment fracture was observed [25]. Kyphoplasty may actually decrease risk of adjacent segment fracture if percutaneous augmentation reestablishes the natural alignment of the spine and eliminates unequal weight-bearing between adjacent vertebrae [24].

Pharmacologic Management: Currently Available Agents

A number of agents exist to treat osteoporosis but due to possible side effects, they should be carefully considered depending on the clinical comorbidities of each patient (Table 1). In addition, the efficacy of the various agents differs based on duration and populations studied within a given clinical trial (Table 2). To assist the clinician with initiating osteoporosis medications based on risk and benefits to an individual patient, the NOF has created guidelines for initiating pharmaceutical

Table 2 Effect of osteoporosis medications on bone mineral density

Drug	Increase in BMD	Population studied	Study cited
Alendronate	Lumbar spine: 4.8 %	487 postmenopausal women with low bone density received either alendronate 70 mg once weekly and daily placebo identical to raloxifene or raloxifene 60 mg daily and weekly placebo identical to alendronate for 12 months	Sambrook, *J Intern Med* 2004 [41]
	Total hip: 2.3 %		
Ibandronate	Lumbar spine: 4.27 %	158 postmenopausal osteoporotic women either received 2 mg IV ibandronate once every three months or 70 mg oral alendronate once per week	Li M, *J Bone Miner Metab* 2010 [43]
	Femoral neck: 3.48 %		
Zoledronic acid	Lumbar spine: 6.71 %	3,889 patients (mean age, 73 years) received a single 15-min infusion of zoledronic acid (5 mg) and 3,876 received placebos	Black D, *NEJM* 2007 [39]
	Total hip: 6.02 %		
	Femoral neck: 5.06 %		
Denosumab	Lumbar spine: 5.7 %	228 ambulatory men between the ages of 30 and 85 years with low BMD	Orwoll, *J Clin Endocrinol Metab.* 2012 Sep [46]
	Total hip: 2.4 %		
	Femoral neck: 2.1 %		
Raloxifene	Lumbar spine: 2.2 %	487 postmenopausal women with low bone density received either alendronate 70 mg once weekly and daily placebo identical to raloxifene or raloxifene 60 mg daily and weekly placebo identical to alendronate for 12 months	Sambrook, *J Intern Med* 2004 [41]
	Total hip: 0.8 %		
Teriparatide	Lumbar spine: 6.4 %	578 postmenopausal women and older men received a once weekly injection of 56.5 μg of teriparatide over the course of 72 weeks	Sonea, Teruki et al. *Bone* 2014 [42]
	Total hip: 3.0 %		
	Femoral neck: 2.3 %		

agents in postmenopausal women. The qualifying group should have one of the criteria listed in Table 3.

Bisphosphonates, denosumab, selective estrogen receptor modulators (SERMs), calcitonin, and parathyroid hormone (PTH) constitute the approved pharmacologic agents for prevention and treatment of osteoporosis in women. With the exception of PTH, they all act to inhibit the activity of osteoclasts, effectively reducing bone

Table 3 NOF guidelines for treatment initiation in postmenopausal women [31]

Previous vertebral hip fracture
T-score below -2 by hip DXA
T-score below -1.5 by hip DXA and 1 or more of the risk factors
Personal history of fracture as an adult
History of fragility fracture in first-degree relative
Low body weight (less than 127 lbs)
Current smoking
Oral corticosteroids (more than three months)

Source: National Osteoporosis Foundation [31]

resorption; for a transient period, formation outpaces resorption. PTH, commercially sold as teriparatide, acts as an anabolic agent to directly stimulate bone formation.

Three bisphosphonates—alendronate (Fosamax), risedronate (Actonel), and zoledronic acid (Reclast)—have been found to improve bone mineral density (BMD), reduce the risk of hip and other nonvertebral fractures, and prevent vertebral fractures. Both alendronate and risedronate are recommended if osteoporosis is caused by overuse of steroid medications, but risedronate also prevents steroid-induced osteoporosis [28]. Because both medications reduce the occurrence of vertebral and nonvertebral fractures by about 50 %, they are currently termed "agents of choice." Comparative studies of the anti-fracture efficacy of the two drugs have not been conducted and are unlikely to be carried out, given the need to obtain statistical data from more than 500,000 subjects in order to detect even a 10 % difference between alendronate and risedronate [29]. Although both medications have been shown to reduce fracture risk, outcomes are compromised by noncompliance with daily or weekly oral medications [30].

Another bisphosphonate, ibandronate, reduces the incidence of vertebral fractures by approximately 50 % over three years. Whereas these drugs can be taken orally, zoledronic acid (ZA) is administered intravenously which may help to increase adherence to therapy.

Several bisphosphonates can be used for primary and corticosteroid-induced osteoporosis. The long half-life of these medications allows for intermittent dosing on a weekly, monthly, semiannually, and, in the case of ZA, yearly basis [31, 32]. Associated dyspepsia, nausea, fever, or transient bone or muscle pain may occur, depending on the route of administration.

If a patient is affected by hip more than spine osteoporosis, certain bisphosphonates are preferable to others. The Health Outcomes and Reduced Incidence with Zoledronic Acid Once Yearly Recurrent Fracture Trial (HORIZON-RFT) found no difference in nonunion rates between zoledronic acid and placebo when ZA was administered within two weeks, 2–4 weeks, 4–6 weeks, or six weeks after hip fracture repair [33]. An annual infusion of ZA following hip fracture does not result in the additional morbidity and cost of delayed healing. Similar findings have also been found with risedronate [34]. Bone mineral density is improved in osteoporotic postmenopausal women who take alendronate, risedronate, and ZA which have reduced the risk of hip and other nonvertebral fractures [31, 32, 35, 36]; another bisphosphonate, ibandronate, has been shown to be more effective at the spine than the hip [35].

Zoledronic acid is the most potent of the bisphosphonates and has demonstrated significantly better reduction in bone turnover markers relative to alendronate [37]. Patient satisfaction questionnaires found that despite flu-like symptoms associated with ZA for the first three days after infusion, patients preferred this once annual treatment to weekly alendronate doses [38]. In an early large-scale investigation using 5 mg of once yearly intravenous ZA, Black et al. [39] found a 77 % reduction in clinical vertebral fractures after three years, as well as a 41 % decrease in hip fractures. Although risedronate and alendronate have been shown to reduce fracture risk, outcomes are compromised by noncompliance with daily or weekly oral medications [39].

One of the newest treatments for osteoporosis is denosumab (Prolia), a monoclonal antibody that is given subcutaneously to neutralize the receptor activator of nuclear factor-kB ligand (RANKL), linked to bone resorption. Because osteoclasts require RANKL to support their formation and ultimate survival, an antibody added to their existence results in reduction of bone turnover markers. Compliance is also favorable with this agent, given its twice annual administration in a doctor's office. Unlike zoledronic acid, denosumab is not cleared renally and therefore can be safely administered to those with renal insufficiency [40] (see also Table 2).

Estrogen prevents or delays bone loss in postmenopausal women; however it is associated with an increased risk of breast cancer and is no longer FDA approved for treatment unless other agents cannot be used. Selective estrogen receptor modulators (SERMs) have dual actions as estrogen agonists and antagonists [44] and provide the same benefits as estrogen without its adverse effects. The only SERM thus far sanctioned by the FDA for osteoporotic women is raloxifene which decreases the risk of spine fractures but, as yet, has not been shown to affect hip fracture risk and may not be as effective in preventing bone loss as bisphosphonates [45]. Tamoxifen, a SERM used to treat breast cancer, has been shown to preserve BMD in postmenopausal women [46] and older men [47] but has yet to receive federal approval.

Calcitonin, secreted by thyroid parafollicular cells, acts to suppress osteoclastic activity that leads to small increases in bone mass and reduction in vertebral, but not hip or distal extremity, fracture risk. Approved for women who are at least five years postmenopausal, it is administered intranasally, with potential adverse effects of congestion or epistaxis. Given its limited effect, calcitonin is not considered a first-line treatment.

Parathyroid hormone (teraparatide/Forteo), approved by the FDA as a daily injection in men and women over 28 days, has been demonstrated to increase BMD as well as reduce the likelihood of vertebral and nonvertebral fractures in women. Unlike other treatments, it is an anabolic agent that stimulates bone formation. Reported side effects include hypercalciuria, causing acute gout, leg cramps, or dizziness with orthostatic hypotension [48, 49]. Early studies suggested that concomitant use of bisphosphonates and parathyroid hormone (PTH) would diminish the anabolic effect of

PTH. However, the timing of initiation of the respective agents, as well as the population studied, clouded the interpretation of early findings [50].

In contrast, later reports demonstrated that there are gains in combining antiresorptive agents with PTH but primarily for the hip rather than the spine, with two notable exceptions. Zoledronic acid plus subcutaneous daily teriparatide, a form of PTH, resulted in BMD gains in the lumbar spine of 7.5 % after three years. Gains in BMD for patients receiving ZA alone were 7.0 % over three years versus 4.4 % for those receiving teriparatide alone [51]. Although ZA is the only bisphosphonate that thus far produces favorable outcomes in combination with PTH, denosumab combined with PTH has also demonstrated positive gains in spine BMD [50].

Only four of these medications—alendronate, risedronate, zoledronic acid, and teriparatide—have been approved for men (see chapter on male osteoporosis). Head-to-head trials of bisphosphonates have produced insufficient evidence to prove or disprove any single agent's superiority in preventing fractures; similarly head-to-head trials of bisphosphonates compared to teriparatide or raloxifene have produced insufficient evidence to prove or disprove relative superiority [52].

Although improvement in BMD is an important factor when considering osteoporosis medications, fracture prevention is the ultimate goal. The currently available osteoporosis medications and their effects on fracture prevention are compared in Table 4.

Pharmacologic Agents on the Rise

Strontium Ranelate

Antiresorptive and anabolic agents remain the two primary drugs of choice for prevention and treatment of osteoporosis. Although antiresorptive agents reduce the rate of bone remodeling, they do not increase BMD. Restoration of BMD and bone formation is not achieved through antiresorptives alone but rather requires the use of anabolic drugs [53]. Strontium ranelate (SR) is a relatively new, orally active drug that has shown positive results in reducing the risk of vertebral fractures in osteoporotic, postmenopausal women [54]. SR has a significant advantage because it decreases bone resorption, and its mechanisms are similar to those of PTH in that it stimulates bone formation and increases BMD.

Vertebral Fractures

In the early 2000s, four randomized placebo-controlled clinical trials emerged that paved the way for introducing SR into osteoporosis treatment and prevention [53, 55–57]. In 2002, Meunier et al. were the first to demonstrate SR efficacy on vertebral osteoporosis in a controlled clinical trial [53]. The study population included 353 postmenopausal women with diagnoses of osteoporosis as well as a past

Table 4 Comparison of medication effects on vertebral, nonvertebral, and hip fractures

Generic name	Brand name	Reduced risk of vertebral fractures	Reduced risk of nonvertebral fractures[a]	Reduced risk of hip fracture
Bisphosphonates				
Alendronate	Fosamax	Y	Y	Y
Risedronate	Actonel, actonel with calcium, atelvia	Y	Y	Y
Ibandronate	Boniva	Y	Unknown	Limited to date
Zoledronic acid	Reclast	Y	Y	Y
Biologicals				
Denosumab	Prolia	Y	Y	Y
Hormone therapy				
Estrogen	Premarin	N	N	N
SERMs				
Raloxifene	Evista	Y	N	N
PTH				
Teriparatide	Forteo	Y	Y	Potentially[b]

Source: Adapted from: Agency for Healthcare Research and Quality, US Department of Health and Human Services, Reducing the risk of bone fracture: a review of the research for adults with low bone density. 2012. http://effectivehealthcare.ahrq.gov/index.efm/search-for-guides-reviews-and-reports/prod

[a]Nonvertebral fractures affect bones of the appendicular skeleton apart from the hip. Includes distal femur, tibia, humerus, radius

[b]Weekly injections of 56.5 μg teriparatide may have the potential to reduce the risk of hip fracture. Studies that are designed to determine the effect of teriparatide to reduce the incidence of hip fracture are unavailable and are not likely to be conducted. The human bone biopsy information obtained from the iliac crest may not be representative of the effects of teriparatide at the hip

medical history positive for a vertebral fracture. The double-blind study compared placebo to three groups receiving SR in doses of 0.5, 1, and 2 g daily for two years. Results effectively demonstrated a dose-dependent increase in BMD in these groups versus a decrease in the placebo-controlled group. Although the primary efficacy measure was lumbar BMD, results also demonstrated a 44 % decreased incidence of fracture in the group receiving 2 g per day SR, compared to the placebo group. Similarly, Meunier et al.'s 2004 study supported findings that over a period of three years, fewer patients treated with SR, as opposed to those given the placebo, experienced new vertebral fractures [54].

Nonvertebral Fractures

Reginster et al. [55] showed that 1 g per day SR for 24 months significantly increased BMD in lumbar spine, femoral neck, and total hip in 160 early postmenopausal women, with no known prior history of osteoporosis. Any dose less than 1 g per day showed no significant effect on BMD. In another clinical trial of 5,091 postmenopausal females given 2 g per day SR for five years, a 19 % relative risk (RR) reduction of major osteoporotic nonvertebral fractures was observed in patients with average risk [56]. In a population identified as high risk, a 36 % RR reduction of hip fracture was exhibited in those receiving 2 g per day SR.

In the above studies, no significant difference in adverse effects occurred in SR as compared with control groups. The dosages of SR administered ranged from 125 mg/day to 2 g per day with the higher dosages demonstrating the most significant improvements in outcomes. The most prevalent reported adverse events consistent among the four studies were gastrointestinal issues including nausea, diarrhea, and headache.

Subsequently, however, the French Agency for the Safety of Health Products (AFSSAPS, now termed the National Agency for the Safety of Medicines and Health Products (MSNA)) conducted a review of the primary side effects of SR. From January 2006 (the date of commercialization of the product) to March 31, 2009, the AFSSAPS examined data from 31 pharmaceutical vigilance monitoring centers. The most common serious adverse events (SAEs) were cardiovascular related, equaling 52 %. Thromboembolic events (venous thrombosis, pulmonary embolism (PE), stroke, central retinal artery or vein occlusion, supraventricular tachycardia (SVT), or peripheral edema) contributed to two out of the three deaths attributable to SR use [57]. In a 2014 public statement, the European Medicines Agency recommended that patients with a history of venous thromboembolism (VTE), temporary or permanent immobilization due to a medical condition, or reduced mobility due to postoperative precautions, not use SR. The agency stipulated that use of SR be restricted in patients with cerebrovascular disease, peripheral arterial disease, and ischemic heart disease, due to risk of heart attacks or obstruction of blood vessels [58].

Cathepsin K Inhibitors

One key to improving bone density is to eliminate the undesired coupling that occurs between bone formation and bone resorption. Although bisphosphonates, SERMs, and denosumab reduce bone resorption, they correspondingly inhibit formation. Agents currently under development promise to inhibit bone resorption without affecting bone formation. Cathepsin K is a cysteine protease expressed in osteoclasts located at the ruffled border, the active portion of the cell that resorbs bone. Cathepsin K inhibitors have been explored in phase II and III clinical trials. Early results demonstrate significant reduction in N-telopeptide and C-telopeptide (NTX and CTX) and similar markers of bone loss, but no effect on markers of bone formation such as bone-specific alkaline phosphatase. In terms of clinical trials, odanacatib is the agent with the most advanced data. It is dosed weekly and administered orally. Unlike potent bisphosphonates such as zoledronic acid, the half-life of odanacatib is about one week, and it is reversible in a similar time frame, should adverse symptoms occur after use [59, 70].

Results of a phase III long-term odanacatib fracture trial (LOFT) were released in early 2015; the study population consisted of 16,713 women age 65 and older who had BMD of ≤2.5 at the hip or femoral neck, or, alternatively, a *T*-score of ≤1.5 in total hip or femoral neck in the presence of existing vertebral fracture. Findings in comparison with placebo indicate that a 50 mg per week dose inhibits bone resorption and increases BMD, with only a temporary decline in bone markers. A planned interim analysis, conducted by an independent committee, brought this study to an early halt, due to the striking efficacy and favorable risk/benefit of odanacatib compared with placebo. More than 8,000 patients (presumed to be taking the placebo) dropped out of the trial due to excessive bone loss, and a subsequent, still blinded extension study of 8,256 women includes only subjects remaining on odanacatib. The sponsor of the study plans to follow those subjects in the extension trial that will focus on the long-term safety and efficacy of odanacatib [61].

Wnt Signaling Targets: Sclerostin Inhibitors

Given the limitations of current antiresorptive therapies, particularly the uncertainly about their long-term effects, researchers are focusing on the development of anabolic treatments to increase bone formation and bone mass. Teriparatide is currently the only anabolic agent FDA approved for treating osteoporosis in both men and women. Efforts to neutralize inhibitors of Wnt signaling shows promise of enhancing bone formation. Wnt's are secreted glycoproteins that communicate by signals involving seven transmembrane receptors and a number of co-receptors; they, in turn, utilize low-density lipoprotein receptor proteins (LDLRP) five and six to facilitate gene transcription and subsequent bone mass accrual. Ectopic Wnt signaling influences osteoprogenitor cells toward the osteoblast lineage. Future pharmacologic agents that stimulate Wnt signaling would favor osteoblast formation and net bone density increase [62].

Wnt signaling is inhibited by sclerostin, which binds to the LDLRP five and six complex, halting the steps needed to influence the osteoprogenitor cells which, in turn, form osteoblasts that produce bone tissue; consequently there is a growing interest in the use of agents that inhibit sclerostin [60]. Preclinical studies of sclerostin inhibition in monkeys and ovariectomized rats have shown a substantial increase in bone formation, particularly in trabecular bone at the femoral neck and lumbar spine. Because no increase in bone resorption markers occurred, the net result was an overall increase in bone mass, confirmed by a corresponding increase in osteocalcin [63]. Inasmuch as the majority of the prior trials have focused on estrogen loss correction, this study was designed specifically to examine a possible anabolic mechanism of bone formation in men.

A phase I study in humans using three escalating doses of a sclerostin antibody, romosozumab [AMG 785], resulted in dose-dependent increases of bone formation markers yet showed a decrease in resorption marker, serum CTX. Although increases in spine BMD of 5.3 % and total hip BMD of 2.8 % occurred, six patients receiving the highest of the three doses developed antibodies to the drug with two patients demonstrating neutralizing antibodies. The presence of antibodies did not appear to compromise the effectiveness of the drug [64, 65]. Adverse effects including injection-site hemorrhage or site erythema, back pain, headache, dizziness, and hepatitis were noted in 28 % of subjects who received the drug versus 11 % of placebo subjects.

Following the phase I study, a phase II multicenter international randomized controlled trial examined 419 postmenopausal women ages 55–85 with low BMD over a 12-month period. Subjects received 70, 140, or 210 mg of subcutaneous romosozumab monthly or an every three-month dose of either 140 or 210 mg romosozumab. Other groups received placebo, alendronate orally, or subcutaneous daily teriparatide (PTH) [66]. Those subjects in the monthly 210 mg group demonstrated an 11.3 % increase in BMD in the lumbar spine, far exceeding the 4 and 6 % increases seen at six months with alendronate or teriparatide [65, 66]. A phase III study, now in progress, will clarify long-term adverse effects enabling healthcare professionals to use appropriate risk stratification in prescribing sclerostin inhibitors when they are released for use by regulatory agencies.

Nonpharmacologic Interventions

Bracing

To provide mechanical support in the osteoporotic spine, braces are prescribed in cases of acute compression fracture or symptomatic chronic vertebral fractures. The use of an orthosis supports weakened soft tissue structures, maintains anatomical alignment of the spine to promote healing, helps prevent further fractures within the affected area, and improves pain management enabling mobilization and deterring bed rest [67]. The acuity and the type of vertebral fracture are two factors that determine whether bracing should be employed.

A thoracic lumbar sacral orthosis (TLSO) may be indicated when immobilization of the spine is necessary in all planes: coronal, transverse, and frontal. Less restrictive braces, which are more comfortable, easier to fit, but do not restrict motion as fully in all three planes of motion, are prescribed when spinal fractures are considered stable and not at risk for progression [68].

Biomechanically, the objectives of a brace are to decrease axial loading on the anterior bodies of the spine and prevent flexion of the spine. Thus, braces are often designed to promote hyperextension of the spine in order to reduce pressure on the vertebral bodies. Common braces that achieve this hyperextension goal are the Jewett (Fig. 9) and Taylor braces as well as the cruciform anterior spinal hyperextension (CASH) brace (Fig. 10). All three orthoses prevent flexion and facilitate hyperextension; the restriction in other planes of motion is limited [69]. The Jewett brace may place too much force on the posterior elements of the

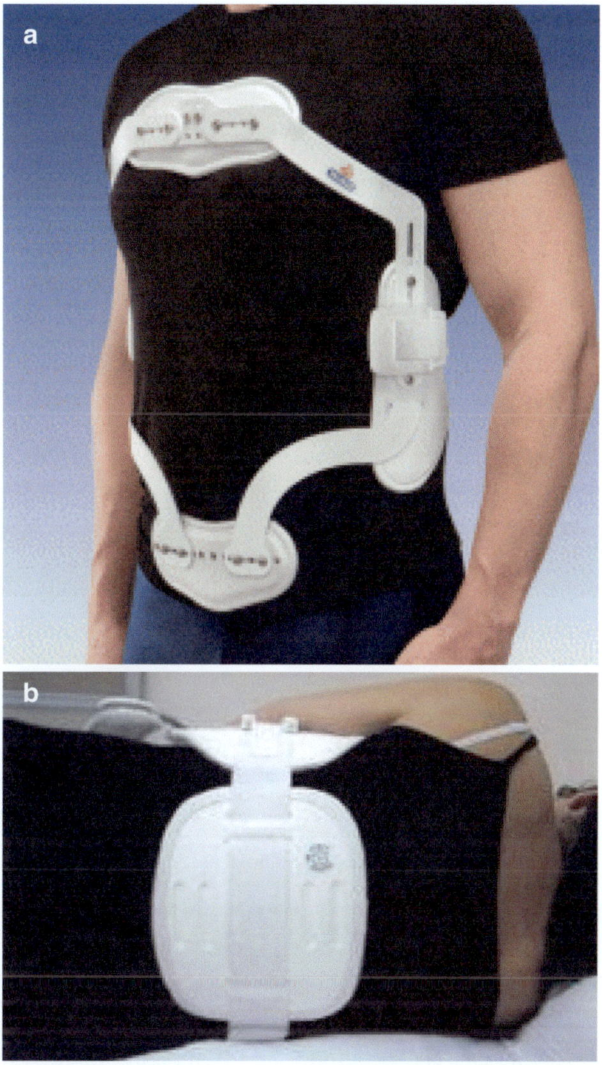

Fig. 9 Two views of the Jewett brace. (**a**) Shows the anterior view in stance and (**b**) illustrates the posterior view in the side lying position. (*Source*: Courtesy of Orthotics Department Teaching Files, Thomas Jefferson University, Philadelphia PA)

spine and thus should be avoided in cases of already established osteoporosis. Although the Jewett and CASH braces restrict flexion and promote extension, their effect in preventing spinal movement in other planes is limited [69, 70].

Bracing is often cumbersome, with several studies demonstrating decreased compliance with brace wear as compared to alternative osteoporosis treatments [69, 71]. Biomechanically, the spinal orthosis inhibits axial muscle use because the brace provides support to the spine passively rather than actively. Most osteoporosis experts agree that a brace should be discontinued as soon as the pain is resolved to prevent atrophy of axial muscles [67]. Few studies quantify the effectiveness of orthotics in the scope of osteoporosis. However, Pfeifer and colleagues did find a correlation between decreased pain and increased back extensor strength [72, 73].

Fig. 10 Photograph of an individual wearing a CASH brace (*Source*: Adapted from WPD. Accessed 23 Nov 2015)

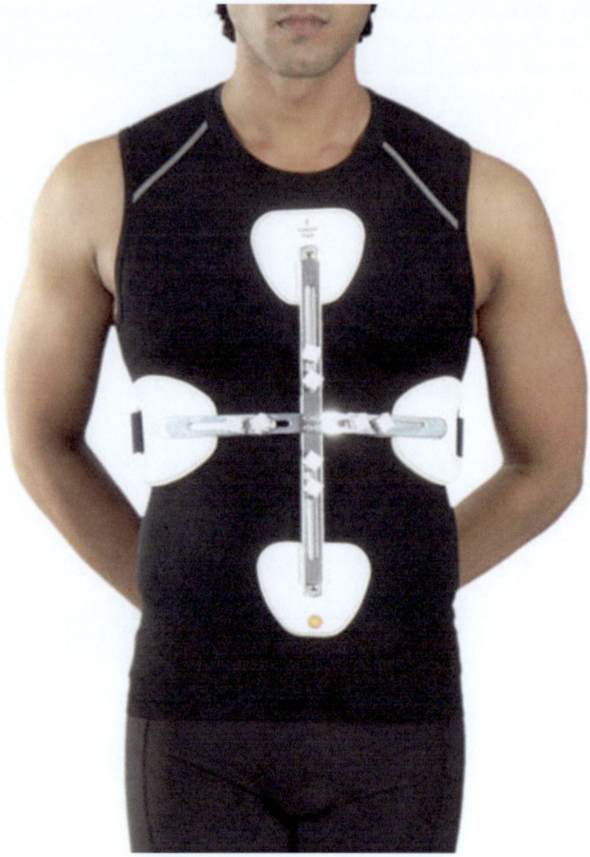

Therapy Interventions

Gait Retraining and Fall Prevention Techniques

Dynamic exercise programs are often recommended when proprioceptive deficits are identified. One method of proprioception remediation, specific to the osteoporotic population with increased kyphosis, is the application of a weighted kypho-orthosis. Unlike braces to limit flexion through the use of anterior restraints, a kypho-orthosis employs gravity to improve spinal alignment, thereby encouraging the use of axial muscles instead of inhibiting the muscles with bracing [71, 74, 75].

The weighted kypho-orthosis resembles a soft backpack with a weight present at the thoracic spine, just caudal to the inferior angles of the scapula (Fig. 11). Determination of orthosis weight varies; some studies employ a percentage of body weight, whereas others demonstrate results with a uniform weight of 1 kg [68, 71, 75, 76]. Ideally, the device should be worn 20–30 minutes for multiple sessions per day, while the patient is concomitantly performing spine extension exercises [68].

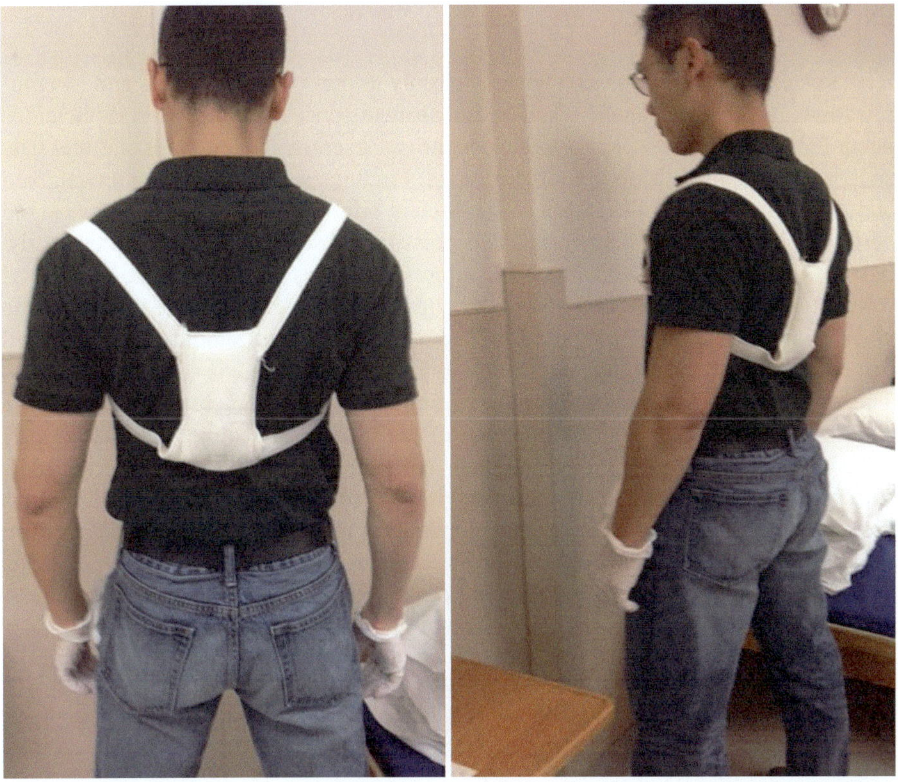

Fig. 11 Photograph of an individual with a kypho-orthotic brace (*Source*: Courtesy of Thomas Jefferson University, Department of Rehabilitation Medicine and the Office of Hospital Volunteers, Philadelphia, PA)

Kaplan et al. suggest that the kypho-orthosis reduces compression fractures with two mechanisms. The first is passive: the weight produces a force posteriorly below the inferior angles of the scapula, thus reducing anterior compressive forces on the spine. With the second, the weight produces proprioceptive input, which in turn promotes activation of back extensors and, over time, results in improved posture and back extensor strength [71].

A number of researchers have examined the benefits of a proprioceptive exercise program for patients with osteoporosis [1, 76–78]. The spinal proprioceptive extension exercise dynamic (SPEED) program, developed by M. Sinaki, combines the use of weighted kypho-orthosis, muscle and facet joint reeducation with postural, as well as resistance exercises [67, 79]. Patients were instructed in a 4-week spinal proprioception extension exercise program, performed at home while wearing a weighted kypho-orthosis. Results demonstrated reduced back pain, improved lumbar strength, reduced risk of falls based on the Falls Efficacy Scale, and increased level of overall physical activity. Significant changes were achieved in the computerized dynamic posturography score for gait and self-reported "fear of falls" [80].

Exercise Principles

Research exists on exercise as a means not only to prevent osteoporosis and its complications but also to manage resultant impairments once osteoporotic complications occur [81]. With a known history of osteoporosis, exercises making use of either passive or active spine flexion are to be avoided. Findings suggest that even unweighted and low velocity spinal flexion creates sufficient biomechanical loading of the fragile vertebra [79, 82], increasing intradiskal pressure substantially and heightening the risk of fracture. Damage occurs when compressive forces on the spine are transferred to structurally fragile vertebral bodies in conjunction with compressive loading of the anterior spinal column [83]. Abdominal and back musculature should be strengthened in neutral spinal positioning, with progression toward spine extension as tolerated. This technique allows for core muscle reinforcement without increasing force on the anterior column of the spine. An objective of exercise in the treatment of osteoporosis is to improve axial stability by gradually activating spinal extensor muscles [84]. Rudins et al. calculated that the relative risk for compression fracture is 2.7 times greater in subjects who did not perform extension exercises than in a back exercise group [85]. At the physiological level, exercise increases BMD, with greater changes noted in patients undergoing exercise in combination with pharmacologic treatment than in those undergoing pharmacologic treatment alone [68].

Weight-bearing exercise is paramount because it helps to stimulate osteoblasts to form bone. Selecting the proper physical exercise can increase muscle strength and BMD thereby decreasing the risk of appendicular fractures and related mortalities in the elderly [1]. Weight-bearing exercises, such as walking, are important for maintenance of BMD of the hips and lower extremities.

As patients age, the presence of stenosis or spondylosis creates a challenge. Kinematically, extension-based spinal exercises cause approximation of facet joints and reduction of the intervertebral foramen [86]. Repetitive extension can irritate the nerve root passing through the foramen, causing localized or radicular symptoms. Extension-based exercises may be contraindicated if osteoporosis is present and spondylosis is severe [84]. In the presence of stenosis, neither flexion nor extension exercises may be appropriate due to severe pain, but core strengthening and pelvic stabilization exercises, performed isometrically in a neutral spine position, are indicated [81, 83, 85]. Also, lower extremity flexibility should be addressed as tight leg muscles can produce tension on the axial skeleton, influencing the angle of pelvis and lumbosacral spine. Before prescribing an exercise program in either an inpatient or outpatient setting, knowledge of spondylosis, stenosis, or compression fractures is essential. Moreover, rehabilitation physicians and therapists must be made aware of any spinal precautions before instituting a treatment plan, so that safe and appropriate therapies are undertaken.

Whole Body Vibration Exercise

Whole body vibration (WBV) exercise is a forced oscillation that transfers energy from a vibration platform to the body [87]. Vibration exercise has been identified as a successful countermeasure against the loss of bone mineral in animal populations, including those with conditions similar to menopause in humans [85, 86]. Research conducted on athletes and healthy adults demonstrate some benefits from WBV therapy, especially in terms of strength and decreased BMI.

Many studies of WBV have expanded to include older populations but have frequently excluded patients with osteoporosis [88]. In previous investigations [85–88], patients receiving WBV demonstrated slight increases in BMD at the hip, but not in the spine [89–91]. Other trials with a similar subject population showed improvements in lower extremity muscle strength, BMI, pain, and balance without resultant increase in BMD [88–98]. However, two investigations included patients with osteoporosis. Ruan et al. found increases in both femoral and lumbar BMD at six months after WBV; in contrast, matched subjects without WBV therapy exhibited decreases in both femoral and lumbar BMD [92]. A second investigation found a significant reduction in back pain but no improvement in BMD [93].

WBV platforms have not been approved by the FDA for medical purposes. Disadvantages of the therapy include unknown long-term safety considerations and out-of-pocket costs to the patient. Vibration may result in loss of balance and vestibular dysfunction. Moreover the vibratory effect may compromise postoperative spinal stability or recent cataract surgery. Thus clearance from the patient's individual surgeon is strongly recommended before prescribing vibratory therapy [97, 99–101]. Further research on patients with osteoporosis is needed, with extended follow-up times to assess any long-term adverse or therapeutic effects of vibration therapy [88].

Monitoring Osteoporosis Therapy

Adherence to a prescribed treatment plan is one of the major challenges facing physicians and other healthcare providers dealing with osteoporosis patients. Since most people cannot detect whether bones are growing stronger or weaker, they have no way of knowing whether their condition has changed unless they are examined on a regular basis. One of the principal reasons for the examination is simply to review the patient's basic needs including adequate intake of calcium and vitamin D, compliance with a prescribed exercise program, maintenance of height and recommended weight, and cessation of smoking and excessive alcohol use.

In addition, the National Osteoporosis Foundation has outlined goals for the assessment of both antiresorptive and anabolic medications. In the case of antiresorptives including bisphosphonates, calcitonin, estrogen agonists/antagonists, and denosumab, the objective is to prevent additional bone loss and reduce fracture risk. A patient has a favorable response to treatment if bone density remains stable or improves and if no broken bones occur. In the case of the anabolic medicine, teriparatide, the goal is to rebuild bone, increase bone mass, and reduce fracture risk. A patient's progress is considered good if the rate of bone formation as well as bone density improves and, again, no broken bones occur [102]. In consultation with patients, healthcare providers need to determine the length of treatment with antiresorptive medicines; for example, studies show that postmenopausal women treated with alendronate or raloxifene may lose BMD in the first year, yet gain BMD if treatment is continued in year two [103]. In the case of teriparatide, however, the FDA stipulates that it should not be taken for more than two years [102].

DXA testing of the hip and lumbar spine and the use of biochemical markers of bone formation and resorption are the standard techniques for monitoring the efficacy of osteoporosis treatment. Although BMD measurements are generally performed every two years, recent studies indicate that changes in bone density may take up to three years to detect and even then may not predict a reduction in fracture risk [104]. In addition, these changes tend to be small and may vary depending on such factors as the instruments used, the position of the patient, and the technicians ability to analyze the results, all of which may introduce errors and result in mistaken interpretations, either positive or negative [27]. Since bone turnover markers are noninvasive, inexpensive, and able to detect turnover rates earlier than DXA, they may be more effective monitoring tools, but, as Compston points out, the variability in their measurement significantly limits their value in clinical practice [104]. Ultimately, neither DXA testing nor bone turnover markers improve compliance to treatment. Quite apart from test results, continuing interaction with a healthcare professional remains the key to successful osteoporosis therapy.

References

1. Sinaki M. Falls, fractures, and hip pads. Curr Osteoporos Rep. 2004;2(4):131–7.
2. Michelson JD, Myers A, Jinnah R, Cox Q, Van Natta M. Epidemiology of hip fractures among the elderly: risk factors for fracture type. Clin Orthop Relat Res. 1995;311:129–35.
3. Grimes JP, Gregory PM, Noveck H, Butler MS, Carson JL. The effects of time-to-surgery on mortality and morbidity in patients following hip fracture. Am J Med. 2002;112(9):702–9.
4. Poh KS, Lingaraj K. Complications and their risk factors following hip fracture surgery. J Orthop Surg. 2013;21(2):154–7.
5. Casaletto JA, Gatt R. Post-operative mortality related to waiting time for hip fracture surgery. Injury. 2004;35(2):114–40.
6. Dorotka R, Schoechtner H, Buchinger W. The influence of immediate surgical treatment of proximal femoral fractures on mortality and quality of life. Operation within 6 hours of the fracture versus later than 6 hours. J Bone Joint Surg (Br). 2003;85(8):1107–13.
7. Karagas MR, Lu-Yao GL, Barrett JA, Beach ML, Baron JA. Heterogeneity of hip fracture: age, race, sex, and geographic patterns of femoral neck and trochanteric fractures among the US elderly. Am J Epidemiol. 1996;143(7):677–82.
8. Wheeless CR. Fractures of the lesser and greater trochanter. Wheeless Textbook of Orthopedics. http://www.wheelessonline.com/ortho/fractures_of_the_lesser_and_greater_trochanter. Accessed 25 Jan 2015.
9. Koval KJ, Zuckerman JD. Hip fractures: II. Evaluation and treatment of intertrochanteric fractures. J Am Acad Orthop Surg. 1994;2(3):150–6.
10. Koval KJ, Zuckerman JD. Hip fractures: I. Overview and evaluation and treatment of femoral-neck fractures. J Am Acad Orthop Surg. 1994;2(3):141–9.
11. Parker MJ, Gurusamy K. Internal fixation versus arthroplasty for intracapsular proximal femoral fractures in adults. Cochrane Database Syst Rev. 2006;18(4), CD001708.
12. Yoon BH, Baek JH, Kim MK, Lee YK, Ha YC, Koo KH. Poor prognosis in elderly patients who refused surgery because of economic burden and medical problem after hip fracture. J Korean Med Sci. 2013;28(9):1378–81.

13. Siebens HC, Sharkey P, Aronow HU, Horn SD, Munin MC, De Jong G, et al. Outcomes and weight-bearing status during rehabilitation after arthroplasty for hip fractures. PM&R. 2012;4(8):548–55.
14. Ariza-Vega P, Jiménez-Moleón JJ, Kristensen MT. Non-weight-bearing status compromises the functional level up to 1 yr after hip fracture surgery. Am J Phys Med Rehabil. 2014;93(8):641–8.
15. Koval KJ, Hoehl JJ, Kummer FJ, Simon JA. Distal femoral fixation: a biomechanical comparison of the standard condylar buttress plate, a locked buttress plate, and the 95-degree blade plate. J Orthop Trauma. 1997;11(7):521–4.
16. Mont MA, Maar DC. Fractures of the ipsilateral femur after hip arthroplasty: a statistical analysis of outcome based on 487 patients. J Arthroplasty. 1994;9(5):511–9.
17. Petersen MM, Lauritzen JB, Pedersen JG, Lund B. Decreased bone density of the distal femur after uncemented knee arthroplasty: a 1-year follow-up of 29 knees. Acta Orthop Scand. 1996;67(4):339–44.
18. Moatz B, Ludwig SC, Tortolani PJ. Fixation in osteoporotic patients. Cont Spine Surg. 2013;14(1):1–7.
19. Dahdaleh NS, Dlouhy BJ, Hitchon PW. Percutaneous pedicle screw fixation for the treatment of thoracolumbar fractures. Cont Neurosurg. 2011;33(14):1–8.
20. Vaccaro AR, Kim DH, Brodke DS, Harris M, Chapman JR, Schildhauer T, et al. Diagnosis and management of thoracolumbar spine fractures. J Bone Joint Surg. 2003;85-A(12): 2456–70.
21. Campbell SE, Phillips CD, Dubovsky E, Cail WS, Omary RA. The value of CT in determining potential instability of simple wedge-compression fractures of the lumbar spine. AJNR Am J Neuroradiol. 1995;16(7):1385–92.
22. McGroy BJ, VanderWilde RS, Currier BL, Eismont FJ. Diagnosis of subtle thoracolumbar burst fractures. A new radiologic sign. Spine. 1993;18(15):2282–5.
23. Baron EM, Zeiller SC, Vaccaro AR, Hilibrand AS. Surgical management of thoracolumbar fractures. Cont Spine Surg. 2006;7(1):1–7.
24. Truumees E, Hilibrand AS, Vaccaro AR. Percutaneous vertebral augmentation. Spine J. 2004;4(2):218–29.
25. Garfin SR, Yuan HA, Reiley MA. New technologies in spine: kyphoplasty and vertebroplasty for the treatment of painful osteoporotic compression fractures. Spine. 2001;26(14):1511–5.
26. Rousing R, Andersen MO, Jespersen SM, Thomsen K, Lauritsen J. Percutaneous vertebroplasty compared to conservative treatment in patients with painful acute or subacute osteoporotic vertebral fractures: three-months follow-up in a clinical randomized study. Spine. 2009;34:1349–54.
27. Grados F, Depriester C, Cayrolle G, Hardy N, Deramond H, Fardellone P. Long-term observations of vertebral osteoporotic fractures treated by percutaneous vertebroplasty. Rheumatology. 2000;39(12):1410–4.
28. Camacho PM. Osteoporosis drugs and medications. In: EndocrineWeb. 2014. http://www.endocrineweb.com/conditions/osteoporosis/osteoporosis-drugs-medications. Accessed 8 Jul 2015.
29. Grey A, Reid IR. Differences between the bisphosphonates for the prevention and treatment of osteoporosis. Ther Clin Risk Manag. 2006;2(1):77–86.
30. Blouin J, Dragomir A, Moride Y, Ste-Marie LG, Fernandes JC, Perreault S. Impact of noncompliance with alendronate and risedronate on the incidence of nonvertebral osteoporotic fractures in elderly women. Br J Clin Pharmacol. 2008;66(1):117–27.
31. National Osteoporosis Foundation. Clinician's guide to prevention and treatment of osteoporosis. Washington, DC: National Osteoporosis Foundation; 2013. p. 31–2
32. McClung M, Geusen P, Miller P, Zippel H, Bensen WG, Roux C, et al. Effect of risedronate on the risk of hip fracture in elderly women. N Engl J Med. 2001;344(5):333–40.
33. Cummings SR, Black DM, Thompson DE, Applegate WB, Barrrett-Connor E, Musliner TA, et al. Effect of alendronate on risk of fracture in women with low bone density but without vertebral fractures: results from the Fracture Intervention Trial. JAMA. 1998;280(24): 2077–82.

34. Colón-Emeric C, Nordsletten L, Olson S, Major N, Boonen S, Haentjens P, et al. Association between timing of zoledronic acid infusion and hip fracture healing. Osteoporos Int. 2011;22(8):23–9.
35. Kim TY, Ha YC, Kang BJ, Lee YK, Koo KH. Does early administration of bisphosphonate affect fracture healing in patients with intertrochanteric fractures? J Bone Joint Surg (Br). 2012;94(7):956–60.
36. Freemantle N, Cooper C, Diez-Perez A, Gitlin M, Radcliffe H, Shepherd S, Roux C, et al. Results of indirect and mixed treatment comparison of fracture efficacy for osteoporosis treatments: a meta-analysis. Osteoporos Int. 2013;24(1):209–17.
37. Lyles KW, Colón-Emeric CS, Magaziner JS, Adachi JD, Pieper CF, Mautalen C, et al. Zoledronic acid and clinical fractures and mortality after hip fracture. N Engl J Med. 2007;357(18):1799–809.
38. Saag K, Lindsay R, Kriegman A, Beamer E, Zhou W. A single zoledronic acid infusion reduces bone resorption markers more rapidly than weekly oral alendronate in postmenopausal women with low bone mineral density. Bone. 2007;40(5):1238–43.
39. Black DM, Delmas PD, Eastell R, Reid IR, Boonen S, Caualey JA, et al. Once-yearly zoledronic acid for treatment of postmenopausal osteoporosis. N Engl J Med. 2007;356(18): 1809–22.
40. Yee AJ, Raje NS. Denosumab, a RANK ligand inhibitor, for the management of bone loss in cancer patients. Clin Interv Aging. 2012;7:331–8.
41. Sambrook PN, Geusens P, Ribot C, Solimano JA, Ferrer-Barriendos J, Gaines K, Verbruggen N, Melton ME. Alendronate produces greater effects than raloxifene on bone density and bone turnover in postmenopausal women with low bone density: results of EFFECT (Efficacy of FOSAMAX versus EVISTA Comparison Trial) International. J Intern Med. 2004;255(4): 503–11.
42. Sone T, Itob M, Fukunagac M, Tomomitsud T, Sugimotoe T, Shirakif M, Yoshimurag T, Nakamurah Y. The effects of once-weekly teriparatide on hip geometry assessed by hip structural analysis in postmenopausal osteoporotic women with high fracture risk. Bone. 2014;64:75–81.
43. Li M, Xing XP, Zhang ZL, et al. Infusion of ibandronate once every 3 months effectively decreases bone resorption markers and increases bone mineral density in Chinese postmenopausal osteoporotic women: a 1-year study. J Bone Miner Metab. 2009; (3):299–305.
44. Gennar L, Merlotti D, Nuti R. Selective estrogen receptor modulator (SERM) for the treatment of osteoporosis in post-menopausal women: focus on lasofoxifene. Clin Interv Aging. 2011;5:19–29.
45. Rosen HN. Patient information: osteoporosis prevention and treatment (beyond the basics). In: UpToDate. 2014. http://www.uptodate.com/contents/osteoporosis-prevention-and-treatment-beyond-thebasics. Accessed June 2015.
46. Ramaswamy B, Shapiro CL. Osteopenia and osteoporosis in females with breast cancer. Semin Oncol. 2003;30(6):763–75.
47. Snyder PJ, Peachey H, Hannoush P, Berlin JA, Loh L, Holmes JH, et al. Effect of testosterone therapy on bone mineral density in men over 65 years of age. J Clin Endocrinol Metab. 1999;84(6):1966–72.
48. Neer RM, Arnaud CD, Zanchetta JR, Prince R, Gaich GA, Reginster J-Y, et al. Effect of parathyroid hormone (1–34) on fractures and bone mineral density in postmenopausal women with osteoporosis. N Engl J Med. 2001;344(19):1434–41.
49. Orwoll E, Scheele W, Paul S, Adami S, Syversen U, Diez-Perez A, et al. Brief therapy with recombinant human parathyroid hormone (1–34) increases lumbar spine bone mineral density in men with idiopathic or hypogonadal osteopenia or osteoporosis. J Bone Miner Res. 2001;16(1):S221.
50. Cosman F. Combination therapy for osteoporosis: a reappraisal. Bonekey Rep. 2014;3:518. doi:10.1038/bonekey.2014.13.

51. Cosman F, Eriksen EF, Recknor C, Miller PD, Guanabens N, Kaspeck C, et al. Effects of intravenous zoledronic acid plus subcutaneous teriparatide [rhPTH(1–34)] in postmenopausal osteoporosis. J Bone Miner Res. 2011;26(3):503–11.
52. Crandall CJ, Newberry SJ, Diamant A, Lim Y-W, Gellad WF, Suttorp M, et al. Treatment to prevent fractures in men and women with low bone density or osteoporosis: update of a 2007 report, Comparative Effectiveness Review No. 53. Rockville: Agency for Healthcare Research and Quality; 2012. p. ES-13–22.
53. Meunier PJ, Slosman DO, Delmas PD, Sebert JL, Brandi ML, Albanese C, et al. Strontium ranelate: dose-dependent effects in established postmenopausal vertebral osteoporosis—a 2-year randomized placebo controlled trial. J Clin Endocrinol Metab. 2002;87(5):2060–6.
54. Meunier PJ, Roux C, Seeman E, Ortolani S, Badurski JE, Spector TD, et al. The effects of strontium ranelate on the risk of vertebral fracture in women with postmenopausal osteoporosis. N Engl J Med. 2004;350:459–68.
55. Reginster JY, Deroisy R, Dougados M, Jupsin I, Colette J, Roux C. Prevention of early postmenopausal bone loss by strontium ranelate: the randomized, double-masked, dose-ranging, placebo-controlled PREVOS trial. Osteoporos Int. 2002;3(12):925–31.
56. Reginster JY, Seeman E, DeVernejoul MC, Adami S, Compston J, Phenekos C, et al. Strontium ranelate reduces the risk of nonvertebral fracture in postmenopausal women with osteoporosis: Treatment of Peripheral Osteoporosis (TROPOS) study. J Clin Endocrinol Metab. 2005;90(5):2816–22.
57. Jonville-Bera AP, Autret-Leca E. Adverse drug reactions of strontium ranelate (Protelos® in France). Presse Med. 2011;40(10):e453–62. doi:10.1016/j.lpm.2011.0.010.
58. Protelos/Osseor to remain available but with further restrictions. In: European medicine agency, Committee on Medicinal Products for Human Use (CHMPP), pharacovigilance risk assessment committee. 2014. http://www.ema.europa.eu/ema/index.jsp?curl=pages/news_and_events/. Accessed 15 Apr 2015.
59. Eisman JA, Bone HG, Hosking DJ, McClung MR, Reid IR, Rizzoli R, et al. Odanacatib in the treatment of postmenopausal women with low bone mineral density: three-year continued therapy and resolution of effect. J Bone Miner Res. 2011;26(2):242–52. doi:10.1002/jbmr.212.
60. Ng KW, Martin TJ. Future therapies of osteoporosis. In: Rosen CJ, editor. Primer on metabolic bone diseases. 8th ed. Ames: Wiley-Blackwell; 2013. p. 461–67.
61. Bone HG, Dempster DW, Eisman JA, Greenspan SL, McClung MR, Nakamura T, et al. Odanacatib for the treatment of postmenopausal osteoporosis; development and participant characteristics of LOFT, the long-term odanacatib fracture trial. Osteoporos Int. 2015;26(2):699–712.
62. Canalis E. Wnt signaling in osteoporosis: mechanisms and novel approaches. Nat Rev Endocrinol. 2013;9(10):575–83. doi:10.1038/nrendo.2013.154.
63. Li X, Warmington KS, Niu QT, Asuncion FJ, Barrero M, Grisanti M, et al. Inhibition of sclerostin by monoclonal antibody increases bone formation, bone mass, and bone strength in aged male rats. J Bone Miner Res. 2010;25(12):2647–56. doi:10.1002/jbmr.182.
64. Padhi D, Jang G, Stouch B, Fang L, Posvar E. Single dose, placebo-controlled randomized study of AMG 785. J Bone Miner Res. 2011;26(1):19–26.
65. Clarke BL. Anti-sclerostin antibodies: utility in treatment of osteoporosis. Maturitas. 2014;78(3):199–204. doi:10.1016/jmaturitas.2004.04.016.
66. McClung MR, Grauer A, Boonen S, Bolognese MA, Brown JP, Diez-Perez A. Romosozumab in postmenopausal women with low bone mineral density. N Engl J Med. 2014;370:412–20. doi:10.1056/NEJMoa1305224.
67. Sinaki M. Critical appraisal of physical rehabilitation measures after osteoporotic vertebral fracture. Osteoporos Int. 2003;14(9):773–9.
68. Lin JT, Lane JM. Nonpharmacologic management of osteoporosis to minimize fracture risk. Nat Clin Pract Rheum. 2008;4(1):20–5.

69. Prather H, Watson JO, Gilula LA. Nonoperative management of osteoporotic vertebral compression fractures. Injury. 2007;38(3):S40–8.
70. Buchalter D, Kahanovitz N, Viola K, Dorsky S, Nordin M. Three-dimensional spinal motion measurements. Part 2: a noninvasive assessment of lumbar brace immobilization of the spine. J Spinal Disord Tech. 1988;1(4):284–6.
71. Kaplan RS, Sinaki M, Hameister MD. Effect of back supports on back strength in patients with osteoporosis: a pilot study. Mayo Clin Proc. 1996;71(3):235–41.
72. Pfeifer M, Begerow B, Minne HW. Effects of a new spinal orthosis on posture, trunk strength, and quality of life in women with postmenopausal osteoporosis: a randomized trial. AJPMR. 2004;83:177–86.
73. Pfeifer M, Kohlwey L, Begerow B, Minne HW. Effects of two newly developed spinal orthoses on trunk muscle strength, posture, and quality-of-life in women with postmenopausal osteoporosis: a randomized trial. Am J Phys Med Rehabil. 2011;90(10):805–15.
74. Sinaki M, Brey RH, Hughes CA, Larson DR, Kaufman KR. Balance disorder and increased risk of falls in osteoporosis and kyphosis: significance of kyphotic posture and muscle strength. Osteoporos Int. 2005;16(8):1004–10.
75. Sinaki M, Lynn S. Reducing the risk of falls through proprioceptive dynamic posture training in osteoporotic women with kyphotic posturing: a randomized pilot study. Am J Phys Med Rehabil. 2002;81(4):241–6.
76. Kaplan RS, Sinaki M. Posture training support: preliminary report on a series of patients with diminished symptomatic complications of osteoporosis. Mayo Clin Proc. 1993;68:1171–6.
77. Sinaki M, Wollan PC, Scott RW, Gelczer RK. Can strong back extensors prevent vertebral fractures in women with osteoporosis? Mayo Clin Proc. 1996;71(10):951–6.
78. Sinaki M. Exercise for patients with osteoporosis: management of vertebral compression fractures and trunk strengthening for fall prevention. Am J Phys Med Rehabil. 2012;4(11):882–8.
79. Sinaki M, Brey RH, Hughes CA, Larson DR, Kaufman KR. Significant reduction in risk of falls and back pain in osteoporotic-kyphotic women through a Spinal Proprioceptive Extension Exercise Dynamic (SPEED) program. Mayo Clin Proc. 2005;80(7):849–55.
80. Sinaki M, Pfeifer M, Preisinger E, Itoi E, Rizzoli R, Boonen S, et al. The role of exercise in the treatment of osteoporosis. Curr Osteoporos Rep. 2010;8(3):138–44.
81. Sinaki M, Itoi E, Wahner HW, Wollan P, Gelzcer R, Mullan BP, et al. Stronger back muscles reduce the incidence of vertebral fractures: a prospective 10 year follow-up of postmenopausal women. Bone. 2002;30(6):836–41.
82. Sinaki M, Mikkelsen BA. Postmenopausal spinal osteoporosis: flexion versus extension exercises. Arch Phys Med Rehabil. 1984;65(10):593–6.
83. Sinaki M. Nonpharmacologic interventions: exercise, fall prevention, and role of physical medicine. Clin Geriatr Med. 2003;19(2):337–59.
84. Sinaki M, Nwaogwugwu NC, Phillips BE, Mokri MP. Effect of gender, age, and anthropometry on axial and appendicular muscle strength. Am J Phys Med Rehabil. 2001;80(5):330–8.
85. Rudins A, Sinaki M, Miller JL, Piper SM, Bergstrahl EJ, et al. Significance of back extensors versus back flexors in truncal support. Arch Phys Med Rehabil. 1991;72(10):824.
86. Inufusa A, An HS, Lim TH, Hasegawa T, Haughton VM, Nowicki BH. Anatomic changes of the spinal canal and intervertebral foramen associated with flexion-extension movement. Spine. 1996;21(21):2412–20.
87. Ezenwa B, Yeoh HT. Multiple vibration displacements at multiple vibration frequencies stress impact on human femur computational analysis. J Rehabil Res Dev. 2011;48(2):179–90.
88. Wysocki A, Butler M, Shamliyan T, Kane R. Whole-body vibration therapy for osteoporosis, Comparative Effectiveness Technical Briefs. No. 10. Rockville: Agency for Healthcare Research and Quality (US); 2011.
89. Gusi N, Raimundo A, Leal A. Low-frequency vibratory exercise reduces the risk of bone fracture more than walking: a randomized controlled trial. BMC Musculoskelet Disord. 2006;7(1):92.

90. Verschueren S, Roelants M, Delecluse C, Swinnen S, Vanderschueran D, Bonner S, et al. Effect of 6-month whole body vibration training on hip density, muscle strength, and postural control in postmenopausal women: a randomized controlled pilot study. J Bone Miner Res. 2004;19(3):352–9.
91. Slatkovska L, Alibhai SM, Beyene J, Cheung AM. Effect of whole-body vibration on BMD: a systematic review and meta-analysis. Osteoporos Int. 2010;21(12):1969–80.
92. Ruan X, Jin F, Liu Y, Peng ZL, Sun YG. Effects of vibration therapy on bone mineral density in postmenopausal women with osteoporosis. Chin Med J (Engl). 2008;121(13):1155–8.
93. Iwamoto J, Takeda T, Sato Y, Uzawa M. Effect of whole-body vibration exercise on lumbar bone mineral density, bone turnover, and chronic back pain in post-menopausal osteoporotic women treated with alendronate. Aging Clin Exp Res. 2005;17:157–63.
94. Bemben DA, Palmer IJ, Bemben MG, Knehans AW. Effects of combined whole-body vibration and resistance training on muscular strength and bone metabolism. Bone. 2010;47(3):650–6.
95. Lau RW, Liao LR, Yu F, Teo T, Chung RC, Pang MY. The effects of whole body vibration therapy on bone mineral density and leg muscle strength in older adults: a systematic review and meta-analysis. Clin Rehabil. 2011;25(11):975–88.
96. Sitjà-Rabert M, Rigau D, Fort Vanmeerghaeghe A, Romero-Rodriguez D, Bonastre Subirana M, Bonfill X. Efficacy of whole body vibration exercise in older people: a systematic review. Disabil Rehabil. 2012;34(11):883–93.
97. Rittweger J. Vibration as an exercise modality: how it may work, and what its potential might be. EJAP. 2010;108(5):877–904.
98. Torvinen S, Kannus O, Sievanan H, Jarvinen TA, Pasanen M, Kontulainen S, et al. Effect of 8-month vertical whole body vibration on bone, muscle performance, and body balance: a randomized controlled study. J Bone Miner Res. 2003;18(5):352–9.
99. Lings S, Leboeuf-Yde C. Whole-body vibration and low back pain: a systematic, critical review of the epidemiological literature 1992–1999. Int Arch Occup Environ Health. 2000;73(5):290–7.
100. Seidel H, Harazin B, Pavlas K, Stroka C, Richter J, Bluthner R, et al. Isolated and combined effects of prolonged exposures to noise and whole-body vibration on hearing, vision and strain. Int Arch Occup Environ Health. 1988;61(1–2):95–106.
101. Dandanell R, Engström K. Vibration from riveting tools in the frequency range 6 Hz-10 MHz and Raynaud's phenomenon. Scand J Work Environ Health. 1986;12(4):338–42.
102. National Osteoporosis Foundation. Types of osteoporosis medications. Washington, DC: National Osteoporosis Foundation. http://nof.org/articles/22. Accessed 6 June 2015.
103. Cummings SR, Palermo L, Browner W, Marcus R, Wallace R, Pearson J, et al. Monitoring osteoporosis therapy with bone densitometry: misleading changes and regression to the mean. JAMA. 2002;283(10):1318–21. doi:10.1001/jama.283.10.1318.
104. Compston J. Monitoring osteoporosis treatment. Best Prac Res Clin Rheumatol. 2009;23(6):781–8. doi:10.1016/j.berh.2009.09.007.

Chapter 6
Osteoporosis in Men

Christina V. Oleson

In 2008, the American College of Physicians observed that osteoporosis in men is "substantially underdiagnosed, undertreated, underreported, and inadequately researched" [1]. To a considerable extent, that statement remains true, yet there are signs of increasing clinical and public recognition of the impact of osteoporosis on men, as evidenced in a growing number of research studies on the epidemiology, prevention, and treatment of male osteoporosis as well as in reports of the US National Osteoporosis Foundation and other public agencies. Worldwide, the International Osteoporosis Foundation (IOF) chose to place men at the center of its World Osteoporosis Day in 2014, with the publication of an in-depth report: *Osteoporosis in Men—Why Change Needs to Happen* [2].

The report emphasizes that by 2050 more than 900 million men worldwide will have lived beyond age 60. As life expectancy has increased and medical advances have brought a decline in male deaths attributable to heart disease, cancer, and stroke, men have become more susceptible to chronic disease including osteoporosis. Moreover, in the case of hip fractures and most fragility fractures, men have a higher mortality rate than women—as high as 37 % in the year following a hip fracture. The fact that men experience hip fractures later in life may account for this higher mortality rate [3].

In the United States, it is projected that between the years 2010 and 2030, the number of hip fractures in men will increase 51.8 %, compared with a decrease of 3.5 % in women. As the elderly population increases over the next two decades, the anticipated rise in the total number of hip fractures will be affected, on the one hand, by the decreasing percentage of hip fracture rates in women and, on the other, by the much higher percentage of fractures in men [4]. This chapter will focus on the risk factors, diagnosis, prevention, and treatment of osteoporosis specific to men, recognizing that previous chapters have dealt with these issues in a broader context.

C.V. Oleson, *Osteoporosis Rehabilitation*, DOI 10.1007/978-3-319-45084-1_6

Causes and Consequences

Like women, men experience both primary and secondary osteoporosis. *Primary osteoporosis* in men includes both *idiopathic*, or osteoporosis of unknown etiology, and *age-related osteoporosis* (also called senile osteoporosis). In men under the age of 65–70, idiopathic osteoporosis is evidenced by one or more fractures as well as by a low bone formation rate and low bone mass. Proposed etiologies include familial history and genetic factors, not only because risk of fractures can be inherited but also because between 50 % and 85 % of the variance in peak bone mass is genetically determined [5–7].

Whereas the occurrence of idiopathic osteoporosis is uncommon, age-related osteoporosis, particularly skeletal fragility, is *the major precipitating factor in male osteoporosis*. As discussed earlier in this volume, childhood and adolescence are crucial periods for the accumulation of bone size and strength. Sex hormones play a significant role in bone growth; in contrast to estrogen, testosterone during puberty contributes to the development of a larger skeleton by reducing bone resorption and enhancing bone tissue formation [6]. Growth hormone (GH) and insulin-like growth factor 1 (IGF-1) in male adolescence also contribute to the development of thicker cortices, larger bones, and consequently greater bone strength than in women.

Exercise is another critical factor in bone formation, with recent evidence demonstrating that its value can persist well beyond adolescence into old age. A study by Nilsson et al. indicates that exercise during growth is independently associated with greater cortical bone size and bone strength in elderly men [8], whereas Warden and Roosa's study of former MLB players found that even inactive players in their 80s retained 56 % of bone size, and 34 % of bone strength benefits in their throwing arms, despite the fact that they had not thrown for over 50 years [9].

Other studies demonstrate that by the age of 18, men have higher lean mass (92 %) than women (79 %); they also have greater bone mineral content (BMC), bone area (BA) at the femoral neck and total femur, as well as 8 % higher hip bone mineral density (BMD) and 5.30 total tibia BMD [10]. Peak bone mass is generally achieved by age 30 and sustained until the early 40s [2].

Although men do not experience the rapid bone loss associated with female menopause, their trabecular bone begins to thin in midlife, possibly in association with decreases in IGF-1 [2]; subsequently, the cortical bone also thins and increases in porosity. Concurrently, however, the *outer* (periosteal) bone formation (which is greater in men than in women), coupled with expansion of the marrow cavity, offsets bone loss on the *inner* surface, resulting in an enlargement of bone diameter and, to some extent, an increase in bone strength. This balancing process persists until the age of 65–70, when bone loss in the marrow cavity is no longer compensated by periosteal bone formation. At that stage, the rate of bone loss in men equals that in women [11, 12].

For many years, it was thought that a decrease in androgens was the principal cause of age-related osteoporosis in men. Declining sex steroid levels are associated with an age-related increase in sex hormone-binding globulin (SHBG) levels, resulting in a decrease in bioavailable testosterone (T) by 64 % and in estrogen (E) by 47 % [13]. In a study of healthy men 40 years and older, Sartorius et al. reported that low serum testosterone levels may not be caused by age itself, but instead are the result of comorbidities related to age [14]. However, other studies maintain that advancing age apart from comorbidities is a determining factor [15].

There is no definitive evidence supporting an assertion that a decrease in testosterone is the most immediate cause of male age-related osteoporosis. Indeed, findings indicate that increased BMD in younger men and decreased BMD in older are more closely associated with bioavailable estradiol (E2) levels than with testosterone. Here again, however, a correlation should not be equated with a cause. The most direct evidence for a causal effect of estrogen and testosterone on male bone health is described by Falahati-Nini et al. [16]. In research entailing pharmacologic suppression of T and E production replaced with topical T and E, they found that the absence of both T and E led to a significant increase in bone resorption, which was completely preventable with T and E therapy. Whereas treatment with estrogen alone prevented an increase in bone resorption, testosterone had a much more limited effect, leading to the conclusion that estrogen is the primary androgen in determining bone health [16].

However, testosterone does contribute to maintenance of balance and muscle strength in men—a critical factor in decreasing the risk of fracture. Although studies are limited, there are also indications that testosterone is related to sarcopenia, the age-related loss of skeletal muscle mass and strength; further research will elaborate on this relationship and serve to increase awareness of the need for treatment [17].

In addition to bone loss and the impact of sex steroids, male osteoporosis can be traced to a number of factors, including medications, diseases, and lifestyle behaviors, classified as *secondary osteoporosis*. Among the most common are hypogonadism and glucocorticoid excess. Male hypogonadism is generally defined as the reduction or absence of hormone secretion by the testes or a serum testosterone level of less than 300 (ng/dl); it occurs in two-thirds of American men who have suffered a hip fracture and are residents in nursing homes [5, 6]. Primary hypogonadism, originating in an inherent testicular defect, may be caused by Klinefelter syndrome (which is marked by an additional X chromosome, 47xxy), mumps, chemotherapy or radiation therapy, and injuries to the testicles. In secondary hypogonadism, the defect lies outside the testicles and is related to Kallmann syndrome (abnormal development of the hypothalamus which controls pituitary hormone secretion), other pituitary disorders, obesity, and normal aging [18]. Differences in primary and secondary osteoporosis are given in Table 1 [5].

Special attention should be given to the adverse effects of androgen deprivation therapy (ADT) administered for prostate cancer. Not only is bone loss, ranging from 6.5 % to 17.3 %, accelerated with ADT but in the first year of treatment alone, bone loss of 2–4 % occurs at the lumbar spine and hip [19]. A 2013 Swedish study of the link between ADT, hip fracture, and risk of death demonstrated that hip fractures result in an additional 30 deaths per 1,000 person-years for men with prostate cancer on ADT compared to all men with prostate cancer, particularly in

Table 1 Causes of osteoporosis and bone loss in men

Osteoporosis classification	Causes
Primary osteoporosis	Aging
	Idiopathic
Secondary osteoporosis	Hypogonadism
	Excess glucocorticoid
	Alcohol abuse
	Tobacco abuse
	Renal insufficiency
	Hepatic disorders
	Gastrointestinal disorders/malabsorption
	Hyperparathyroidism
	Hypercalciuria
	Anticonvulsants
	Thyrotoxicosis
	Chronic respiratory disorders
	Homocystinuria
	Systemic mastocytosis

Source: Orwoll [5]

the first months following fracture—a finding that underlies the need for greater awareness of this interaction [20].

Another drug-induced form of osteoporosis stems from glucocorticoid medications: steroids used to treat inflammatory, allergic, and immunological illnesses, ranging from asthma to rheumatoid arthritis. For men, glucocorticoid therapy is used particularly in cases of chronic obstructive pulmonary disease (COPD), inflammatory bowel disease, and organ transplantation. A UK general practice database study revealed that even a small dose of 5 % mg prednisolone daily can lead to an increased fracture risk in as little as three months [21]. Bone loss, primarily in the ribs and vertebra, increases until cessation of treatment and may be attributed to several factors, including direct effect of steroids on bone, muscle weakness or immobility, reduced absorption of calcium, decrease in testosterone levels, or a combination of these [3]. Again, recognition of the risk of glucocorticoid therapy is the key to successful treatment.

Many of the other secondary causes of osteoporosis including excessive alcohol use, smoking, and calcium and vitamin D deficiency have been discussed in an earlier chapter. Gastrointestinal disorders that hinder absorption of essential nutrients, hypercalciuria that results in loss of too much calcium through urine, and prolonged bed rest or immobility must also be considered in the diagnosis of male osteoporosis. Below is a list of risk factors [5, 22]:

- Increased age (especially after 70 years)
- Low body weight (body mass index less than 20–25)
- Weight loss of more than 10 % body weight
- Physical inactivity

- Corticosteroid use
- Androgen deprivation therapy
- Previous fragility fracture
- Spinal cord injury
- Chronic obstructive pulmonary disease

Screening and Diagnosis

Although interest in male osteoporosis is growing, there is still a serious lack of awareness, on the part of both healthcare professionals and men themselves, of the threat posed by the disease. A delayed diagnosis of male osteoporosis is further exacerbated by the fact that bone mass density persists longer in men than in women and that osteoporosis may present with no symptoms until a fracture occurs. The American College of Physicians (ACP) was among the first organizations to develop a set of risk factors for identifying male osteoporosis, including age 70 and over (50 and over if a fracture has occurred); low body weight defined as body mass of <20–25 kg/m^2, weight loss of >10 % compared with adult weight or weight loss in recent years, lack of physical activity as well as other risk factors discussed above. Based on a meta-analysis, it proposed that periodic individualized risk assessment in men be initiated before the age of 65. In addition to a complete physical exam and history, it also endorsed measurement of bone density with a dual-energy x-ray absorptiometry (DXA) scan of the spine and hip for men who are at increased risk of osteoporosis and are candidates for drug treatment [1]. The results of a DXA scan are reported in terms of a *T*-score: the number of standard deviations that bone density is above or below that of a young healthy adult.

By using a simple, relatively new (2007) clinical prediction rule, primary care physicians are in a key position to advance early recognition of osteoporosis and thereby determine whether men 50–70 years might benefit from a DXA scan. The Male Osteoporosis Risk Estimation Score (MORES) incorporates three variables: ≤55 to ≥75 years of age; weight of ≤154 to ≥176 lb; history of COPD as well as both controllable and noncontrollable risk factors [23]. In an analysis of a nationally representative sample of men (n=2,995) aged 50 and older who participated in the National Health and Nutrition Examination Survey (NHANES), Shepard et al. identified 93 % of men with previously unrecognized osteoporosis and 44 % of men who would benefit from a confirmatory DXA scan [23]. See Table 2. Another testing model, the Osteoporosis Self-Assessment Tool (OST) uses self-reporting age and weight, subtracting the age from the weight in kilograms and multiplying the result by 0.2 [24]. A subsequent study employing MORES, conducted in a primary care setting with a smaller number of men (n=346) ≥60 years, found a slightly lower prevalence of osteoporosis compared with the earlier study: 80 % in contrast to 93 % of men identified with osteoporosis and 33 % in contrast to 44 % referred for a DXA scan [25]. Possible limitations included a more confined geographical area (the Texas Gulf Coast), the smaller cohort, and a potential bias toward more robust older men.

Table 2 Male Osteoporosis Risk Estimation Score (MORES)

Risk factor	Points
Age ≤55 years	0
Age 56–74 years	3
Age ≥75 years	4
Presence of chronic obstructive pulmonary disease	3
Weight ≤154 lb	6
Weight 155–176 lb	4
Weight >176 lb	0

Source: Shepherd et al. [24]
Male Osteoporosis Risk Estimation Score (MORES) is used to evaluate the need for osteoporosis screening. A total score ≥6 points is the threshold to screen for dual-energy x-ray absorptiometry

Nonetheless, MORES is an inexpensive, easily administered and calculated tool applicable in a clinical setting, with the prospect of identifying male osteoporosis at an early stage [26].

Recommendations regarding testing for male osteoporosis lack uniformity. The US Preventive Screening Task Force (USPSTF) finds insufficient evidence for assessing the risks and benefits of screening for male osteoporosis. However, the Endocrine Society in 2012 [26] and NOF in 2014 [27] have issued indicators for BMD testing including (1) men age 70 and older, regardless of clinical risk factors, (2) men age 50–69 with clinical risk factors for fracture, (3) all adults with a fracture after age 50, and (4) adults with conditions or medications associated with low bone mass or bone loss.

Reduced BMD in men is generally quantified by a *T*-score of −1.0 to −2.5 for osteopenia and −2.5 or less for osteoporosis, a grading system analogous to that used for women. As would be expected, the initial criteria for diagnosing osteoporosis, issued by the World Health Organization in 1994, were developed for women. Whether a male specific or a female specific *T*-score should be used for men has come under question. As Adler points out, for some time, DXA machines in the United States and most of the world used a male normative base for determining male *T*-scores. However, in recent years, the World Health Organization, the International Osteoporosis Foundation (IOF), and the International Society for Clinical Densitometry(ISCD) have endorsed the use of a white female database (NHANES III, Caucasian women aged 21–29) to obtain a BMD value at the femoral neck for both men and women [28]. To obtain the most accurate reading, DXA results should be used in combination with the FRAX tool, which predicts a 10-year hip fracture rate based on a series of risk factors including age, gender, previous fragility fracture, *T*-score of ≤ −2.5 at the femoral neck or spine, low bone mass as indicated by a *T*-score between −1.0 and −2.5 at the femoral neck or spine, glucocorticoid treatment, smoking, excessive alcohol intake, other causes of secondary osteoporosis, and a 10-year probability of high fracture of ≥3 % [29]. When DXA and FRAX are used together, it is likely that a larger number of older men will be identified for treatment under the new NOF guidelines. However, as Adler points out, while more men may be identified, there is no evidence indicating that men who show no signs of osteoporosis through DXA but have a high fracture risk by FRAX will respond to therapy [20].

Although other bone densitometry techniques exist, there is insufficient evidence that quantitative computer tomography (QCT), peripheral QCT (pQCT), or peripheral dual-energy x-ray absorptiometry (pDXA) can predict fracture risk in men [27]. However, Bauer et al. found that validated heel quantitative ultrasound densitometry (QUS) mechanisms predict risk of hip and nonvertebral fracture in men 65 and older almost as well as does BMD [30].

In addition to the history, physical examination, BMD measurement, and FRAX assessment, a series of laboratory tests may be performed to determine correctable causes of bone loss. See Chapter 2. They include a complete blood count; serum chemistry levels, specifically calcium to detect hyperparathyroidism or hypocalcemia; phosphate, alkaline phosphatase and 25(OH) vitamin D to assess osteomalacia; creatinine levels for renal function; magnesium for calcium absorption and metabolism; liver function tests for alcohol abuse; thyroid-stimulating hormone (TSH) levels for thyroid dysfunction; and 25-(OH) vitamin D levels for vitamin D deficiency [31]. See Table 3.

It has long been recognized that men have a higher prevalence of secondary osteoporosis than do women; for example, a recent study of 234 men at a mean age of 70.6 years found secondary osteoporosis in 75 % of the cohort [32]. Tests for secondary causes include 24-hour urine calcium level for hyper-and hypocalciuria, indicating possible vitamin D deficiency, parathyroid hormone level for hyperparathyroidism, and testosterone and gonadotropic levels in younger men with reduced bone mass for sex hormone deficiencies [31].

Table 3 Suggested basic and advanced laboratory testing for osteoporosis in men

Initial laboratory tests	Advanced laboratory tests
Serum calcium, phosphorus, BUN, and creatinine	24 h urine cortisol and urine creatinine
Liver enzymes including alkaline phosphatase	Markers of bone formation: Bone specific alkaline phosphatase; procollagen N-1 terminal propeptide
Serum vitamin D25 OH and intact parathyroid hormone (PTH)	Markers of bone loss: Urine N-terminal telopeptide Serum C-telopeptide
Serum testosterone and luteinizing hormone	Immunological tests for sprue
Thyroid-stimulating hormone	Full panel of thyroid function tests

Source: Bethel et al. [31]

All men should have the panel of basic laboratory tests done. However, if high suspicion of osteoporosis exists or osteoporosis is found by DXA without a clear etiology, laboratory studies in the advanced testing list should be pursued

Biochemical markers of bone formation and resorption have been examined to determine their value in predicting fracture risk in men; however, given available evidence, they are not considered to be a replacement for DXA measurements. Although NOF guidelines state that biochemical markers *may* predict risk of fracture, the results of other studies are promising but inconclusive and conflicting. For example, in the Dubbo Osteoporosis Epidemiology Study, only one bone turnover marker, carboxyterminal cross-linked telopeptide of type 1 collagen (S-ICTP), was associated with high bone resorption and increased risk of fracture, independent of BMD [33]. Bauer et al. conducted a sub analysis of the Osteoporosis Fracture in Men (MrOS) study cohort ($n=947$ randomly selected from the original 5,995 men), focusing on the relation between elevated bone turnover markers (BTMs) and the risk of hip and other nonspine fractures. Bone markers used were formation marker PINP, resorption marker βCTX, and osteoclast number marker (TRACP5b). Findings indicated that elevated serum levels of these markers were related to a higher rate of hip bone loss in older men, but the link was insufficient to predict fracture accurately. Moreover, after accounting for baseline BMD, none of the relationships between BTMs and fracture were statistically significant, leading to their conclusion that BTMs should not be included in risk stratification tools for men [34]. The MINOS study, reported a year earlier, also found no association between high bone turnover and increased fracture risk in men ≥50 and stressed that BTMs cannot be used to predict male fractures in clinical practice [35].

In the absence of additional research and despite their seeming advantages in terms of low cost and noninvasiveness, BTMs are contraindicated as a predictive tool for male osteoporosis in routine clinical practice. Current efforts to establish and implement international consensus reference standards, using s-PINP as the bone formation marker and s-βCTX as the resorption marker in all clinical trials, are an important steps in advancing the clinical utility of BTMs in both predicting and managing osteoporosis [36].

Because vertebral fracture is consistent with a diagnosis of osteoporosis quite apart from BMD measurement, the NOF recommends vertebral imaging in men age 80 and older if BMD *T*-score at the spine, hip, and femoral neck is ≤ −1.0; at age 70–79 if BMD *T*-score is ≤ −1.5, and −3.0; and at age 50 and older with low-trauma fracturing during adulthood, height loss of 1.5 inches or more; prospective height loss of 0.8 inches or more; and recent or ongoing long-term glucocorticoid treatment. Since most densitometers can also perform vertebral imaging, the tests can be done concurrently.

Prevention

Strategies to prevent osteoporosis are not significantly different in men and women, but just as male osteoporosis is not as widely recognized, preventative and therapeutic measures are not broadly prescribed and implemented. Here the healthcare professional plays a key role in ensuring that risk factors for osteoporosis are an important part of regular physical examinations. Adequate calcium and vitamin D are key factors in preventing osteoporosis. In terms of calcium intake, the NOF recommends a daily dose of 1,000 mg for men aged 50–70, with 1,200 mg daily for men 71 and older. For vitamin D, the NOF recommendation is 800–1,000 international units (IU) for all adults age 50 and older, while the Institute of Medicine advocates a lower dose of 600 IU per day until age 70, and then 800 IU per day for ages 71 and older. In a 1997 study, Dawson-Hughes et al. demonstrated that in both men and women age 65 and older, calcium and vitamin D supplementation reduced bone loss moderately over a 3-year period and reduced the incidence of nonvertebral fractures; in men, a significant effect at the hip, spine, and total body was evident [37]. A subsequent study involving 2017 men and 649 women, aged 65–85, confirmed these findings, with results indicating a 22 % reduction in total fracture incidence and a 33 % reduction in fractures at major osteoporotic sites [38]. For patients at risk of a vitamin D deficiency, the goal is to maintain serum 25 (OH) levels at or above 30 ng/ml to ensure optimal skeletal health [27].

Smoking cessation, whether undertaken individually or in monitored cessation programs, alcohol intake of no more than two drinks per day, and weight-bearing exercise programs, including jogging, walking, weight lifting, dancing, and other aerobic sports are all recommended preventative measures for males. In terms of smoking, a 1996 analysis of the Framingham Heart Study cohort (which at that point had prospectively collected 40 years of data on smoking) determined that smoking at any stage of life produced adverse effects on the male skeleton. In particular, men who smoked at any point in life had a lower BMD at all skeletal sites; male smokers who had quit <10 years prior to the study had lower BMD than those who had quit ≥10 years prior [39]. A more recent study confirms that smoking is a much stronger risk factor for fracture in men than in women, as well as a stronger and more lasting risk factor than previously determined. However, the risk is reversible: in the first 10 years following cessation, the risk is cut in half and no independent association has been found between risk fracture and duration of smoking [40].

Excessive alcohol not only reduces the body's calcium reserves and increases cortisol levels but also results in the production of less testosterone which, in turn, restricts bone formation. Chronic alcoholism in men induces lower bone density in the femoral neck and trochanter with a significant inverse correlation between the amount of alcohol consumed and the degree of bone loss [41]. Alcohol can also compromise balance and gait, leading to increased risk of falls and fractures.

Lack of physical exercise, application of casts to treat fractures, prolonged bed rest, and various forms of immobilization, from stroke and other types of paralysis to weightlessness in space, can be precipitating factors for what is generally known as "disuse osteoporosis" [42]. As calcium leaches out of the bone, calcium excretion in the urine becomes four to six times higher than normal within three weeks of immobility. Because bones are no longer engaged in weight-bearing, they lose density; indeed, bone density of the vertebral column decreases by 1 % per week of bed rest, which is nearly 50 times greater than that of normal age-related bone loss [43].

Regular and lifelong exercise can help to ensure bone strength, improve balance, and halt or slow the progression of osteoporosis. Exercise for even a half hour per day strengthens muscles, works to preserve and increase bone mass, and improves coordination and balance. The three basic types of exercise for male osteoporosis are weight-bearing, resistance, and flexibility. High-impact weight-bearing exercises, including hiking, jogging, jumping, dancing, tennis, and aerobic sports, more generally, build and maintain bone strength, whereas swimming and cycling are not as effective. Running improves BMD but can be detrimental in cases of high mileage. A study by Hetland et al. indicates that male long-distance runners ($N=120$, 19–56 years old) who logged up to 100 miles per week had reduced bone mass and increased bone turnover compared to controls [44]. It confirms similar findings by MacDougall et al. [45] that bone density in long-distance male runners with mileage at 60–70 miles/week is lower than in men in a 15–20 mile group—the so-called endurance paradox. Mussolino et al. demonstrated that jogging is also associated with significantly higher femoral BMD in young and middle-aged men—a finding that may be of public health importance because femoral BMD is a strong predictor of hip fracture. The similarity in femoral BMD between those who jogged more than nine times a month and those who jogged less frequently again underscored the existence of a ceiling effect on the distance needed to improve BMD [46].

For those unable to undertake high-impact exercise, the NOF recommends brisk walking, low-impact aerobics, and the use of stair-step and elliptical training machines. The elderly can also benefit from such weight-bearing exercises as squats and leg presses, yoga and Tai Chi, and standing on one leg. In a study of elderly women but with results applicable to men, Finnish researchers identified a number of "impact exercises" to slow the progression of osteoporosis, including jumping, feet stomping, knee bends, leg lifts, and stair climbing [47]. Resistance exercises ranging from lifting weights and using elastic exercise bands to functional movement such as rising up on your toes preserve bone calcium and increase muscle strength. Flexibility exercises such as yoga, Pilates, and Tai Chi can strengthen legs and improve balance; combined with evidenced-based fall prevention efforts and hip protectors, they can decrease risk of falls and fractures [48].

Finally prevention of male osteoporosis should take into account underlying medical conditions and medications such as glucocorticoid treatment that is known to cause bone loss. Early recognition can lead to effective treatment.

Treatment

A judgment on when treatment for osteoporosis should be initiated is based on the series of factors determined by the physical examination and history, DXA findings, and FRAX results, and, to a limited extent, BTM levels.

Bisphosphonates

As FDA recommendations demonstrate, it cannot be assumed that anti-osteoporotic drugs for women will be equally effective in men, and indeed thus far the FDA has approved only five medications for men—the bisphosphonates: alendronate, risedronate, and zoledronic acid; the anabolic agent: parathyroid hormone (teriparatide) and, most recently, the monoclonal antibody to RANKL: denosumab. Bisphosphonates have a high affinity for bone mineral but not for other tissues. They attach to bone surfaces, are incorporated into sites of bone remodeling, and suppress bone resorption [49]. Although bisphosphonates have been shown to reduce fragility fractures in women, males experience positive effects primarily in terms of an increase in BMD and a decrease in both bone resorption and bone formation markers; nonetheless, these findings serve as the basis for justifying the use of bisphosphonates in men [50]. Bisphosphonates also produce BMD changes in men with low testosterone levels as well as in those with normal levels.

In one of the key studies of alendronate therapy for male osteoporosis, Orwoll et al. found that 10 mg of alendronate over two years decreased bone turnover and increased bone density of the spine, hip, and total body—results that were evident within six months of initiating treatment. Moreover, using quantitative methods, they also found an incidence of vertebral fractures in only 0.8 % of the alendronate group as opposed to 7.1 % of men in the placebo group—an outcome consistent with the results of similar studies in postmenopausal women. A positive relationship between alendronate and hip fractures in men has yet to be determined. Because alendronate increases BMD in patients with low testosterone as well as in those with normal levels, it may be effective in hypogonadal and gonadal men. The ability of alendronate to reduce height loss—a nonsignificant 0.6 mm in alendronate group compared to 2.4 mm in placebo group—is also consistent with anti-fracture efficacy [51].

Alendronate is effective in cases of androgen deprivation therapy (ATP) for prostate cancer, glucocorticoid-induced osteoporosis (GC), and immobilization. To counteract the risk of bone loss and fracture in ATP patients with severe osteopenia or osteoporosis, a dose of 70 mg/week significantly increased BMD at the lumbar spine and femoral neck and markedly decreased the risk of femoral risk fracture [52]. In an analysis of the benefits of early and sustained therapy, Greenspan and colleagues determined that treatment with 70 mg/week should be initiated early in the course of ADT and continued for at least two years [53].

Glucocorticoids are immunosuppressive drugs generally prescribed for men with inflammatory bowel disease, chronic obstructive pulmonary disease, organ transplantation, and, should the need arise, inflammatory arthritis. However, they inhibit bone formation and increase the risk of spine and hip fracture. In addition to adequate amounts of calcium and vitamin D, alendronate 70 mg/week for a year significantly increased lumbar spine (2.45 %), trochanter (1.27 %), total hip (0.75 %), and total body BMD (1.70 %) in patients taking glucocorticoids compared with placebo; biochemical markers of bone remodeling also decreased [54]. Finally, the efficacy of alendronate has been proven in cases of disuse immobilization both on the ground and in space. A ground-based test of men consigned to bed rest for 17 weeks revealed no loss of BMD, decreased bone formation markers, and decreased or only slightly elevated bone resorption markers in the treated group as opposed to an untreated group [55]. An analogous study of International Space Station crew members indicated that alendronate, in combination with exercise devices, lessened anticipated losses in bone mineral density of the spine, hip, and pelvis as well as in trabecular and cortical bone mass in the hip—a benefit applicable to patients on earth [56].

Second to alendronate in terms of prescribed bisphosphonates is risedronate. Risedronate tablets are prescribed for men with osteoporosis, particularly for those on. In a 2-year study of the use of risedronate 5 mg daily (coupled with calcium and vitamin D supplementation) by men with primary and secondary osteoporosis, the incidence of new vertebral fractures in the risedronate group was significantly reduced (9.2 %) compared to control (23.6 %), and the occurrence of nonvertebral fractures also declined (11.8 %) versus control (22.3 %). BMD at the lumbar spine, femoral neck, and total hip improved markedly, while loss of height and back pain decreased—all indicating that risedronate can be effective for a term of at least two years [57]. Using risedronate 35 mg/week and comparable calcium and vitamin D supplementation, a double-blind 2-year study with placebo demonstrated the rapid efficacy of risedronate, with significant BTM decreases as early as three months and BMD increases as early as six months. In an open-label, 2-year extension of this study, risedronate continued to be well tolerated and to produce significant increases in lumbar spine BMD (7.87 % from baseline) in those patients who took the drug for four years—a finding similar to that of postmenopausal women treated with risedronate for the same time period. The generally accepted term is now 3–5 years.

With respect to corticosteroid-induced osteoporosis, treatment with risedronate 5 mg for 12 months increases BMD in both men and women receiving high doses of the treatment, with a 2.5 mg dose being less effective; combined data for both the 2.5 and 5 mg groups reveals a 70 % reduction in vertebral fracture incidence [58]. A subsequent study indicated that daily treatment with risedronate decreased vertebral fracture risk within one year in men receiving corticosteroids [59]. Further studies are needed to provide clarification on the comparative effectiveness of not only alendronate versus risedronate but of all medications used for osteoporosis.

Although prescribed for women to prevent and treat postmenopausal osteoporosis, the bisphosphonate, ibandronate, is not FDA approved for men. In a 2010 trial, the STudy Researching Osteoporosis iN Guys (STRONG), conducted over a 1-year period, men receiving oral ibandronate experienced a significantly greater increase in lumbar spine BMD than those taking placebo (3.5 % vs. 0.9 %) as well as increases at the total hip, femoral neck, and trochanter [60]. However, ibandronate can cause serious problems in the stomach and esophagus and requires the patient to sit upright or stand for one hour after administration. Despite their effectiveness, oral bisphosphonates have several disadvantages; they can cause gastrointestinal distress in some patients and require frequent dosing. These factors potentially contribute to a detrimental effect on drug adherence.

The most studied of the intravenous bisphosphonates, zoledronic acid, was approved by the FDA in 2008 as, thus far, the only treatment shown to reduce the incidence of fracture and mortality in patients with a previous low-trauma hip fracture. The FDA cited the results of the HORIZON Recurrent Fracture Trial in which men ≥50 years of age comprised 24 % of a cohort of 2,126 patients: all had experienced low-trauma hip fracture and could not tolerate oral bisphosphonates. A once yearly 5 mg dose of zoledronic acid age administered 90 days after surgical repair of a hip fracture reduced the rate of a new clinical, but not hip, fracture, by 35 %, while increasing total hip and femoral neck BMD after 36 months in both men and women compared with the placebo group. It also decreased the all-cause mortality by 28 %, perhaps in part because of the reduction in new fractures [61]. Further research determined that the optimal time for zoledronic acid infusion was 2–12 weeks following fracture repair [62]. In the first male osteoporosis trial with fracture as an end point, participants experienced primary osteoporosis or osteoporosis due to hypogonadism, with one or more vertebral fractures at baseline; results showed that two annual infusions of zoledronic acid reduced the risk of new morphological vertebral fractures by 67 %—a result similar to that for postmenopausal women [63]. Further evidence is needed to determine the efficacy of bisphosphonates for nonvertebral and hip fractures in men.

Teriparatide

Unlike the antiresorptive therapies outlined above, the parathyroid hormone, teriparatide, is the only approved agent that increases bone formation in male osteoporosis. It is self-injected in a recommended dose of 20 mcg/day for no more than 24 months. A study ($\underline{n}$=437) indicating higher BMD at the spine and femoral neck for those on teriparatide [64] was followed by an analysis of a portion of the same population (n=355) at 30 months posttreatment. Following discontinuation of teriparatide, BMD gradually decreased but lumbar spine and total hip values remained higher than at baseline; although the risk of vertebral fractures fell by a nonsignificant 51 %, the incidence of moderate or severe fractures was significantly reduced by 83 %. It is important to note that the administration of bisphosphonates following withdrawal from teriparatide maintains and even leads to increased BMD [65].

Combination therapies involving teriparatide and antiresorptive agents designed to increase bone mass and strength have yet to be proven safe and effective. Thus far, it is known that alendronate combined with teriparatide hinders the ability of teriparatide to induce bone formation at the lumbar spine and femoral neck [66], whereas risedronate combined with teriparatide increases BMD at the total hip and femoral neck to a greater extent than either therapy alone; at 18 months, lumbar spine BMD increased for all three groups but with no significant difference among them [67]. Forthcoming research on fracture outcomes should provide greater insight into the potential efficacy of combination therapies for osteoporosis.

Teriparatide has been identified as a principal therapy for men with glucocorticoid-induced osteoporosis (GIO), outpacing risedronate in treating bone loss associated with inflammatory, autoimmune, and allergic disorders (specifically chronic respiratory and inflammatory bowel disease) associated with GIO. In a 36-month study of men and women with GIO, teriparatide proved to be significantly more effective than alendronate in increasing BMD at the lumbar spine (11.0 % vs. 5.3 %), total hip (5.2 % vs. 2.7 %), and femoral neck (6.3 % vs. 3.4 %), tracking similar findings for women; moreover, fewer vertebral fractures occurred with teriparatide (0.6 %) than with alendronate (6.1 %) [68]. In another trial, comparing the results of teriparatide and risedronate in men with GIO over a 18-month period, greater increases in BMD at the lumbar spine were found with teriparatide than with risedronate (from baseline, 16.3 % vs. 3.8 %); teriparatide also produced significant increases in bone formation markers (PINP) as well as a trend toward fewer vertebral fractures [69]. Given the capacity of teriparatide to increase bone formation and cortical thickness in the total skeleton, these trials strongly indicate, but do not definitively prove, that teriparatide can prevent hip fracture. Unfortunately adherence to teriparatide is severely challenged by the need for daily self-injection over two years, adverse effects including the potential risk for osteosarcoma, and an extremely high cost, excluding insurance or special payment plans.

Denosumab

Most recently, the FDA approved an alternative antiresorptive agent to bisphosphonates, denosumab, to increase bone mass in men at high risk of fracture, particularly those on androgen deprivation therapy (ADT). Denosumab inhibits the action of RANKL, a protein that regulates the formation, function, and survival of osteoclasts which, in turn, stimulate bone resorption. Approval was based on data from the international, 12-month ADAMO (acronym for *A* multicenter, randomized, double-blind, placebo-controlled study to compare the efficacy and safety of *D*enosum*A*b 60 mg every 6 months vs. placebo in *M*ales with *O*steoporosis) study which provided strong evidence of significant increases in BMD at the lumbar spine, total hip, femoral neck and one-third distal radius as well as reduction in bone resorption, regardless of age, geographic region, testosterone levels, or estimated fracture risk [70]. A follow-up study at 24 months affirmed that increased BMD and decreased bone resorption continued into a second year [71].

In a trial involving men receiving ADT treatment, denosumab at 60 mg twice yearly resulted in a 5.6 % increase in BMD at lumbar spine at the 24-month mark, with increases evident at one month and sustained through 36 months [72]. At each time point, increases in BMD occurred at the total hip, femoral neck, and one-third distal radius—a site of cortical bone that has not been positively affected by bisphosphonates or estrogen receptor modulators. By 36 months, a decreased incidence of new vertebral fractures (1.5 % vs. 3.9 % placebo) in men with ADT also occurred but was limited in comparison with the effect of estrogen receptor modulator, toremifene, which reduced fractures by 50 %, increased BMD at the lumbar spine, hip, and femoral neck, and decreased bone turnover markers [73].

In 2013, the FDA-approved denosumab for giant cell tumor of bone (GCTB) in adults and skeletally mature adolescents. GCTB produces bone fractures and destroys normal bone as it grows; often it cannot be removed surgically or only with surgery that threatens severe morbidity, including loss of limbs or joint removal. Recent studies have demonstrated the efficacy of denosumab in treating

GCTB. Thomas et al. recorded an 86 % tumor response rate, defined as nearly complete elimination of giant cells, as evident in a biopsy after treatment or radiographic stabilization of the disease at six months; in addition, 84 % of patients experienced clinical benefits including reduced pain and improved functional status [74]. In another trial, focusing on both safety and efficacy, 74 out of 100 patients who had originally contemplated surgery for GCTB no longer required the procedure, while 16 of 26 patients who underwent surgery by the analysis cutoff point, now required a less morbid procedure than initially anticipated [75].

Although all of the above are approved treatments, they each have adverse side effects. Bisphosphonates may produce atypical femur fractures, osteonecrosis of the jaw, hypercalcemia, and oversuppression of bone turnover; oral bisphosphonates may lead to esophageal cancer. Teriparatide can cause fainting, muscle weakness, and hypercalcemia, while denosumab can result in numbness, trouble breathing, neck and joint pain, hypercalcemia, and osteonecrosis of the jaw. These drugs must be administered on the basis of a thorough physical examination, medical history, and confirmed diagnosis of osteoporosis and should be accompanied by nonpharmacological therapy including calcium and vitamin D supplementation, good nutrition, and exercise. Although repeat bone density tests are not recommended for routine monitoring of osteoporosis therapy, physicians must be aware of both the continuing impact of adverse effects on patients and the increasing concerns about the optimal duration of treatment. For example, in the case of bisphosphonates, FDA analyses have raised questions about whether continuous treatment beyond five years provides additional fracture prevention benefits compared with cessation of treatment at that point [76].

Alternative Therapies: Old and New

Testosterone

Testosterone is not regarded as a standard treatment for male osteoporosis. There is no evidence of its efficacy in reducing fracture risk, but testosterone undecanoate (1,000 mg/12 weeks for up to six years) does normalize serum testosterone levels, thereby increasing BMD and improving *T*-scores in osteoporotic men, with significant progression over the duration of treatment [77]. As Haider et al. point out, men diagnosed with osteoporosis at the outset of the study achieved *T*-scores classified as osteopenia by its conclusion; moreover, risks of testosterone administration to elderly men were acceptable and manageable for the term of the study, but risks are uncertain over a longer term.

Testosterone treatment increases spine BMD, trabecular connectivity, and bone turnover markers in men with both hypogonadism and osteoporosis [78]. Analysis of a potential combined testosterone-bisphosphonate therapy is yet to come, but a 2013 study postulates that bisphosphonates could restore eugonadal status without adversely affecting testosterone therapy for men at high fracture risk [79].

Selective Estrogen Receptor Modulators (SERMS)

Although not yet FDA approved, a relatively new group of drugs—selective estrogen receptor modulators (SERMs), specifically raloxifene and toremifene—are now being investigated as potential treatments for males receiving gonadotropin-releasing hormone (GnRH) agonists—the most commonly used ADT—to counter prostate cancer. In such cases, low estradiol levels, rather than testosterone deficiency, increase the risk of clinical, vertebral compression and hip fractures, leading to severe disability or even death. By replicating the effects of estrogen without incurring its harmful side effects, raloxifene stimulates estrogen receptors in bone and has the potential of becoming a new therapy to prevent bone loss in hypogonadal men. To determine its efficacy, Smith et al. randomly assigned raloxifene (60 mg/day) and no raloxifene to 48 men on GnRH agonists, finding that BMD of the total hip increased significantly, with modest increases in lumbar spine and decreases in bone turnover markers in the raloxifene group [80].

Toremifene, another type of SERM, has also produced promising results for men on ADT therapy. A study focusing on bone loss revealed that, in comparison with placebo, toremifene (60 mg/day) significantly increased BMD and reduced hot flashes after only six months of therapy [81]. Two subsequent trials conducted by Smith et al. confirmed toremifene's ability to reduce fracture risk in men receiving ADT. In the first, smaller ($n = 847$), 24-month study of men under the age of 80, toremifene (80 mg/day) increased BMD and significantly decreased the relative risk of new vertebral fractures by 79.5 % (new fracture incidence was 1.0 % for toremifene vs. 4.8 % for placebo), as well as the occurrence of nontraumatic fracture or greater than 7 % bone loss by end of study. In this trial, the rate of venous thromboembolic events was similar in the toremifene and placebo group [82].

In a second, much larger ($n = 1{,}284$), 24-month study, toremifene (80 ng/day) resulted in a significant relative risk reduction of 50 % (new fracture incidence at 2.5 % for toremifene vs. 4.9 % for placebo), along with increased BMD at the lumbar spine, hip, and femoral neck and a decrease in bone turnover markers. However, venous thromboembolic events (blood clots) occurred more frequently with toremifene than with placebo [73]. Because both raloxifene and toremifene entail the risk of venous thromboembolism, pulmonary embolism, and death due to stroke, they are contraindicated in patients who have a past or active history of these conditions or are at risk of developing them.

Selective Androgen Receptor Modulators (SARMS)

Whereas SERMs act by blocking estrogen receptors, another, even newer class of drugs—selective androgen receptor modulators (SARMS)—work by preventing the enzyme, aromatase, from changing other hormones into estrogen enzymes, thereby decreasing estrogen levels in the body and hindering the ability of estrogen receptors to grow. They are a potential alternative to oral testosterone applications currently on the market. Negro-Vilar has characterized the "ideal" SARM as orally active, administered daily, and capable of exerting anabolic effects on bone and muscle with little or no effect on the prostate [83]. As one of the initial steps in developing these drugs for humans, tests have been conducted on male rats (serving as models for male hypogonadism) to determine the effect of an investigational SARM, LGD2226, on bone and muscle. Evidence revealed its ability to prevent bone loss, stimulate bone formation, inhibit bone turnover, and exert anabolic activity on the levator ani muscle, indicating that SARMs may have the potential to treat elderly, hypogonadal men. In an early clinical trial for the SARM, bicalutamide (150 mg/day), BMD was maintained in lumbar spine and hip for patients who require long-term ADT for prostate cancer [84].

SERMs and SARMs are available in the form of bodybuilding dietary supplements (not subject to FDA action); none of the substances in either category have received FDA approval as a medication for men. The mechanisms underlying their action, the possibility of adverse side effects, and the efficacy of individual compounds compared with others in their category, as well as with other approved therapies, require more extensive study.

Agents Approved in Selected Countries

The metallic element, strontium, has been translated into drug form as strontium ranelate (SR), not to be confused with a performance-enhancing nutritional supplement under the name, strontium citrate. Approved for use by men in Europe and Australia but not in the United States, SR has been associated with a 22 % greater increase in BMD at the lumbar spine and 23 % increase at the total hip when compared with alendronate—a finding similar to that for postmenopausal women [85]. A more recent trial, known as MALEO (MALE osteoporosis), was the first to examine the efficacy and safety of SR in men with low BMD. It confirmed increases in BMD at all skeletal sites as well as lower vertebral fracture incidence, again comparable to results for postmenopausal osteoporosis. A few cases of coronary artery disorders occurred but were confined to patients with a history of the disease.

It is important to note that the European Union's recommendation of SR (Protelos/Osseor in Europe) is restricted to patients, both men and women, who are at high risk for fractures and cannot be treated with other approved osteoporosis medications. Patients must be monitored regularly and treatment halted if heart or circulatory problems, such as high blood pressure or angina, develop. SR is contraindicated in those with a history of heart or circulatory issues, including stroke and heart attack [86]. Because SR acts by replacing calcium in bone, it can affect interpretation of BMD testing results. With a heavier atomic weight than calcium, it may cause misleading readings indicating that bones may be stronger than they actually are. DXA scans generally based on calcium readings must be adjusted to account for the presence of strontium in bones [87].

Calcitonin

Finally, calcitonin, a synthetic hormone that mimics the action of the natural hormone produced by the thyroid, is of limited use in treating male osteoporosis. It inhibits osteoblastic activity, slowing the rate of bone removal and improving BMD in the spine; on a short-term basis, it also relieves acute pain associated with vertebral collapse. Calcitonin is FDA approved in an injectable form and, more recently, as a nasal spray which is more effectively absorbed into the bloodstream, causes fewer side effects and is recommended for use by men with normal testosterone levels and those who cannot tolerate testosterone therapy [88].

In a year-long trial of the effect of nasal spray salmon calcitonin (SCT-200 IU/day) on men, the increase in lumbar spine BMD was significantly greater in the calcitonin group compared with placebo, but there were no significant changes in the femoral neck or trochanter BMD [89]. Overall calcitonin is less effective than bisphosphonates in treating male osteoporosis. The drug's more important contribution may be its effect on nontraumatic osteoporotic vertebral crush fractures (OVCF). Men and postmenopausal women ($n = 100$), taking SCT 200 IU/day for four weeks, experienced a sharp decrease in spinal pain as well as earlier mobilization and restoration of locomotive functions compared with placebo [90]. A review of 13 trials examining the analgesic efficacy of calcitonin for OVCF determined that although it significantly reduced the severity of acute pain in recent OVCFs, evidence for reduction of chronic pain from older fractures is lacking [91]. Recent concerns about a potential link between calcitonin and cancer, coupled with the limited efficacy of the drug compared with other osteoporotic medications, have led experts to question its use and, if prescribed, to advocate individualized monitoring on a regular basis.

Monitoring of Treatment

Once a therapeutic approach has been adopted, clinicians must assess the response to treatment in terms of both the efficacy of the drugs used and the patient's capacity for adherence. As described in more detail in Chaps. 5 and 20, management may involve serial DXA BMD testing and the use of bone turnover markers. However, both have serious drawbacks. Changes in BMD, brought about by antiresorptive agents, occur so slowly that they will not exceed the measurement error of the machine until two or more years after therapy is initiated; only then can a change be deemed significant. In addition, BMD may decrease in the first year of treatment only to rebound and gain in the second [92]. In contrast to BMD scans, changes in bone turnover markers are observable within 3–6 months of initiating treatment, potentially permitting early intervention and a possible change in treatment. While they are difficult to collect and demonstrate considerable variability, they may be used to measure treatment efficacy, and possibly increased adherence, before a change in BMD can be assessed [93].

In an aging population, the risk of male osteoporosis, its serious consequences, and the costs involved—physical, mental and financial—have become a public health priority. The rising incidence of its worldwide occurrence has engendered an increasing body of research on the prevention and treatment of what is still widely regarded as a "woman's" disease. But, unless more effective measures can be adopted to engender wider recognition of the short-and long-term effects of male osteoporosis, research findings may be confined to journals and medical conferences. The adoption of national clinical guidelines and their routine implementation by physicians; the expansion of educational programs such as those developed by Fracture Liaison Services; and the power of print and social media to convey accessible medical information to a broad audience must all be invoked to ensure that scientific research is translated into individualized care.

References

1. Qaseem A, Snow V, Shekelle P, Hopkins Jr R, Forciea MA, Owens DK. Screening for osteoporosis in men: a clinical practice guideline from the American College of Physicians. Ann Intern Med. 2008;148(9):680–4.
2. Eberling P. Osteoporosis in men: why change needs to happen. In: International Osteoporosis Foundation. 2014. http://www.iofbonehealth.org/data-publications/reports/osteoporosis-men-why-change-needs-happen. Accessed 15 Apr 2015.
3. National Institute of Arthritis and Musculoskeletal and Skin Diseases. Osteoporosis in men. Washington, DC: 2012. http://www.niahs.nih.gov/health_infor/bone/osteoporosis.men/asp. Accessed 16 Apr 2015.
4. Steven JA, Rudd RA. The impact of decreasing U.S. hip fracture rates on future hip fracture estimates. Osteoporos Int. 2013;24(10):2725–8.
5. Orwoll E. Osteoporosis in men. In: Rosen CJ, editor. Primer on the metabolic bone diseases and disorders of mineral metabolism. Ames: Wiley; 2013. p. 510.
6. Willson T, Nelson SD, Newbold J, Nelson RE, LaFleur J. The clinical epidemiology of male osteoporosis: a review of the recent literature. Clin Epidemiol. 2015;7:65–76.
7. Ralston SH, de Crombrugghe B. Genetic regulation of bone mass and susceptibility to osteoporosis. Genes Dev. 2006;20(18):2492–506.
8. Nilsson M, Sundh D, Ohlsson C, Karlsson M, Mellstrom, Lorentzon M. Exercise during growth and young adulthood is independently associated with cortical bone size and strength in old Swedish men. J Bone Miner Res. 2014;29(8):1798–804.
9. Warden SJ, Mantilla Roosa SM. Physical activity completed when young has residual bone benefits at 94 years of age: a within-subject controlled study. J Musculoskelet Neuronal Interact. 2014;14(2):239–43.
10. Nieves JW, Formica C, Ruffing J, Zion M, Garrett P, Lindsay R, et al. Males have larger skeletal size and bone mass than females, despite comparable bone size. J Bone Miner Res. 2005;20(2):529–35.
11. Seeman E. Pathogenesis of bone fragility in women and men. Lancet. 2002;359(9320):1841–50.
12. Sutton RAL, Dian L, Guy P. Osteoporosis in men: an underrecognized and undertreated problem. B C Med J. 2011;53(10):535–40.
13. Giusti A, Bianchi G. Treatment of primary osteoporosis in men. Clin Interv Aging. 2014;10:105–15.
14. Sartorius G, Spasevska S, Idan A, Turner L, Forbes E, Zamojska A. Serum testosterone, dihydrotestosterone, and estradiol concentrations in older men self-reporting very good health: the healthy man study. Clin Endocrinol (Oxf). 2012;77(5):755–63.

15. Wu FCW, Tajar A, Beynon J, Pye SR, Silman AJ, Finn JD. Identification of late-onset hypogonadism in middle-aged and elderly men. N Engl J Med. 2010;363:123–35.
16. Falahati-Nini A, Riggs BL, Atkinson EJ, O'Fallon WM, Eastell R, Khosla S. Relative contributions of testosterone and estrogen in regulating bone resorption and formation in normal elderly men. J Clin Invest. 2000;106(12):1553–60.
17. Tenover JS. Androgen replacement therapy to reverse and/or prevent age-associated sarcopenia in men. Baillieres Clin Endocrinol Metab. 1998;12(3):419–25.
18. Mayo Clinic. Male hypogonadism: causes. http://www.mayoclinic.org/diseases-conditions/male-hypogonadism/basics/causes/con-20014235. Accessed 16 Apr 2015.
19. Banu J. Causes, complications, and treatment of osteoporosis in men. Drug Des Devel Ther. 2013;7:849–60.
20. Van Henelrijck M, Garmo H, Michaelsson K, Thorstenson A, Akra O, Stattin P, et al. Mortality following hip fracture for men with prostate cancer. PLOSone. 2013;8(9), e74492. doi:10.1371/journalpone.0074492.
21. Adler RA, Hochberg MC. Glucocorticoid-induced osteoporosis in men. J Endocrinol Invest. 2011;34(6):481–4.
22. Rao SS, Budhwar N, Ashfaque A. Osteoporosis in men. Am Fam Physician. 2010;82(5):503–8.
23. Shepherd AJ, Cass AR, Carlson CA, Ray L. Development and internal validation of male osteoporosis risk evaluation score. Ann Fam Med. 2007;5(6):540–6.
24. Skedros JG, Sybrowsky CL, Stoddard GJ. The osteoporosis self-assessment screening tool: a useful tool for the orthopaedic surgeon. J Bone Joint Surg Am. 2007;89(4):765–72.
25. Cass AR, Shepherd AJ. Validation of the male osteoporosis risk estimation score (MORES) in a primary care setting. J Am Board Fam Med. 2013;26(4):436–44. doi:10.3122/jabfm.2013.04.120182.
26. Watts NB, Adler RA, Bilezikian JP, Drake MT, Eastell Y, Orwoll ES, et al. Osteoporosis in men: an Endocrine Society clinical practice guideline. J Clin Endocrinol Metab. 2012;97(6):1802–22.
27. Clinician's guide to prevention and treatment of osteoporosis. National Osteoporosis Foundation. 2013. p. 20. doi:10.1007/s00198-014-2794-2.
28. Kanis JA, Bianchi G, Bilezikian JP, Kaufman J-M, Khosla S, Orwoll E, et al. Towards a diagnostic and therapeutic consensus in male osteoporosis. Osteoporos Int. 2011;22(11):2789–98.
29. World Health Organization Collaborative Centre for Metabolic Bone Diseases. FRAX: WHO fracture risk assessment tool. University of Sheffield, UK. https://www.shef.ac.uk/FRAX/tool.jsp. Accessed 08 Aug 2015.
30. Bauer DC, Ewing SK, Cauley JA, Ensrud KE, Cummings SP, Orwoll ES, et al. Quantitative ultrasound predicts hip and non-spine fracture in men: the MrOS study. Osteoporos Int. 2007;18(6):771–7.
31. Bethel M, Machua W, Carbone LD, Lohr KM. Osteoporosis workup: laboratory studies. http://emedicine.medscape.com/article/330598-workup. Accessed 5 May 2015.
32. Ryan CS, Petkov VI, Adler RA. Osteoporosis in men: the value of laboratory testing. Osteoporos Int. 2011;22(6):1845–53.
33. Meier C, Nguyen TV, Center JR, Seibel MJ, Eisman JA. Bone resorption and osteoporotic fractures in elderly men: the Dubbo osteoporosis epidemiology study. J Bone Miner Res. 2005;20(4):579–87.
34. Bauer DC, Garnero P, Harrison SL, Cauley JA, Eastell R, Ensrud K, et al. Biochemical markers of bone turnover, hip bone loss, and fracture in older men: the MrOS study. J Bone Miner Res. 2009;24(12):2032–8.
35. Szulc P, Montella A, Delmas PD. High bone turnover is associated with accelerated bone loss but not with increased fracture risk in men aged 50 and over: the prospective MINOS study. Ann Rheum Dis. 2008;67(9):1249–55.
36. Vasikaran S. Bone turnover markers: the impact of assay standardization on assessing and monitoring osteoporosis. In: American Association for Clinical Chemistry. 2013. https://www.aacc.org/publications/cln/articles/2013/july/bone-turnover-markets. 10 Aug 2015.

37. Dawson-Hughes B, Harris SS, Krall EA, Dallal GE. Effect of calcium and vitamin D supplementation on bone density in men and women 65 years of age or older. N Engl J Med. 1997;337(10):670–6.
38. Trivedi DP, Doll R, Khaw KT. Effect of four monthly oral vitamin D_3 (cholecalciferol) supplementation on fractures and mortality in men and women living in the community: randomized double blind controlled trial. BMJ. 2003;326(7387):469. doi:10.1136/bmj.326.7387.469.
39. Kiel DP, Zhang Y, Hannan MT, Anderson JJ, Baron JA, Felson DT. The effect of smoking at different life stages on bone mineral density in elderly men and women. Osteoporos Int. 1996;6(3):240–8.
40. Olofsson H, Byberg L, Mohsen R, Mehus H, Lithell H, Michaelsson K. Smoking and the risk of fracture in older men. J Bone Miner Res. 2005;20(7):1208–15.
41. Kim MJ, Shim MS, Kim MK, Lee Y, Shim YG, Chung CH, et al. Effect of chronic alcohol ingestion on bone mineral density in males without liver cirrhosis. Korean J Intern Med. 2003;18(3):174–80.
42. Takata S, Yasui N. Disuse osteoporosis. J Med Invest. 2001;48(3–4):147–56.
43. Nigram Y, Knight J, Jones A. Effects of bedrest: musculoskeletal and immune systems, skin and self-perception. Nurs Times. 2009;105(23):18–22.
44. Hetland H, Haarbo J, Christiansen C. Low bone mass and high bone turnover in male long distance runners. J Clin Endocrinal Metab. 1993;77(3):770–5.
45. MacDougall JD, Webber CE, Martin J, Ormerod S, Chesney A, Younglai EV, et al. Relationship among running mileage, bone density, and serum testosterone in male runners. J Appl Physiol. 1992;73(3):1165–70.
46. Mussolino ME, Looker AC, Orwell ES. Jogging and bone mineral density in men: results from NHANES III. Am J Public Health. 2001;91(7):1056–9.
47. Reents S. Exercise and osteoporosis. In: AthleteInMe.com. 2007–2014. http://www.athleteinme.com/ArticleView.aspx?id=283. 10 Aug 2015.
48. Herrera A, Lobo-Escolar A, Mateo J, Gil J, Ibarz, Gracia L. Male osteoporosis: a review. World J Orthop. 2012;3(12):223–340.
49. Drake MT, Clarke B, Khosla S. Bisphosphonates: mechanism of action and role in clinical practice. Mayo Clin Proc. 2008;83(9):1032–45.
50. Sim IW, Eberling PR. Treatment of osteoporosis in men with bisphosphonates: rationale and latest evidence. Ther Adv Musculoskelet Dis. 2013;5(5):259–67.
51. Orwoll E, Ettinger M, Weiss S, Miller P, Kendler D, Graham J. Alendronate for the treatment of osteoporosis in men. N Engl J Med. 2000;343(9):604–10.
52. Planas J, Trilla E, Raventos C, Cecchini L, Orsola A, Salvador C. Alendronate also decreases the fracture risk in patients with prostate cancer on androgen-deprivation therapy and with severe osteopenia or osteoporosis. BJU Int. 2009;104(11):1637–40.
53. Greenspan S. Protecting bone health in men with prostate cancer undergoing ADT. In: Review of endocrinology. 2009. http://bmctoday.net/reviewofendo/2009/02/article.asp?f=review0209_04.php 20 Aug 2015.
54. Stoch SA, Saag KG, Greenwald M, Sebba AI, Cohen S, Verbruggen N, et al. Once-weekly oral alendronate 70 mg in patients with glucocorticoid-induced bone loss: a 12-month randomized, placebo-controlled clinical trial. J Rheumatol. 2009;36(8):1705–14.
55. Le Blanc AD, Driscol TB, Shackelford LC, Evans HJ, Rianon NJ, Smith SM. Alendronate as an effective countermeasure to disuse induced bone loss. J Musculoskelet Neuronal Interact. 2002;2(4):335–43.
56. LeBlanc A, Matsumoto T, Jones J, Shapiro J, Lang T, Shackelford L. Bisphosphonates as a supplement to exercise to protect bone during long-duration space flight. Osteoporos Int. 2013;24(7):2105–14.
57. Ringe JD, Farahmand P, Faber H, Dorst A. Sustained efficacy of risedronate in men with primary and secondary osteoporosis: result of a 2 year study. Rheumatol Int. 2009;29(3):311–5.
58. Reid DM, Hughes RA, Laan RFJM, Sacco-Gibson NA, Wenderoth DH, Adami S, et al. Efficacy and safety of daily risedronate in the treatment of corticosteroid-induced osteoporosis in men and women: a randomized trial. J Bone Miner Res. 2000;15(6):1006–13.

59. Reid DM, Adam S, Devogelaer JP, Chines AA. Risedronate increases bone density and reduces vertebral fracture risk within one year in men on corticosteroid therapy. Calcif Tissue Int. 2001;69(4):242–7.
60. Orwoll ES, Binkley NC, Lewiecki EM, Gruntmanis U, Fries MA, Dasic G. Efficacy and safety of monthly ibandronate in men with low bone density. Bone. 2010;46(4):970–6.
61. Lyles K, Colon-Emetic CS, Magazine JS, Adachi JD, Pieper CF, Matalan C, et al. Zoledronic acid in reducing clinical fracture and mortality after hip fracture. N Engl J Med. 2007;357:1799–809. doi:10.1056/NEJMoa074941.
62. Erikson EF, Lyles KW, Colon-Emetic CS, Pieper CFR, Magazine JS, Adachi J, et al. Antifracture efficacy and reduction of mortality in relation to timing of the first dose of zoledronic acid after hip fracture. J Bone Miner Res. 2009;24(7):1308–13.
63. Boonen S, Reginster J-V, Kaufman J-M, Lippunar K, Zanchetta J, Langdahl B, et al. Fracture risk and zoledronic acid therapy in men with osteoporosis. N Engl J Med. 2012;367(18):1714–23.
64. Orwoll ES, Scheele WH, Paul S, Adami S, Syversen U, Diez-Perez A, et al. The effect of teriparatide [human parathyroid hormone (1-34)] therapy on bone density in men with osteoporosis. J Bone Miner Res. 2003;18(1):9–17.
65. Kaufman JM, Orwoll E, Goemaere S, San Martin J, Hossain A, Dalsky GP, et al. Teriparatide effects on vertebral fractures and bone mineral density in men with osteoporosis: treatment and discontinuation of therapy. Osteoporos Int. 2005;16(5):510–6.
66. Finkelstein JS, Hayes A, Hunzelman JL, Wyland JJ, Lee H, Neer RM. The effects of parathyroid hormone, alendronate, and both in men with osteoporosis. N Engl J Med. 2003;349(13):1216–26.
67. Walker MD, Cusano NE, Sliney Jr J, Romano M, Zhang C, McMahon DJ, et al. Combination therapy with risedronate and teriparatide in male osteoporosis. Endocrine. 2013;44(1):237–46.
68. Saag KG, Zanchetta JR, Devogelaer JP, Adler RA, Eastell R, See K, et al. Effects of teriparatide versus alendronate for treating glucocorticoid-induced osteoporosis: thirty-six month results of a randomized, double-blind, controlled trial. Arthritis Rheum. 2009;60(11):3346–55.
69. Gluer CC, Marin F, Ringe JD, Hawkins F, Moricke R, Papaioannu N, et al. Comparative effects of teriparatide and risedronate in glucocorticoid-induced osteoporosis in men: 18-month results of the EuroGIOPs trial. J Bone Miner Res. 2013;28(6):1355–68.
70. Orwoll E, Teglbjaerg CS, Langdahl BL, Chapuriat R, Czerwinski E, Kendler DL, et al. A randomized, placebo-controlled study of the effects of denosumab for treatment of men with low bone mineral density. J Clin Endocrinol Metab. 2012;97(9):3161–9.
71. Langdahl BL, Teglbjaerg CS, Ho PR, Chapuriat R, Czerwinski E, Kndler DL, et al. A 24-month study evaluating the efficacy and safety of denosumab for the treatment of men with low bone mineral density: results from the ADAMO trial. J Clin Endocrinol Metab. 2015;100(4):1335–42.
72. Smith MR, Egerdie B, Hernandez Toriz N, Feldman R, Tammela TLJ, Saad F, et al. Denosumab in men receiving androgen–deprivation therapy for prostate cancer. N Engl J Med. 2009;361(8):745–55.
73. Smith MR, Morton RA, Barnette KG, Sieber PR, Malkowicz SB, Rodriquez D, et al. Toremifene to reduce fracture risk in men receiving androgen deprivation therapy for prostate cancer. J Urol. 2013;189(1 Suppl):45–50. 2013.
74. Thomas D, Henshaw R, Skubitz K, Chawla S, Staddon A, Blay JL, et al. Denosumab in patients with giant-cell tumour of bone: an open-label, phase 2 study. Lancet Oncol. 2010;11(3):275–80.
75. Chawla S, Henshaw R, Seeger L, Choy E, Blay JY, Farrari S, et al. Safety and efficacy of denosumab for adults and skeletally mature adolescents with giant cell tumour of bone: interim analysis of an open-label, parallel-group, phase 2 study. Lancet Oncol. 2013;14(9):901–8.
76. Whitaker M, Guo J, Kehoe T, Benson G. Bisphosphonates for osteoporosis—where do we go from here? N Engl J Med. 2012;366(22):2048–51.
77. Haider A, Meergans U, Traish A, Saad F, Doros G, Lips P, et al. Progressive improvement of T-scares in men with osteoporosis and subnormal serum testosterone levels upon treatment with testosterone over six years. Int J Endocrinol. 2014. doi:10.1155/2014/496948.

78. Dandona P, Rosenberg MT. A practical guide to male hypogonadism in the primary care setting. J Clin Pract. 2010;64(6):682–96.
79. Ie-Wen S, Ebeling PR. Treatment of osteoporosis in men with bisphosphonates: rationale and latest evidence. Ther Adv Muscoloskelet Dis. 2013;5(5):259–67.
80. Smith MR, Fallon MA, Lee H, Finkelstein JS. Raloxifene to prevent gonadotropin-releasing hormone agonist induced bone loss in men with prostate cancer. J Clin Endocrinol Metab. 2004;89(8):3841–6.
81. Steiner MS, Patterson A, Israeli R, Barnette KG, Boger R, Price D. Toremifene citrate versus placebo for treatment of bone loss and other complications of androgen deprivation therapy in patients with prostate cancer. J Clin Oncol: Proc 2004 Am Soc Clin Oncol Annu Meet. 2004;22(14S):4597.
82. Smith MR, Malkowicz SB, Brawer MK, Hancock ML, Morton RA, Steiner MS. Toremifene decreases vertebral fractures in men younger than 80 years receiving androgen deprivation therapy for prostate cancer. J Urol. 2011;186(6):2239–44.
83. Negro-Vilar A. Selective androgen receptor modulators (SARMs): a novel approach to androgen therapy for the new millennium. J Clin Endocrinol Metab. 1999;84(10):597–617.
84. Sieber PR, Keiller DL, Kahnoski RJ, Gallo J, McFadden S. Bicalutamide 150 mg maintains bone mineral density during monotherapy for localized or locally advanced prostate cancer. J Urol. 2004;171(6.1):2272–6.
85. Ringe JD, Dorst A, Farahmand P. Efficacy of strontium ranelate on bone mineral density in men with osteoporosis. Arzneimittelforschung. 2010;60(5):267–72.
86. European Medicines Agency. Protelos/Osseor to remain available but with further restrictions. 2014. http://www.ema.europa.eu/ema/index.jsp?curl=pages/medicines/human/referrals/Protelos_and_Osseor/human_referral_prac_000025.jsp&mid=WC0b01ac05805c516f. Accessed 20 Aug 2015.
87. Berkeley Wellness. A new supplement for old bones. 2015. http://www.berkeleywellness.com/supplements.mineral/articles/new-supplement-old-bones. Accessed 21 Aug 2015.
88. Drugs for the treatment of osteoporosis: calcitonin and bisphosphonates. Endocrineweb. 2014. http://www.endocrineweb.com/conditions/osteoporosis/newest-drugs-treatment-osteoporosis. 21 Aug 2015.
89. Trovas GP, Lyritis GP, Galanos A, Raptou P, Constantelou E. A randomized trial of nasal spray salmon calcitonin in men with idiopathic osteoporosis: effects of bone mineral density and bone markers. J Bone Miner Res. 2002;17(3):521–7.
90. Lyritis GP, Paspati I, Karachalios T, Ioakimidis D, Skarantavos G, Lyritis PG. Pain relief from nasal salmon calcitonin in osteoporotic vertebral crush fractures. A double blind, placebo-controlled clinical study. Acta Orthop Scand Suppl. 1997;276:112–4.
91. Knopp-Sihota JA, Newburn-Cook CV, Homik J, Cummings GG, Voaklander D. Calcitonin for treating acute and chronic pain of recent and remote osteoporotic vertebral compression fractures: a systematic review and meta-analysis. Osteoporos Int. 2012;23(1):17–38.
92. Cummings SR, Palermo L, Browner W, Marcus R, Wallace R, Pearson J, et al. Monitoring osteoporosis therapy with bone densitometry: misleading changes and regression to the mean. Fracture Intervention Trial Research Group. JAMA. 2000;283(10):1318–21.
93. Wheater G, Elshahaly M, Tuck SP, Datta HK, van Laar JM. The clinical utility of bone marker measurements in osteoporosis. J Transl Med. 2013;11:201.

Chapter 7
Bone Disorders with Brain and Behavioral Conditions

Christina V. Oleson, Tracy E. Ransom, and Akinpelumi A. Beckley

Traumatic Brain Injury

In the past decades, traumatic brain injury (TBI) was more common among younger adults due to motor vehicle accidents, violence, and sports-related injuries. Over the last 10–15 years, the percentage of older individuals experiencing TBI has been steadily rising, primarily due to falls. The older population of Americans experiencing TBI may be at particular risk for fractures, given the cognitive deficits, ataxia, and impulsivity that may follow TBI. Even the younger individuals experiencing TBI have risk factors for osteoporotic fractures, including physical and functional immobility; medications to control behavior, headaches, seizures, or pain; posttraumatic seizures; and poor overall nutrition [1]. While the preceding factors put patients at increased risk of fracture after TBI, some patients have preexisting reasons for low BMD, even before developing their injury. A significant percentage of younger individuals experiencing TBI have partially treated or unrecognized depression, anxiety, and substance abuse [1, 2]. The above considerations should be incorporated when designing an optimal rehabilitation program and when offering anticipatory guidance for ongoing bone health after TBI.

Epidemiology

Banham-Hall and colleagues [1] examined 51 TBI subjects (80 % male) who were receiving treatment at a behaviorally focused neuro-rehabilitation center. The majority of subjects in the study had a number of known risk factors for osteoporosis. In their investigation, the most reliable risk factors were advancing age, smoking, low body weight or recent weight loss, current fracture, and immobility. Less reliable predictors were height loss, family history, current physical activity, muscle strength, and alcohol or calcium intake (Table 1). This study found 36 % prevalence

C.V. Oleson, *Osteoporosis Rehabilitation*, DOI 10.1007/978-3-319-45084-1_7

Table 1 Risk factors for osteoporosis in TBI patients

Factor	Description
Mobility:	
1. Nonmobile	Wheelchair used indoors and outdoors, requirement of physical assistance of another person, with or without a walking aid, to walk short distances indoors
2. Walks with assistance	Wheelchair used to mobilize outdoors but independently mobile indoors without aid
Smoking history	Determined by number of packs per day and years at that rate
Medication history	Includes current and previous prescriptions for antipsychotic or antiepileptic drugs
Fragility fracture history	Relates to additional fracture risk and increased osteoporosis because may cause decreased mobility
Age	>60
Gender	Higher risk in females over males
Ethnicity	Higher risk in those with darker skin

Source: Banham-Hall et al. [1]. Used with permission

of osteopenia and 8 % osteoporosis at the tibia. The radius did not demonstrate osteoporosis in any subjects but did show osteopenia in 18 % of the population.

Pathophysiology of Bone Metabolism After TBI

Inflammatory Mediators

Most of the investigations of bone metabolic abnormalities following TBI have not focused on osteoporosis but rather on heterotopic ossification (HO), a process by which new bone is formed along with bone marrow in locations and tissues that normally do not ossify. These areas are typically found near but not within joints, generally the hip and shoulder following traumatic brain injury. Measures of bone formation including osteocalcin, bone-specific alkaline (B-ALK) phosphatase, and procollagen N1 terminal propeptide (P1NP) have been noted to be lower in persons immediately following TBI relative to subjects with new fractures absent of TBI [3], but these levels may be higher than those of healthy uninjured subjects. Osteocalcin remained low over the 7-day observation period but P1NP increased after three days, findings similar to those observed in patients with fractures alone.

The accelerated fracture healing and osteogenesis in the form of HO is thought to be centrally regulated, perhaps accentuated in the presence of inflammatory markers like IL-6 [4]. In an animal model that compared TBI without fracture to experimentally induced TBI, no pattern of enhanced osteogenesis was found, but rather a predisposition toward osteoporosis [5]. At the time of injury, markers of bone formation and resorption were not significantly increased in TBI patients without associated fractures. However, both P1NP and CTX were higher in those with TBI one week after injury ($p=0.053$ and $p=0.059$) but levels failed to reach statistical significance. While small sample sizes could account for lack of significance, these factors may be only part of the cause. Radiographic evidence of the lumbar spine and both distal femurs had a significant decline in BMD at only one week, suggesting a very rapid bone loss brought on by immobilization and potential biochemical and endocrine changes that remain undefined [5].

In both adults [6] and children [7], interleukin 6 (IL-6) stimulates vasopressin secretion in the posterior pituitary, causing elevated levels of antidiuretic hormone (ADH). The syndrome of inappropriate antidiuretic hormone (SIADH) is prevalent after TBI [8] and results in hyponatremia. SIADH may adversely affect functional outcomes, depending on the severity, persistence, and response to treatment. Dimopoulou et al. [6] assessed morning samples of baseline IL-6 and tumor necrosis factor alpha (TNF-α) in participants who received a low-dose cortisol stimulation test once critical care issues had stabilized sufficiently for such a test. All 40 subjects met definitions of moderate to severe head injury. Results found that 15 % of subjects were classified as nonresponders to the low-dose stimulation test. The responders had levels of IL-6 that were nearly double the responders, indicating that IL-6 levels are fundamentally altered in those with pituitary dysfunction. In contrast, TNF-α levels did not differ statistically between responders and nonresponders. Adrenocorticotrophic hormone (ACTH) function was also assessed, and CT of the adrenals was obtained, with primary and secondary adrenal failure noted in the absence of direct adrenal trauma. Medications inducing a similar type of picture, but instead suggesting inflammatory cytokines including IL-6 could be responsible for alterations in hypothalamic–pituitary–adrenal (HPA) axis.

The relationship of IL-6 and its link to SIADH is critical if not clinically corrected early in the hospital course. Hyponatremia is one consequence of sustained SIADH. A recent study examined 5,122 men from the Osteoporotic Fractures in Men study and found statistically significant increases in both vertebral and hip fractures among those with hyponatremia, defined as serum sodium <135 [9]. Specifically, the fully adjusted model accounting for all confounders found that prevalent morphometric vertebral fractures, incident morphometric vertebral fracture, hip fracture, and other nonspine fracture were all increased in men with hyponatremia. An earlier large prospective study from Rotterdam showed that even mild hyponatremia can increase risk of nonvertebral fractures, but a relationship to vertebral fractures was less certain [10]. This investigation differed from that of Jamal in that the study population was 50 % female and 8 % male. The lower percentage of males may explain why only 1.6 % of the study group demonstrated hyponatremia [9].

There are a number of possible explanations for why hyponatremia may increase risk of fractures. Falls have been linked to hyponatremia by causing gait instability, balance issues, and decreased attention. In the investigation by Jamal and colleagues [9], 31 % of the men with hyponatremia reported falls in the 12 months prior to assessment, compared to 21 % of those with normal serum sodium levels. Animal data has shown that sustained hyponatremia of longer than 90 days resulted in a 30 % reduction in femoral BMD in rats, relative to animals with normal sodium levels [11]. Findings demonstrating a relationship between hyponatremia and osteoporosis, with and without the presence of fractures, have also been shown in human studies [12–16] but are subject to many confounding variables including thiazide diuretic use, other medications predisposing to falls, uncertain cardiac conditions with arrhythmias contributing to falls, and underreported drug or alcohol use.

Endocrine Conditions

Endocrine factors also predispose to bone loss following TBI. Posttraumatic hypopituitarism (PTHP) is a frequent occurrence following TBI. Recent estimates are that PTHP affects 28–35 % of newly injured patients [17, 18] and 36–68 % of those with chronic TBI of 3–30 years [19–21]. Dysfunction in the hypothalamic–pituitary axis contributes not only to compromised bone health but also to control of emotion, regulation of body temperature, blood glucose control, muscle strength, cognition, and reproductive function [22]. PTHP results in a number of secondary endocrine abnormalities, many of which lead to increasing bone loss or predispose a patient to fracture. Because a number of the deficits are similar to the conditions seen in patients with TBI absent of PTHP, it can be difficult to determine the primary cause of functional, cognitive, and emotional outcome measures. Table 2 [6, 8, 9, 22–25, 41, 51] summarizes the specific endocrine abnormalities patients experience due to PTHP. These studies discuss PTHP in several contexts, unrelated to TBI.

Nonpharmacologic Treatment

Given the challenges of decreased balance, aggression, impulsivity, and unpredictable muscle weakness, patients with acute TBI are clearly at increased risk for falls. Exercise programs may contribute to prevention efforts, but to be most effective for osteoporosis prevention, they must be easy to follow, incorporate weight-bearing as well as aerobic fitness, and recognize cognitive and physical endurance limitations of these patients. Schwandt and colleagues found that aerobic exercise with hand cycles had a positive impact on depression reduction in subjects with TBI [26]. Other authors have found similar results [26, 27]. Many of the studies selected modes of exercise that did not involve weight-bearing such as seated bicycling, hand cycle ergometry, or swimming [26, 28]. In general, aerobic exercise properly chosen may have benefits in physical and emotional health following TBI.

Banham-Hall and colleagues [1] recommend that an exercise program in TBI patients to decrease osteoporosis should have the following elements:

1. Intensity of exercise should be moderate to high.
2. Exercises should target sites of common fracture (hips, spine, ankles, wrists).
3. Exercises should have low impact such that one leg is firmly on the ground at all times.
4. Exercise should progress gradually from a comfortable level to a more intense level.

Table 2 Endocrine abnormalities following PTHP

Endocrine abnormality	Frequency after TBI	Study specific notes	Relation to osteoporosis or fractures	Source
Glucocorticoid deficiency/ACTH deficiency	11.8 % (range 0–47 % with varying definitions and times of evaluation)	Acute: first month Chronic: years after TBI	Life threatening (bed rest immobility) Fatigue, weakness, decreased attention and concentration, predisposition to falls due to inattention, lack of strength	Bonadenelli M. et al. [22]
Gonadotropin deficiency	28.8 % (range 2–62 %)	Men: low testosterone Women: low estrogen Starts at day two post TBI and lasts at least two months but persists in many patients	Accelerated osteoporosis in combination with reduced peak bone density in younger men and women; in addition low testosterone is associated with fatigue, muscle atrophy, anhedonia, decreased estrogen with reduced motor processing speed, reaction time, and vigilance	Dimpopoulo I. et al. [6] Clark JD. et al. [23] Woolf PD. et al. [24]
Growth hormone deficiency	30 % (range 14.6–60 %)	Generally seen in acute phase	Muscle atrophy, fatigue, poor concentration—leading to greater fall risk	Masel BE.et al. [25]
Hypothyroidism	18.5 % (range 3.6–31 %)	Review article summarizing several studies	Fatigue, muscle wasting, decreased attention and memory	Misra M. et al. [41]
Hyperprolactinemia	>50 %	Review article summarizing several studies	Stimulated bone resorption	Powner DJ. et al. [8] and Filipek PA. et al. [51]
SIADH (if associated with hyponatremia)	20 ± 10 %	Review article summarizing several studies	Increased fracture risk	Powner DJ. et al. [8] and Jamal SA. et al. [9]

In addition to the above features, duration of exercise must take into consideration each patient's physical and emotional tolerance, particularly in those with tendency toward violent or impulsive behavior. The exercise regimen should be simple and time limited. Doing an activity for hours at one time may not be conducive to learning or participation. Although variety may help patients with practicing cognitive goals of divided attention and task switching, a more basic program involving a component of repetition is frequently preferred, particularly given difficulties with new learning in patients with TBI. Some aspect of vestibular retraining is also advisable since TBI may impair a patient's ability to utilize normal righting reactions in an effort to prevent fall.

One of the greatest challenges with any exercise program is compliance. Short-term memory deficits and psychological resistance based on mood could deter participation on any given day. Secondly, finding an appropriate venue in which to undertake an exercise program can be problematic. A gym or training center with loud music or many people could be too stimulating for some patients and lead to increased anxiety, agitation, and panic. Home settings may not be safe due to inadequate space for moving around, inappropriate flooring for seated stretching activities, or lack of devices for support during standing balance activities. Finally, the TBI patient benefits best from similar daily activities, so a twice weekly program may be inadequate. A daily program would be preferred, but available help for such a program is limited by family skill set and availability and by insurance caps for outpatient therapy visits. If chosen and accessible to patients, an outpatient therapy center should assist the patient with attendance by phone call reminders or text messages prior to each meeting.

Pharmacologic Treatment

Given the benefits of hormonal correction for subjects experiencing panhypopituitarism, supplementation with estrogen, progesterone, or testosterone would favor a preservation of bone density. Adopting a strategy of giving one of the above hormones in an effort to prevent a "future health problem" of osteoporosis and fracture prevention is a difficult task for patients to accept given the many other medications they take for immediate medical concerns. If supplementation with progesterone or estrogen has benefits for recovery of TBI while also protecting bones, patients may be more willing to consider their use in the weeks and months immediately following injury.

Selective Estrogen Receptor Modulators

Selective estrogen receptor modulators (SERMs) have been successfully used as a treatment for osteoporosis in women. Raloxifene, one of the older and most tested SERMs, can reduce reactive gliosis after TBI [29] and, in one report, improved sensorimotor function and reduced working memory deficits after bilateral cortical contusions [30]. Evidence from studies on postmenopausal women, without a TBI, also suggests raloxifene may help in preventing cognitive decline [31] and improving verbal memory [32].

In terms of actual neuroprotection following TBI, a number of animal models suggest that selected SERMs including raloxifene promote axonal growth and the expression of synaptic markers, with the thought that such actions may contribute to health of functional circuitry and repair of damaged neural connections following injury from TBI [33]. In additional models, examining levels of endorphin and tetrahydroprogesterone are increased in rats who receive raloxifene. While it is unclear if similar mechanisms exist in humans, basic science studies by Genazzani et al. as well as Bernardi et al. [34–36] imply that raloxifene can modulate local levels of neuroactive substances in the brain and, in doing so, influence synaptic function of neurons [33].

Progesterone

Along with estrogen, progesterone plays an important role in maintaining bone health in post- and perimenopausal women. Progesterone and estradiol control actions of both RANK and RANKL which independently play an essential part in bone metabolism. Reduced levels of progesterone stimulate RANK ligand to bind to RANK in a manner that upregulates osteoclastic function and promotes bone resorption. In this manner, progesterone plays a role in prevention of secondary osteoporosis. Following injury, some have proposed that progesterone prevents inflammation through inhibiting inflammatory cytokine production, reducing levels of complement factor C3, blocking activation of inflammatory-mediated microglial cells, and regulating vasogenic edema [37]. Preclinical trials of progesterone in humans demonstrated promise in reducing mortality if administered within hours of injury [38, 39]. However, a follow-up investigation by Skolnick [37] did not demonstrate any significant difference in mortality outcome between those subjects receiving placebo and those receiving progesterone. Given this outcome, it is unlikely that patients with TBI will be eager to undertake progesterone as a treatment among other choices for osteoporosis prevention.

Bisphosphonates and Denosumab

Among bisphosphonates, denosumab, and other less potent options such as SERMs, practitioners may wish to strongly consider a treatment modality in which compliance can be effectively guaranteed. Options would include annual zoledronic acid 5 mg IV, denosumab 60 mg given twice annually via subcutaneous injection, or ibandronate 3 mg IV given every three months. All of the above are done in physician offices, ensuring that treatment is successfully achieved. Lack of compliance is a significant factor in outcomes of treatment programs among the patients without neurological disorders. For those with memory deficits, consistently taking medication and following directions for usage are even greater challenges.

Impact of Psychiatric Diseases on Bone Health

Prevalence, Pathophysiology, and Risk Factors

Psychiatric disorders as well as medications to treat psychiatric conditions are indicated in bone health conditions such as osteoporosis and osteopenia [40, 41]. Conditions such as autism spectrum disorders, bipolar disorders, borderline personality disorder, depressive disorders, and thought disorders such as schizophrenia have been studied and indicate risk factors for a decrease in bone mineral density (BMD) [41–43]. Medical treatments for these conditions, such as antidepressants, benzodiazepines, and antipsychotics, carry several side effects, including decreases in BMD [44–46]. In addition to BMD loss, other complications of psychotropic use include dyskinesias, orthostatic hypotension, as well as sedation, which can lead to an increase in risk of falls [41].

Many additional factors also affect BMD including age, race, gender, nutrition, and genetics other than psychiatric conditions and medications [47]. Halbreich and Palter [40] also report that BMD may be due to decreased levels of estrogen and testosterone, decreased calcium, smoking, alcoholism, polydipsia, increased interleukin activity, impaired electrolyte and fluid balances, dietary imbalances, hypercortisolemia, and hyperprolactinemia. Comorbidities of these conditions in the psychiatric population can be quite high, especially due to immobility, poor health choices, lack of sunshine, and substance use [43, 46, 48]. The relationship between psychiatric conditions, medications, and bone health is unclear, but the neuroendocrine system has been shown to be impacted due to low bone turnover [49].

Autism Spectrum Disorders

Autism spectrum disorders (ASD) are a classification of disorders defined and characterized by behavioral disturbances including repetitive or restrictive interests or activities and difficulty with social communication [50]. Attentional disorders, mental retardation, anxiety, depression, epilepsy, and obsessive-compulsive disorders occur frequently with ASD [51]. These conditions can range from mild to severe impairment of functioning. Hediger et al. [52] studied 75 boys aged 4–8 years for metacarpal bone cortical thickness (BCT) and found that casein-free diet use, supplements, and medications had an impact on bone development. In particular, while study subjects and controls showed BCT levels to increase incrementally with age, there appeared to be a sharp deviation between the ages of seven and eight, indicating that dietary intake, specifically calcium and vitamin D (which are low in dairy-free casein diets), was almost twice that of controls with less restrictive diets. Researchers also concluded that other factors including lack of sunlight, low levels of physical activity, and other GI disorders led to a slowing of bone growth for this population [52–55].

Neumeyer et al. [56] also confirm that lower BMD in autistic children and adults leads to a significant increase in the hip, forearm, and spine fractures as studied from a large database of emergency departments in the United States. Their study concluded that factors such as lower amounts of physical activity, reduced vitamin D intake, as well as use of antipsychotic medications contributed to the findings. Roke et al. [57] add that long-term use of antipsychotic treatments for boys between the ages of 10 and 20 years with ASD shows an increase in hyperprolactinemia on BMD. This antipsychotic-induced hyperprolactinemia may affect bone turnover by the stimulation of bone resorption over bone formation as well as diminishing the development of sex hormones which leads to changes in bone metabolism. Filipek et al. [51] add that besides poor nutrition, medications to treat ASD often interfere with bone metabolism and suppress the appetite. Vitamin D deficiency was also found in studies of autistic children [58–60], and because of this, production of serum anti-MAG autoantibodies was implicated, leading to an autoimmunity concern for the study groups.

Bipolar Disorder

Bipolar disorders are classified as mood conditions that feature the presence of an occurrence of a manic episode and often a major depressive episode. Manic episodes are defined by a specific period of a persistently elevated, irritable, or expansive mood and at least three other symptoms including increased self-esteem or grandiosity, decreased need for sleep, pressure speech, flight of ideas or racing thoughts, being easily distracted, and an increase in goal-directed activity and risky behaviors. Depressive symptoms such as feeling sad or empty, anhedonia, weight loss, insomnia, fatigue, and feelings of worthlessness are often present. A mixed episode for bipolar disorders indicates that criteria are met for both a manic episode and a major depressive episode for nearly every day lasting at least one week [50]. Several medications that are used to treat bipolar disorder have an impact on bone metabolism [41]. In particular, lithium has a well-known association with hyperparathyroidism which leads to a suppression in thyroid-stimulating hormone (TSH) that impairs bone metabolism [41] as well as increases bone turnover and bone reabsorption [61]. Misra et al. [41] also point out that anticonvulsants, often used as mood stabilizers to treat bipolar conditions, frequently show an association with osteopenia. Yang et al. [49] also support these studies showing that both lithium and mood stabilizers such as valproate reduce BMD. Their study of 19 subjects with bipolar disorder and therapy with valproate demonstrated that 47.4 % of the subjects showed a decreased BMD on DEXA scans and 22.3 % had osteoporosis in premenopausal women.

Borderline Personality Disorder

Borderline personality disorder (which is often diagnosed with major depressive disorder) shows a pattern of instability in personal relationships, poor self-image, marked impulsivity, and fears of real or imagined abandonment [50]. There is no specific medical treatment for personality disorders, and borderline personality disorder often requires years of psychotherapy, including dialectical behavior therapy [62]. Few studies have shown impact on BMD in individuals with psychiatric personality disorders. However, Kahl et al. [63, 64] researched bone loss in patients with borderline personality disorder along with major depressive disorder and show a possible association between cytokines that were able to activate osteoclastic cells. The researchers studied 22 patients with borderline personality disorder with and without comorbid major depressive disorder as well as 20 healthy volunteers. BMD was measured, and bone turnover and endocrine and immune determinations were included in the study. The results indicated that the subjects with borderline personality disorder along with major depressive disorder have significantly lower BMD than healthy subjects or those study participants with borderline personality alone. In particular, osteocalcin, serum cortisol, tumor necrosis factor (TNF), and interleukin-6 were significantly higher for the group with borderline personality disorder plus major depressive disorder versus the other two groups.

The researchers concluded that young women with borderline personality disorder along with comorbid major depressive disorder are at high risk for the development of osteoporosis and that borderline personality alone is not indicated as an independent risk for bone health. They further propose that immune and endocrine imbalances are the contextual factors for these findings [63, 64]. The researchers suggest their findings do not support previous hypotheses of vitamin D or estradiol deficiencies as well as alterations of bone metabolism as contributing factors to loss in BMD. They do, however, offer support for factors such as poor nutrition, neglect in childhood, and lack of support which are often contributing factors in major depressive disorder to overall health and possibly linked to lower BMD.

Depressive Disorders

Affective disorders, including depression, can affect 5–10 % of the general population and are the most commonly described condition seen in clinical practice, second to hypertension [41, 65]. Aloumanis and Mavroudis [66] further add that depression and osteoporosis affect a large part of the population and the two have an impact on quality of life, morbidity, and life expectancy. Interestingly, these researchers also provide further evidence that depression impacts bone health at a higher degree than osteoporosis, affecting mood. Cizza et al. [65] support this concept by indicating that depression induces bone loss and fractures, due to immune and endocrine changes. Gebara et al. [67] also review criteria to summarize causation between depression and decreased bone density and show the influence of the neurotransmitter serotonin on bone health as well as a gradient of worsening bone health in correlation with worsening depression. Conversely, Wu et al. [68] report that depressive disorders and loss of BMD have inconsistent reports. They, in turn, completed a meta-analysis of 14 studies which found that decreased BMD and depression showed clinical significance, especially when related to bone loss of the spine and hip for women diagnosed with clinical depression. Misra et al. [41] show a strong association between lower BMD in both men and women who have affective disorders with neuroendocrine implications. Adjusting for conditions such as age, gender, activity, hormones, substance use, and lifestyle, depressive symptoms accounted for lower levels of osteocalcin and deoxypyridinoline (indicators for bone formation and reabsorption).

Furthermore, depression leads to an increasing level of the hormone cortisol over time which results in increasing levels of loss of bone as well as reduction in bone turnover [41]. The hypothalamic–pituitary–adrenal (HPA) axis and role of cortisol often leads to hypercortisolemia which is a causal factor in loss of BMD [65]. In addition, immune factors and cytokine activity, such as IL-1, IL-6, and TNF-α, stimulate the HPA axis and may contribute to higher cortisol levels [65, 69, 70]. It should be noted that appetite and weight loss commonly occur with affective disorders, many times leading to eating disorders such as anorexia nervosa, which can correlate with loss of BMD. However, even when controlling for body mass index (BMI), Misra et al. [41] show that major depressive disorder, as an independent risk factor, leads to lower BMD. Lower physical activity reduces biomechanical forces on the bone and excessive activity can also impact BMD [41]. Depressive disorders should be considered as a risk factor for bone health and osteoporosis [67, 68].

Thought or Psychotic Disorders/Schizophrenia

Research has shown increases in bone loss and changes in bone metabolism with thought disorders including schizophrenia. Thought disorders (or disorders of psychosis) have characteristic symptoms including delusions, hallucinations, disorganized speech, catatonic behavior, or negative symptoms (i.e., flat affect, alogia, or avolition) [50]. Schizophrenia affects approximately 1 % of the population, but accounts for one of the top ten reasons for long-term disability [47]. Psychotic disorders and related conditions such as schizophrenia and schizoaffective disorders impact BMD in two ways—hypogonadism due to the disease process and prolactin elevations with neuroleptic medication use which is a common treatment for thought disorders. In a meta-analysis of 160 peer-reviewed articles [41], Hummer et al. [71] show that a significant concern with antipsychotic medications used for thought disorders is related to prolactin. In particular, Bishop et al. [72] indicate prolactin secretion increases when antipsychotic medication blocks dopamine D2 receptors. Adjusting for age-related decline, the authors show men have significantly lower BMD in the lumbar region if they are treated for schizophrenia with neuroleptic medications. Women, on the other hand, were found to have higher bone turnover but normal BMD.

In addition, factors such as nutrition, smoking, and hypogonadotropic hypogonadism are found in this population [41]. Levine et al. [73] studied a group of young schizophrenic males and found elevated plasma homocysteine levels, which are thought to be related to osteoporotic bone fractures. In particular, close to 85 % of people with schizophrenia are reported tobacco users, and smoking has been implicated as a toxic effect on osteoblasts as well as protective effects of estrogen on bone health [41, 72]. Kinon et al. [43] and Takahashi et al. [74] further support elevated prolactin levels as common concerns for patients treated with antipsychotic medications, and therefore a decrease in BMD due to elevated prolactin. Okita et al. [46] studied not only prolactin but also testosterone, estradiol, and bone resorption makers (TRACP-5b) on bone health in 167 patients with schizophrenia along with a control group of 60. Patients with schizophrenia showed significantly higher levels of prolactin along with lower levels of TRACP-5b compared to the control group. Wang et al. [47] support this research and studied effects of both conventional and atypical antipsychotic treatments for 163 patients who took medication as prescribed for 12 months. The results indicate that post 12-month treatment, BMD values in patients who took both types of antipsychotic medications were significantly lower than healthy controls, with conventional antipsychotic medications showing more significant BMD loss. Causes for bone change are usually encountered with atypical neuroleptics due to lowering levels of prolactin in the body.

Medication and Treatment Effects

Antipsychotic Treatments

As previously discussed, antipsychotic treatments create a higher risk of osteoporosis and osteopenia [46]. Researchers propose that prolactin and TRACP-5b are compromised, along with sex hormone suppression which impacts bone health [46, 74] In particular, prolactin-sparing medications such as aripiprazole was helpful in normalizing prolactin levels when combined with higher-risk antipsychotics such as haloperidol and risperidone [74]. Wang et al. [47] compared subjects in two groups using conventional antipsychotics (perphenazine, sulpiride, and chlorpromazine) or atypical antipsychotics (clozapine, quetiapine, and aripiprazole). In their research, the BMD values for subjects utilizing conventional antipsychotic medications were significantly lower than with atypical treatments. Wang et al. [47] further add that the metabolism of antipsychotics can impact liver function, and therefore a reduction of vitamin D occurs and calcium absorption decreases in the gastrointestinal system. The sedative effects of treatment also likely contribute to increases in anhedonia [47] which relates to lower activity levels and lack of natural sunlight. In addition, schizophrenia is believed to be related to the hyperactivity of both dopamine and serotonin function, and serotonin (5-HT) receptors in particular can promote prolactin release. All antipsychotic medications block dopamine D2 receptors, which impact prolactin release, leading to hyperprolactinemia [61].

Antidepressant Medications

The effects of antidepressant medications on bone mass and fracture have been indicated in medical psychiatric patients for the last 30 years, according to Cizza et al. [65]. Antidepressant medications, such as selective serotonin reuptake inhibitors (SSRIs) and tricyclic antidepressants (TCAs), do not cause significant hyperprolactinemia as indicated in antipsychotic treatments [41]. Although some elevations of prolactin can be shown with TCA treatment (such as with trimipramine, desipramine, and clomipramine), imipramine does not appear to increase prolactin along with a similar medication, tianeptine. Older monoamine oxidase inhibitors (MAOI) such as pargyline and moclobemide showed only minor changes in prolactin levels [41]. SSRIs such as fluoxetine, paroxetine, fluvoxamine, sertraline, and citalopram are widely used as treatments for depressive disorders. Interestingly, Misra et al. [41] find some increase in prolactin levels in short term or beginning stages of SSRI treatment, but in contrast, long-term treatment appears to level off cortisol, prolactin, and growth hormone changes in general. Aloumanis and Kostanitos [66] indicate an associated increase of fracture risk, especially in older adults with antidepressants including barbiturates and SSRIs when controlling for potential confounds. However, Cizza et al. [65] suggest that cardiac arrhythmias or orthostatic hypotension may be factors from SSRI use, leading to falls and fracture risk. Furthermore, Cizza et al. [69] add that syncope, dizziness, vertigo, ataxia, somnolence, and blurred vision are common side effects from antidepressants, hypnotics, and sedatives and can in turn relate to falls and specifically hip fractures. Gebara et al. [67] suggest that bone turnover rates in two small studies showed a decrease in bone resorption marker beta-CTX in treatment with SSRI escitalopram and serotonin–norepinephrine reuptake inhibitor (SNRI) venlafaxine, but only when antidepressant medications do not remit depressive symptoms.

From a biological standpoint, Cizza et al. [65] offer that serotonin transporter receptors have been indicated in osteoblast development. Hodge et al. [75] suggest that SSRIs sequester in bone marrow at a higher degree than in brain tissue or blood, therefore increasing the risk of bone development, but the relation between osteoblast and osteoclast development is unclear. Diem et al. [42] further add that blocking serotonin reuptake can affect bone metabolism and BMD in a large cohort of over 2,700 older women (mean age, 78.5 years). After adjusting for confounds, the depressed group who utilized SSRI treatments had a hip BMD decrease of 0.82 % per year compared to 0.47 % in both TCA and nonusers, respectively. However, Diem et al. [76] examined a large cohort of middle-aged women and found that the use of SSRIs and TCAs was not associated with a higher degree of lower BMD as compared to controls, therefore contributing to the uncertainty that SSRI and TCA use impacts BMD. Haney et al. [77] also showed mixed results in a large cohort of men: BMD was lower for those utilizing SSRI therapy, but not significantly altered among men using other antidepressant treatments. Winterhalder et al. [78] add that younger depressive patients utilizing SSRI treatments appear to have stable BMD over a 12-month period. In particular, Haney et al. [77] showed that serotonin and antidepressant treatment are implicated in

Table 3 Psychiatric disorders and bone health

Disorder	Effect on bone health
Autism spectrum disorders	
Classification of disorders characterized by behavioral disturbances. Attentional disorders, mental retardation, anxiety, depression, epilepsy, and OCD can occur with ASD	Vitamin D deficiency due to low levels of physical activity and lack of sunlight leads to slowing of bone growth
Bipolar disorder	
Classified as mood conditions that feature the presence of a manic episode and often a major depressive episode as well	Lithium leads to suppression of TSH, impairing bone metabolism
	Anticonvulsants that are used as mood stabilizers are associated with osteopenia
Borderline personality disorder	
Mental illness marked by behaviors, moods, and relationships that are unstable	Cytokines used to activate cytokines do not function optimally, resulting in low BMD
	Impaired immune function due to disorder is cause for poor bone health
Depressive disorders	
Classified as affective disorders and are the most commonly described conditions witnessed in clinical practices	Can induce decreased bone health and decreased secretion of the neurotransmitter serotonin
	The increased level of cortisol caused by depression also leads to a reduction in bone turnover
Thought or psychotic disorders/schizophrenia	
These disorders are characterized by delusions, hallucination, disorganized speech, catatonic behavior, and negative symptoms	Hypogonadism
	Prolactin elevation

bone health outcomes and BMD and that those who take SSRIs may be indicated for screening for bone loss, but lifestyle choices are strong confounding factors that should not be overlooked.

Bone health and psychiatric conditions (Table 3), as well as treatment with psychiatric medications, present a compelling concern for clinicians. While the research indicates many lifestyle factors at play for the populations discussed here, contributing factors (i.e., lack of physical exercise, lower amounts of natural sunlight, inadequate nutrition, alcohol and substance use, etc.) appear to play a large, complimentary role in bone health and BMD and present challenges for further research in this area.

References

1. Banham-Hall N, Kothwal K, Pipkin J, Bentley J, Dickens GL. Prevalence of low bone mineral density in inpatients with traumatic brain injury receiving neurobehavioral rehabilitation: a postoperative, observational study. Physiotherapy. 2013;99(4):328–34. doi:10.1016/j.physio.2012.12.009.
2. Chan J, Parmenter T, Stancliffe R. The impact of traumatic brain injury on the mental health outcomes of individuals and their family carers. Aus e-J Adv Ment Health. 2009;8(2):155–64.

3. Trentz OA, Handschin AE, Bestmann L, Hoerstrup SP, Trentz OL, Platz A. Influence of brain injury on early posttraumatic bone metabolism. Crit Care Med. 2005;33(2):399–406.
4. Beeton CA, Chatfield D, Brooks RA, Ruston N. Circulating levels of interleukin-6 and its soluble receptor in patients with head injury and fracture. J Bone Joint Surg Br. 2004;86(6):912–7.
5. Lee JI, Kim JH, Kim HW, Choi ES, Lim SH, Ko YJ, et al. Changes in bone metabolism in a rat model of traumatic brain injury. Brain Inj. 2005;19(14):1207–11.
6. Dimopoulou I, Tsagarakis S, Kouyialis AT, Roussou P, Assithianakis G, Christoforaki M, et al. Hypothalamic-pituitary-adrenal axis dysfunction in critically ill patients with traumatic brain injury: incidence, pathophysiology, and relationship to vasopressor dependence and peripheral interleukin-6 levels. Crit Care Med. 2004;32(2):404–8.
7. Gionis D, Ilias I, Moustaki M, Mantzos E, Papadatos I, Koutras DA, et al. Hypothalamic-pituitary-adrenal axis and interleukin-6 activity in children with head trauma and syndrome of inappropriate secretion of antidiuretic hormone. J Pediatr Endocrinol Metab. 2003;169(1):49–54.
8. Powner DJ, Boccalandro C, Alp MS, Vollmer DG. Endocrine failure after traumatic brain injury in adults. Neurocrit Care. 2006;5(1):61–70.
9. Jamal SA, Arampatzis S, Harrison SL, Bucur RC, Ensrud K, Orwoll ES, et al. Hyponatremia and fractures: findings from the MrOS study. J Bone Miner Res. 2015;30(1):970–5.
10. Hoorn EJ, Rivadeneira F, van Meurs JB, Ziere G, Stricker BH, Hofman A, et al. Mild hyponatremia as a risk factor for fractures: the Rotterdam Study. J Bone Miner Res. 2011;26(8):1822–8.
11. Verbalis JG, Barsony J, Sugimura Y, Tian Y, Adams DJ, Carter EA, et al. Hyponatremia-induced osteoporosis. J Bone Miner Res. 2010;25(3):554–63. doi:10.1359/jbmr.090827.
12. Gankam KF, Andres F, Sattar C, Melot L, Decaux C. Mild hyponatremia and risk of fracture in the ambulatory elderly. QJM. 2008;101(7):583–8.
13. Tolouian R, Alhamad T, Farazmand M, Mulla ZD. The correlation of hip fracture and hyponatremia in the elderly. J Nephrol. 2012;25(5):789–93.
14. Sandhu HS, Gilles E, DeVita MV, Panagopoulos G, Michellis MF. Hyponatremia associated with large-bone fracture in elderly patients. Int Urol Nephrol. 2009;41(3):733–7.
15. Arapatzis S, Gaetcke LM, Funk GC, et al. Diuretic-induced hyponatremia and osteoporotic fractures in patients admitted to the emergency department. Maturitas. 2013;75(1):81–6.
16. Kinsella S, Moran S, Sullivan MO, Molloy MG, Eustace JA. Hyponatremia independent of osteoporosis is associated with fracture occurrence. Clin J Am Soc Nephrol. 2013;5(2):275–80.
17. Aimaretti G, Ambrosia MR, Di Somma C, Fusco A, Cannavo S, Gasperi M, et al. Traumatic brain injury and subarachnoid haemorrhage are conditions at high risk for hypopituitarism: screening study at 3 months after the brain injury. Clin Endocrinol (Oxf). 2004;61(3):320–6.
18. Agha A, Rogers B, Sherlock M, O'Kelly P, Tormey W, Phillips J, et al. Anterior pituitary dysfunction in survivors of traumatic brain injury. J Clin Endocrinol Metab. 2004;89(10):4929–36.
19. Bondanelli M, De Marinis L, Ambrosio MR, Monesi M, Valle D, Zatelli MC, et al. Occurrence of pituitary dysfunction following traumatic brain injury. J Neurotrauma. 2004;21(5):685–96.
20. Lieberman SA, Oberoi AL, Gilkison CR, Masel BE, Urban RJ. Prevalence of neuroendocrine dysfunction in patients recovering from traumatic brain injury. J Clin Endocrinol Metab. 2001;86(2):2752–6.
21. Kelly DF, Gonzalo IT, Cohan P, Berman N, Swerdloff, Wang C. Hypopituitarism following traumatic brain injury and aneurysmal subarachnoid hemorrhage: a preliminary report. J Neurosurg. 2000;93(5):743–52.
22. Bondanelli M, Ambrosio MR, Zatelli MC, De Marinis L, degli Uberti EC. Hypopituitarism after traumatic brain injury. Eur J Endocrinol. 2005;152(5):679–91.
23. Clark JD, Raggatt PR, Edwards OM. Hypothalamic hypogonadism following major head injury. Clin Endocrinol (Oxf). 1988;29(2):153–65.
24. Woolf PD, Hamill RW, McDonald JV, Lee LA, Kelly M. Transient hypogonadotrophic hypogonadism after head trauma: effects on steroid precursors and correlation with sympathetic nervous system activity. Clin Endocrinol (Oxf). 1986;25(3):265–74.

25. Masel BE. Rehabilitation and hypopituitarism after traumatic brain injury. Growth Horm IGF Res. 2004;14(Suppl A):S108–13.
26. Schwandt M, Harris JE, Thomas S, Keightley M, Snaiderman A, Colantonio A. Feasibility and effect of aerobic exercise for lowering depressive symptoms among individuals with traumatic brain injury: a pilot study. J Head Trauma Rehabil. 2012;27(2):99–103. doi:10.1097/HTR.0b013e31820e6858.
27. Ströhle A. Physical activity, exercise, depression and anxiety disorders. J Neural Transm (Vienna). 2009;116(6):777–84. doi:10.1007/s00702-008-0092-x.
28. Gordon WA, Sliwinski M, Echo J, McLaughlin M, Sheerer MS, Meili TE. The benefits of exercise in individuals with traumatic brain injury: a retrospective study. J Head Trauma Rehabil. 1998;13(4):58–67.
29. Barreto G, Santos-Galindo M, Diz-Chaves Y, Pernia O, Carrero P, Azcoitia I, et al. Selective estrogen receptor modulators decrease reactive astrogliosis in the injured brain: effects of aging and prolonged depletion of ovarian hormones. Endocrinology. 2009;150(11):5010–5. doi:10.1210/en.2009-0352.
30. Kokiko ON, Murashov AK, Hoane MR. Administration of raloxifene reduces sensorimotor and working memory deficits following traumatic brain injury. Behav Brain Res. 2006;170(2):233–40.
31. Yaffe K, Krueger K, Cummings SR, Blackwell T, Henderson VW, Sarkar S, et al. Effect of raloxifene on prevention of dementia and cognitive impairment in older women: the Multiple Outcomes of Raloxifene Evaluation (MORE) randomized trial. Am J Psychiatry. 2005;162(4):683–90.
32. Jacobsen DE, Samson MM, Emmelot-Vonk MH, Verhaar HJ. Raloxifene improves verbal memory in late postmenopausal women: a randomized, double-blind, placebo-controlled trial. Menopause. 2010;17(2):309–14. doi:10.1097/gme.0b013e3181bd54df.
33. Arevalo MA, Santos-Galindo M, Lagunas N, Azcoitia I, Garcia-Segura LM. Selective estrogen receptor modulators as brain therapeutic agents. J Mol Endocrinol. 2011;46(1):R1–9. doi:10.1677/JME-10-0122.
34. Genazzani AR, Bernardi F, Stomati M, Rubino S, Giardina L, Luisi S, et al. Raloxifene analog LY 117018 effects on central and peripheral beta-endorphin. Gynecol Endocrinol. 1999;13(4):249–58.
35. Genazzani AR, Benardi F, Stomati M, Monteleone P, Luisi S, Rubino S, et al. Effects of estradiol and raloxifene analog on brain, adrenal and serum allopregnanolone content in fertile and ovariectomized female rats. Neuroendocrinology. 2000;72(3):162–70.
36. Bernardi F, Pluchino N, Stomati M, Pieri M, Genazzani AR. CNS: sex steroids and SERMs. Ann N Y Acad Sci. 2003;997:378–88.
37. Skolnick BE, Maas AI, Narayan RK, van der Hoop RG, MacAllister T, Ward JD, et al. A clinical trial of progesterone for severe traumatic brain injury. N Engl J Med. 2014;371(26):2467–76. doi:10.1056/NEJMoa1411090.
38. Wright DW, Kellermann AL, Hertzberg VS, Clark PL, Frankel M, Goldstein FC, et al. ProTECT: a randomized clinical trial of progesterone for acute traumatic brain injury. Ann Emerg Med. 2007;49(4):391–402.
39. Xiao G, Wei J, Yan W, Wang W, Lu Z. Improved outcomes from the administration of progesterone for patients with acute severe traumatic brain injury: a randomized controlled trial. Crit Care. 2008;12(2):R61. doi:10.1186/cc6887.
40. Halbreich U, Palter S. Accelerated osteoporosis in psychiatric patients: possible pathophysiological processes. Schizophr Bull. 1996;22(3):447–54.
41. Misra M, Papakostas GI, Klibanski A. Effects of psychiatric disorders and psychotropic medications on prolactin and bone metabolism. J Clin Psychiatry. 2004;65(12):1607–18.
42. Diem SJ, Blackwell TL, Stone KL, Yaffe K, Haney EM, Bliziotes MM, et al. Use of antidepressants and rates of hip bone loss in older women: the study of osteoporotic fractures. Arch Intern Med. 2007;167(12):1240–5.
43. Kinon BJ, Liu-Seifert H, Stauffer VL, Jacob J. Bone loss associated with hyperprolactinemia in patients with schizophrenia. Clin Schizophr Relat Psychoses. 2013;7(3):115–23.

44. Haney EM, Warden SJ, Bliziotes MM. Effects of selective serotonin reuptake inhibitors on bone health in adults: time for recommendations about screening, prevention and management? Bone. 2010;46(1):13–7. doi:10.1016/j.bone.2009.07.083.
45. Aman MG, Lam KSL, Van Bourgondien ME. Medication patterns in patients with autism: temporal, regional, and demographic influences. J Child Adolesc Psychopharmacol. 2005;15(1):116–26.
46. Okita K, Kanahara N, Nishimura M, Yoshida T, Yasui-Furukori N, Niitsu T, et al. Second-generation antipsychotics and bone turnover in schizophrenia. Schizophr Res. 2014;157(1–3):137–41. doi:10.1016/j.schres.2014.05.009.
47. Wang M, Hou R, Jian J, Mi G, Qiu H, Cao B, et al. Effects of antipsychotics on bone mineral density and prolactin levels in patients with schizophrenia: a 12-month prospective study. Hum Psychopharmacol. 2014;29(2):183–9.
48. Pack AM, Gidal B, Vazquez B. Bone disease associated with antiepileptic drugs. Cleve Clin J Med. 2004;71 Suppl 2:S42–8.
49. Yang J, Joe SH, Lee MS, Ko YH, Jung IK, Kim SH. Effects of long-term combination treatment with valproate and atypical antipsychotics on bone mineral density and bone metabolism in premenopausal patients with bipolar disorder: a preliminary study. Psychiatry Investig. 2011;8(3):256–61. doi:10.4306/pi.2011.8.3.256.
50. American Psychiatric Association. Diagnostic and statistical manual of mental disorders. 5th ed. Arlington: American Psychiatric Publishing; 2013.
51. Filipek PA, Accardo PJ, Baranek GT, Cook Jr EH, Dawson G, Gordon B, et al. The screening and diagnosis of autistic spectrum disorders. J Autism Dev Disord. 1999;29(6):439–84.
52. Hediger ML, England LJ, Molloy CA, Yu KF, Manning-Courtney P, Mills JL. Reduced bone cortical thickness in boys with autism or autism spectrum disorder. J Autism Dev Disord. 2008;38(5):848–56. doi:10.1007/s10803-007-0453-6.
53. Millward C, Ferriter M, Calver S, Connell-Jones G. Gluten- and casein-free diets for autistic spectrum disorder. Cochrane Database Syst Rev. 2004;16(2):CD003498. doi:10.1002/14651858.CD003498.
54. Schreck KA, Williams K, Smith AF. A comparison of eating behaviors between children with and without autism. J Autism Dev Disord. 2004;34(4):433–8.
55. Williams PG, Dalrymple N, Neal J. Eating habits of children with autism. Pediatr Nurs. 2000;26(3):259–64.
56. Neumeyer AM, O'Rourke JA, Massa A, Lee H, Lawson EA, McDougle CJ, et al. Brief report: bone fractures in children and adults with autism spectrum disorders. J Autism Dev Disord. 2015;45(3):881–7. doi:10.1007/s10803-014-2228-1.
57. Roke Y, van Harten PN, Buitelaar JK, Tenback DE, Quekel LG, deRijke YB, et al. Bone mineral density in male adolescents with autism spectrum disorders and disruptive behavior disorder with or without antipsychotic treatment. Eur J Endocrinol. 2012;167(6):855–63. doi:10.1530/EJE-12-0521.
58. Mostafa GA, Al-Ayadhi LY. Reduced serum concentrations of 25-hydroxy vitamin D in children with autism: relation to autoimmunity. J Neuroinflammation. 2012;9:201.
59. Knivsberg AM, Reichelt KL, Høien T, Nødland M. A randomised, controlled study of dietary intervention in autistic syndromes. Nutr Neurosci. 2002;5(4):251–61.
60. Knivsberg AM, Reichelt KL, Nødland M. Reports on dietary intervention in autistic disorders. Nutr Neurosci. 2001;4(1):25–37.
61. Gyulai L, Jaggi J, Bauer MS, Younkin S, Rubin L, Attie M, et al. Bone mineral density and L-thyroxine treatment in rapidly cycling bipolar disorder. Biol Psychiatry. 1997;41(4):503–6.
62. Linehan MM. Cognitive-behavioral treatment of borderline personality disorder. New York: Guilford Press; 1993.
63. Kahl K, Rudolf S, Stoeckelhuber BM, Dibbelt L, Gehl HB, Markhof K, et al. Bone mineral density, markers of bone turnover, and cytokines in young women with borderline personality disorder with and without comorbid major depressive disorder. Am J Psychiatry. 2005;162(1):168–74.
64. Kahl K, Greggesen W, Rudolf S, Stoeckelhuber BM, Bergmann-Koester CU, Dibbelt L, et al. Bone mineral density, bone turnover, and osteoprotegerin in depressed women with and without borderline personality disorder. Psychosom Med. 2006;68(5):669–74.

65. Cizza G, Primma S, Csako G. Depression as a risk factor for osteoporosis. Trends Endocrinol Metab. 2000;20(8):367–73.
66. Aloumanis K, Mavroudis K. The "depressive" face of osteoporosis and the "osteoporotic" face of depression. Hormones. 2013;12(3):350–62.
67. Gebara MA, Shea ML, Lipsey KL, Teitelbaum SL, Civitelli R, Müller DJ, et al. Depression, antidepressants, and bone health in older adults: a systematic review. J Am Geriatr Soc. 2014;62(8):1434–41.
68. Wu Q, Magnus JH, Liu J, Bencaz AF, Hentz JG. Depression and low bone mineral density: a meta-analysis of epidemiologic studies. Osteoporos Int. 2009;20(8):1309–20. doi:10.1007/s00198-009-0918-x.
69. Cizza G, Ravn P, Chrousos GP, Gold PW. Depression: a major, unrecognized risk factor for osteoporosis? Trends Endocrinol Metab. 2001;12(4):198–203.
70. Cizza G. Major depressive disorder is a risk factor for low bone mass, central obesity, and other medical conditions. Dialogues Clin Neurosci. 2011;13(1):73–87.
71. Hummer M, Malik P, Gasser R, Hofer A, Kemmler G, Moncayo Naveda RC, et al. Osteoporosis in patients with schizophrenia. Am J Psychiatry. 2005;162(1):162–7.
72. Bishop JR, Alexander B, Lund BC, Klepser TB. Osteoporosis screening and treatment in women with schizophrenia: a controlled study. Pharmacotherapy. 2004;24(4):515–21.
73. Levine J, Stahl Z, Ami B, Slava S, Ruderman GV, Belmaker RH. Elevated homocysteine levels in young male patients with schizophrenia. Am J Psychiatry. 2002;159:1790–2.
74. Takahashi T, Uchida H, John M, Hirano J, Watanabe K, Mimura M, et al. The impact of prolactin-raising antipsychotics on bone mineral density in patients with schizophrenia: findings from a longitudinal observational cohort. Schizophr Res. 2013;147(2–3):383–6. doi:10.1016/j.schres.2013.04.015.
75. Hodge JM, Wang Y, Berk M, Collier FM, Fernandes TJ, Constable MJ, et al. Selective serotonin reuptake inhibitors inhibit human osteoclast and osteoblast formation and function. Biol Psychiatry. 2013;74(1):32–9.
76. Diem SJ, Ruppert K, Cauley JA, Lian Y, Bromberger JT, Finkelstein JS, et al. Rates of bone loss among women initiating antidepressant medication use in midlife. J Clin Endocrinol Metab. 2013;98(11):4355–63. doi:10.1210/jc.2013-1971.
77. Haney EM, Benjamin KS, Chan MS, Diem SJ, Ensrud KE, Cauley JA, et al. Association of low bone mineral density with selective serotonin reuptake inhibitor use by older men. Arch Intern Med. 2007;167(12):1246–51.
78. Winterhalder L, Eser P, Widmer J, Villiger PM, Aeberli D. Changes in volumetric BMD of radius and tibia upon antidepressant drug administration in young depressive patients. J Musculoskelet Neuronal Interact. 2012;12(4):224–9.

Chapter 8
Osteoporosis in Stroke and Seizure Disorders

Christina V. Oleson

Osteoporosis is recognized as a frequent consequence following cerebrovascular events. Not only is there an increased incidence of fractures primarily in the hip, but there are complications from fractures that lead to increased morbidity and mortality; increased healthcare costs, pain, and discomfort; and increased burden of care on the family members ultimately responsible for stroke patients. The causes of osteoporosis post stroke include preexisting osteoporosis, immobility, medications, and poor balance, leading to reduced weight-bearing activity and reduced maintenance of current bone density. In terms of falls, decreased strength, balance, proprioception, and cognition all play an important role. This chapter will review unique causes of osteoporosis in the stroke population, illustrate both functional and biological risk factors for falls, and discuss approaches to treatment.

The leading cause of disability, stroke is the most common diagnosis among patients admitted to inpatient rehabilitation hospitals and to subacute nursing facilities that offer rehabilitation [1]. In acute rehabilitation facilities, stroke admissions in the United States annually account for the diagnosis of disability and functional deficits more than any other single diagnosis [2]. Remarkably, osteoporosis has received little attention as a consequence of stroke. Early recognition must be given to consideration of premorbid risk factors for osteoporosis, prior to the first stroke. Additionally, evaluation of ongoing factors following the stroke that might increase the risk of falls and efforts to prevent future falls must be undertaken. Should osteoporosis develop in the first year following stroke, when resorption of bone is aggressive and rapid, treatment must be initiated as soon as possible.

Epidemiology of Osteoporosis After Stroke

While osteoporosis is highly prevalent in the elderly, once a stroke has occurred, it is very important to recognize the presence of any preexisting osteoporosis. A Korean study from 2008 describes baseline BMD and fracture presence in patients

C.V. Oleson, *Osteoporosis Rehabilitation*, DOI 10.1007/978-3-319-45084-1_8

at the time of diagnosis of a new stroke. Kim et al. [3] evaluated 48 patients within the first 30 days of a stroke, specifically looking at bone density in both the total hip, femoral neck, and lumbar spine. Plain x-rays were also obtained for both thoracic and lumbar spine. Results indicated osteoporosis at the total hip in 37.5 %, 39.8 % at the femoral neck, and 31 % at the lumbar spine. Overall 43.8 % of the 48 subjects had established osteoporosis at the onset of the stroke, while 39.6 % were osteopenic. In addition, 25 % had at least one thoracic or lumbar vertebral body (VB) fracture, and 16.7 % had two or more VB fractures.

Moreover, of the 12 individuals in the study that had established fractures, only four were aware of these fractures. Given anticipated further bone loss and functional deficits following stroke, it is imperative that initial screening for BMD and at least a basic thoracolumbar spine image be performed. As described in earlier chapters, osteoporotic compression fractures of the spine are commonly painless and often go undetected. However, if a patient were to fall following a stroke, this type of fracture could result in additional fractures or angulation of the current fracture and potentially compromise to the spinal cord, leading to devastating consequences. Early screening for osteoporosis is essential in building a safe and effective rehabilitation program for these patients.

A number of prior studies have documented the incidence of osteoporosis post stroke. A large cohort study of 78,461 patients in Germany over six years found an increased risk of osteoporotic fractures among stroke subjects without functional deficits relative to healthy controls [4]. Yet it did not find an increase in osteoporosis for patients with functional deficits, above what a comparable non-stroke reference group of subjects with equivalent functional deficits demonstrated. Relative risk of fractures for the stroke patients remaining with good overall function was higher in the lower extremities than upper extremities. In terms of absolute risk, data clearly demonstrate higher fracture rates in nonfunctional patients due to paresis on the affected side, but the unusual increase seen even among those who regained function warrants closer analysis. The reasons the stroke patients had increased risk of fractures even in the absence of functional deficits are unclear. Stroke patients share a number of common medical conditions also seen in patients with established osteoporosis, including higher than desirable alcohol consumptions, smoking, and suboptimal diet with poor calcium intake [5–7]. Studies have demonstrated a possible association of vascular calcifications and vascular cerebral events leading to ischemia, oxidative stress factors, and chronic inflammation [8].

Additional studies have illustrated a relationship between stroke and bone loss at 6–12 months following the stroke. Liu et al. [9] studied 69 men and 35 women with stroke at baseline with a follow-up at seven months post stroke. Their findings indicate a 15.2 % loss in the total arm, 11.6 % BMD decline in the humerus and 15.6 % in the distal radius, 5 % in the total femur, and 7.4 % in the proximal femur. A more common time for follow-up has been 12 months post stroke. Multiple investigations have demonstrated bone loss in the upper extremities (humerus or distal radius) ranging from 12 to 16 % and in the lower extremities (total leg or femoral neck) from 5 to 12 % [10–14]. Bone loss is typically on the side affected by the stroke and more in the upper than lower extremity [15]. Sato observed not only a decline in the upper more than lower limb bone density on the hemiplegic limb and a greater decline in the upper extremity BMD than lower but also the presence of a decline over the first year after stroke in the unaffected side [16]. This unexpected decrease in BMD may be the result of reduced weight-bearing following hemiplegia; the relative absence of sunlight exposure if going outdoors is less frequent or nonexistent; limited sun exposure due to placement in short- or long-term nursing facilities if functional deficits are substantial; and changes in diet with less calcium or vitamin D if dysphagia is present or if depression leads to anorexia.

In comparing the Liu study performed at an average of 203 days post stroke to the many other studies with one year follow-up, it is clear that, much like spinal cord injury, bone loss on the hemiparetic side following stroke occurs rapidly following the loss of motor function [15, 16]. The precise pathophysiology of bone loss is a function of five factors: (1) partial or complete paralysis, reduced mobility, and reduction in bone loading, (2) endocrine changes promoting bone loss, (3) nutritional causes, (4) older age, and (5) pharmacologic influences [9, 15].

Paralysis, Reduced Mobility, and Bone Load Reduction

The mechanism of rapid bone loss in the paretic side following stroke is a function of the extent of weakness, the duration of time the limb remains weak, and the time for reinitiation of activity in the affected limb. The sooner and more complete the recovery occurs, the less potent the metabolic forces that resorb bone. Following acute reduction of mobility and weight-bearing, osteoclastic upregulation occurs, leading to bone loss. Whereas in the case of fracture there is compensatory upregulation of osteoblastic activity, in patients with immobility, the unloading of bone leads to a decrement of osteoblastic activity and results in cortical thinning [17]. The early initiation of functional activity post stroke and the intensity of treatment actively mobilizing the affected limb have implications not only for osteoporosis prevention but also for facilitating more complete motor recovery [18, 19]. Also, Liu et al. [9] found the loss of bone in the humerus quantified by DXA correlated with increase in bone turnover markers: urinary pyridinoline and deoxypyridinoline.

Endocrine Changes and Nutrition

Reduced sunlight exposure, poor intake of foods with high percentages of vitamin D, and potential post stroke inhibition of PTH secretion may all contribute to osteoporosis. Hypercalcemia due to bone unloading will block and/or reduce PTH secretion, thereby blocking the renal synthesis of 1,25$(OH)_2$ vitamin D3. The prevention of the active form of vitamin D from being formed contributes to post stroke osteoporosis [15]. Sato [20] in his review of factors contributing to osteoporosis in post stroke patients found significant decrements in vitamin D, especially among inpatients relative to outpatients. An older report by Sato and colleagues [21] found that 64 % of outpatients with long-standing stroke had serum vitamin D25-OH concentrations of below 10 ng/ml, in the range of osteomalacia, and 82 % of patients with long-standing stroke admitted to the hospital for other new medical reasons had deficits in this range. In fact, 17 % and 47 %, respectively, actually had levels below 5 ng/ml. In addition, Sato [20] indicated that many patients who are older have less access to outdoor activities following stroke, and others have levels of vitamin D low enough to cause secondary hyperparathyroidism which will favor additional bone resorption.

Vitamin K is critical to the construction of the bone matrix due to its utilization by G1a protein carboxylation. Increased hip fracture rates are seen in stroke patients with reduced G1a protein levels [15]. Sato [20] also found a correlation between serum vitamin K levels and stroke patients in the first year following the onset of paralysis. Their investigation also demonstrated improvement in BMD after supplementation with vitamin K.

Those with stroke as well as TBI and various forms of paraneoplastic syndromes are susceptible to the syndrome of inappropriate antidiuretic hormone (SIADH), the treatment for which is generally fluid restriction but in some cases also salt tablets orally. In this context, observations by Antonios and colleagues [22] that higher salt intake produces increased hydroxyproline excretion are noteworthy. Hydroxyproline is one of several bone breakdown products. It is conceivable that bone breakdown occurs in the context of a high-sodium diet, through alterations of calcium balance in a mechanism involving sodium–calcium exchange.

The Impact of Spasticity

Whereas in SCI, spasticity has been shown to have either a neutral or positive effect on BMD [23], there is clearly a negative effect on the bone after stroke. In a study of radial BMD in 47 partially ambulatory chronic (> one year) stroke patients ages 50 or older, significant side to side differences in BMD were observed. Spasticity, along with chronic disuse and muscle weakness, had an adverse effect on several parameters of bone quality. Based on the Modified Ashworth Scale (MAS), regression analysis demonstrated that spasticity alone accounted for 23.2 % of the variance in bone mineral content and BMD, determined by quantitative CT between the paretic and non-paretic sides. Spasticity was independent of motor weakness and disuse in individual regression models, although a cumulative effect of all three factors was also found [24].

In a study examining hip BMD one year after stroke, no significant correlation of MAS to BMD at the proximal femur was seen between the affected and unaffected limbs of 58 subjects. There was a trend of increasing spasticity corresponding to lower BMD, but the relationship failed to reach statistical significance, in part due to the relatively preserved ambulatory status of low spasticity scores. Spastic subjects reported a median score of 1 on the MAS scale which ranges from 0 to 4. In this case, neither the lack of ground reaction force due to impaired active or passive range of motion (ROM) from spasms nor the relative preservation of muscle mass from spasms, sufficient to translate to muscle pulling on the bone in a positive manner, would affect BMD [25]. Another study investigated BMD in the distal tibia and found that BMD in this location was negatively associated with spasticity; the higher the spasticity was, the lower the BMD [26].

Spasticity can be classified in terms of "positive" symptoms and "negative" symptoms, which characterize the activity and potency of the upper motor neuron system activity. These terms do not refer to a beneficial (positive) or detrimental (negative) effect on the patient. Rather, both types of symptoms can cause functional problems in stroke patients with spasticity. Table 1 gives the positive and negative symptoms of spasticity.

Because spasticity can increase falls, decrease ability of the patient to perform transfers, and contribute to osteoporosis by limiting functional activities including ambulation and weight-bearing, treatment should be considered that promotes the above tasks without causing side effects that compromise safety, function, and quality of life. Many pharmacologic agents, including baclofen, benzodiazepines like diazepam and clonazepam, and even alpha-2 agonists such as tizanidine, can cause fatigue, postural instability, unintended weakness, hypotension, confusion, and inattention, all of which may lead to falls [27].

For stroke patients with widespread spasticity in multiple muscles of the upper and lower hemiparetic limbs, system oral medications are appropriate. Baclofen acts on GABA-B receptors but has the adverse effects of moderate hypotension, muscle fatigue, and weakness with increasing activities. It is most suitable for patients with tonic spasticity, characterized by muscle tension that inhibits active and passive range of motion. It can be problematic because a dose high enough to assist with increased tone in one limb may adversely affect the uninvolved limb or a patient's core strength.

Diazepam, a long-acting benzodiazepine, and clonazepam, a benzodiazepine of intermediate duration, are helpful with phasic or episodic spasticity and clonus. Both agents enhance the action of the GABA-A receptor whose action reduces muscle spasms and jerking. These agents often cause sedation, worsen confusion, and may exacerbate depression in patients who already have or are prone to this

Table 1 Positive and negative symptoms of spasticity

Positive symptoms of spasticity	Negative symptoms of spasticity
Exaggerated deep tendon reflexes	Reduced deep tendon reflexes
Rigidity	Flaccidity
Dystonia	Fatigue
Flexor spasms	
Extensor spasms	
Contractures from excessive tone	Contractures from lack of range of motion

condition [28]. They can also increase ataxia leading to potential falls. Because of adverse effects on alertness and mental processing, benzodiazepines are best used at night. Advantages of benzodiazepines include their ability to help promote sleep and generally last the full eight hours of sleep time [29]. Because of the above concerns, slower renal clearance and prolonged half-life of 20–60 hours for clonazepam and 35–100 for diazepam, the use of these medications is particularly problematic in elderly patients [28]. Moreover, regular use of benzodiazepines leads to rebound insomnia [28] and chemical dependency, requiring need for slow taper when discontinued [30].

Tizanidine, a centrally acting alpha-2 adrenergic agonist, has a rapid onset as well as a short half-life of only 2.5 hours, the smallest of all the common oral spasticity agents. Benefits of this agent include its lack of clinical dependency and the absence of abuse potential. However, tizanidine has significant sedative properties, may cause confusions or hallucinations, and even low doses can lead to profound hypotension. Another concern, although uncommon, is elevation of liver enzymes. The doses needed to cause liver damage are generally not tolerable in stroke patients, from the perspective of sedation or blood pressure regulation, so this side effect is rarely observed. Another disadvantage is its contraindication with the use of fluoroquinolone antibiotics, a class of antibacterial agents, often used in hospital settings due to their once or twice a day oral usage and their effectiveness and tolerance.

Finally, dantrolene is a common agent of choice to treat spasticity in stroke patients because it acts peripherally at the level of the calcium channels in muscle spindles and has significantly lower risk of cognitive side effects, but fatigue, muscle weakness, hypotension, and elevated liver enzymes have been reported with daily use. The risk of hepatotoxicity is higher than that seen with other antispasticity agents [27].

Due to the above concerns with oral medications, focal treatment with bracing in conjunction with therapy should be the first approach. Localized injections with botulinum toxin (botox) type A to the muscle or alcohol versus phenol to either the nerve or motor point have the benefit of targeted therapy delivered to the spastic extremity of concern, while avoiding systemic adverse effects that oral antispasticity medications can produce. Injections with alcohol or phenol create neurolysis or soft tissue lysis, thereby blocking transmission of excessive nerve impulses to muscles, but side effects can include painful dysesthesias. One benefit of alcohol or phenol is a longer duration of action, up to six months, and significantly lower cost in comparison to botulinum toxin.

Botulinum toxin (botox) type A causes reversible muscle relaxation when directly injected into the most active region of spastic muscles, best identified under electromyographic (EMG) guidance. While botox A is most commonly used in bicep, elbow, and wrist to facilitate ADLs after stroke, it can also be beneficial from a weight-bearing standpoint in stroke patients with equinovarus of the ankle [27]. If reduction of ankle tone permits weight-bearing and standing, this intervention may significantly affect bone density over time.

Pharmacologic Influences

With the exception of severe hemorrhagic stroke, as part of ongoing stroke prophylaxis from a second event, minimizing future risks of stroke from conditions such as irregular heart rhythms (atrial fibrillation, premature contractions), oral anticoagulants are instituted as soon as practitioners feel the risk of a thrombotic event exceeds the risk of post stroke bleeding. In addition, heparins in subcutaneous form are often given for deep vein thrombosis (DVT) prophylaxis until levels of oral anticoagulants are therapeutic. Heparin inhibits osteoblast differentiation and compromises osteoblast function, resulting in decreased bone formation [31, 32]. In the setting of heparin, osteoprotegerin (OPG) upregulates RANKL that promotes osteoclastic differentiation which, in turn, increases bone resorption. Generally, heparin is used only as a bridge to warfarin following stroke, a duration lasting generally 14–30 days depending on bleeding risk. Most studies demonstrating a relationship of heparin use to bone loss describe longer use in terms of either months or years [33]. In contrast, warfarin is used for long-term protection against future strokes. This medication has been shown to decrease the carboxylation of osteocalcin and compromise the calcium-binding capacity of osteocalcin [31].

Warfarin reduces stores of vitamin K, important in the maintenance of bone density. In 1998, Sato et al. [34] supplemented chronic stroke patients that did not require warfarin with vitamin K and observed an improvement in bone density. With the creation of newer anticoagulants such as apixiban and Xarelto that do not deplete levels of vitamin K, bone density may be affected to a lesser extent in future years as these newer agents gain acceptance in the medical community and with third-party payers. Few controlled studies exist on the newer anticoagulants, although preliminary reports indicate their effects are less harmful on BMD than many traditional anticoagulants.

Nonpharmacologic Treatment

Reduction of Falls

The majority of acute fractures following stroke occur from falling, primarily to the paretic side. Ramnemark et al. [35] found that among 1,139 patients with stroke within the last three years, 154 fractures were seen in 120 patients, with 84 % occurring from falls. Hip fracture was the most common type of fracture observed. Moreover, the majority of the 154 fractures observed (13.5 % of the sample) happened within 24 months, when the onset of osteoporosis on the affected side has had adequate time to develop. Stroke patients have multiple reasons for falls, apart from established osteopenia or osteoporosis:

- Weakness
- Ataxia or motor planning deficits

- Poor vision or visual neglect of one side
- Impaired cognition
- Agitation or impulsivity
- Urinary incontinence
- Forgetting to use or lack of immediate access to wheelchair, walker, or cane
- Forgetting to wear or inability to reach orthotics needed for gait stability

Prevention of falls in relation to prevention of osteoporosis is intimately linked in a number of nonpharmacologic interventions and is accomplished through physical therapy measures, working on strengthening, balance skills, and anticipatory planning of motor activities and those skills of daily living where falls frequently occur, such as during transfers to and from toilet, while getting dressed, and during bathing.

Apart from direct instruction on these skills, the use of mechanical hip protectors has been advocated as a means of minimizing the impact of a fall in high-risk patients. By this same measure, the use of seizure pads on the ground at the bedside and choosing a low bed rather than one of standard height may be helpful if a confused patient awakens and attempts to get out of bed without assistance. Falling out of bed and attempts to walk at night are common in elderly patients or in those with cognitive deficits who may also be impulsive.

The Role of Exercise

Exercise has been recently adopted as an additional intervention to facilitate osteoporosis rehabilitation in patients with stroke, independent of the role of exercise in treating muscle weakness, pain, spasticity, and balance deficits. Exercise serves a role in not only reducing the incidence of falls but also in maintaining bone health. As Eng et al. point out, because the greatest amount of rapid bone loss occurs in the first six months following stroke, early intervention with exercise therapy is essential [36]. Because the number of falls that also result in a bone fracture is relatively small (approximately 10 % of total falls), large samples are needed for high statistical power, ensuring the accurate evaluation of exercise [36] in reducing fractures. In a study that examined 560 stroke patients, the authors found a 64 % reduction in the risk of hip fractures with a power of 80 % *p*-value 0.05 % for a structured program of exercise. Eng and colleagues found a number of benefits after a 19-week fitness program with mobility exercises. Known as the "FAME" program, skills such as repeated practice of sit to stand transfers, stepping onto risers, brisk walking, and other tests of walking endurance resulted in improved aerobic capacity, muscle strength, stamina, tolerance to activity, and retention of bone mineral density in the hip. The intervention group lost only 0.7 % of bone mineral density in the femoral neck, whereas the control group lost 2.5 %. This stands in contrast to comparably aged adults without stroke who lose only 0.5–0.9 % per year.

Pharmacologic Treatment

Given the anticipated rapid bone loss in the immediate months following stroke, prevention of increased bone turnover and osteoclastic upregulation can be addressed by the use of oral bisphosphonates. Several studies have examined the use of oral bisphosphonates following stroke. Sato et al. [37] studied subjects who received 2.5 mg of daily risedronate for one year versus placebo, with onset of treatment beginning two days after an acute stroke. The 375 Asian women who were examined showed reduced hip fracture risk and improved BMD. A very similar study was performed in Asian males [38]. Of the 280 subjects examined, ten subjects in the placebo group and only two in the risedronate group experienced a fracture in the 18-month assessment time. The BMD at 18 months post stroke after using 2.5 mg daily risedronate versus placebo was 2.5 % higher in the hip of those receiving the drug but 3.5 % decreased in the placebo patients. Despite the limitations of the use of lower than standard doses of risedronate and potential lack of applicability to other ethnic groups, the study showed good promise for subjects able to take oral medications so soon following stroke. Two studies examined the effects of etidronate which is a less potent oral bisphosphonate, but outcomes in both were limited to BMD improvement in the metacarpal region only and used computer x-ray densitometry rather than the more accepted DXA technology as a tool to assess BMD [15].

Oral bisphosphonates have several disadvantages if used following acute stroke. Because a number of the pills that must be swallowed are large, patients with dysphagia or reflux have difficulty. If patients must have medications crushed, once weekly or monthly bisphosphonates, such as alendronate or ibandronate, must be avoided. A daily form of alendronate still exists but has the same lifestyle requirements of sitting upright 30–60 minutes after ingestion and abstaining from food two hours prior to consumption [17].

Intravenous bisphosphonates eliminate the concern for dysphagia as well as compliance. Most are given once or twice annually in a doctor's office so reliability of a patient with cognitive impairments is not a concern. Poole and colleagues [17] examined 27 acute stroke patients within 35 days of the onset of neurological event. Patients received either 4 mg of intravenous zoledronic acid or placebo. On the affected side, the mean BMD in the total hip was changed by 0 % in the group receiving the drug but declined by 5.5 % in the total hip and 8.1 % in the subtrochanteric region in the placebo group. On the unaffected side, those stroke patients who received zoledronic acid improved by 1.0 % but declined by 2.7 % in the placebo group. Interestingly, 72 % of patients in the study experienced a fall in the follow-up time, but no subjects in either group experienced a fracture.

Limited research has been published on outcomes of intravenous bisphosphonates. Careful risk benefit assessment should be done before initiating intravenous bisphosphonates in terms of hydration and renal function, especially in elderly patients [39]. Given the challenges of dysphagia and compliance with oral medications, alternative intravenous or subcutaneous forms of osteoporosis prevention and treatment deserve further study.

Epilepsy and Chronic Seizure Disorders

Patients with neurological conditions inclusive of seizures disorders experience an increased incidence of osteoporosis. Seizures and epilepsy are not synonymous. An epileptic seizure is a transient event caused by abnormal excessive neuronal activity, synchronous in nature. In the United States, epilepsy affects 2.4 million adults (1.8 % of the population aged 18 and older) and 460,000 children (1 % of the population aged 0–17) [40]. It involves multiple recurrent unprovoked seizures, characterized by an ongoing predisposition to generate excessive neuronal activity in the brain, leading to long-term neurobiological, cognitive, psychological, and social consequences [41]. This general definition, developed in 2005 by the International League Against Epilepsy (ILAE) [42], was revised in 2014. To be classified as epileptic, an individual must now meet any one of the following conditions [43, 44]:

1. At least two unprovoked seizures occurring more than 24 hours apart
2. One unprovoked or reflex seizure and a probability of further seizures over the next 10 years, equivalent to the probability of the general recurrence risk (60 %), typically seen after two unprovoked seizures
3. Diagnosis of an epilepsy syndrome: individuals who have had an age-dependent syndrome but are now past the applicable age (generally 16–21 years) or those who have been seizure-free for 10 years and off medications for five years

The new definition effectively classifies epilepsy as a disease rather than a disorder, underlying its serious nature and incorporating the concept of "resolved epilepsy," meaning that although epilepsy may return, the likelihood is small and individuals may consider themselves to be free of the disease.

Individuals who do not meet the pure definition of epilepsy can nonetheless have a seizure condition that contributes to osteoporosis and related metabolic bone diseases such as osteomalacia. Persons with increased intracranial pressure following a large stroke, those with hemorrhagic stroke or other nontraumatic brain dysfunction such as cerebral aneurysms, or those with brain tumors can experience repeated seizures. However, seizures among these groups are most often considered to be provoked and, with few exceptions, do not fall within the accepted definition of epilepsy. Epilepsy in its pure form can begin in childhood, but bone disease may only manifest itself years later. A subsequent chapter of this book will include a section on seizure disorders in that select population and discuss the long-term effects these young adults face.

Epidemiology of Osteoporosis in Seizure Disorders

The development of low BMD and osteoporosis in patients with seizure disorders contributes to the risk of fractures but is only one of many factors leading to fractures in this population. Low BMD in the hip, spine, and other bones in both hospitalized and ambulatory patients with seizure disorders has been recognized and described in a number of trials. Among patients taking conventional antiepileptic drugs (AEDs) such as carbamazepine (CBZ) and valproate (VPA), Hamed et al. [45] found statistically significant changes in BMD of the lumbar spine and femoral neck among male and female adults with seizure disorders ranging in duration from 6 to 25 years, with more men affected than women. Pack et al. [46] conducted a retrospective cross-sectional study of 141 patients with enzyme-inducing AED use of >3 years. Men and women were analyzed together in this sample given the lack of significant differences in other baseline characteristics. Relative to healthy postmenopausal females under age 50 with presumed osteopenia of 15.3 % and osteoporosis of less than 1 %, those who took AEDs had 40.2 % osteopenia and 10.3 % osteoporosis at the femoral neck, with 32.7 % osteopenia and 13.7 % osteoporosis at the lumbar spine. For patients over age 50, the findings were even more striking. At the femoral neck, 50.9 % of subjects had osteopenia and 22.6 % had osteoporosis, while at the spine, 35.3 % had osteopenia and 25.5 % showed osteoporosis.

Duration of use of AEDs has also been cited as a causal factor for increased loss of BMD [45, 47]. But other trials focusing on valproate illustrate a conflict in outcome data. Whereas Triantafyllou et al. [48] found that valproate monotherapy duration and dosage did not correlate with BMD in patients who had taken the drug for at least two years, a 6-month prospective study by Boluk et al. [47] showed that valproate monotherapy led to significant decreases in BMD. In both trials, patients were from an ambulatory, community-based practice. In addition, ages studied were similar. Because sodium valproate is not among the traditional enzyme-inducing AEDs, it should theoretically be a better option for preserving BMD than some agents, yet multiple investigations have found reduced BMD and increased fracture risk with this nonenzyme-inducing medication.

Epidemiology of Fractures

Sheth [41] has suggested that AED treatment for at least five years places patients age 50 years or older at twice the risk for osteoporotic fractures. Many studies over the last three decades have described increased risks of fracture for those with seizure disorders, but to what extent these medications are the cause of fractures remains controversial. In 2005, Vestergaard [49] conducted one of the most comprehensive evaluations of osteoporosis and fracture risk associated with epilepsy. In his review of 12 studies of BMD, varying markedly in terms of ages studied, exposures to AEDs, and comorbidities, he demonstrated not only a significant decrease in spine as well as hip BMD (based on *Z*-scores of −0.38 and −0.56, respectively) but a heightened fracture risk as well, with the relative risk (RR) of spine fractures at 6.2 and that of hip fractures at 5.3. Most of the investigations examined, both those involving enzyme-inducing AEDs as well as those using nonenzyme AEDs, reported modest reductions in BMD. While the BMD values were lower than those of age-matched controls, low BMD alone cannot account for the marked elevation in fracture rates. Other factors, both pharmacologic and functional, clearly contributed to increased fall risk which, in turn, increased fracture rates.

A decade after the Vestergaard review, a second meta-analysis [50] reexamined the relationship between use of AEDs and fracture risk, using RR calculations for case-control, cross-sectional, and cohort studies. It encompassed studies that evaluated "any fracture" or isolated hip fractures in adults over age 50; none of the studies chosen considered spine fractures specifically. Relative risk of any osteoporotic fracture for those using AEDs of any subtype was 1.86. The RR of persons using enzyme-inducing AEDs was 1.6, while the RR for those on nonenzyme-inducing AEDs was 1.27; those using AEDs of any subtype demonstrated an RR of 1.9 for isolated hip fractures. The strong association between AEDs and loss of BMD cannot be disputed, and there are further indications that some AEDs may entail greater risks than others.

Pathophysiology

Metabolic and Pharmacological Mechanisms of Altered Bone Biology

Decreased bone mineralization is not a direct outcome of seizures. Rather, it is multifactorial and often occurs as a result of decreased vitamin D levels attributed to the use of antiepileptic drugs (AEDs). The more potent enzyme-inducing AEDs (carbamazepine, phenobarbital, phenytoin) contribute to increased fracture risk more than do weak enzyme-inducing AEDs (oxcarbazepine and topiramate) or nonenzyme-inducing AEDs (gabapentin, levetiracetam, lamotrigine) [51, 52]. See Table 2 [53, 54].

Vitamin D is essential for calcium absorption and strong bones, and vitamin D deficiency is considered to be another cause of bone loss. Such AEDs as carbamazepine, phenobarbital (PB), and phenytoin (PHT) increase the metabolic rate of the liver, causing a reduction in vitamin D. They act by inducing the P450 enzyme system, precipitating increased hepatic hydroxylation of vitamin D to polar inactive metabolites, and reducing bioavailable vitamin D [55]. The result is secondary hyperparathyroidism, which, in turn, increases bone turnover and lowers bone density, both of which are key factors in the development of osteoporosis. Moreover, interference with vitamin D metabolism leads to osteomalacia, or the abnormal mineralization of bone, which is distinctly different from osteoporosis [56]. Both osteomalacia and osteoporosis are associated with fractures.

At the same time, recent cross-sectional studies of patients taking enzyme-inducing AEDs have found reduction in bone density even in the absence of vitamin D deficiency [57–59]. This finding is consistent with the results reported in the meta-analyses of Vestergaard and of Sheth et al. [49, 57].

Table 2 Fracture risk of common seizure medications

Drug	Liver-inducing AED Nicholas et al. [53]	Effect on fracture risk Jette et al. [54]	Population studied Jette et al. [54]
Carbamazepine	Y	1.81 (1.46–2.23)	Odds ratios and 95 % confidence intervals were calculated for association between current AED use and fractures. Model was adjusted for sociodemographic variables + homecare use + comorbidities and all AEDs simultaneously
Clonazepam	N	1.24 (1.05–1.47)	
Levetiracetam	N	N/A	
Gabapentin	N	1.49 (1.10–2.02)	
Phenobarbital	Y	1.60 (1.16–2.19)	
Phenytoin	Y	1.91 (1.58–2.30)	
Valproate sodium	N	1.10 (0.70–1.72)	

Sources: Adapted from Nicholas et al. [53] and Jette et al. [54]

Alternative mechanisms of bone loss due to use of AEDs also exist, including indirect metabolic effects on other vitamins or calcium. Studies evaluating agents and their actions [41, 60] found that long-term therapy with phenytoin and carbamazepine may lead to low BMD through a direct adverse effect on human osteoblast-like cells. Impaired calcium absorption can occur through either inadequate oral consumption of calcium-rich foods or by a scenario in which there is sufficient calcium intake but the presence of a superimposed wasting syndrome from medications such as proton pump inhibitors. These agents block acid production in the stomach, creating a chemical environment that is not conducive to absorption of calcium in the gut. Kruse and Kracht [61] propose that inhibition of calcitonin secretion may also contribute to bone loss, possibly as a result of the release of dopamine from nerve tracts in the hypothalamus.

Radiographic evidence of osteoporosis illustrates the association with long-term sodium valproate, phenytoin carbamazepine, and phenobarbital treatments [41]. However, although radiographs may demonstrate an end result of osteoporosis, they do not establish a direct cause and effect relationship. For example, among the AEDs noted above, sodium valproate does not induce the hepatic drug metabolizing enzymes of the P450 system, implying that other mechanisms are also involved and relevant for osteoporosis.

A number of common metabolic causes of osteoporosis in patients with chronic seizure disorders are outlined below [62]:

- The use of enzyme-inducing AEDs causing accelerated hepatic vitamin D metabolism
- Lowered calcitonin levels due to use of AEDs
- Inhibition of calcium absorption by other medications
- Poor intake of calcium from diet
- Poor absorption of calcium due to simultaneous use of H+ inhibitors or H2 blockers
- Poor intake of vitamin D from diet

- Altered vitamin K metabolism from medications
- Reduced IGF-binding protein 1 or 3 from hormonal changes
- Reduced sunlight levels due institutionalization
- Reduced levels of estrogen, testosterone, or sex hormone-binding globulin from endocrine changes

In terms of diagnosing osteoporosis in epilepsy, BMD assessment with dual photon x-ray absorptiometry (DXA) remains the gold standard. However, markers of bone remodeling have emerged as valuable tools to assess the rate of bone formation and resorption and to help clinicians intervene in a timely manner to predict fracture risk and ideally prevent fractures. As described in earlier chapters of this book, the ligand of receptor activator of nuclear factor kappa (RANKL) is elevated in settings of heightened osteoclastic activity. RANKL stimulates RANK located on the surface of osteoclasts to further their promotion and differentiation. Osteoprotegerin (OPG) is a decoy protein for RANK such that RANK accepts OPG's binding, rather than that of RANKL. In the latter scenario, osteoclastic activation does not occur because RANKL could not bind to RANK to form the unit required to stimulate action of bone resorbing cells [63].

In the Hamed et al. study [45], significant differences were observed between patients with epilepsy or ongoing seizure disorders and control subjects: markers of bone formation (OPG) and nutrients that work to promote bone formation (serum calcium and serum vitamin D25-OH) were lower in patients with seizure disorders, whereas markers involved in bone resorption including RANKL and RANKL/OPG ratios were elevated Moreover, findings showed no relation between DXA scores and the type of AED used but did show an association between BMD and serum vitamin D25-OH levels, OPG levels, RANKL levels, duration of AED use (of any type), and total duration of illness. Relative to controls, patients with seizures had significantly lower BMD at the femoral neck and in lumbar spine between L2-4.

Nonpharmacologic Causes of Osteoporosis and Fractures

Aside from pharmacologic agents, patients with a recent or long-term history of seizures may be at risk for osteoporosis. Disuse resulting from mobility limitations and decreased weight-bearing through long bones can lead to decreased bone mineralization. Poor nutrition may also be contributory to overall BMD. Lower socioeconomic status may be related to nutrition and has been linked to more emergency room visits, poor adherence to medications, and the use of less expensive medications rather than the agent prescribed for optimal seizure control [64]. Moreover, those with compromised funding may be forced to take generic equivalents of seizure medications, which are among the few classes of pharmaceuticals in which prescription brand and generic options differ substantially in quality and effectiveness. Because medications ultimately issued may be less effective at preventing seizures and because even appropriate agents may be taken inconsistently, seizures are less well controlled and patients may have breakthrough symptoms, leading to falls. Sudden losses of balance often result in unexpected falls, which may be severe enough to cause fractures, pain, or additional injury due to the osteoporotic fragility of bones.

In patients with epilepsy or other conditions leading to frequent seizures, factors associated with duration of muscle disuse and reduced weight-bearing activity become relevant. Patients with seizures have elevated risks of fractures due to forceful muscle contractions on the skeleton during convulsions. In this scenario, sudden increased loading of the spine or an extremity can trigger joint dislocation, particularly if the onset of seizure is sudden. The dislocation would cause balance loss and falls. A second reason for fracture is the general lack of awareness during the immediate seizure or postictal state, characterized by decreased responsiveness, delayed reaction times, and confusion. During this time, ambulatory patients may experience a loss of balance and increased fatigue. Finally, falls in chronic seizure patients can occur if repeated parenchymal damage and chemical alterations occur from accumulating seizure events.

Pharmacologic Treatment

Bisphosphonates

Only a limited number of investigations have explored osteoporosis drug treatment to prevent further bone loss in patients using long-term antiepileptic agents. Lazzari et al. [65] looked at the effect of risedronate versus placebo treatment in 80 male veterans who had taken one of several AEDs—carbamazepine, phenytoin, phenobarbital, or sodium valproate—for a minimum of two years. Imaging with DXA was performed at 1- and 2-year follow-up times for both groups, who simultaneously received calcium and vitamin D supplementation. At year one, a significant increase in BMD by 3.5 % was evident in the risedronate subjects compared with a nonsignificant decrease in bilateral proximal femoral BMD in placebo subjects. For the spine, again there was a significant BMD increase of 5.2 % in the risedronate subjects with no effective change in the placebo group. Findings were similar for outcomes at year two, except by this time, the total body BMD in placebo subjects demonstrated a significant decline.

At the end of the study, significant improvement in BMD at any of the evaluated sites was evident in the placebo group, a finding that may be attributable to calcium and vitamin D supplementation. However, the percentages of bone gain were far better in the risedronate group with a significant increase in BMD observed in 70 % of these patients, particularly at L1–4, where the increase significantly exceeded that of the placebo group. Moreover, the risedronate subjects had no occurrence of fracture, as opposed to five fractures in the placebo group.

Calcium and Vitamin D

Trials involving treatment with vitamin D and calcium in the absence of other medications directed at bone loss (bisphosphonates, denosumab, SERMs, or other agents) have produced mixed results. In the Lazzarri et al. study, 65 % of the placebo group had significant improvement in BMD at one site or another in the setting of supplemental vitamin D and calcium [65]. Other studies have found a similar positive correlation [66]. Yet in a large trial involving 3,303 veterans with prolonged seizure disorders, Espinosa and colleagues [67] found that supplementation failed to affect fracture prevalence. Meier and Kraenzlin advise that patients on enzyme-inducing AEDs receive 2,000–4,000 international units (IU) supplemental vitamin D daily and those taking nonenzyme-inducing AEDs take 1,000–2,000 IU daily [55]. For the individual patient, there may be a benefit and rarely is there a disadvantage to such supplementation [68]. Drezner further advises that at the time patients are started on any AED, they simultaneously begin supplemental vitamin D, with doses starting as high as 2,000 IU in patients who are on multiple AEDs, institutionalized, or have limited outdoor activity. In patients with established osteoporosis by BMD, doses may need to be as high as 4,000 IU daily [69].

In all cases, serum calcium and PTH levels should be followed to monitor for secondary hyperparathyroidism. Supplemental calcium should not be given without careful monitoring of serum electrolytes (calcium and phosphorous), vitamin D25-OH levels, and PTH. If the vitamin D deficiency and bone biopsy suggest osteomalacia, doses of supplemental vitamin D may need to be between 5,000 and 15,000 IU daily for 3–4 weeks, during which time calcium and phosphorous levels must be closely followed. It often takes more than a month for serum levels to normalize and all such patients should be monitored by an endocrinologist or rheumatologist with specialized training in this area [68].

Nonpharmacologic Treatment

Any patient who has been on long-standing AEDs for clinical management should undergo basic screening for osteoporosis including serum vitamin D25-OH level, calcium, and PTH. If significantly abnormal serum levels in any of the above measures are identified, ongoing outpatient care with a bone specialist at the time of discharge from acute care or inpatient rehabilitation should be initiated. Patients who meet clinical definitions of epilepsy or who have neurological conditions such as hemorrhagic stroke or brain tumors with edema, leading to ongoing risk for seizures, may require AEDs chronically. Consequently, an intervention plan should be created taking into account the ongoing presence of medications that will further compromise osteoporosis. Coordinating this plan with the patient's neurologist is also strongly advised.

Dedicated training of balance and gait stability are potential avenues of optimization in the effort to decrease falls. Reinforcement of skills learned in inpatient rehabilitation or at a skilled nursing facility can be carried out short term with a home therapist in the weeks following a patient's transition home. However, this form of individualized therapy is limited, and after 30–60 days, patients are left with a home exercise regimen. Ongoing balance and endurance activities must be emphasized and, if possible, supervised by family or caregivers to ensure these skills are maintained. Loss of function in terms of balance and strength due to lack of practice and failure to repeat safe transfers and proper gait technique translates to an increased fall risk to these patients.

Surgical techniques to control seizures are rapidly advancing in the effort to provide better disease control and reduce the need for medications that may be intermittently rather than consistently effective, cause undesirable side effects, and burden families and patients with high cost. Nowell and colleagues describe several new approaches to improving traditional surgery outcomes [70]. Surgical outcomes for seizure control have been limited by suboptimal imaging for planning procedures. Better imaging of the epileptogenic zone will enable surgeons to more completely ablate an area of seizure focus. A better contoured brain map of seizure probability can help advise surgeons of the risk benefit ratio in attempting to ablate areas closer to essential brain function. A newer imaging modality in the form of 3D magnetic resonance technology may assist clinicians to identify unique differences from patient to patient which may not be as visible in two-dimensional films.

As an alternative to conventional brain surgery for neuroablation of seizures, two types of electrical stimulation, vagus nerve stimulation and deep brain stimulation, have been initiated in both the United States and Canada. These procedures are considered in patients that have seizures in a site of non-resectable brain tissue and for patients in whom conventional antiseizure medications fail to control symptoms or cause such severe side effects that the medications are intolerable [71]. While the procedures are costly and not without risk, they may be beneficial for seizure reduction and quality of life. If deep brain stimulation or vagal nerve stimulation permits the discontinuation of seizure medications that damage the bone, a benefit of improved BMD and reduced fracture risk may be seen over time.

Future Directions

Ultimately, the challenge of metabolic bone disease in patients with seizure disorders including traditional epilepsy will depend on the duration of treatment, agents chosen, and commitment of the whole treatment team to include continued bone health as a focus of the long-term care plan. Too often, patients and practitioners are overwhelmed with management of immediate medical concerns, and in the case of seizure patients, funds and resources are directed largely at pharmacologic treatment and testing for the seizure condition itself. Medications for seizures are enormously expensive with potentially significant out-of-pocket costs. Funds for other potentially expensive medications to maintain bone health and testing to diagnose early osteoporosis, including laboratory studies and DXA imaging, are limited or nonexistent. Moreover, initiating discussions about a future health problem may not be well received or even recalled during a time when other medical issues are more pressing. Adopting bone health as a strategy of prevention when patients are first put on AEDs, initiating prevention doses of vitamin D at that time, and optimizing their physical functioning and mobility from the onset of diagnosis may be the best approach to preserving bone health in patients with epilepsy and related seizure disorders.

References

1. Duncan PA, Zorowitz R, Bates B, Choi JY, Glasberg JJ, Graham GD et al. Management of adult stroke rehabilitation care: a clinical perspective. Stroke. 2005; 36:e100–e143. doi:10.1161/01.STR.0000180861.54180.FF.
2. Centers for Medicare & Medicaid Services, U.S. Department of Health and Human Services. Report to Congress: Post-Acute Care Payment Reform Demonstration (PAC–PRD). 2012. http://www.medpac.gov/documents/reports/mar13_entirereport.pdf?sfvrsn=0.
3. Kim HW, Kang E, Im S, Ko YJ, Im SA, Lee JI. Prevalence of pre-stroke low bone mineral density and vertebral fracture in first stroke patients. Bone. 2008;43:183–6.
4. Benzinger P, Rapp K, König HH, Bleibler F, Globas C, Beyersmann J, et al. Risk of osteoporotic fractures following stroke in older persons. Osteoporos Int. 2015;26:1341–9. doi:10.1007/s00198-014-3005-x.
5. Palomäki H, Kaste M. Regular light-to-moderate intake of alcohol and the risk of ischemic stroke. Is there a beneficial effect? Stroke. 1993;24(12):1828–32.
6. Abbott RD, Curb JD, Rodriguez BL, Sharp DS, Burchfiel CM, Yano K. Effect of dietary calcium and milk consumption on risk of thromboembolic stroke in older middle-aged men. The Honolulu Heart Program. Stroke. 1996;27(5):813–8.
7. Gillum RF, Mussolino ME, Ingram DD. Physical activity and stroke incidence in women and men. The NHANES I epidemiologic follow-up study. Am J Epidemiol. 1996;143(9):860–9.
8. Lampropoulos CE, Papaioannou I, D'Cruz DP. Osteoporosis: a risk factor for cardiovascular disease. Nat Rev Rheumatol. 2012;8(10):587–98.
9. Liu M, Tsuji T, Higuchi Y, Domen K, Tsujiuchi K, Chino N. Osteoporosis in hemiplegic stroke patients as studied with dual-energy X-ray absorptiometry. Arch Phys Med Rehabil. 1999;80(10):1219–26.
10. Jørgensen L, Crabtree NJ, Reeve J, Jacobsen BK. Ambulatory level and asymmetrical weight bearing after stroke affects bone loss in the upper and lower part of the femoral neck differently: bone adaption after decreased mechanical loading. Bone. 2000;27(5):701–7.
11. Lazoura O, Groumas N, Antoniadou E, Papadaki PJ, Papadimitriou A, Thriskos P, et al. Bone mineral density alterations in upper and lower extremities 12 months after stroke measured by peripheral quantitative computed tomography and DXA. J Clin Densitom. 2008;11(4):511–7. doi:10.1016/j.jocd.2008.05.097.
12. Ramnemark A, Nyberg L, Lorentzon R, Englund U, Gustafson Y. Progressive hemiosteoporosis on the paretic side and increased bone mineral density in the nonparetic arm the first year after severe stroke. Osteoporos Int. 1999;9(3):269–75.
13. Jørgensen L, Jacobsen BK. Changes in muscle mass, fat mass, and bone mineral content in the legs after stroke: a 1 year prospective study. Bone. 2001;28(6):655–9.
14. Jørgensen L, Jacobsen BK. Functional status of the paretic arm affects the loss of bone mineral in the proximal humerus after stroke: a 1-year prospective study. Calcif Tissue Int. 2001;68(6):11–5.
15. Carda S, Cisari C, Invernizzi M, Bevilacqua M. Osteoporosis after stroke: a review of the causes and potential treatments. Cerebrovasc Dis. 2009;28(2):191–200.

16. Sato Y, Maruoka H, Honda Y, Asoh T, Fujimatsu Y, Oizumi K. Development of osteopenia in the hemiplegic finger in patients with stroke. Eur Neurol. 1996;36(5):278–83.
17. Poole KE, Reeve J, Warburton EA. Falls, fractures, and osteoporosis after stroke: time to think about protection? Stroke. 2002;33(5):1432–6.
18. Boake C, Noser EA, Ro T, Baraniuk S, Gaber M, Johnson R, et al. Constraint-induced movement therapy during early stroke rehabilitation. Neurorehabil Neural Repair. 2007;21(1): 14–24.
19. Tanaka N, Sonoda S, Arita M, Suzuki M, Chino N. Biochemical markers of bone turnover in hemiplegic patients relation to time from stroke onset and grip strength of the affected side. Jpn J Rehabil Med. 1997;34(5):332–6.
20. Sato Y. Abnormal bone and calcium metabolism in patients after stroke. Arch Phys Med Rehabil. 2000;81(1):117–21.
21. Sato Y, Maruoka H, Oizumi K, Kikuyama M. Vitamin D deficiency and osteopenia in the hemiplegic limbs of stroke patients. Stroke. 1996;27(12):2183–7.
22. Antonios TF, MacGregor GA. Deleterious effects of salt intake other than effects on blood pressure. Clin Exp Pharmacol Physiol. 1995;22(3):180–4.
23. Löfvenmark I, Werhagen L, Norrbrink C. Spasticity and bone density after a spinal cord injury. J Rehabil Med. 2009;41(13):1080–4. doi:10.2340/16501977-0469.
24. Pang MY, Ashe MC, Eng JJ. Muscle weakness, spasticity and disuse contribute to demineralization and geometric changes in the radius following chronic stroke. Osteoporos Int. 2007;18(9):1243–52.
25. Pang MY, Eng JJ, McKay HA, Dawson AS. Reduced hip bone mineral density is related to physical fitness and leg lean mass in ambulatory individuals with chronic stroke. Osteoporos Int. 2005;16(12):1769–79.
26. Pang MY, Ashe MC, Eng JJ. Compromised bone strength index in the hemiparetic distal tibia epiphysis among chronic stroke patients: the association with cardiovascular function, muscle atrophy, mobility, and spasticity. Osteoporos Int. 2010;21(12):997–1007. doi:10.1007/s00198-009-1038-3.
27. Esquenazi A. Falls and fractures in older post-stroke patients with spasticity: consequences and drug treatment considerations. Clinical Great. 2004; 12 (8) In: Consultant360.com. 2004. http://www.consultant360.com/articles/falls-and-fractures-older-post-stroke-patients-spasticity-consequences-and-drug-treatment. Accessed 06 Dec 2015.
28. Riss J, Cloyd J, Gates J, Collins S. Benzodiazepines in epilepsy: pharmacology and pharmacokinetics. Acta Neurol Scand. 2008;118(2):69–86. doi:10.1111/j.1600-0404.2008.01004.x.
29. Wuis EW, Dirks MJ, Termond EF, Vree TB, Van der Kleijn E. Plasma and urinary excretion kinetics of oral baclofen in healthy subjects. Eur J Clin Pharmacol. 1989;37(2):181–4.
30. Lee-Chiong T. Sleep medicine: essentials and review. New York: Oxford University Press; 2008.
31. Panday K, Gona A, Humphrey MB. Medication-induced osteoporosis: screening and treatment strategies. Ther Adv Musculoskelet Dis. 2014;6(5):185–202. doi:10.1177/1759720X14546350.
32. Rajgopal R, Bear M, Butcher MK, Shaughnessy SG. The effects of heparin and low molecular weight heparins on bone. Thromb Res. 2008;122(3):293–8.
33. Hirsh J, Bauer KA, Donati MB, Gould M, Samama MM, Weitz JI, et al. Parenteral anticoagulants: American College of Chest Physicians Evidence-Based Clinical Practice Guidelines (8th edition). Chest. 2008;133(6 Suppl):141S–59. doi:10.1378/chest.08-0689.
34. Sato Y, Honda Y, Kuno H, Oizumi K. Menatetrenone ameliorates osteopenia in disuse-affected limbs of vitamin D-and K-deficient stroke patients. Bone. 1998;23:291–6.
35. Ramnemark A, Nyberg L, Borssén B, Olsson T, Gustafson Y. Fractures after stroke. Osteoporos Int. 1998;8(1):92–5.
36. Eng JJ, Pang MY, Ashe MC. Balance, falls, and bone health: role of exercise in reducing fracture risk after stroke. J Rehabil Res Dev. 2008;45(2):297–313.
37. Sato Y, Iwamoto J, Kanoko T, Satoh K. Risedronate therapy for prevention of hip fracture after stroke in elderly women. Neurology. 2005;64(5):811–6.

38. Sato Y, Iwamoto J, Kanoko T, Satoh K. Risedronate sodium therapy for prevention of hip fracture in men 65 years or older after stroke. Arch Intern Med. 2005;165(5):1743–8.
39. Myint PK, Poole KE, Warburton EA. Hip fractures after stroke and their prevention. QJM. 2007;100(9):539–45.
40. Centers for Disease Control and Prevention. Epilepsy fast facts. Centers for Disease Control and Prevention. 2015: http://www.cdc.gov/epilepsy/basic/fast-facts.html. Accessed 08 Dec 2015.
41. Sheth RD. Bone health in epilepsy. Epilepsia. 2002;43(12):1453–4.
42. International League Against Epilepsy. Definition of epilepsy. West Hartford: International League Against Epilepsy; 2015. http://www.ilae.org. Accessed 08 Dec 2015.
43. Epilepsy Foundation. What is epilepsy? Landover: Epilepsy Foundation; 2015. http://www.epilepsy.com/. Accessed 08 Dec 2015.
44. Fisher RS, Acevedo C, Arzimanoglou A, Bogacz A, Cross JH, Elger CE, Engel Jr J, et al. ILAE official report: a practical clinical definition of epilepsy. Epilepsia. 2014;55(4):475–82. doi:10.1111/epi.12550.
45. Hamed SA, Moussa EM, Youssef AH, Abd ElHameed MA, NasrEldin E. Bone status in patients with epilepsy: relationship to markers of bone remodeling. Front Neurol. 2014;5:142. doi:10.3389/fneuro.2014.00142.
46. Pack AM, Olarte LS, Morrell MJ, Flaster E, Resor SR, Shane E. Bone mineral density in an outpatient receiving enzyme-inducing antiepileptic drugs. Epilepsy Behav. 2004;4(2): 169–74.
47. Boluk A, Guzelipek M, Savli H, Temel I, Ozişik HI, Kaygusuz A. The effect of valproate on bone mineral density in adult epileptic patients. Pharmacol Res. 2004;50(1):93–7.
48. Triantafyllou N, Lambrinoudaki I, Armeni E, Evangelopoulos EM, Boufidou F, Antoniou A, et al. Effect of long-term valproate monotherapy on bone mineral density in adults with epilepsy. J Neurol Sci. 2010;290(1–2):131–4. doi:10.1016/j.jns.2009.12.015.
49. Vestergaard P. Epilepsy, osteoporosis and fracture risk – a meta-analysis. Acta Neurol Scand. 2005;112(5):277–86.
50. Shen C, Chen F, Zhang Y, Guo Y, Ding M. Association between use of antiepileptic drugs and fracture risk: a systematic review and meta-analysis. Bone. 2014;64:246–53. doi:10.1016/j.bone.2014.04.018.
51. Teagarden DL, Meador KJ, Loring DW. Low vitamin D levels are common in patients with epilepsy. Epilepsy Res. 2014;108(8):1352–6. doi:10.1016/j.eplepsyres.2014.06.008.
52. Kim SH, Lee JW, Choi KG, Chung HW, Lee HW. A 6-month longitudinal study of bone mineral density with antiepileptic drug monotherapy. Epilepsy Behav. 2007;10(2):291–5.
53. Nicholas JM, Risdale L, Richardson MP, Grieve AP, Gulliford MC. Fracture risk with use of liver enzyme inducing antiepileptic drugs in people with active epilepsy: cohort study using the general practice research database. Seizure. 2012;22(1):37–42.
54. Jette N, Lix LM, Metge CJ, Prior HJ, McChesney J, Leslie WD. Association of antiepileptic drugs with nontraumatic fractures. Arch Neurol. 2011;68(1):107–12.
55. Meier C, Kraenzlin ME. Antiepileptics and bone health. Ther Adv Musculoskelet Dis. 2011;3(5):235–43. doi:10.1177/1759720X11410769.
56. Fitzpatrick LA. Pathophysiology of bone loss in patients receiving anticonvulsant therapy. Epilepsy Behav. 2004;5:S3–15.
57. Sheth RD, Wesolowski CA, Jacob JC, Penney S, Hobbs GR, Riggs JE, et al. Effect of carbamazepine and valproate on bone mineral density. J Pediatr. 1995;127(2):256–62.
58. Andress DL, Ozuna J, Tirschwell D, Grande L, Johnson M, Jacobson AF, et al. Antiepileptic drug-induced bone loss in young male patients who have seizures. Arch Neurol. 2002;59(5):781–6.
59. Farhat G, Yamout B, Mikati MA, Demirjian S, Sawaya R, El-Hajj Fuleihan G. Effect of antiepileptic drugs on bone density in ambulatory patients. Neurology. 2002;58(9):1348–53.
60. Feldkamp J, Becker A, Witte OW, Scharff D, Scherbaum WA. Long-term anticonvulsant therapy leads to low bone mineral density—evidence for direct drug effects of phenytoin and carbamazepine on human osteoblast-like cells. Exp Clin Endocrinol Diabetes. 2000;108:37–43.

61. Kruse K, Kracht U. Inhibitory effect of calcium on serum prolactin. Acta Endocrinol (Copenh). 1981;98:339–44.
62. Bartl R, Frisch B. Osteoporosis and drugs. In: Osteoporosis: diagnosis, prevention and therapy. 2nd ed. Berlin: Springer; 2009.
63. Sattler AM, Schoppet M, Schaefer JR, Hofbauer LC. Novel aspects on RANK ligand and osteoprotegerin in osteoporosis and vascular disease. Calcif Tissue Int. 2004;74(1):103–6.
64. Szaflarski M. Social determinants of health in epilepsy. Epilepsy Behav. 2014;41:283–9. doi:10.1016/j.yebeh.2014.06.013.
65. Lazzari AA, Dussault PM, Thakore-James M, Gagnon D, Baker E, Davis SA, et al. Prevention of bone loss and vertebral fractures in patients with chronic epilepsy—antiepileptic drug and osteoporosis prevention trial. Epilepsia. 2013;54(11):1997–2004. doi:10.1111/epi.12351.
66. Mikati MA, Dib L, Yamout B, Sawaya R, Rahi AC, Fuleihan G-H. Two randomized vitamin D trials in ambulatory patients on anticonvulsants: impact on bone. Neurology. 2006;67(11): 2005–14.
67. Espinosa PS, Perez DL, Abner E, Ryan M. Association of antiepileptic drugs, vitamin D, and calcium supplementation with bone fracture occurrence in epilepsy patients. Clin Neurol Neurosurg. 2011;113(7):548–51. doi:10.1016/j.clineuro.2011.03.011.
68. Drezner MK. Treatment of anticonvulsant drug-induced bone disease. Epilepsy Behav. 2004;5(Suppl2):S41–7.
69. Collins N, Maher J, Cole M, Baker M, Callaghan N. A prospective study to evaluate the dose of vitamin D required to correct low 25-hydroxyvitamin D levels, calcium, and alkaline phosphatase in patients at risk of developing antiepileptic drug-induced osteomalacia. Q J Med. 1991;78(286):113–22.
70. Nowell M, Miserocchi A, McEvoy AW, Duncan JS. Advances in epilepsy surgery. J Neurol Neurosurg Psychiatry. 2014;85(11):1273–9. doi:10.1136/jnnp-2013-307069.
71. Chambers A, Bowen JM. Electrical stimulation for drug-resistant epilepsy: an evidence-based analysis. Ont Health Technol Assess Ser. 2013;13(18):1–37.

Chapter 9
Osteoporosis in Spinal Cord Medicine

Christina V. Oleson

Acute traumatic spinal cord injury (SCI) can result in abrupt motor loss and inability to ambulate. Due to sudden immobility, increased bone turnover and eventual osteoporosis become prevalent in the first several months post injury [1]. Forms of nontraumatic spinal cord injury also exist and are discussed briefly in this chapter, as well as in areas of this text that cover the primary reasons for motor and sensory loss in these patients, including metastatic lesions to the spine with cord compression or demyelinating lesions in the spinal cord. In complete contrast to the rapid development of bone loss evident in both adult and pediatric traumatic spinal cord injuries, spina bifida occurs at birth and demonstrates very different mechanisms. The distinctions among these conditions and the divergent approaches to treatment are discussed in this chapter.

Traumatic Spinal Cord Injury

Traumatic spinal cord injury affects approximately 12,500 persons in the United States annually, with an approximate prevalence of 276,000 [2]. Motor vehicle accidents followed by falls are the two most common causes of acute traumatic SCI. Whereas acts of violence, including gunshot wounds, have decreased among the total percentage of spinal cord injuries, a rapid rise has occurred in injuries resulting from falls, consistent with the increase in the elderly population. For persons over the age of 60, falls are now the most common source of injury.

Traumatic SCI can be described by *neurological level of injury* (NLI), from cervical to thoracic or lumbar, and by *severity*, graded from A to E with "A" representing complete injuries and the absence of motor and sensory function below the level of the spinal cord lesion and "E" signifying minimal deficits. The levels of injury and regions tested in the body to determine the level and severity are described in Fig. 1 [3].

C.V. Oleson, *Osteoporosis Rehabilitation*, DOI 10.1007/978-3-319-45084-1_9

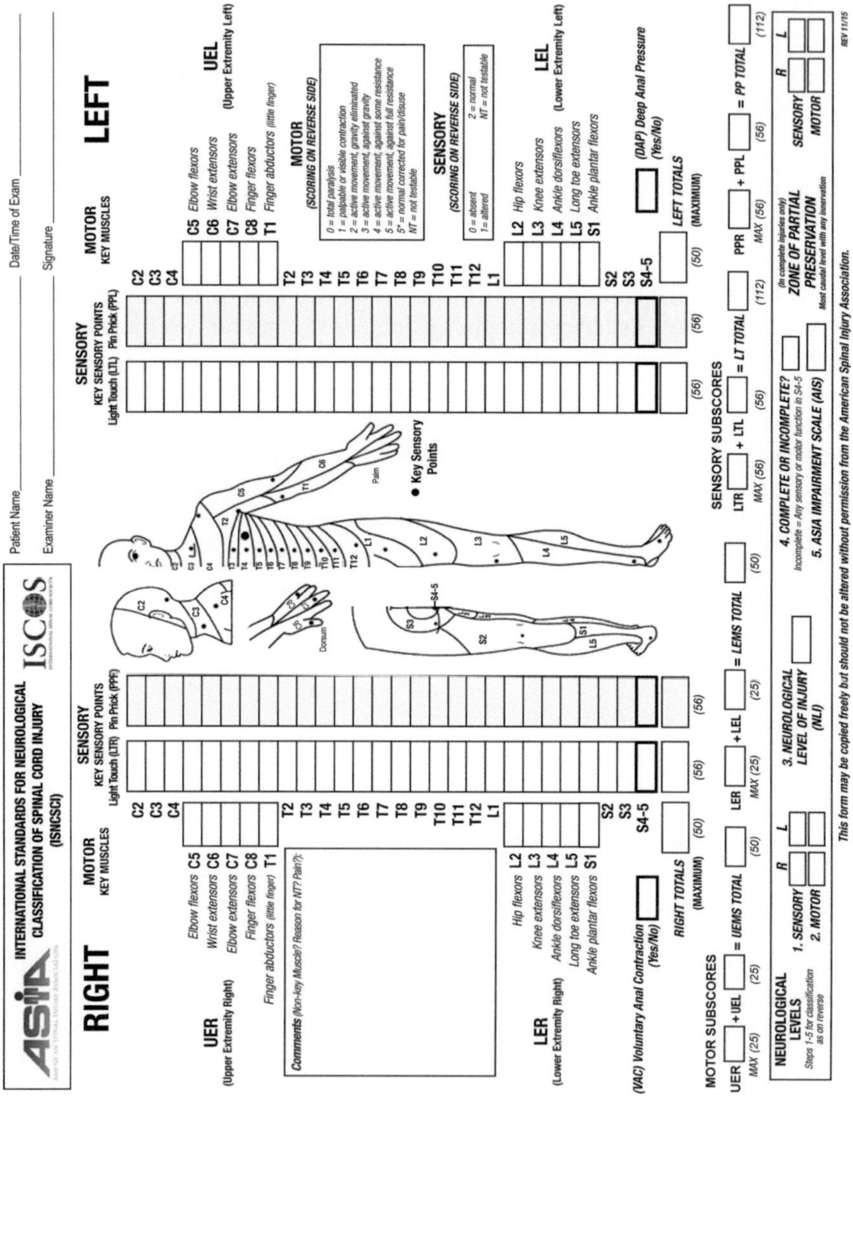

Fig. 1 Official grading sheet for the International Standards of Neurological Classification of Spinal Cord Injury (*Source:* Courtesy of American Spinal Injury Association, Atlanta, Georgia)

Muscle Function Grading

0 = total paralysis
1 = palpable or visible contraction
2 = active movement, full range of motion (ROM) with gravity eliminated
3 = active movement, full ROM against gravity
4 = active movement, full ROM against gravity and moderate resistance in a muscle specific position
5 = (normal) active movement, full ROM against gravity and full resistance in a functional muscle position expected from an otherwise unimpaired person
5* = (normal) active movement, full ROM against gravity and sufficient resistance to be considered normal if identified inhibiting factors (i.e. pain, disuse) were not present
NT = not testable (i.e. due to immobilization, severe pain such that the patient cannot be graded, amputation of limb, or contracture of > 50% of the normal ROM)

Sensory Grading

0 = Absent
1 = Altered, either decreased/impaired sensation or hypersensitivity
2 = Normal
NT = Not testable

When to Test Non-Key Muscles:

In a patient with an apparent AIS B classification, non-key muscle functions more than 3 levels below the motor level on each side should be tested to most accurately classify the injury (differentiate between AIS B and C).

Movement	Root level
Shoulder: Flexion, extension, abduction, adduction, internal and external rotation **Elbow:** Supination	C5
Elbow: Pronation **Wrist:** Flexion	C6
Finger: Flexion at proximal joint, extension. **Thumb:** Flexion, extension and abduction in plane of thumb	C7
Finger: Flexion at MCP joint **Thumb:** Opposition, adduction and abduction perpendicular to palm	C8
Finger: Abduction of the index finger	T1
Hip: Adduction	L2
Hip: External rotation	L3
Hip: Extension, abduction, internal rotation **Knee:** Flexion **Ankle:** Inversion and eversion **Toe:** MP and IP extension	L4
Hallux and Toe: DIP and PIP flexion and abduction	L5
Hallux: Adduction	S1

ASIA Impairment Scale (AIS)

A = Complete. No sensory or motor function is preserved in the sacral segments S4-5.

B = Sensory Incomplete. Sensory but not motor function is preserved below the neurological level and includes the sacral segments S4-5 (light touch or pin prick at S4-5 or deep anal pressure) AND no motor function is preserved more than three levels below the motor level on either side of the body.

C = Motor Incomplete. Motor function is preserved at the most caudal sacral segments for voluntary anal contraction (VAC) OR the patient meets the criteria for sensory incomplete status (sensory function preserved at the most caudal sacral segments (S4-S5) by LT, PP or DAP), and has some sparing of motor function more than three levels below the ipsilateral motor level on either side of the body.
(This includes key or non-key muscle functions to determine motor incomplete status.) For AIS C – less than half of key muscle functions below the single NLI have a muscle grade ≥ 3.

D = Motor Incomplete. Motor incomplete status as defined above, with at least half (half or more) of key muscle functions below the single NLI having a muscle grade ≥ 3.

E = Normal. If sensation and motor function as tested with the ISNCSCI are graded as normal in all segments, and the patient had prior deficits, then the AIS grade is E. Someone without an initial SCI does not receive an AIS grade.

Using ND: To document the sensory, motor and NLI levels, the ASIA Impairment Scale grade, and/or the zone of partial preservation (ZPP) when they are unable to be determined based on the examination results.

AMERICAN SPINAL INJURY ASSOCIATION

INTERNATIONAL STANDARDS FOR NEUROLOGICAL CLASSIFICATION OF SPINAL CORD INJURY

INTERNATIONAL SPINAL CORD SOCIETY

Steps in Classification

The following order is recommended for determining the classification of individuals with SCI.

1. Determine sensory levels for right and left sides.
The sensory level is the most caudal, intact dermatome for both pin prick and light touch sensation.

2. Determine motor levels for right and left sides.
Defined by the lowest key muscle function that has a grade of at least 3 (on supine testing), providing the key muscle functions represented by segments above that level are judged to be intact (graded as a 5).
Note: in regions where there is no myotome to test, the motor level is presumed to be the same as the sensory level, if testable motor function above that level is also normal.

3. Determine the neurological level of injury (NLI)
This refers to the most caudal segment of the cord with intact sensation and antigravity (3 or more) muscle function strength, provided that there is normal (intact) sensory and motor function rostrally respectively.
The NLI is the most cephalad of the sensory and motor levels determined in steps 1 and 2.

4. Determine whether the injury is Complete or Incomplete.
(i.e. absence or presence of sacral sparing)
If voluntary anal contraction = ***No*** *AND all S4-5 sensory scores =* ***0*** *AND deep anal pressure =* ***No,*** *then injury is* ***Complete.***
Otherwise, injury is ***Incomplete.***

5. Determine ASIA Impairment Scale (AIS) Grade:
Is injury **Complete?** **If YES, AIS=A** and can record ZPP (lowest dermatome or myotome on each side with some preservation)
NO ↓
Is injury Motor **Complete?** **If YES, AIS=B**
NO ↓ (No=voluntary anal contraction OR motor function more than three levels below the motor level on a given side, if the patient has sensory incomplete classification)

Are at least half (half or more) of the key muscles below the neurological level of injury graded 3 or better?
NO ↓ **AIS=C**
YES ↓ **AIS=D**

If sensation and motor function is normal in all segments, AIS=E
Note: AIS E is used in follow-up testing when an individual with a documented SCI has recovered normal function. If at initial testing no deficits are found, the individual is neurologically intact; the ASIA Impairment Scale does not apply.

Fig. 1 (continued)

Regionalization and Pathophysiology of SCI-Associated Osteoporosis

Traumatic SCI is one of several neurological disorders leading to disuse osteoporosis and resultant fractures, but it differs from many other clinical conditions in the rate of osteoporosis development. Approximately two weeks after acute spinal cord injury, a rapid process of bone resorption exceeding that of bone formation begins to occur, primarily due to upregulation of the osteoclasts [4, 5]. Given its faster turnover rate [6, 7], trabecular bone is more commonly affected than cortical bone in the first four months following SCI. During the first six months following acute SCI, markers of bone formation range from mildly depressed to slightly elevated, depending on the study cited [5, 8, 9]. Even if markers of formation are slightly increased, this compensatory process is not sufficient to counteract the significant bone resorption that occurs concurrently. Roberts and colleagues [9] observed a rapid rise in urinary values of total and free deoxypyridinoline, total pyridinoline, and NTX in the immediate period following injury. Elevations in bone resorption markers began at one week post injury, peaked at 16–20 weeks, and then gradually declined. At their highest value, some markers measured ten times the upper limit of normal. Given that bone loss begins shortly after injury, with the bulk of loss in BMD occurring within 4–6 months, aggressive steps should be undertaken to prevent bone loss shortly after injury [10–12].

Radiographic evidence suggests that an estimated 25 % of BMD below the level of injury is lost within the first four months following acute SCI, progressing to a 33 % loss by 16 months post injury [1, 13] and leaving patients at or near the fracture threshold [1]. Additional investigations extending the time from injury to two years estimate a BMD reduction of 30–40 % at the femoral neck, 37–52 % at the distal femur [14, 15], and 50–70 % at the proximal tibia [8, 15], with the majority of this loss occurring during the first 12 months. Bone loss subsequent to SCI occurs specifically below the level of injury. In some regions, it progresses at 1 % per week in the acute phases post injury [16]. Relative to other conditions including space travel, where losses are 0.25 % per week [17], and bed rest in otherwise neuro-intact patients, where bone loss is 0.1 % per week [18], bone loss due to acute SCI is 10–40 times greater and to date, appears to be more resistant to treatment. Intervention is needed early after injury to halt the rapid progression of bone loss, but such measures are difficult to implement given the complex metabolic factors leading to accelerated bone loss as well as medical comorbidities that may exist during the acute care phase of hospitalization.

Specifically, individuals with SCI develop sublesional osteoporosis, namely, bone loss below the level of paralysis [14]. Bone abnormalities after SCI develop at an increased rate in the following areas: proximal femur, distal femur, and proximal tibia [8, 9]. In contrast, persons without SCI exhibit higher rates of osteoporotic fractures in the axial skeleton. Areas of the appendicular skeleton in the SCI population are highly susceptible to bone demineralization due to decreased weight-bearing affecting these areas when patients are in lying and sitting positions [14].

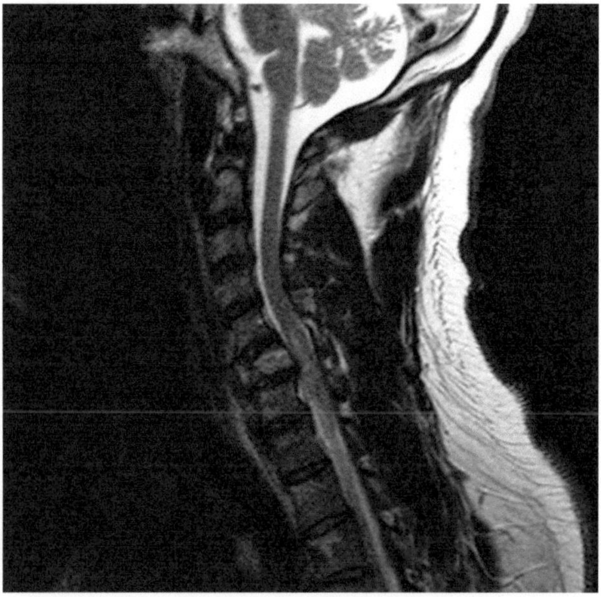

Fig. 2 MRI of a complete cervical SCI. MRI in sagittal view of a 30-year-old male with traumatic C6 ASIA impairment A spinal cord injury due to a motor cycle accident. The image shows a C6 burst fracture with retropulsion of fragments resulting in spinal cord contusion and narrowing of central canal (*Source*: Courtesy of Thomas Jefferson University, Department of Radiology)

The regional BMD in the area below the injury, rather than the overall BMD, is among the strongest predictors of future "fragility fractures" or ones that occur under conditions of minimal or low impact in the absence of trauma [19, 20]. The most significant risk factor for osteoporosis after SCI is the completeness of injury by American Spinal Cord Injury Association (ASIA) grades A through E [21], with patients who have complete injuries at greater risk than those with motor preservation below the injury level. Those with ASIA impairment A (complete) injuries as shown in Fig. 2 are more likely to experience sublesional bone loss than those with motor incomplete injuries (ASIA impairment C or D) who have retained some ability to move their lower extremities. However, having an incomplete SCI (Fig. 3) does not imply the ability to walk or even bear weight on the lower extremities. Originally developed by ASIA, this grading scheme has been adopted as the International Standards for Neurological Classification of Spinal Cord Injury. A higher incidence of sublesional osteoporosis is also observed with increasing number of years post injury [6, 22], increasing age [21, 23], female gender [24] and onset of SCI prior to age 16, when peak bone mass has not yet been achieved [14].

Epidemiology of Osteoporosis Following SCI

SCI patients with more severe injuries (complete or near-complete) are at heightened risk of developing osteoporosis, particularly if an individual is older and has a cervical level of injury, minimal spasticity, and a longer chronicity of injury [8]. The

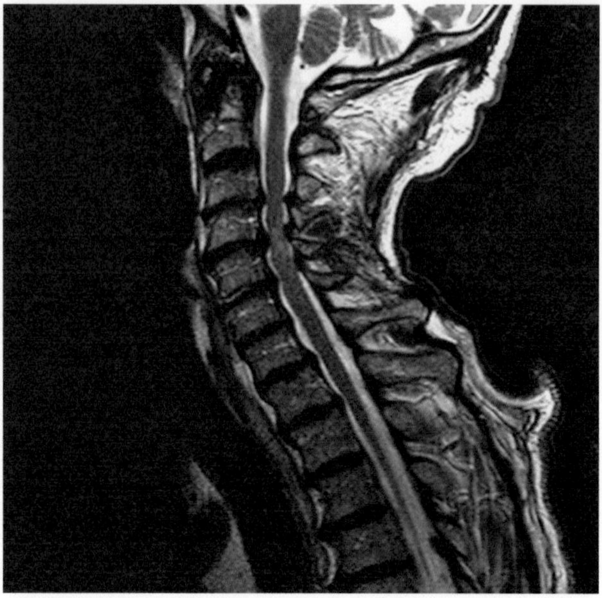

Fig. 3 MRI of an incomplete cervical SCI, shown in sagittal view of an 81-year-old male with a traumatic C4 ASIA impairment C spinal cord injury, due to a fall. There are multi-level degenerative changes in the cervical spine most noticeable at the C4–5, where abnormal cord signal is also seen. In addition, increased T2 signal is seen within the disk space at C5–6, contiguous with prevertebral fluid (*Source*: Courtesy of Thomas Jefferson University, Department of Radiology)

percentage of patients affected with osteoporosis is also dependent on the years since injury, gender, and neurological level of injury (cervical, thoracic or lumbar, complete or incomplete). Although bone loss inevitably occurs in the vast majority of individuals with motor complete as well as substantial numbers of motor incomplete patients with SCI, additional factors contribute to the rate and extent of bone loss below the level of injury. Apart from the severity of SCI and neurological level of injury, nutrition, lifestyle/activity levels, smoking, and family history must also be taken into account. However, these factors may be more relevant in contributing to pre-injury BMD than in preventing bone loss after SCI. The greater the deficiency in an individual's bone density at the time of injury, the more bone a patient could theoretically lose before becoming osteoporotic.

Gifre and colleagues have developed a prediction model for development of osteoporosis 12 months after injury [25]. Their examination of 35 patients with a diagnosis of motor complete SCI of six months or less revealed that total femur BMD <1 g/cm^2 (RR 3.61) and lumbar BMD <1.2 g/cm^2 (RR 2.83) were the strongest predictive factors for development of osteoporosis by one year post injury. Both factors together suggested a probability of 96.8 % that a given individual would develop osteoporosis. Although the authors based this model on a relatively small sample, it included primarily young males with a mean age of 30, likely healthier than some populations of patients, with many still young enough not to have reached peak BMD. Overall, 52 % of their sample developed osteoporosis by one year. Other studies suggest a wide range of percentages by the first year. By patient self-report covering over 1,000 Canadians (approximately 55 % with complete injuries), 21 % stated that they had received a diagnosis of osteoporosis [26]. Given the self-report study design, this estimate is likely to be low; the results were further influenced by the inability to define the timeline of development of osteoporosis from the onset of SCI. In other investigations, prevalence of osteoporosis in SCI patients was found to be much higher; many subjects who do not reach threshold by DXA for −2.5 standard deviations below young normal by a *T*-score are categorized as osteopenic (*T*-score of −1.5 to −2.49).

In a survey by Hammond et al. involving 115 female and 264 male chronic SCI patients seen in an outpatient clinic, 34.9 % met the clinical definition of osteoporosis, while another 46.7 % were classified as osteopenic [27]. Lazo and colleagues reported a high incidence of osteoporosis in a sample of male veterans at an average of 15 years post SCI (median age of 55). In their trial, 61 % met the definition of osteoporosis, while another 19.5 % were osteopenic [28]. Perhaps the highest percentage of osteoporosis was evident in a study by Shojaei et al. of SCI veterans in Iran. In this investigation, 81.5 % demonstrated osteoporosis in the femoral neck, and another 13.1 % were found to have osteopenia. As in similar studies, the lumbar spine had lower degrees of osteoporosis due to loading in the lower back during transfers. In the lumbar lateral spine, a view which is more sensitive than the anterior–posterior view (as described in earlier chapters of this book), 16.7 % were osteoporotic while 18.2 % were osteopenic [29]. Table 1 summarizes the many investigations that have shown sublesional osteoporosis in SCI, with a mix of prospective and cross-sectional studies [15, 22, 24, 30–36].

The Role of Vitamin D in SCI

In addition to the nutritional prevention strategies outlined earlier in this book, spinal cord injury patients have some specific risk factors for malnutrition. Low levels of serum 25-hydroxy vitamin D occur in substantial numbers of persons with acute and chronic SCI [37–41]. In humans, sunlight is the primary source of vitamin D and typically provides up to 90 % of the daily requirement [42, 43]. The capacity of a spinal cord-injured person to absorb vitamin D from the sun is limited by seasonal and related extremes of heat, cold, humidity, or dryness; skin pigmentation; functional mobility; and availability of assistance from caregivers. Individuals with tetraplegia frequently depend on others to get them out of bed, but such assistance may not be available at desired times of peak sunlight. In addition, those with injures above T6 face thermoregulatory challenges and are highly sensitive to extreme heat and humidity, while others with respiratory issues are adversely affected by very dry climates.

All persons with insensate skin are at risk of developing sunburn and those with complete spinal cord injuries are at particular risk. Although use of sunscreen with SPF >8 will block harmful ultraviolet rays and prevent such burns, cutaneous production of vitamin D3 is reduced by more than 95 % [42–44]. In most climates of the United States, exposure to sunlight for only 15 minutes between 10 am and 3 pm in spring, summer, and early fall is sufficient to obtain adequate vitamin D in persons

Table 1 Sublesional bone mineral density in spinal cord-injured patients (arranged by prospective/cross-sectional studies)

Author	Type of study	Duration after injury	Male/female	Age (years)	Skeletal site measured	BMD (Z-score, SD, or % loss or reduction of BMD)
Biering et al. [30]	Prospective	Nine days–53 months	8:0		Femoral neck	−30 to 40 %
					Distal femur	−48 %
					Proximal tibia	−45 %
					Femur diaphysis	−25 %
					Tibia diaphysis	−25 %
Garland et al. [31]	Prospective		6:0		Distal femur	−27 %
					Proximal tibia	−32 %
Uebelhart et al. [32]	Prospective	> Six months	6:0		Lower extremity	−6.4 %
Warden et al. [33]	Prospective	1–6 months	15:0	19–40	Calcaneus	−7.5 ± 3.0 %
					Proximal Tibia	−5.3 ± 4.2 %
Dauty et al. [15]	Cross-sectional	>One year	31:0	18–60	Femoral neck	−30 %
					Femoral trochanter	−39 %
					Distal femur	−70 %
					Proximal tibia	−52 %
Finsen et al. [34]	Cross-sectional	Seven months –33 years	19:0	15–64	Tibia distal diaphysis	−26 %
					Tibia distal metaphysic	−45 %
Zehnder et al. [22]	Cross-sectional	< One year	16:0	18–60	Femoral neck	−0.03 ± 0.25 SD
		< One year	16:0		Tibia epiphysis	−0.34 ± 0.22 SD
		1–9 years	38:0		Femoral neck	−1.65 ± 0.17 SD
		1–9 years	38:0		Tibia epiphysis	−3.81 ± 0.13 SD
		10–19 years	31:0		Femoral neck	−1.76 ± 0.25 SD
		10–19 years	31:0		Tibia epiphysis	−4.00 ± 0.21 SD
		20–29 years	13:0		Femoral neck	−1.76 ± 0.28 SD
		20–29 years	13:0		Tibia epiphysis	−4.12 ± 0.24 SD

Garland et al. [24]	Cross-sectional	2–8 years	0:6	20–30	Knee	−37.90 %
					Hip	−17.50 %
		3–30 years	0:16	31–50	Knee	−41.30 %
					Hip	−25 %
		9–44 years	0:9	53–77	Knee	−47 %
					Hip	−25.50 %
Jones et al. [35]	Cross-sectional	7–372 months	20:0	17–52	Femur	−27 %
					Hip	−37 %

Source: Adapted with permission from Jiang et al. [36]

Table 2 Vitamin D levels in acute traumatic SCI patients according to season

Vitamin D levels in summer and winter in acute traumatic SCI patients		
Serum 25-OH vitamin D (ng/ml)	Summer (% total/season)	Winter (% total/season)
Therapeutic (≥32 ng/ml)	34.5	15.4
Subtherapeutic (20–31.99)	31.0	30.8
Insufficient (13–19.99)	27.6	23.0
Deficient (0–12.99)	6.9	30.8

The population studied in the above report consisted of adults, male and female, 2–6 months post-traumatic SCI. The sample was taken from patients in Birmingham, Alabama, a region of the country where sunlight is more plentiful during summer and, in a relative sense, winter months. Summer levels were drawn between June and September and winter ones between December and February (*Source*: Adapted from Oleson et al. [39])

with fair skin. Persons living in far northern states would incur this benefit only later in the spring or in early fall [45]. Although such limited time will not result in sunburn, some with cervical or upper thoracic neurologic levels of SCI cannot tolerate even this short period, due to temperature dysregulation related to alterations in the autonomic nervous system.

Research examining levels of vitamin D in SCI patients according to season and ethnicity has demonstrated that only 35 % of acute SCI patients injured in summer months and 16 % in winter months actually have therapeutic levels of vitamin D (>32 ng/ml). The remainder required supplementation to achieve therapeutic levels. Findings are summarized in Table 2 [39].

Epidemiology of Insufficiency Fractures Subsequent to SCI

Frequency and Location of Fractures

Patients with complete as opposed to incomplete SCI are at exceptionally high risk of developing fractures in the years subsequent to injury, with the most common sites being the distal femur and proximal tibia [16]. While Bauman et al. focused on hip fractures caused by falls to the ground from wheelchairs or during wheelchair sports, the majority of fractures occur in the lower extremity in the absence of, or with minimal trauma, often as a result of transferring to a car from a wheelchair; a low velocity fall on an outstretched knee; bumping into unforeseen objects [26]; or the sudden stopping of a moving vehicle, prompting rapid forward flexion of the femur, even while the patient remains belted in a sitting position. In a study by Akhigbe and colleagues, the four fractures attributable to motor vehicle accidents occurred in the femur. Similar to other studies, most fractures arose from wheelchair-related activities (43 %) which included transfers, although transfers not involving the chair also accounted for 22 % of fractures [46].

The likelihood of fracture occurrence without antecedent trauma is closely related to the level of BMD in the area at risk (sublesional). According to Garland, the threshold for increased fracture risk is achieved when BMD has declined by 36 % [47]. However, this percentage cannot be taken as an absolute measure of fracture risk, since the initial BMD of a given patient is of paramount importance [25].

While there has been more extensive research on osteoporosis following SCI, fewer studies on fracture incidence have been published. Many investigations involve not only a wide range of years since SCI but also heterogeneous ages and levels of injury. Pelletier et al. [26] studied a 1-year fracture incidence in patients with SCI, with both baseline status and the follow-up findings obtained by phone/website questionnaire. Among the entire cohort of 1,137 patients, 84 or 7.8 % experienced a fracture over the study period. Only 55 % of the subjects had a complete SCI. Factors strongly associated with increased fracture risk were motor and sensory complete SCI (OR = 2.2) and motor complete but sensory incomplete SCI with OR of 1.7, and the presence of three or more of the following risk factors: neurological level of injury, age at injury, duration of injury, or female gender. Since this was only a 1-year evaluation, fracture incidence was lower than other studies. Gifre et al. examined incidence of fracture in the initial 10 years following SCI and found that 25 % of those with complete injuries had experienced at least one fracture since leaving the inpatient rehabilitation unit, with most occurring 6–10 years after injury—a finding that was four times the rate of fracture among the incomplete patients in their study.

In the study above by Akhigbe and colleagues [46], fracture incidence in a group of veterans studied for five years was 13.7 % in the years of evaluation, but over one-third had a fracture that occurred following their SCI but before initiation of the study observation period. In an examination of 3,125 patients over a 6-month interval, Morse et al. reported that approximately 10 % had experienced low-impact fractures below the level of their SCI (study excluded high impact fractures) [20]. Notable findings from this investigation were a longer than normal length of hospitalization (35 days) due to the complications linked to the fracture including non-union/delayed healing, increased muscle spasms as well as pain (in incomplete SCI patients), autonomic dysreflexia, and heterotopic ossification at the fracture site. The authors further stated that no individual with a fracture-related admission underwent an evaluation for osteoporosis during that hospital stay. In 83 % of patients studied by Akhigbe et al., the presence of a new fracture prompted the need for modified or costly new adaptive equipment in the form of wheelchairs, transfer equipment, or lower limb braces.

Regrettably, the majority of patients examined by Pelletier et al. [26] and Gifre et al. (the 2016 study) failed to receive proper diagnostic workup in the form of a DXA scan subsequent to the fracture. Also, both investigations indicate a sharp discordance between those individuals diagnosed with osteoporosis along with those diagnosed with an SCI-related osteoporotic fracture and the actual number of patients who were referred for and received treatment. For example, the study by Morse et al. [20] indicated that in the year prior to the low-impact fracture, 13 % of patients were taking calcium supplements, 33 % took vitamin D, and 2 % were prescribed bisphosphonates, with no patients on teriparatide. In the first year after the fracture, no substantial changes to prescription medications for osteoporosis were seen. Calcium intake increased to 30 %; vitamin D intake went from 33 % to 38 %; bisphosphonate prescriptions increased from 2 % to 7 %; and no patients were prescribed teriparatide. The above data suggests large numbers of the study sample remained untreated.

Fractures and Their Effects on Quality of Life and Mortality

In the investigation by Pelletier [26], those who experienced a fracture commented on how their overall functioning and activities of daily living have been affected. While 22.6 % reported the fracture affected them "not at all" or "very little," 21.4 % admitted the their life was affected to some extent, while a concerning 56 % declared that fracture affected their life either "completely" or "to a great extent." Other findings indicated that medical complications including increased pain in those with residual feeling, heighted lower extremity spasticity, and muscle contractures causing obliquity and risk of pressure ulcers impacted functional mobility and participation in activities of daily living. Independence is compromised by the above factors. Moreover, if pressure ulcers develop, prolonged bed rest may be needed, leading to further medical complications such as deep vein thrombosis, orthostatic hypotension, and potentially depression [20, 25, 26, 46, 48].

In addition to quality of life, fractures can alter life expectancy. Carbone et al. [48] investigated the mortality associated with lower extremity fracture and determined that the hazard ratio (HR) for all SCI participants was 1.38 (complete and incomplete patients) and 1.46 for SCI veterans of all ages with exclusively complete SCI. However, for older men (≥age 50) with complete SCI, the hazard ratio is significantly higher at 3.13. In contrast, younger men (<age 50) with complete SCI had a comparatively lower HR of 1.71. The above reports indicate that not only the quality of life but also its duration can be impacted by fractures subsequent to SCI-related osteoporosis.

Management of Osteoporotic Fractures

In patients with SCI, the primary goal is fracture prevention. Among those with chronic SCI, 25–49 % ultimately experience a fragility fracture [49, 50]. For patients who are unlikely to ambulate, conservative treatment with a soft splint has given way to more aggressive intervention. Untreated fractures in all sites below the level of spinal cord injury can be complicated by increased spasticity, autonomic dysreflexia, and limb deformity after healing that make transfers more difficult not just during the fracture recovery period but long afterward [51]. Femoral neck fractures heal poorly and are among the most challenging to treat. Healing is complicated by bone instability and migration of the pelvis proximally, causing pelvic obliquity, altered sitting balance, and ultimately ischial pressure ulcer development. Plaster casts have been shown to cause skin breakdown unknown to the patient or vascular compromise [50]. Since pinning often results in nonunion, endoprosthetic replacement is recommended but can be compromised by subluxation for adductor spasticity. If prosthetic replacement seems most beneficial for the patient, the physiatrist may wish to consider inpatient rehabilitation admission after the procedure, specifically to provide spasticity management along with prevention of autonomic dysreflexia. Pressure mapping to prevent pressure ulcers and review of safety with functional mobility, particularly transfers, would be additional goals of a rehabilitation stay.

The proximal tibia and distal femur are the locations with the greatest degree of bone loss from immobilization following spinal cord injury. In a series of nine patients with spinal cord disorders of mixed etiologies, each with at least one lower extremity long bone fracture, Sugi et al. [52] demonstrated superior patient outcomes relative to earlier studies. All nine subjects returned to their prior functional baseline at their final post-op outpatient visit. No participants experienced a perioperative or postoperative complication, including nonunion or infection. Significant improvement in life satisfaction was observed postoperatively, using the spinal cord injury quality of life measure. With the combined effects of an increased life expectancy after SCI and greater fracture incidence in persons over age 55, the cost physically and emotionally to the patient and financially to the patient and healthcare system will rise in the coming years [10–12, 53, 54]. Given the increasing availability of robotic ambulation devices and assisted-walking technologies involving full-body bracing, patients with complete paraplegia may be candidates for a walking program. Participation will be possible only for those subjects with reasonable bone density who have no contraindications of active unstable fractures.

Treatment

Nonpharmacologic Interventions

A number of nonpharmacologic interventions have been explored to prevent and treat bone loss secondary to SCI. Effects of gravity, mechanical and electrical stimulation, and other forms of exercise or positioning are utilized in an effort to improve BMD. Multiple studies have found no significant change in bone density post static weight-bearing (standing frame) [55, 56] or partial body weight-supported treadmill training [57, 58]. Researchers have produced mixed results in their investigations of functional electrical stimulation (FES) [32, 59, 60]. Recent years have shown more promise with the latter modality, but the onset of therapy, in relation to the time from acute SCI, the age and health of the population tested, and the duration of weeks of treatment, has varied, contributing to inconclusive results when a number of studies are taken into account. Table 3 summarizes the results of a number of investigations using FES in patients with acute SCI [61–65].

Table 3 Studies using FES/EMS to improve BMD in acute SCI patients

Source	Modality studied	Number and demographics of patients studied	Outcomes/findings
Arija-Blazquez et al. [61]	Electromyostimulation (EMS) for 47 minutes/day, five days/week	$n=8$, male patients with acute SCI, ASIA A, eight weeks post injury. Control versus EMS	EMS produced no significant difference in bone biomarkers or BMD changes compared to control
Eser et al. [62]	FES cycling Ergometry for 30 minutes, three days/week for duration of rehabilitation (mean six months)	$n=38$, para- and tetraplegic patients 4–5 weeks post injury	Both control and FES showed reduced tibial cortical BMD within 3–10 months. FES did not significantly attenuate bone loss
Clark et al. [63]	Discontinuous FES to lower limb muscles 15 minutes, 2× day, five days/week over five months	$n=23$, SCI (C4-T12) patients (ASIA A-D) FES versus control	FES and control differed significantly at three months but not thereafter
Lai et al. [64]	FES cycling Ergometry for up to 30 minutes, three days/week, three subsequent months	$n=24$ SCI (C5-T8) patients 26–52 days post injury (control vs. FES). Mean age 28 years	BMD decrease rate in distal femur was significantly less in FES group than the control group during first three months. No significant difference after three months
Sheilds et al. [65]	NMES on one leg, other leg as control. Exercise for ≥two years	$n=7$, ASIA A, above T12. SCI injury within six weeks	31 % higher trabecular BMD in trained limbs versus untrained limbs

Pharmacologic Treatment

Initial interventions often involve supplemental calcium and vitamin D, but these measures are insufficient to prevent fractures or enhance bone density in the absence of additional forms of treatment. Multiple investigations have demonstrated that avoidance of calcium in the acute phase following acute SCI is not a risk factor for the development of kidney disease; in fact, in most cases, eliminating or restricting dietary calcium will only predispose patients to additional early bone loss [16].

Thiazide Diuretics

Thiazide diuretics may be a new avenue of prevention of osteoporosis through their mechanism of preventing urinary calcium excretion, therefore promoting increased BMD. A meta-analysis of 21 observational studies, comprising over 400,000 patients with SCI of all severities who were prescribed thiazide diuretics for other medical conditions, showed a 24 % reduction in risk of hip fractures [66]. Carbone et al. [48] examined thiazide use in a 5-year cohort study of 6,969 veterans with varying levels of SCI. Of the 1,433 who used thiazides (HR = 0,750) for medical purposes other than bone preservation, a one-quarter risk reduction was observed, particularly in patients who were also prescribed vitamin D supplements.

Oral Bisphosphonates

Several groups have explored the use of various bisphosphonates for prevention of bone loss in acute and chronic SCI. Zehnder et al. focused on the use of oral alendronate plus calcium and demonstrated that this combination resulted in maintenance of pretreatment BMD, while the group receiving calcium alone had a steady decline in BMD [67]. Another trial found that subjects receiving weekly alendronate administration experience a less notable decline in BMD than those given a placebo [68]. However, giving oral alendronate in the setting immediately following SCI poses a number of challenges. Limitations to achieving an upright posture include postoperative spinal stability precautions, delay in brace fitting needed to maintain stability in sitting position, autonomic effects of orthostasis, and pain. Erosive esophagitis may occur following consumption of oral bisphosphonates, unless patients are able to sit fully upright after administration of medications [67, 68]. Because IV formulations can be administered in the supine position, investigators have explored the use of IV bisphosphonates in the setting of acute SCI.

Intravenous Bisphosphonates

Nance and colleagues conducted one of the first investigations using an IV bisphosphonate, specifically pamidronate, which was given every four weeks for six months. Although BMD improved in incomplete ASIA impairment scale D patients at the end of the trial and marginally improved at the 6-month follow-up in complete SCI patients, benefits were not maintained at one year [69]. These findings were supported by a later study by Bauman et al. [70].

Zoledronic acid (ZA) is an agent in the treatment of osteoporosis for individuals after SCI which works by suppressing activity of the osteoclast. This pharmacologic intervention has been shown to regulate enzyme activity (farnesyl diphosphate synthetase) more effectively than other bisphosphonates and thus produces more robust effects in BMD for the general population [71, 72]. Research has been completed in patients with subacute SCI while further research is ongoing to determine the effectiveness of ZA in those with acute SCI.

Four small investigations have explored the use of ZA in subacute SCI. The first was a double-blind placebo-controlled trial by Shapiro et al. who examined the effect of intravenous (IV) ZA in 17 patients with ASIA impairment grade A or B SCI given at 10–12 weeks post injury [73]. Four subjects received 4 mg IV ZA, four received 5 mg ZA, and the remaining nine received placebo. Both the intertrochanteric region and the cortical shaft in the ZA-treated group maintained BMD near baseline values up to 12 months, while BMD declined in the control group. In contrast, the femoral neck showed an increased BMD from baseline to six months, but fell back to baseline by 12 months in the ZA group.

In the second trial, Bubbear et al. completed a randomized, open-label study of 14 patients with acute SCI, all of whom received either 4 mg IV ZA or standard medical treatment within three months (mean of 58 days of injury) [74]. Neurological levels of participants ranged from C4 to L3 and included 11 complete (five experimental, six control) and three incomplete subjects (two experimental, one control). Twelve months after the study of drug administration, the ZA-treated subjects had significantly higher BMD than the controls in three areas: 3 % for the lumbar spine ($p<0.05$), 12 % for the total hip ($p<0.05$), and 11 % ($p<0.05$) at the greater trochanter. The 5 % increase for the femoral neck was not significant. In the ZA group, BMD at the total hip and greater trochanter was maintained from baseline, but the area of the femoral neck still lost 10 % of the original BMD. In both of the above studies, pharmacologic intervention did not occur until 2–3 months post injury, when a notable amount of bone mass has already been lost. Furthermore, neither study evaluated BMD at the distal femur and proximal tibia, two high-risk areas for sublesional fractures after SCI.

The third investigation was a nonrandomized clinical trial performed in veterans within 16 weeks of SCI [75], six patients received IV ZA while seven received placebo. BMD at the hip and proximal femoral shaft was preserved but not at the distal femur or proximal tibia. This study was however limited by the use of high-dose steroids in 71 % of controls but only in 33 % of treatment subjects. In addition, ASIA grades were heterogeneous among the groups and three patients (two treatment, one control) converted from complete to incomplete SCI during the study. A very recent study by Schnitzer et al. [76] in subacute SCI patients, up to 12 weeks post injury, demonstrated smaller degrees of bone loss at the hip and femoral neck in six patients given ZA, relative to six controls. Less favorable results were seen for BMD at the knee. As with the investigations above, numbers were small. In addition, authors examined a heterogenous SCI population of ASIA Grades of A, B, and C, with outcome assessments at six months.

Monoclonal Antibodies

The first study on the use of the monoclonal antibody, denosumab, specifically in SCI patients, was recently published by Gifre et al. [77] but involved only 14 patients who were 12–18 months post injury, by which time significant amounts of bone have already been lost. In terms of demographics, all subjects were male, mean age 39, NLI C4-8, with 12 classified as ASIA impairment A. Of the remaining two subjects, one was ASIA impairment B and the other C. To enroll in the study, the patients had to have already met the definition of osteoporosis based on outpatient clinical screening by DXA. Although relative to baseline the SCI patients who participated did improve, it is doubtful if they ever came close to recovering their pre-injury bone density. Results did show encouraging gains in the lumbar spine of 7.8 % (although this is an area where bone is not typically lost after SCI) and in the total hip of 2.4 % and in the femoral neck of 3.5 %, following two treatments of denosumab, six months apart. Because this agent can predispose patients to skin and urinary tract infections, administration at this later time could be more acceptable to spine surgeons and treating physicians. The above study suggests denosumab may be a good option for patients who were not treated with other forms of osteoporosis medications in the acute phase of injury.

Parathyroid Hormone

One trial in chronic SCI patients by Gordon et al. [78] published in 2013 examined 12 patients who were treated with robotic-assisted stepping three times a week combined with 20 μg of daily teriparatide for six months, followed by a subsequent six months of teriparatide without robotic therapy. All patients had low bone mass at the outset of the study, but not so low that weight-bearing in a robot was unsafe. Levels of SCI were from C1 to T10 but no information about ASIA grades was provided, other than nonambulatory status. Results at 12 months found that BMD in lumbar spine was numerically but not statistically increased, while no significant changes in BMD at the hip were observed. Since the osteoclastic function is increased acutely but may decline chronically, addition of an anabolic agent seems appropriate theoretically; however this particular trial was unable to demonstrate a benefit in the SCI population. Admittedly, one major drawback of this agent is its form of delivery—a subcuticular daily injection for 1–2 years—which is likely to compromise patient compliance. Secondly, the base cost of teriparatide is nearly $12,000 annually, relative to $1,000–1,200 for annual zoledronic acid.

Future Treatments

At the time of publication of this book, anti-sclerostin antibody agents are still in preclinical trials, but they may represent a potential agent for bone salvage in SCI patients given their combined benefits of anti-catabolic and pro-anabolic actions. A recent publication of preclinical findings in postmenopausal women demonstrated improved gains in the lumbar spine, femoral neck, and total hip [79]. Unfortunately, the same atypical femur fractures seen in oral bisphosphonates have recently been reported by the manufacturer of romosozumab [80]. As noted in earlier chapters, strontium ranelate, currently used in some European countries, is unlikely to be prescribed to SCI patients given the heightened risk of venous thromboembolism or deep vein thrombosis (DVT) with this drug, particularly in patient population.

Finally, participation in clinical trials of FDA-established medications for osteoporosis, without a specific indication for SCI, and involvement in trials of newer agents not yet FDA approved may be precluded in favor of participation in competing drug trials, such as those that are meant to achieve neurorecovery. Many patients find they must choose between competing trials, even at the risk of receiving a placebo. A future goal is to make osteoporosis prevention medications part of "usual and customary care," because these agents are available in hospitals and could be paid for by third parties, without the patient needing to enroll in clinical trials to receive optimal care.

Spina Bifida in Children

Spina bifida, meaning "split spine," is a birth defect characterized by the incomplete development of the brain, spinal cord, and their protective covering known as the meninges. The most common neural defect in the United States, it affects 1,500–2,000 of more than four million children born annually, currently an estimated 166,000 individuals in this country. In the first month of pregnancy, the neural tube—a narrow, hollow tube of ectodermal tissue—begins to develop, eventually evolving into the brain, spinal cord, and nervous system. A malformation in this development results in an incomplete closing at any point along the tube, exposing the spinal cord [81].

Causes and Symptoms

The cause of spina bifida is unknown although it is generally attributed to a combination of inherited, environmental, and nutritional factors. Because low levels of folic acid have been implicated as an underlying factor in the development of spinal bifida, the Centers for Disease Prevention and Control recommend that all women of childbearing age take 0.4 mg of folic acid daily and that those with a previous pregnancy affected by spina bifida take 4.0 mg for 1–3 months before and during the first trimester [82]. However, even if women adhered to this recommendation, some 30 % of spina bifida cases would still occur [83].

Spina bifida is generally divided into three categories, each with specific characteristics and symptoms. These are illustrated in Fig. 4.

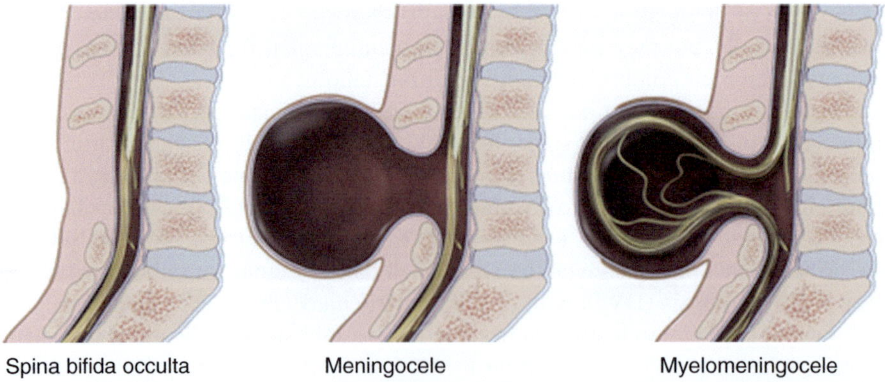

Fig. 4 The anatomic changes that occur in spina bifida occulta, meningocele, and myelomeningocele (*Source*: Courtesy of Centers of Disease Control, Atlanta, Georgia, public domain)

1. Myelomeningocele: The most severe form and the type most often referred to when the term "spina bifida" is used, myelomeningocele is characterized by the presence of a sac of fluid that protrudes through an opening in the child's back and contains damaged parts of the spinal cord and nerves. This form of spina bifida is associated with a Chiari II malformation, a protrusion of the brain stem and cerebellum into the neck or spinal canal which interferes with the flow of cerebrospinal fluid to and from the skull and spinal cord. The result is hydrocephalus, an accumulation of the fluid in and around the brain causing damaging pressure that leads to difficulties in breathing, eating, and swallowing. Hydrocephalus occurs in as many as 90 % of the affected children. Myelomeningocele may also involve a "tethering" or abnormal stretching of the spinal cord, causing nerve impingement and loss of motor and sensory function. Other complications include bowel and urinary incontinence and/or retention, moderate to severe disabilities ranging from paralysis to cognitive problems, learning impairments, deficient physical coordination, and poor language processing.
2. Meningocele: A sac of fluid, sometimes covered by skin, comes through the child's back but contains no parts of the spinal cord and no neural elements. Symptoms range from minor disabilities to serious outcomes including paralysis and bladder and bowel dysfunction.
3. Spina Bifida Occulta ("Hidden" Spina Bifida): The mildest and most common form of the disease, it is identified by a dimple, tuft of hair, or birthmark at the back part of the pelvis, with no opening in the vertebrae and no sac. With few or no neurological symptoms, it may remain undiscovered until later in childhood or even in adulthood [81, 84].

Diagnosis and Treatment

To determine the likelihood of myelomeningocele, a series of tests can be performed during the second trimester of pregnancy. A prenatal maternal serum alpha-fetoprotein (AFP) screening, indicating an usually high level of AFP in the mother, may indicate that she is carrying a child with an open neural tube defect. However, AFP levels alone cannot provide a definitive diagnosis. Recent evidence indicates that the primary screening tool should be an ultrasound of the fetus with the serum AFP level as a secondary screening modality. With its advanced detection sensitivity and safety, ultrasound can screen for multiple congenital anomalies and is not affected by fetal movement. Another diagnostic option, particularly for high-risk pregnancies, is amniocentesis, involving the removal of fluid from the amniotic sac to test for chromosomal abnormalities. Prenatal magnetic resonance imaging (MRI) may also be useful if further assessment of the fetal CNS is needed to inform parents and counselors faced with deciding whether or not to terminate or continue the pregnancy [81, 85].

With no cure, spina bifida is treated primarily with surgery but also with physiotherapy and assistive devices, as well as with medications and procedures to alleviate urinary and bowel incontinence. In children with myelomeningocele, surgery is performed within days of birth to close the defect, protecting the nerves and tissue from trauma and preventing infection. To test the hypothesis that prenatal repair may result in better neurologic function than post-birth repair, a prospective, randomized study compared the children of women who underwent prenatal surgery with those who had standard postnatal repair [86]. In utero surgery improved motor function at 30 months, reduced the need to shunt fluid away from the brain, and increased the possibility that the child could walk without orthotics or devices. However, it was also associated with risk of preterm delivery, uterine dehiscence, and maternal and fetal morbidity. Continued follow-up of the children in the study is needed to assess whether the early benefits will be durable.

In terms of physical activity, the CDC recommends that depending on the severity of the disease, patients should engage in 60 minutes of physical activity daily by playing with friends, engaging in appropriate sports, walking, and undertaking exercises recommended by a physical therapist [87]. The use of assistive devices varies with the location of the defect. In general, those with a defect high on the spine will have more extensive paralysis and require a wheelchair, whereas those with a lower defect may be able to use braces and walkers. In Fig. 5, an illustration of neurological levels of injury, muscles affected, and associated functional deficits is given in relation to risk of osteoporosis and potential adaptive equipment to enhance remaining function.

Osteoporosis in Children with Spina Bifida

Epidemiology of Osteoporosis

Lower extremity motor and sensory loss, decreased ambulation and disuse of lower limbs, and physical inactivity are among the factors underlying the increased risk of fractures and osteoporosis in children with myelomeningocele. Research indicates that low bone density, which correlates with fracture incidence, is prevalent in these children. In a study of 35 patients aged 6–19 years, both ambulatory and nonambulatory, Quan et al. demonstrated that BMD of the distal radius was 1–2 standard deviations below normal, a finding that may explain the higher incidence of bone fractures in these patients. In nonambulators more than ambulators, elevated urinary pyridinoline levels (indicating higher bone resorption) and higher urinary calcium excretion were both present, contributing to decreased BMD in nonambulators. The BMD of the eight patients who developed multiple fractures was significantly lower than in patients without fractures [88]. A subsequent study confirmed that reduced BMD represents a serious threat to children with myelomeningocele, emphasizing

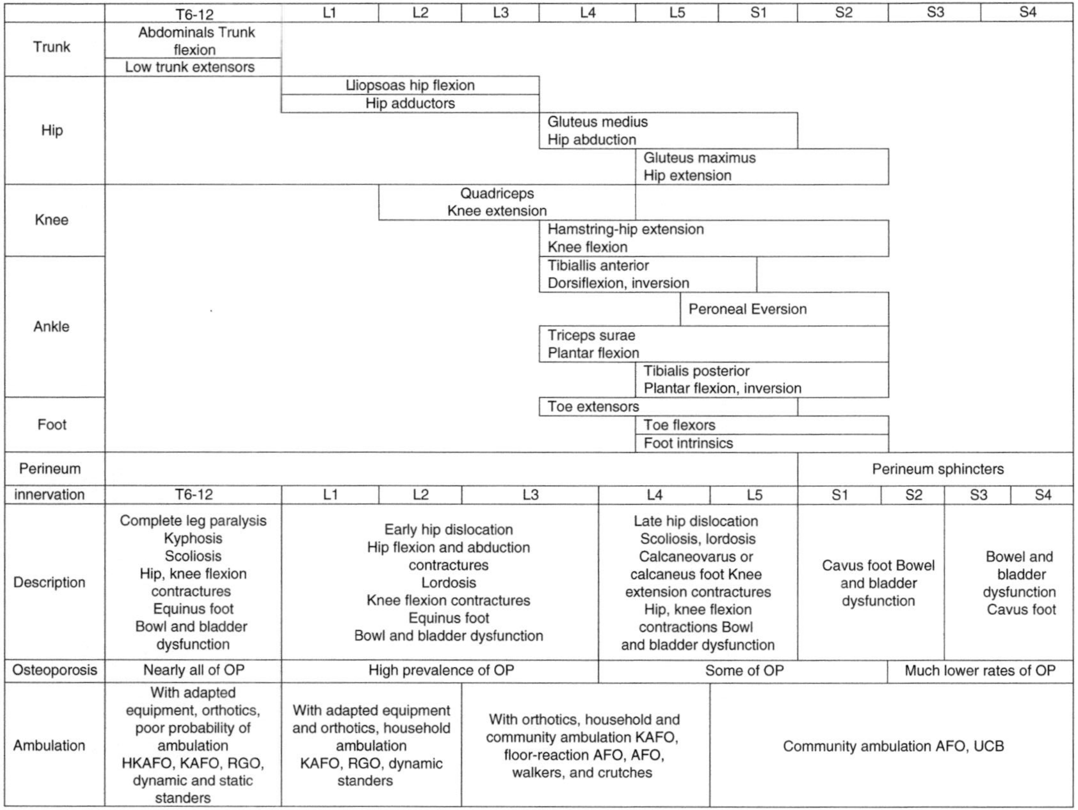

Fig. 5 Segmental innervation in spina bifida in comparison to functional deficits and osteoporosis. In the level of the vertical column, body areas are matched to segmental innervation and the specific muscle groups associated with neurological levels. The mid-lower portion of the figure compares the percentage of patients likely to experience osteoporosis with each neurological level of injury. In the bottom row, potential for ambulation is given with or without assisted devices and lower extremity braces. Abbreviations used: *HKAFO* (hip knee ankle foot orthoses), *KAFO* (knee ankle foot orthoses), *RGO* (reciprocating gait orthoses), *UCB* University of California, Berkeley. UCB is a support for the heel and arch of the foot, used to correct mild ankle pronation

that ambulatory children have significantly better BMD than do those dependent on wheelchairs. In this investigation, no specific relation was found between fracture and reduced BMD [89].

On the basis of a more recent analysis of 37 children with myelomeningocele, researchers reported similar low *Z*-scores as well as one or more fractures among those patients with previous fracture information. The sample size was too small to correlate *Z*-scores with fracture [90]. The fact that these studies do not indicate a direct (as opposed to a possible) association between low BMD and fracture occurrence suggests that treating low BMD may not improve fracture incidence in this population [91].

Epidemiology of Fractures

The incidence of fractures is much greater in children ages 2–10 (23/1,000) and adolescents ages 11–18 (29/1,000) than in adults ages 19–58 (18/1,000) [92]. With the median age of first fracture at 11 years, Dosa et al. have hypothesized that increased physical activity and less supervision, coupled with inexperience or poor judgment, increased fracture rates. The authors felt that the only other factors independently associated with fractures were younger age and higher defect level: 26 % of patients with a thoracic defect level experienced a fracture as opposed to 25 % with a mid-lumbar motor level and 19 % with low-lumbar functional levels. An association among the mechanism of fracture, the type of ambulation, and the level of the lesions was identified by Marreiros et al. Patients with higher levels of neurological injury were confined to wheelchairs and experienced pathological fractures, whereas patients with lesions at the sacral level had no spontaneous fractures [93].

Treatment of Osteoporosis in Children with Spina Bifida

Given the limited number of studies on the nonpharmacological and pharmacological treatment of osteoporosis in children with spina bifida, there is an understandable motivation to extrapolate from treatments proven effective in other childhood disorders. However, the defining characteristics of spina bifida may obviate direct application of such treatments. In physical therapy, for example, any positive effect anticipated through the use of standing frames and vibrating platforms may be negated by the different bone response in children with spina bifida and flaccid paralysis, as opposed to the response seen in children with spastic cerebral palsy [91]. The results of a study to determine whether patients (ages 12–20) with high-level spina bifida (implying NLI in thoracic region) would benefit from early walking led Mazur et al. to conclude that patients who participated in a walking program had fewer fractures, were more independent, and were better able to transfer than those who were wheelchair-dependent at an early age [94].

Intake of calcium and vitamin D should be routinely monitored in spina bifida children with osteoporosis, again taking into account several additional factors associated with the disease. On the basis of an analysis of 166 subjects, Baum et al. reported that 75 % had suboptimal vitamin D (<30 ng/ml): with 40 % vitamin D deficient (<20 ng/ml) and 35 % insufficient (21–30 ng/ml). They further demonstrated that fractures were more common in non-weight-bearing children than in those who were ambulatory and in children with thoracic lesions as compared to lumbar or sacral lesions [95]. Calcium intake must be carefully measured because supplementation can worsen constipation in spina bifida patients as well as increase hypercalcuria which, in turn, exacerbates metabolic calcuria [91]. Calcium carbonate is far more likely to cause constipation than calcium citrate.

The use of bisphosphonates in children with spina bifida is problematic, especially in the absence of trials specifically related to their impact on this population. In two studies of nonambulatory children, only one child with spina bifida was included in each. Steelman et al. [96] showed that intravenous pamidronate was both well tolerated and efficacious, with spinal BMD *Z*-scores increasing in all patients after six months. In a trial involving ten nonambulatory children taking alendronate, Sholas et al. [97] found only one fracture in the follow-up period compared with 17 prior to alendronate treatment. The potential efficacy of bisphosphonates in spina bifida must not only be derived from studies relating to other childhood diseases but must necessarily be tempered by the uncertainty regarding the amount of dosage and the duration of treatment.

Zoledronic acid is contraindicated in children who are still in the growth phase according to prescribing information. Denosumab has similar precautions in some reports but other studies demonstrated safety in small samples of subjects with other conditions, including giant cell tumors [98] and osteogenesis imperfecta [99, 100]. To date, no clinical trials have been done on patients with any form of spina bifida but denosumab offers a potential future form of treatment which is likely to be safe in the pediatric population, given data on other conditions.

Measures to prevent fracture occurrence in myelomeningocele include a regular program of physiotherapy beginning early in life; vertical loading; fall prevention, dividing structured exercise into several sessions of short intervals, and cast immobilization limited to no more than four weeks [101]. Regardless of their efficacy, medications cannot prevent fractures without adjunctive processes.

Spina Bifida in Adults

For spina bifida patients, the circumstances surrounding the transition from pediatric to adult care are analogous to those observed in cerebral palsy: adult specialists with limited knowledge and interest in caring for this population, failure to review the original diagnosis and current medications, the reluctance of parents to relinquish their “caring” role, and, in general, the lack of preparation to ensure a coordinated, effective transfer from one healthcare system to another. Increasingly, patients are referred to spinal cord injury physiatrists who are potentially better equipped to treat the neurogenic bowel and bladder issues and functional mobility challenges, but may not recognize the retained pediatric aspects of spina bifida. In addition, lifetime caregivers are often not aware of the high mortality rate for individuals born with open myelomeningocele.

In 2009, a cohort study of 117 patients in the United Kingdom with mean age of 40 revealed that 40/117 died before the age of five; another 31/117 died during the following 35 years, over ten times the average for the normal population. The 39 % who remained alive were the least severely affected at birth. The most frequent causes of death after age five were acute hydrocephalus, renal sepsis, pulmonary embolus, and epileptic seizures [102].

Although advances in treatment and relevant technologies may result in improved numbers, patients continue to face a series of medical and rehabilitative challenges. For example, after years of operating without symptoms, shunts to control hydrocephalus may fail due to blockage or infection, requiring replacement; a missed diagnosis can result in chronic morbidity or death. Shunt failure most commonly occurs in the first year after insertion, but it has been observed up to 20 years later when patients are no longer continually monitored for this complication. In their study of shunt malfunction in 110 adults, Tomlinson and Sugarman observed that only 40 % of the cohort underwent regular review, including an assessment of shunt function [103].

Two other complications of spina bifida—Chiari brainstem compression and spinal cord tethering—may be related to shunt failure [104]. Scoliosis, premature arthritis, decreased mobility, obesity, and renal failure (now significantly reduced through the use of clean intermittent bladder catheterization) are further issues confronting adults with spina bifida. These issues underline the need for improved, multidisciplinary healthcare networks for an aging population as well as increased patient responsibility for periodic review of anticipated and unanticipated medical problems.

Osteoporosis in Adults with Spina Bifida

As Valtonen et al. have revealed, early-onset osteoporosis occurs in almost 50 % of adults with spina bifida, primarily between ages 20 and 40 [105]. The assumption is that patients with myelomeningocele will exhibit osteoporosis at a younger age, given their impaired walking ability and reduced physical activity. Another known risk factor for osteoporosis is renal failure resulting from neurogenic bladder dysfunction. Because urinary diversion surgery, once commonly used to treat renal dysfunction, can also cause acidosis and osteoporosis, it has been replaced by bladder augmentation, now regarded as the cornerstone of surgical management of this condition in spina bifida patients [106]. Medications for epilepsy may also contribute to the development of osteoporosis. An examination of 71 ambulatory patients (42 adults, 29 children and adolescents) on anticonvulsant therapy for six months demonstrated that BMD decreased in the adults and that 50 % of the subjects in both groups had low levels of vitamin D25-OH [107]. Finally, oral cortisone treatment for more than three months is yet another risk factor.

Fractures in Adults with Spina Bifida

Fracture prevention is among the major goals of spina bifida patients dealing with osteoporosis. With an incidence rate of 18/1,000 as opposed to 29/1,000 for adolescents, fractures in adults are independently associated only with age and level of defect. In a trial involving 109 adults ages 19–58 with spina bifida, Dosa et al. reported that 8/31 patients with thoracic defect level experienced a fracture, compared with 20/81 patients with mid-lumbar motor defect level and 15/79 patients with low-lumbar motor levels [92]. Fractures were generally attributed to accidental falls and to incidents linked to exercise/physical therapy. These adults with spina bifida may be protected from fractures by better transfer techniques, greater awareness of their physical limitations, and a sedentary lifestyle. Further research, particularly longitudinal studies, on the development of osteoporosis and fracture occurrence is needed to better understand and assess the underlying factors and treatment options in adult osteoporosis with myelomeningocele.

Treatment of Osteoporosis in Adult Spina Bifida

The Valtonen et al. analysis of the *T*-scores for BMD in 21 adults (mean age = 30) with meningomyelocele revealed that three patients had osteopenia and two had osteoporosis at the lumbar spine; 7 of 15 subjects, who could be reliably measured, had osteoporosis in the femoral neck or trochanteric region of the hip. Although the trial was based on the hypothesis that ambulation and physical activity would promote higher BMD, it revealed instead that ambulation alone showed only a "tendency" to result in lower BMD. In contrast, the medical risk factors noted above were shown to decrease BMD at the femoral neck and trochanteric hip region with this effect being stronger in non-ambulators than in ambulators. Regular screening of BMD is recommended [105].

Few treatment options for patients with meningomyelocele and osteoporosis have been identified. Calcium and vitamin D supplementation may exacerbate constipation and nephrolithiasis; given its ability to reduce urinary calcium excretion, hydrochlorothiazide may be a potential treatment option. Table 4 outlines the differences in treatment for spina bifida and related bone disease in adults versus children [87–89, 95, 97, 99, 100, 105]. The effect of standing is unclear and the presence of gastroesophageal reflux in some patients may preclude the use of bisphosphonates. The positive effect of bisphosphonate treatment in CP and SCI patients with osteoporosis indicates that similar results may be possible in adult spina bifida [105].

Table 4 Treatment differences for spina bifida and related bone disease in adults versus children

Treatment	Adults vs. children
Calcium + vitamin D supplementation [87–89, 95]	Adults
	Children
Oral alendronate [97, 105]	Adults: approved but tolerance is limited by GI side effects
	Children: one study demonstrated efficacy but concerns raised regarding safe dosages and duration of treatment
Intravenous pamidronate [96]	Adults: treatment approved but showing limited efficacy
	Children: well tolerated with one study showing benefit after six months. Similar concerns regarding safety as above
Intravenous zoledronic acid	Adults: no publications dedicated to adults with spina bifida
	Children: contraindicated in children who are still growing. No publications
Subcutaneous denosumab [99, 100]	Adults: no trials in adults with spina bifida as of this publication
	Children: no studies in children with spina bifida but efficacy demonstrated in other pediatric disorders

Sources: Centers for Disease Control [87], Quan et al. [88], Apkon et al. [89], Baum et al. [95], Steelman et al. [96], Sholas et al. [97], Yamashita [99], Grasemann et al. [100], and Valtonen et al. [105]

References

1. Garland DE, Stewart CA, Adkins RH, et al. Osteoporosis after spinal cord injury. J Orthop Res. 1992;10(3):371–8.
2. SCI National Statistical Center. Spinal cord injury facts and figures at a glance. J Spinal Cord Med. 2015;39(3):370–1.
3. American Spinal Injury Association. The international standards for the classification of spinal cord injury, examination sheet. 2015. http://asia-spinalinjury.org/wp-content/uploads/2016/02/International_Std. Accessed 5 Jun 2016.
4. Chantraine A, Heynen G, Franchimont P. Bone metabolism, parathyroid hormone, and calcitonin in paraplegia. Calcif Tissue Int. 1979;27(3):199–204.
5. Reiter AL, Volk A, Vollmar J, Fromm B, Gerner HJ. Changes of basic bone turnover parameters in short-term and long-term patients with spinal cord injury. Eur Spine J. 2007;16(6): 771–6.
6. Eser P, Frotzler A, Zehnder Y, Denoth J. Fracture threshold in the femur and tibia of people with spinal cord injury as determined by peripheral quantitative computed tomography. Arch Phys Med Rehabil. 2005;86(3):498–504.
7. Shields RK, Dudley-Javoroski S, Boaldin KM, Corey TA, Fog DB, Ruen JM. Peripheral quantitative computed tomography: measurement sensitivity in persons with and without spinal cord injury. Arch Phys Med Rehabil. 2006;87(10):1376–81.
8. Biering-Sorensen F, Bohr H, Schaadt O. Bone mineral content of the lumbar spine and lower extremities years after spinal cord lesion. Paraplegia. 1988;26(5):293–301.
9. Roberts D, Lee W, Cuneo RC, et al. Longitudinal study of bone turnover after acute spinal cord injury. J Clin Endocrinol Metab. 1998;83(2):415–22.
10. Galea MP. Spinal cord injury and physical activity: preservation of the body. Spinal Cord. 2012;50(5):344–51.
11. Biering-Sorensen F, Hansen B, Lee BSB. Non-pharmacological treatment and prevention of bone loss after spinal cord injury: a systematic review. Spinal Cord. 2009;47(7):508–18.
12. Fattal C, Mariano-Goulart D, Thomas E, Rouays-Mabit H, Verollet C, Maimoun L. Osteoporosis in persons with spinal cord injury: the need for a targeted therapeutic education. Arch Phys Med Rehabil. 2011;92(1):59–67.

13. Minaire P, Neunier P, Edouard C, Bernard J, Courpron P, Bourret J. Quantitative histological data on disuse osteoporosis: comparison with biological data. Calcif Tissue Res. 1974;17(1):57–73.
14. Craven BC, Robertson LA, McGillivray CF, Adachi JD. Detection and treatment of sublesional osteoporosis among patients with chronic spinal cord injury: proposed paradigms. Top Spinal Cord Inj Rehabil. 2009;14(4):1–22.
15. Dauty M, Perrouin Verbe B, Maugars Y, Dubois C, Mathe JF. Supralesional and sublesional bone mineral density in spinal cord injured patients. Bone. 2000;27(2):305–9.
16. Bauman WA, Cardozo CP. Osteoporosis in individuals with spinal cord injury. PM R. 2015;7(2):188–201.
17. Vico L, Collet P, Guignandon A, Lafage-Proust MH, Thomas T, Rehaillia M, et al. Effects of long-term microgravity exposure on cancellous and cortical weight-bearing bones of astronauts. Lancet. 2000;355(9215):1607–11.
18. Leblanc AD, Schneider VS, Evans HJ, Engelbretson DA, Krebs JM. Bone mineral loss and recovery after 17 weeks of bed rest. J Bone Miner Res. 1990;5(8):843–50.
19. Ashe MC, Craven C, Krassioukov A, Eng JJ. Bone health following spinal cord injury. Spinal Cord Inj Rehabil Evid. 2007;9:61–9.
20. Morse LR, Battaglino RA, Stolzmann KL, Hallett LD, Waddimba A, Gagnon D, et al. Osteoporotic fractures and hospitalization risk in chronic spinal cord injury. Osteoporos Int. 2009;20(3):385–92.
21. Garland DE, Adkins RH, Kushwaha V, Stewart C. Risk factors for osteoporosis at the knee in the spinal cord injury population. J Spinal Cord Med. 2004;27(3):202–6.
22. Zehnder Y, Luthi M, Michel D, et al. Long-term changes in bone metabolism, bone mineral density, quantitative ultrasound parameters, and fracture incidence after spinal cord injury: a cross-sectional observational study in 100 paraplegic men. Osteoporos Int. 2004;15(3):180–9.
23. Frisbie JH. Fractures after myelopathy: the risk quantified. J Spinal Cord Med. 1997;20(1):66–9.
24. Garland DE, Adkins RH, Stewart CA, Ashford R, Vigil D. Regional osteoporosis in women who have a complete spinal cord injury. J Bone Joint Surg Am. 2001;83-A(8):1195–200.
25. Gifre L, Vidal J, Carrasco JL, Muxi A, Portell E, Monegal A, et al. Risk factors for the development of osteoporosis after spinal cord injury: a 12-month follow-up study. Osteopath Int. 2015;26(9):2273–80.
26. Pelletier CA, Dumont FS, Leblond J, Noreau L, Giangregorio L, Craven BC. Self-report of one-year fracture incidence of osteoporosis prevalence in a community cohort of Canadians with spinal cord injury. Top Spinal Cord Inj Rehabil. 2014;20(4):302–9.
27. Hammond ER, Metcalf HM, McDonald JW, Sadowsky CL. Bone mass in individuals with chronic spinal cord injury: associations with activity based therapy, neurologic and functional status, a retrospective study. Arch Phys Med Rehabil. 2014;95(2):2342–9.
28. Lazo MG, Shirazi P, Sam M, Giobbie-Hurder A, Blacconiere MJ, Muppidi M. Osteoporosis and risk of fracture in men with spinal cord injury. Spinal Cord. 2001;39(4):208–14.
29. Shojaei H, Soroush MR, Modirian E. Spinal cord injury-induced osteoporosis in veterans. J Spinal Disord Tech. 2006;19(2):114–7.
30. Biering-Sorensen F, Bohr HH, Schaadt OP. Longitudinal study of bone mineral content in the lumbar spine, the forearm and the lower extremities after spinal cord injury. Eur J Clin Invest. 1990;20(3):330–5.
31. Garland DE, Adkins RH, Scott M, Singh H, Massih M, Stewart C. Bone loss at the os calcis compared with bone loss at the knee in individuals with spinal cord injury. J Spinal Cord Med. 2004;27(3):207–11.
32. Uebelhart D, Hartmann D, Vuagnat H, Castanier M, Hachen HJ, Chantraine A. Early modifications of biochemical markers of bone metabolism in spinal cord injury patients. A preliminary study. Scand J Rehabil Med. 1994;26(4):197–202.
33. Warden SJ, Bennell KL, Matthews B, Brown DJ, McMeeken JM, Wark JD. Quantitative ultrasound assessment of acute bone loss following spinal cord injury: a longitudinal pilot study. Osteoporos Int. 2002;13(7):586–92.

34. Finsen V, Indredavik B, Fougner KJ. Bone mineral and hormone status in paraplegics. Paraplegia. 1992;30(5):343–7.
35. Jones LM, Legge M, Goulding A. Intensive exercise may preserve bone mass of the upper limbs in spinal cord injured males but does not retard demineralisation of the lower body. Spinal Cord. 2002;40(5):230–5.
36. Jiang SD, Dai LY, Jiang LS. Osteoporosis after spinal cord injury. Osteoporos Int. 2006;17(2):180–92. doi:10.1007/s00198-005-2028-8.
37. Bauman WA, You-Gon Z, Schwartz E. Vitamin D deficiency in veterans with chronic spinal cord injury. Metabolism. 1995;44(12):1612–6.
38. Vaziri ND, Pandian MR, Segal JL, Winer RL, Eltorai I, Brunnemann S. Vitamin D, parathormone, and calcitonin profiles in persons with long-standing spinal cord injury. Arch Phys Med Rehabil. 1994;75(7):766–9.
39. Oleson CV, Patel PH, Wuermser LA. Influence of season, ethnicity, and chronicity on vitamin D deficiency in traumatic spinal cord injury. J Spinal Cord Med. 2010;33(3):202–13.
40. Heaney RP, Abrams S, Dawson-Hughes B, Looker A, Marcus R, Matkovic V, Weaver C. Peak bone mass. Osteoporos Int. 2000;11(12):985–1009.
41. Heaney RP. Lessons for nutritional science from vitamin D. Am J Clin Nutr. 1999;69(5):825–6.
42. Holick MF. Vitamin D: the underappreciated D-lightful hormone that is important for skeletal and cellular health. Curr Opin Endocrinol Diabetes. 2002;9:87–98.
43. Holick MF. Environmental factors that influence the cutaneous production of vitamin D. Am J Clin Nutr. 1995;61 Suppl 3:638S–45.
44. NOAA's National Weather Service. Network for detection of atmospheric composition change. http://www.ndsc.ncep.noaa.gov/UVSpect_web/Health. Accessed 10 May 2016.
45. Holick MF. Sunlight and vitamin D for bone health and prevention of autoimmune diseases, cancers, and cardiovascular disease. Am J Clin Nutr. 2004;80 Suppl 6:1678S–88.
46. Akhigbe T, Chin AS, Svircev JN, Hoenig H, Burns SP, Weaver FM, et al. A retrospective review of lower extremity fracture care in patients with spinal cord injury. J Spinal Cord Med. 2014;38(1):2–9.
47. Garland DE, Adkins RH, Stewart CA. Fracture threshold and risk for osteoporosis and pathologic fractures in individuals with spinal cord injury. Top Spinal Cord Inj Rehabil. 2005;11(1):61–9.
48. Carbone LD, Chin AS, Burns SP, Svircev JN, Hoenig H, Heggeness M, et al. Mortality after lower extremity fractures in men with spinal cord injury. J Bone Miner Res. 2014;29(2):432–9.
49. McClung M, Geusen P, Miller P, et al. Effect of risedronate on the risk of hip fracture in elderly women. N Engl J Med. 2001;344(5):333–40.
50. Lombardi Jr I, Leda MO, Monterio CR, Confessor YQ, Barros TL, Natour J. Evaluation of physical capacity and quality of life in osteoporotic women. Osteoporos Int. 2004;15(1):80–5.
51. Sobel M, Lyden JP. Long bone fracture in a spinal-cord-injured patient: complication of treatment – a case report and review of the literature. J Trauma. 1991;31(10):1440–4.
52. Sugi MT, Davidovitch R, Montero N, Nobel T, Egol KA. Treatment of lower-extremity long-bone fractures in active, nonambulatory, wheelchair-bound patients. Orthopedics. 2012;35(9):e1376–82.
53. Vestergaard P, Krogh K, Rejnmark L, Mosekilde L. Fracture rates and risk factors for fractures in patients with spinal cord injury. Spinal Cord. 1998;36(11):790–6.
54. Comarr AE, Hutchinson RH, Bors E. Extremity fractures of patients with spinal cord injuries. Top Spinal Cord Inj Rehabil. 2005;11(1):1–10.
55. Dudley-Javoroski S, Shields RK. Muscle and bone plasticity after spinal cord injury: review of adaptations to disuse and to electrical muscle stimulation. J Rehabil Res Dev. 2008;45(2):283–96.
56. Qin W, Bauman W, Cardozo C. Bone and muscle loss after spinal cord injury: organ interactions. Ann N Y Acad Sci. 2010;1211:66–84.

57. Coupaud S, Jack LP, Hunt KJ, Allan DB. Muscle and bone adaptations after treadmill training increase bone mass and reverse muscle atrophy in incomplete spinal cord injury: a case study using peripheral quantitative computed tomography. J Musculoskelet Neuronal Interact. 2009;9(4):288–97.
58. Giangregorio LM, Webber CE, Phillips SM, Hicks AL, Craven BC, Bugaresti JM, et al. Can body weight supported treadmill training increase bone mass and reverse muscle atrophy in individuals with chronic incomplete spinal cord injury? Appl Physiol Nutr Metab. 2006;31(3):283–91.
59. Kunkel CF, Scremin AM, Eisenberg B, Garcia JF, Roberts S, Martinez S. Effect of "standing" on spasticity, contracture, and osteoporosis in paralyzed males. Arch Phys Med Rehabil. 1993;74(1):73–8.
60. Garland DE, Adkins RH, Matsuno NN, Stewart CA. The effect of pulsed electromagnetic fields on osteoporosis at the knee in individuals with spinal cord injury. J Spinal Cord Med. 1999;22(4):239–45.
61. Arija-Blázquez A, Ceruelo-Abajo S, Díaz-Merino M, Godino-Durán J, Martínez-Dhier L, Martin JL, et al. Effects of electromyostimulation on muscle and bone in men with acute traumatic spinal cord injury: a randomized clinical trial. J Spinal Cord Med. 2014;37(3):299–309. doi:10.1179/2045772313Y.0000000142.
62. Eser P, de Bruin ED, Telley I, Lechner HE, Knecht H, Stussi E. Effect of electrical stimulation-induced cycling on bone mineral density in spinal cord-injured patients. Eur J Clin Invest. 2003;33(4):412–9.
63. Clark JM, Jelbart M, Rischbieth H, Strayer J, Chatterton B, Schultz C, et al. Physiological effects of lower extremity functional electrical stimulation in early spinal cord injury: lack of efficacy to prevent bone loss. Spinal Cord. 2007;45(1):78–85.
64. Lai CH, Chang WH, Chan WP, Peng CW, Shen LK, Chen JJ, et al. Effects of functional electrical stimulation cycling exercise on bone mineral density loss in the early stages of spinal cord injury. J Rehabil Med. 2010;42(2):150–4. doi:10.2340/15401977-0499.
65. Shields RK, Dudley-Javoroski S. Musculoskeletal plasticity after acute spinal cord injury: effects of long-term neuromuscular electrical stimulation training. J Neurophysiol. 2006;95(4):2380–90.
66. Aung K, Htay T. Thiazide diuretics and the risk of hip fracture. Cochrane Database Syst Rev. 2011;5(10):CD005185. doi:10.1002/14651858.CD005185.pub2.
67. Zehnder Y, Risi S, Michel D, et al. Prevention of bone loss in paraplegics over 2 years with alendronate. J Bone Miner Res. 2004;19(7):1067–74.
68. Gilchrist NL, Frampton CM, Acland RH, et al. Alendronate prevents bone loss in patients with acute spinal cord injury: a randomized, double-blind, placebo-controlled study. J Clin Endocrinol Metabol. 2007;92(4):1385–90.
69. Nance PW, Schryvers O, Leslie W, Ludwig S, Krahn J, Uebelhart D. Intravenous pamidronate attenuates bone density loss after acute spinal cord injury. Arch Phys Med Rehabil. 1999;80(3):243–51.
70. Bauman WA, Wecht JM, Kirshblum S, Spungen AM, Morrison N, Cirnigliaro C, et al. Effect of pamidronate administration on bone in patients with acute spinal cord injury. J Rehabil Res Dev. 2005;42(3):305–13.
71. Dunford JE, Thompson K, Coxon FP, et al. Structure-activity relationships for inhibition of farnesyl diphosphate synthase in vitro and inhibition of bone resorption in vivo by nitrogen-containing bisphosphonates. J Pharmacol Exp Ther. 2001;296(2):235–42.
72. Coxon FP, Helfrich MH, Van't Hof R, et al. Protein geranylgeranylation is required for osteoclast formation, function, and survival: inhibition by bisphosphonates and GGTI-298. J Bone Miner Res. 2000;15(8):1467–76.
73. Shapiro J, Smith B, Beck T, Ballard P, Dapthary M, BrintzenhofeSzoc K, Caminis J. Treatment with zoledronic acid ameliorates negative geometric changes in the proximal femur following acute spinal cord injury. Calcif Tissue Int. 2007;80(5):316–22.
74. Bubbear JS, Gall A, Meddleton FR, Ferguson-Pell M, Swaminathan R, Keen RW. Early treatment with zoledronic acid prevents bone loss at the hip following acute spinal cord injury. Osteoporos Int. 2011;22(1):271–9.

75. Bauman WA, Cirnigliaro C, LaFountaine MF, Martinez L, Kirshblum S, Spungen AM. Zoledronic acid administration failed to prevent bone loss at the knee in persons with SCI. J Bone Miner Metab. 2015;33(4):410–21.
76. Schnitzer TJ, Kim K, Marks J, Yeasted R, Simonian N, Chen D. Zoledronic acid treatment after acute spinal cord injury: results of a randomized, placebo-controlled pilot trial. PM R. 2016;8(9):831–43.
77. Gifre L, Vidal J, Carrasco JL, Muxi A, Portell E, Monegal A, et al. Denosumab increases sublesional bone mass in osteoporotic individuals with recent spinal cord injury. Osteoporos Int. 2016;27(1):405–10.
78. Gordon KE, Wald MJ, Schnitzer TJ. Effect of parathyroid hormone combined with gait training on bone density and bone architecture in people with chronic spinal cord injury. PM R. 2013;5(8):663–71.
79. McClung MR, Grauer A, Boonen, Bolognese MA, Brown JP, Diaz-Perez A, et al. Romosozumab in postmenopausal women with low bone mineral density. N Engl J Med. 2014;370(5):412–20.
80. Amgen press release. http://www.amgen.com/media/news-releases/2016/02/amgen-and-ucb-announce-positive-top-line-results-from-the-phase-3-study-of-romosozumab-in-postmenopausal-women-with-osteoporosis/. Accessed 15 Jun 2016.
81. National Institute of Neurological Disorders and Stroke. Spina bifida fact sheet. http://www.ninds.nih.gov/disorders/spina_bifida/detail_spina_bifida.htm. Accessed 23 Nov 2015.
82. Centers for Disease Control. Effectiveness in disease and injury prevention use of folic acid for prevention of spina bifida and other neural tube defects – 1983–1991. MMWR Wkly. 1991;40(30):513–6.
83. Brei T, Payne C, Worley G. A guide for medical professionals. Spina Bifida Association National Resource Center: 800-621-3141. http://spinabifidaasssociation.org/infosheets/a-guide-for-medical-proessionals. Accessed 23 Nov 2015.
84. National Center on Birth Defects and Developmental Disabilities, Centers for Disease Control and Prevention. Spina Bifida Facts. 2015. http://www.cdc.giv/ncbddd/spinbifida/facts/htm. Accessed 28 Nov 2015.
85. Wilson RD, SOGC Genetics Committee, Wilson RD, Audibert F, Brock JA, Campagnolo C, et al. Prenatal screening, diagnosis, and pregnancy management of fetal neural tube defects: SOGC clinical practice guideline. J Obstet Gynaecol Can. 2014;36(10):927–42.
86. Adzick NS, Thorn EA, Spong CY, Brock III JW, Burrows PK, Johnson MP, et al. A randomized trial of prenatal versus postnatal repair of myelomeningocele. N Engl J Med. 2011;364(11):993–1004.
87. National Center on Birth Defects and Developmental Disabilities, Centers for Disease Control and Prevention. Spina bifida: health issues & treatments. 2014/2015. http://www.cdc.gov/nncbddd/spinabifida/treatment.html.
88. Quan A, Adams R, Ekmark E, Baum M. Bone mineral density in children with myelomeningocele. Pediatrics. 1998;34(102):e34.
89. Apkon SD, Fenton L, Coll JR. Bone mineral density in children with myelomeningocele. Dev Med Child Neurol. 2008;51(1):63–7.
90. Szalay EA, Cheema A. Children with spina bifida are at risk of low bone density. Clin Orthop Relat Res. 2011;469(5):1253–7.
91. Marreiros HF, Loff C, Calado E. Osteoporosis in paediatric patients with spina bifida. J Spinal Cord Med. 2012;35(1):9–21. doi:10.1179/2045772311Y.0000000042.
92. Dosa NP, Eckrich M, Katz DA, Urk M, Liptak GS. Incidence, prevalence and characteristics of fractures in children, adolescents, and adults with spina bifida. J Spinal Cord Med. 2007;30 Suppl 1:S5–9.
93. Marreiros H, Monteiro L, Loff C, Calado E. Fractures in children and adolescents with spina bifida: the experience of a Portuguese tertiary-care hospital. Dev Med Child Neurol. 2010;52(8):754–9.
94. Mazur JM, Shurtieff D, Menelaus M, Colliver J. Orthopaedic management of high-level spina bifida. Early walking compared with early use of a wheelchair. J Bone Joint Surg Am. 1989;71(1):56–61.

95. Baum M, Stein D, Feldman H, Hobbs N, Gordon C. Vitamin D deficiency in children with spina bifida. Conference presentation at the Second World Congress on Spina Bifida Research and Care 2012. 2012. Las Vegas.
96. Steelman J, Zeitler P. Treatment of symptomatic pediatric osteoporosis with cyclic single-day intravenous pamidronate infusions. J Pediatr. 2003;142(4):417–23.
97. Sholas MG, Tann B, Gaebler-Spira D. Oral bisphosphonates to treat disuse osteopenia in children with disabilities: a case study. J Pediatr Orthop. 2005;25(3):326–31.
98. Federman N, Brien EW, Narasimhan V, Dry SM, Sodhi M, Chawla SP. Giant cell tumor of bone in childhood: clinical aspects and novel therapeutic targets. Paediatr Drugs. 2014;16(1):21–8. doi:10.1007/s40272-013-0051-3.
99. Yamashita S. Bone and joint diseases in children. Bisphosphonates in osteogenesis imperfecta. Clin Calcium. 2010;20(6):918–24. doi: CliCa1006918924.
100. Grasemann C, Schundein MM, Hovel M, Schweiger B, Bergmann C, Herrmann R, et al. Effects of RANK-ligand antibody (denosumab) treatment on bone turnover markers in a girl with Juvenile Paget's disease. J Clin Endocrinol Metab. 2013;98(8):3121–6.
101. Akbar M, Bresch B, Raiss P, Furstenberg CH, Bruckner T, Seyler T, et al. Fractures in myelomeningocele. J Orthop Traumatol. 2010;11(3):175–82.
102. Oakeshott P, Hunt GM, Poulton A, Reid F. Expectation of life and unexpected death in open spina bifida: a 40 year complete, non-selective, longitudinal cohort study. Dev Med Child Neurol. 2010;53(8):749–53.
103. Tomlinson P, Sugarman ID. Complications with shunts in spina bifida. BMJ. 1995;311(7000):286–7.
104. Brei T, Merkens M. Health care issues for adults with spina bifida Presented at the 2003 Evidence-Based Practice in Spina bifida Conference. 2003. http://www.spinabifidasupport.com/adultsbhealthcare.htm. Accessed 1 Dec 2015.
105. Valtonen KM, Goksor LA, Jonsson O, Mellstrom D, Alaranta HT, Viikari-Juntura ER. Osteoporosis in adults with meningomyelocele: an unrecognized problem at rehabilitation clinics. Arch Phys Med Rehabil. 2006;87(12):376–82.
106. Wiener JS, Antonelli J, Shea AM, Curtis LH, Schulman KA, Krupski TL, et al. Bladder augmentation versus urinary diversion in patients with spina bifida in the United States. J Urol. 2011;186(1):161–5.
107. Farhat G, Yamout B, Mikati MA, Demirjian S, Sawaya R, El-Haji Fuleihan G. Effect of antiepileptic drugs on bone density in ambulatory patients. Neurology. 2002;58(9):1348–53.

Chapter 10
Osteoporosis in Multiple Sclerosis

Christina V. Oleson

Multiple sclerosis (MS) is an inflammatory disorder of the central nervous system involving lymphocytes that damage myelin and axons, a process resulting in sensory, motor, and eventual cognitive deficits. This condition results in weakness, increased falls, and in advanced stages interferes with awareness and both motor planning and proprioception. Osteoporosis and fall risk are significantly increased in multiple sclerosis. This chapter will discuss the etiology and pathogenesis of MS, describe the different forms of the disorder, and outline approaches to pharmacologic treatment, as well as physical, psychological, and cognitive rehabilitation.

There are four basic types of multiple sclerosis: relapsing remitting, secondary progressive, primary progressive, and progressive relapsing. Relapsing-remitting multiple sclerosis (RRMS) and secondary progressive multiple sclerosis (SPMS) forms constitute 85 % of cases and are predominantly seen in females (Table 1 and Fig. 1) [1, 2]. In contrast, primary progressive multiple sclerosis (PPMS), characterized by a continual decline without remissions and exacerbations, represents only 10 % of the cases and is seen in equal numbers of males and females. The least common form of MS, representing only 5 % of total cases, is termed progressive-relapsing multiple sclerosis (PRMS). Because PRMS combines steady progression of the disease with occasional exacerbations, it can be difficult to distinguish from PPMS [3, 4].

A number of factors contribute to bone loss and bone abnormalities in multiple sclerosis: decreased physical functioning, fall risk leading to fear of mobility, pain or excessive fatigue, biochemical and autoimmune factors, suboptimal nutrition particularly low vitamin D, and adverse effects of medications such as corticosteroids and antiepileptic agents. Falls remain a primary concern in terms of discouraging a patient from mobilizing due to limited help or apprehensiveness; they also directly contribute to fractures in MS patients. A number of medications have been studied to assist with osteoporosis in MS and MS variants. This chapter will consider each of the above points and will propose functional and pharmacological strategies for osteoporosis management in the patient with MS. Finally, we will propose a

C.V. Oleson, *Osteoporosis Rehabilitation*, DOI 10.1007/978-3-319-45084-1_10

Table 1 The four types of multiple sclerosis

	Prevalence	Gender preferences	Clinical features
Relapsing-remitting multiple sclerosis (RRMS)	In combination with SPMS, constitutes **85** % of all cases	Predominantly seen in females	Characterized by paroxysmal attacks (relapses, flare-ups, or exacerbations) of worsening neurologic function, with a return to prior baseline function or with residual deficit upon recovery which can be somewhat worse than baseline
Secondary progressive multiple sclerosis (SPMS)	In combination with RRMS, constitutes **85** % of all cases	Predominantly seen in females	Begins similarly to an RRMS course but with progression at a variable rate which also includes occasional relapses and minor remissions
Primary progressive multiple sclerosis (PPMS)	**10** % of all cases	Equally affects both males and females	Characterized by a continual decline without remissions and exacerbations. Can have occasional plateaus with temporary, minor improvements
Progressive-relapsing multiple sclerosis (PRMS)	**5** % of all cases	Equally affects both males and females	Combines steady progression of the disease with occasional exacerbations and remissions

Source: Campagnolo and Vollmen [1], National MS Society [2]

strategy for timely assessment and early management of osteoporosis due to MS that can be initiated during inpatient rehabilitation and continued in either long-term inpatient care or in a community setting.

Risk Factors for Bone Loss

Physical Factors

The severity of motor, sensory, bowel, bladder, and cognitive deficits is more advanced in secondary progressive and primary progressive forms of the disease relative to relapsing-remitting MS. An individual's level of function can be described using the Kurtzke Expanded Disability Status Scale (EDSS) [5]. Ranging from 1–10 in increments of 0.5, the scale describes the relative functional deficits of patients and classifies their ability to perform daily tasks with and without needed support in the form of adaptive equipment (Table 2) [6]. Because persons with EDSS scores above 6.5 have limited mobility, they are necessarily at increased risk of developing osteoporosis. Limited mobility and weight-bearing on the lower extremities mean less frequent mechanical loading of bone, thereby attenuating the activity of the bone-building osteoblastic cells. As a result, less bone is laid down.

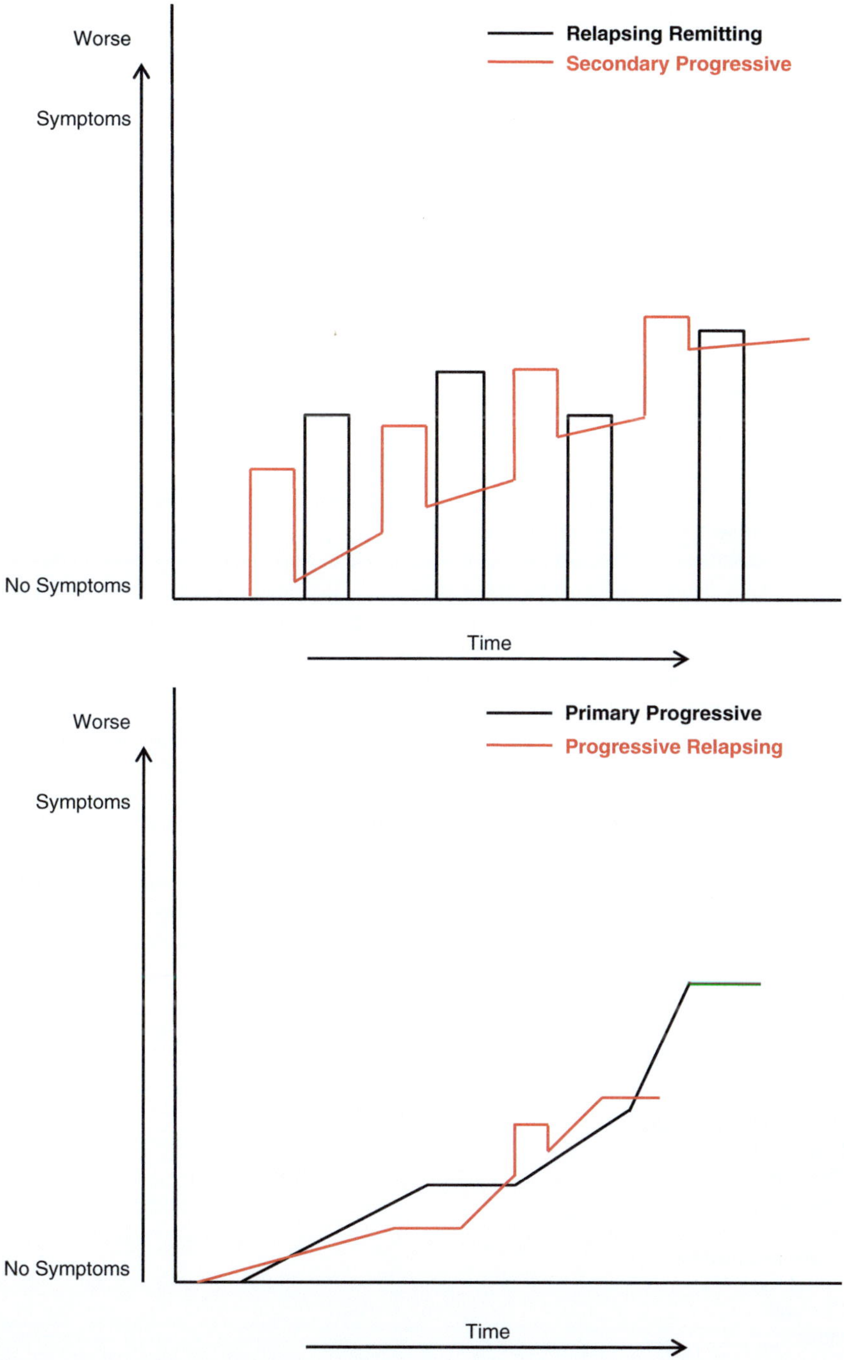

Fig. 1 Clinical course of symptoms (*y*-axis) versus time (*x*-axis) for four different types of multiple sclerosis. On the *top*, a comparison of RRMS (*black*) and SPMS (*red*). On the *bottom*, a comparison of PPMS (*black*) and PRMS (*red*) (*Source*: Adapted from Campagnolo and Vollmen [1])

Table 2 Kurtzke expanded disability status scale

Score	Description
0.0	Normal neurological exam
1.0	No disability, minimal signs in one functional system
1.5	No disability, minimal signs in more than one functional system
2.0	Minimal disability in one functional system
2.5	Mild disability in one functional system or minimal disability in two functional systems
3.0	Fully ambulatory with moderate disability in one functional system or mild disability in multiple functional systems
3.5	Fully ambulatory with moderate disability in one functional system and more than minimal disability in multiple others
4.0	Fully ambulatory without aid; self-sufficient; up and about 12 hours a day despite relatively severe disability in at least one functional system; ambulatory without aid for 500 meters
4.5	Fully ambulatory without aid; self-sufficient; up and about most of the day; able to work a full day but may otherwise have some limitations or need minimal assistance; ambulatory without aid for 300 meters
5.0	Ambulatory without aid for 200 meters; unable to work full day due to severe disability
5.5	Ambulatory without aid for 100 meters; severe disability precludes daily activities
6.0	Intermittent or unilateral constant assistance from cane, crutch, or brace is required to walk about 100 meters with or without resting
6.5	Constant bilateral assistance from canes, crutches, or braces is required to walk about 20 meters without resting
7.0	Restricted to wheelchair; unable to walk more than 5 meters even with aid; uses standard wheelchair and can wheel and transfer self; able to spend 12 hours/day in wheelchair
7.5	Restricted to wheelchair; unable to walk more than a few steps; may require motorized wheelchair and may need help in transfer; unable to stay in wheelchair for full day
8.0	Retains many self-care functions and general effective arm use; essentially restricted to bed or chair or perambulated in wheelchair but may be out of bed for much of the day
8.5	Retains some self-care functions and some effective arm use; essentially restricted to bed activities
9.0	Can communicate and eat but otherwise confined to bed activities
9.5	Unable to eat, swallow or communicate effectively; completely confined to bed
10.0	Death due to multiple sclerosis

Source: Kurtzke [6]
Eight Functional Systems:
Pyramidal
Cerebellar
Brainstem
Sensory
Bowel and bladder
Visual
Cerebral
Other

Moreover, inflammatory forces upregulate osteoclasts which remove bone, leading to an excess of bone resorption relative to bone formation.

Early studies suggested that there is a higher total bone mineral level in persons with MS who remain largely ambulatory, relative to those who demonstrate limited or no ambulation [7–9]. An investigation of premenopausal women ages 26–50, postmenopausal women ages 44–64, and men from age 25–70 demonstrated a significantly greater femoral bone loss and vertebral bone loss in patients with MS relative to controls. This study examined only subjects with EDSS scores between 6 and 7, indicating advanced disease. In addition, fracture rates were 22 % in persons with MS relative to only 2 % among control patients. In one of the largest cohort studies involving 43,832 women ages 55 and older, the second highest incident fracture rates (15 %) were found among women with MS, despite only 272 of the participants having a comorbidity of MS in contrast to over 31,000 with established heart disease [4]. Patients with progressive forms of MS appear to have more extensive bone loss than those with a clinically isolated syndrome or relapsing-remitting forms of the disease [8], a finding that directly relates to overall functional status and EDSS values.

An investigation by Terzi et al. [10] looked specifically at 52 premenopausal females with RRMS having EDSS scores below five, relative to age-matched controls. The MS patients had lower BMD scores overall compared with controls. Group differences demonstrated 10 % with osteoporosis in the MS subjects but 0 % for controls; 38.4 % with osteopenia among MS subjects compared to 20 % for controls; and only 52 % with normal BMD values for the MS patients compared with 72 % of able-bodied subjects. The authors identified a positive relationship between the total Functional Independence Measurement score (FIM) and femoral trochanter BMD, but not in other skeletal areas. They also found a significant negative association between duration of L2–4 BMD and MS, even given the relatively high functional level of MS patients. In addition, higher EDSS scores were associated with FIM scores and with significantly lower BMD in L2-4 of the spine, the greater trochanter of the femur, and the femoral neck.

Cellular and Autoimmune Factors

The number of MS exacerbations driving the frequency of steroid treatment reflects the progression of MS. Each exacerbation may mean a period of bed rest and relative immobility, thereby upregulating osteoclastic function. When patients experience a flare in their disease, a heightened state of inflammation ensues, and osteoclastic function is upregulated. A number of inflammatory molecules activate factors that can stimulate bone resorption. Cytokines, which are products of B cells, T helper cells, and CD8+ T cells have been known to contribute to osteoclastogenesis, leading to bone resorption. Specific cytokines thought largely responsible for this process include interleukins 1, 6, and 11 (IL-1, IL-6, IL-11), and tumor necrosis factor alpha (TNF-α) [11]. Enhanced osteoclastic activity by receptor-activated nuclear factor RANKL occurs independent of the extent of disability. Findings indicate that RANKL is significantly greater in MS patients than controls, even if the degree of disability based on EDSS score is low [12].

Osteopontin (OPN), a protein composed of macrophages, leukocytes, and T cells, is a pro-inflammatory cytokine with actions that specifically increase levels of interferon gamma and selected interleukins that resorb bone [13]. Levels of osteopontin are higher in the cerebrospinal fluid of persons with RRMS relative to controls [12] and actually increase just in advance of a clinical MS exacerbation [13]. Vogt et al. demonstrated a positive correlation between OPN levels and C-terminal telopeptide, a marker of bone degradation. The same study found that RRMS patients with high OPN levels had low serum vitamin D25(OH) levels. Moreover, both vitamin D25(OH) levels and OPN levels were related to immunoglobulin G levels in RRMS patients, suggesting that each could play opposing roles in the inflammatory components of MS [12]. In terms of effects on bone beyond hormonal levels, translational studies have shown that abnormal OPN levels appear to correlate with reduced BMD in the femur, but the results were somewhat contradictory to the findings of basic science studies and require further investigation.

Given its ability to stimulate gastric absorption of calcium, vitamin D is generally regarded as an essential agent to prevent bone loss; however, the active form of vitamin D ($1,25(OH)_2D3$) may also contribute to immunomodulation in the progression of MS [14]. This active form is metabolized through hydroxylation first by the liver and second by the kidney, but is not the storage form that clinicians measure to determine vitamin D status. See Fig. 2 [15]. Also known as dihydroxy vitamin D, this form and its function are regulated by the vitamin D receptor (VDR). Expression of VDR is regulated by a number of cell lines in the central nervous system (CNS).

The role of vitamin D as an immunomodulator was established through confirmation of VDR on macrophages and antigen-presenting cells in the CNS. Findings suggest that low levels of vitamin D are associated with reduced nerve growth factor (NGF) levels in the brain. Conversely, VDR transcription correlates with production of NGF and various neurotrophins as well as factors involved in nerve signaling transmission [16], leading to an overall neuroprotective effect.

Antigen-presenting cells and cytokines are directly involved in the pathogenesis of multiple sclerosis and other inflammatory conditions. Development of antigen-presenting cells and pro-inflammatory cytokine production are both inhibited by levels of $1,25(OH)_2D3$. Production of T lymphocytes needed to preserve myelin and axons is enhanced in the presence of $1,25(OH)_2D3$ [14]. In addition to T lymphocytes, B lymphocytes and their action can be influenced by dihydroxy vitamin D, but it appears only active B lymphocytes are affected. Active forms of vitamin D inhibit adverse immunoglobulin production and induce apoptosis of harmful immunoglobulins resulting in a net effect of reduced inflammation [17].

Interferon beta (INF-β) is a first-line treatment for MS, often prescribed for those subjects with early RRMS. In addition to its effect on the CNS for disease

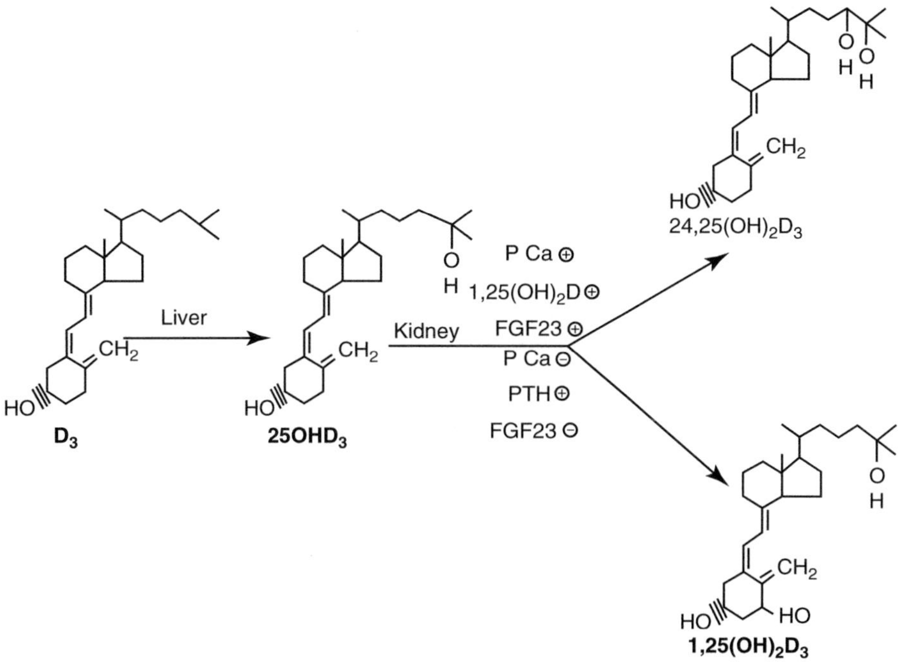

Fig. 2 The metabolism of vitamin D. In the initial step, the liver converts vitamin D_3 to vitamin $25(OH)D_3$. The second step involves the kidney's application of another OH group to form $1,25(OH)_2D_3$ and $24,25(OH)_2D_3$. Elevated parathyroid hormone levels (PTH) with low serum phosphorous, calcium and FGF23 promote formation of $1,25(OH)_2D_3$, while low PTH and high serum phosphorous, calcium and FGF23 favor production of $24,25(OH)_2D_3$ (*Source*: Used with permission from Bikle et al. [15])

modulation, INF-β induces nitric oxide, a substance involved in vascular regulation that also facilitates many positive developments and actions within the CNS. In addition INF-β inhibits osteoclast formation. A negative feedback loop mediated by RANKL signals production of INF-β in the setting of osteoclastogenesis [11].

Increasing evidence suggests that bone markers, including hormones like estrogen and progesterone, cytokines, vitamin D, and PTH, modulate immune function in addition to their individual roles in bone regulation. Growing interest in the field of osteoimmunology is focused on the action of bone in the development and maturation of the immune system within bone marrow as well as on the impact of bone on adaptive immunity. These relationships are pivotal in further investigations of the dual mechanisms of bone modulatory factors as well as on the development of osteoporosis and a parallel upregulation of MS disease progression, frequency of MS exacerbations, and severity of attacks [12, 18]. Many of these attacks involve demyelinating lesions, so periodic monitoring of MRI scans of the brain (Fig. 3) and of the spine (Fig. 4) is recommended, particularly if patients have new symptoms of confusion or weakness.

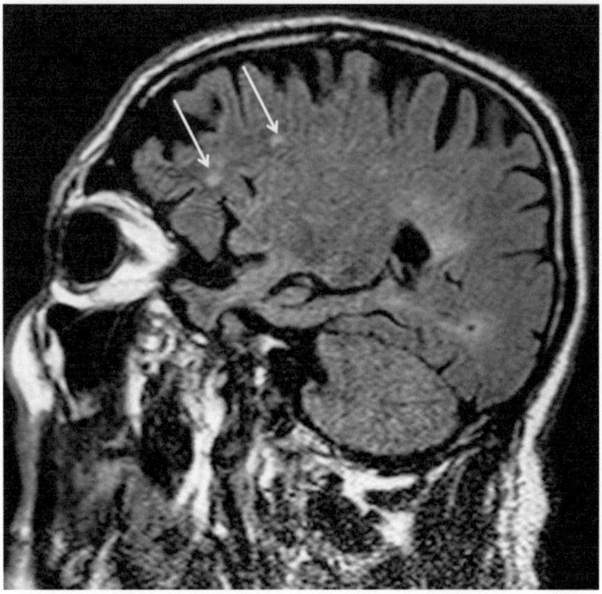

Fig. 3 Demyelinating ovoid lesions seen in brain parenchyma. These are ovoid lesions of T2 enhancement, representing areas of demyelination, in a patient with primary progressive multiple sclerosis (*Source*: Courtesy of Thomas Jefferson University. Used with patient permission)

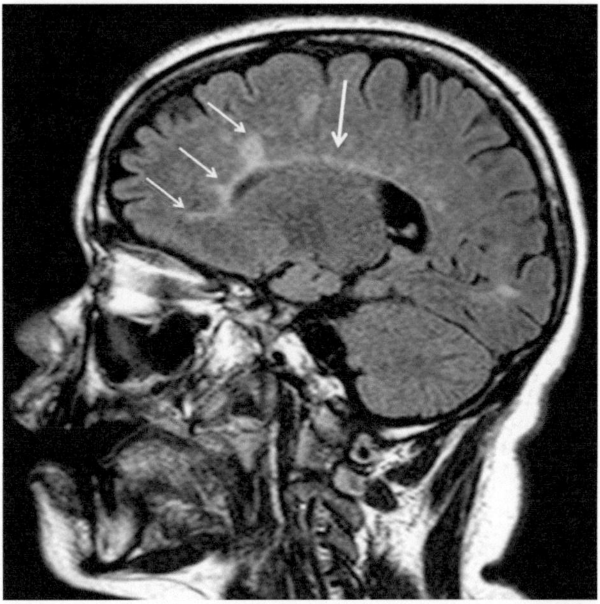

Fig. 4 Classic Dawson's fingers representing demyelinating regions. Enhanced demyelinating regions seen along the roof of the lateral ventricle as well as more extensive areas of T2 hyperintensity with long-axis perpendicular to the callosal septal interface. These regions represent demyelinating disease in a female patient with secondary progressive multiple sclerosis (*Source*: Department of Radiology, Thomas Jefferson University)

Nutritional Issues and Vitamin D Deficiency

Due to a combination of dietary and environmental factors, persons with MS are at risk of low levels of vitamin D [19]. As in the case of persons with spinal cord injury (SCI), those with MS may have issues relating to gastroesophageal reflux or neurogenic bowel, factors which discourage consumption of milk products. Calcium supplements in some forms, such as oyster shell calcium or calcium carbonate, may increase constipation, whereas calcium citrate has a tendency to cause loose stools. Vitamin D does enhance calcium absorption from the gut, but this absorption may be limited by available calcium intake.

Many patients with MS have limited exposure to sunlight, an essential source of natural vitamin D [20]. Heat intolerance discourages MS patients from remaining outdoors long enough to absorb adequate vitamin D from solar sources. Fear of falling may also deter patients from going outdoors for recreation or daily activities unless assistance is available. Those with higher functional deficits may be unable to leave home for medical visits due to lack of personnel needed for transport and monitoring and the costs involved in the face of insurance barriers. In the study described above, Terzi et al. also examined vitamin D25(OH) and parathyroid hormone (PTH) levels. As serum D25(OH) levels fall, parathyroid hormone (PTH) is upregulated in a secondary feedback mechanism. Elevated levels of PTH stimulate osteoclasts to resorb additional bone [10].

Although MS patients have established serum vitamin D25(OH) levels, this factor is unlikely to be solely responsible for osteoporosis in MS [20]. However, inadequate dietary intake of calcium and vitamin D or decreased exposure to sunlight limits adequate absorption for epithelial and gastrointestinal mechanisms. Low calcium and indirectly low serum levels of vitamin D induce hyperparathyroidism that promotes bone resorption in favor of bone formation.

Medications

Medications given for MS exacerbations and long-term prevention have adverse effects on bone health. It was initially felt that steroids prescribed for management of acute exacerbations were more harmful to bone health than medications for secondary prevention of MS, but the latter category has not been well investigated due to patients shifting from one disease modifying agent to another, thereby confounding interpretation of long-term outcomes. In addition, many new medications for disease progression are emerging while others are in the later phases of clinical trials; however, most of these agents have not been examined with specific reference to their effect on bone health.

Glucocorticoids

The adverse effects of glucocorticoids on bone have been extensively documented [21, 22]. Persons with multiple sclerosis receive 3–5 days of intravenous or oral glucocorticoids during an acute exacerbation. While ongoing administration of steroids is known to increase fracture rates and osteoporosis in other populations, evidence for an association of fractures with pulsed steroids given for periodic MS flares is limited. Doses in excess of 15 mg/day for multiple days with repeated cycles of administration increase the risk of osteoporosis [23]. In contrast, increased fracture rates have been seen in MS patients who are on continuous steroids [24]. Some investigations [8, 25] indicate a correlation between cumulative steroid dosing and BMD in the greater trochanter. Ayatollahi et al. [26] found that femoral BMD but not lumbar BMD was reduced among MS patents relative to age-matched controls but found no relationship of BMD to glucocorticoids. Many of these findings can be influenced by age of the participants, number of years with MS, and EDSS scores [10].

Tuzun et al. [27] demonstrated lower BMD in MS patients relative to controls at multiple sites throughout the femur and lumbar spine as well as lower BMD at the femur in women with greater duration of MS, but no effect, positive or negative, on BMD in relation to glucocorticoids. Schwid [28] found BMD was higher if steroids were given to persons with an EDSS below five, but lower if a subject's EDSS was more than five. In Terzi's investigation of MS patients whose EDSS values were all less than five, no effect of short courses of steroids was observed. Steroids may help higher-functioning MS individuals to resume a least partial if not full ambulation and to mitigate the secondary effects of adverse inflammatory molecules such as interleukins that increase osteoclastic function and bone resorption. In this sense, the steroids may be able to help those whose EDSS scores are in the range for ambulation. However, steroids are unlikely to help regain functional capacity in persons who have previously lost the ability to ambulate, and under these conditions, the adverse effects of steroids on bone will be observed.

Antiepileptic Drugs

Due to inflammation in the brain as well as the presence of lesions, persons with MS are at increased risk of seizures. Patients with history of seizure as well as those with many intraparenchymal lesions are often prescribed agents to prevent seizures, with treatment that extends from six months to many years. A number of studies indicate the presence of reduced BMD with ongoing use of some of the older antiepileptic agents, specifically phenytoin, carbamazepine, and phenobarbital [11]. They induce a biochemical cascade involving cytochrome P450, which promotes inactivation of vitamin D, making it less available to assist with calcium absorption through the gut. This mechanism thus predisposes patients to secondary hyperparathyroidism [29]. In addition, animal studies imply direct adverse effects on the osteoblast as well as reduction of carboxylated osteocalcin that leads to incomplete bone mineralization. Valproic acid, a nonenzyme-inducing antiepileptic, is associated with fractures due to hypophosphatemia, again affecting bone mineralization.

Of greater concern is the finding that other nonenzyme-producing antiepileptics are also associated with fractures, yet many of these antiseizure agents are not used for seizures but rather for neuropathic pain, which is a significant clinical issue in the MS population. While agents such as gabapentin, pregabalin, and lamotrigine as well as valproic acid are associated less with fractures than are older antiepileptics like phenytoin and phenobarbital, there remains an increased risk. Brazelier et al. [30] have advised reduction of antidepressants and anticonvulsants among other lifestyle measures such as limiting or eliminating alcohol intake and quitting smoking if the patient is an active smoker. Those with neuropathic pain often use alcohol or smoking as a means of coping with stress, but such maladaptive measures will adversely affect bones over time. Moreover, nicotine depresses appetite, has direct toxic effects on bone, and, in a similar population of SCI patients, was found to actually worsen neuropathic pain [31].

Because many of the traditional antiepileptic agents such as phenytoin require monitoring of blood levels, they are used more often in the hospital for an acute MS exacerbation but less often in the community. Patients have difficulty maintaining therapeutic drug levels if they require the use of intermittent antibiotics, ongoing use of other medications that alter metabolism of anticonvulsants, or changes in diet. Many lack the appropriate ongoing follow-up mechanisms to ensure therapeutic blood levels. Low levels may result in increased seizure risk, whereas supratherapeutic values can cause toxicity in other organ systems. Newer agents such as levetiracetam do not require blood level monitoring and have the advantage of a neutral effect on bone.

Antidepressants

As with many other chronic medical conditions, especially disorders in which functional decline is inevitable, depression is highly prevalent among persons with multiple sclerosis. One study reported a figure as high as 15.7 % over 12 months [32], a figure which exceeds that in the general population by two to threefold [32, 33]. The prevalence jumps to 67–77 % among patients experiencing chronic pain. Depression is frequently seen when the diagnosis is first made and when a significant functional decline has occurred. Examples of the latter include transition from a walker to a wheelchair, needing assistance to facilitate transfers, loss of vision, and onset or progression of neurologic bowel and bladder function.

Medications prescribed for depression have an adverse effect on bone density, most notably selective serotonin reuptake inhibitors (SSRIs) and serotonin–norepinephrine reuptake inhibitors (SNRIs). Because SSRIs were developed a number of years prior to SNRIs, more research has been done on the former group. Among SSRIs, fluoxetine, sertraline, paroxetine, and citalopram are often prescribed since they are available generically and are the most likely to be covered by third-party payers or Medicare prescription plans. Among SNRIs, duloxetine is commonly recommended for persons with combined symptoms of depression and neuropathic pain, but this agent lacks a generic equivalent and is, accordingly, more expensive. Ensrud et al. [34] demonstrated lower bone density and increased fracture risk among individuals prescribed SSRIs.

The precise mechanism of bone loss caused by agents optimizing serotonin levels is not completely delineated. Two studies suggest that serotonin increases bone resorption by increased osteoclast differentiation [35, 36]. However, since serotonin receptors are found on both osteoblasts and osteoclasts, their effects may extend beyond just the bone-resorbing cells [37]. In fact, many pathways appear to be involved: endocrine, paracrine, autocrine, and neuronal, which may explain why, in the absence of BMD reduction, increased rates of fractures are still detected.

Although psychological evaluation and treatment for adjustment disorder and new disability can be very effective, few patients with MS receive appropriate counseling services after completing acute inpatient rehabilitation [38]. Perhaps more frustrating is the fact that insurance companies will cover selected SSRI medications, yet they make the patient responsible for generally 50–100 % of counseling expenses. Support groups can be helpful, but challenges exist to reaching such sites due to immobility and reliance on caregivers, as well as limited or nonexistent funding for transportation to an appointment that is considered to be "not medically necessary." The alternatives to medication can only go so far; quite often a combination approach is needed for the most severe forms of depression.

Proton Pump Inhibitors

The increased risk of fractures from proton pump inhibitors (PPIs) has been noted in a number of studies among the general population [39–41]. Fractures appear to be more common in patients who have been on PPIs for more than one year. Specifically, Lau and Ahmed [42] reported greater risk of hip fracture of 20–62 % and increased risk of vertebral compression of 40–60 %. Short-term use of PPI medications does not appear to cause a significant risk of fracture [29], yet Pouwels et al. [43] did observe an increased adjusted odds ratio (AOR) for fracture of 1.2 with patients currently on PPIs for the first three months of use and an AOR of 1.26 for users between three and 12 months. In September, 2012, the US Food and Drug Administration issued a warning that cautions prescribers about the increased risk of osteoporosis-related fractures with the use of PPIs, specifically of the hip, spine, and wrist [44].

For stress ulcer prophylaxis during administration of IV steroids in an acute exacerbation, patients with MS are customarily put on proton pump inhibitors or alternative gastrointestinal (GI) prophylaxis such as histamine (H2) blockers. In patients with long-term wheelchair use who are suddenly placed on bed rest, DVT prophylaxis is initiated until they return to their former functional level of sitting in a wheelchair for at least 6–8 hours per day. For patients who are temporarily bedridden as a result of a new diagnosis of MS or sudden decline in function from ambulatory to nonambulatory status, short-term pharmacologic anticoagulation in the form of either unfractionated heparin three times daily or enoxaparin once daily is initiated to prevent venous thromboembolism. During this time, PPIs are given to counteract adverse effects of anticoagulation. General recommendations are to continue deep vein thrombosis (DVT) prophylaxis along with PPIs or H2 blockers until patients are either ambulating at least 200 feet per day or are accustomed to a lower level of wheelchair mobility for at least four weeks. These guidelines were developed from patients with spinal cord injury [45] but are frequently applied to individuals with paraparesis or tetraparesis who have MS.

The duration of anticoagulation is recommended for several days to a few weeks to counteract the reduced level of function. Because anticoagulation predisposes patients to GI bleeding, PPIs or equivalent agents are simultaneously prescribed. For most patients with MS, GI prophylaxis continues only as long as anticoagulation is necessary, often less than a month. Under these circumstances, PPIs will not have a significant long-term effect on bone density unless the dose is extremely high. For those with an active gastrointestinal bleed or occult, heme-positive stools, 40 mg of pantoprazole or omeprazole twice a day is prescribed, while awaiting appropriate cauterization or alternative intervention for the active bleeding. Such treatment is generally continued for a short time thereafter.

The mechanism of increased fractures with the use of PPIs is not entirely clear, but preliminary findings suggest that this class of medication suppresses acid secretion in the stomach and thereby decreases intestinal calcium absorption. In cases where inadequate absorption is significant enough to result in hypocalcemia, secondary hyperparathyroidism may develop, further escalating the risk of fractures. Bisphosphonates are ordinarily given to prevent fractures, but with the above mechanism, they are actually contributing to increased risk of fractures when combined with simultaneous use of PPI agents. Bisphosphonates reduce blood calcium levels by maintaining calcium in the bones. The lack of calcium from sequestration in the bone, in combination with decreased GI calcium absorption, compromises the osteoblast to the point where adequate bone formation is impossible, even when balanced by reduced osteoclastic activity [46, 47].

H2 blockers, also called H2-receptor antagonists, are an alternative to PPIs. They reduce the amount of acid the stomach produces by blocking one important producer of acid—histamine. Based on a similar mechanism of action to PPIs, H2-receptor antagonists may also have an adverse effect on the bone but far less so than the PPIs, and several studies revealed no increased risk. Kwok and colleagues demonstrated that H2 blockers are not associated with fractures of the spine or hip whereas PPIs are associated with both [48]. Data from Pouwels et al. challenge these findings, with adjusted odds ratio of 1.19 for H2 users over several time periods. Although very large ($n=33{,}104$), the study was population-based and as such, its size did not permit assessment of additional factors that either contribute to or prevent bone loss [43]. Most of the H2 blockers are less expensive than PPIs and are available over the counter in the United States. Famotidine is also available intravenously for hospitalized patients unable to swallow pills or intubated and lacking oral access. It is often started in the intensive care unit intravenously, but when patients are able to swallow, the medication is changed to an oral form, often a PPI. Consideration should be given to continuation of the H2 blockers in an oral form rather than switching to a PPI, particularly if the patient has other risk factors such as concomitant use of antiepileptics, anticoagulants, bisphosphonates, or steroids.

Long-term effects of PPIs on bone are concerning. Yang et al. examined a large cohort of 13,556 hip fracture patients over age 50, comparing users of PPI medications versus nonusers [49]. The odds ratio of fracture increased sequentially for years of use: OR 1.22 for PPIs used for one year; two years, 1.41; three years, 1.54; and four years, 1.59. Fractures were also more likely in patients using higher dose daily PPIs. Fortunately, many patients with MS require PPIs or H2 blockers for only short-term use while on anticoagulation or on steroids, and findings do suggest that the increased risk of fractures seen in PPI users declines significantly after discontinuation [40]. The decline may occur because long-term changes in bone density are modest or present only in combination with comorbidities [50]. Targonik et al. examined 8340 patients for changes in BMD at the hip, femoral neck, and lumbar spine and compared findings of users and nonusers of PPIs. Initial analysis demonstrated lower BMD in the hip and femoral neck but not lumbar spine [51]. However, when confounding factors were eliminated, repeat analysis did not find lower BMD among PPI users.

Maggio and colleagues studied 1038 geriatric individuals and found PPI use was associated with lower trabecular BMD. Because the study group consisted only of subjects age 65 or above, many individuals could have had other risk factors, including the use of other medications contributing to osteoporosis. Perhaps the findings of Corley and colleagues [52] best clarify the opposing views. In this cohort study of 33,752 individuals with hip fracture and 130,471 controls, derived from a US integrated health services database, increased risk of fracture was seen only among individuals with more than one risk factor, including diabetes, kidney disease, arthritis, glucocorticoid use, and smoking. Risk for hip fracture was higher if subjects used PPIs for more than two years or were taking higher than standard doses. Unfortunately, persons with MS have inherent risk factors for fracture and bone loss by virtue of their diagnosis and its functional limitations, apart from the use of other potentially harmful medications for bone health. In all likelihood, persons with MS have multiple risk factors and, as such, the use of PPIs would add to the probability of developing a fracture.

Anticoagulants

Risk of venous thromboembolism is increased in MS patients who have a more advanced form of the disease. Higher risk would necessarily be seen in those who are nonambulatory or have significant motor and sensory loss due to lesions in the spinal cord. Risk of DVT is generally much less than in those with SCI, since even advanced MS does not usually result in complete spinal cord injuries. As part of standard hospital protocols, DVT prophylaxis is initiated for patients viewed as having increased risk of clotting. Either unfractionated or low-molecular-weight heparin is initiated shortly after admission for MS patients, many of whom continue on similar treatment until the end of their rehabilitation course. As described in earlier portions of this report, once a patient can ambulate 150–200 feet at once or over several sessions in a 24-hour period, pharmacologic DVT prophylaxis can be discontinued. For those who are unable to achieve that level of function by time of discharge, individual risk–benefit assessment must be made, including evaluating a patient's risk for falls versus other measures to increase mobility.

The mechanism by which unfractionated heparin leads to bone loss is well understood. Heparin inhibits osteoblast differentiation and compromises osteoblast function resulting in decreased bone formation [29, 53]. Secondly, heparins reduce OPG which upregulates RANKL to induce osteoclastic differentiation, thereby increasing bone resorption. A number of reports indicate bone loss in association with heparin treatment [54, 55], but most studies showing elevated risk describe longer-term use in terms of either months or years [56, 57]. Although several smaller studies indicate low molecular weight heparin (LMWH) is associated with fewer low-impact osteoporotic fractures than unfractionated heparin, a large study in pregnant females by Backos et al. [58] revealed no statistical difference in fracture incidence. Of note, pregnant females have many other risk factors for thromboembolic events [54]; the above findings should be interpreted in that context. Newer heparins of oral or subcuticular form, including fondaparinux, do not affect osteoblast differentiation in vitro [29, 59].

Warfarin is among the most common long-term anticoagulants for persons with a new DVT or PE [54] or for chronic heart conditions, including arrhythmias. Patients with MS are at an increased risk of DVT, but their disease does not make them particularly susceptible to cardiac conduction abnormalities. Mechanistically, warfarin would confer a negative effect on BMD since it decreases the carboxylates of osteocalcin (OC) and compromises the calcium-binding capacity of OC [29]. While some earlier studies [60] suggested an association of vertebral and rib fractures as well as lower BMD with prolonged use of warfarin, more recent studies have not demonstrated a relationship [61]. More specific studies for at risk populations with precise analysis of findings according to predisposing factors and medical comorbidities would be valuable.

Falls and Their Role in Fractures

A number of factors can increase fall risk in persons with MS. Interventions can be made in the home and work environment to reduce fall risk including eliminating room clutter, securing rugs or using solid flooring, optimizing lighting, and reducing glare. Placing items that are commonly used in nearby locations eliminates frequent transfers and reduces walking distance which indirectly reduces falls by eliminating risks of balance loss and fatigue. Other factors including weakness, proprioceptive loss, and ataxia are more difficult to treat. Table 3 summarizes the more common reasons for falls.

Table 3 Factors leading to falls in persons with multiple sclerosis

Physical deficits	Proprioceptive deficits
	Autonomic deficits
	Fatigue
	Poor vision
	Hearing deficits
Cognitive deficits	Irritability
	Impulsivity
	Short-term memory loss
Social deficits	Denial of balance and functional deficits by family and caregivers
	Denial of cognitive issues and level of independence by family and caregivers

Proprioceptive Deficits

MS patients have proprioceptive deficits as well as cognitive fatigue. As noted earlier, fall risk is significant and precipitated by deficits in proprioception so that patients are unaware of where their feet are in space and have a greater tendency to fall without warning. Ensuring adequate lighting in an area can partially compensate for proprioceptive deficits. In addition fatigue in combination with autonomic effects of a full bladder can make patients transiently weaker when they do not anticipate it and have no assistive device nearby. Numerous reports of falls are reported when a patient is en route to the bathroom, an action undertaken frequently without time to gather an assistive device or don an orthotic. Placement of a bedside commode and management of urinary frequency at night are strongly advised to decrease nocturnal bathroom visits.

Cognitive Contributions to Falls

Cognitive fatigue can be reduced through appropriate scheduling of activities with rest breaks and by educating the patient on energy conservation techniques for their more physically demanding tasks and activities of daily living. Evidence supports the use of amantadine, a drug that reduces fatigue and muscle stiffness potentially through optimizing dopamine availability. It is also a weak N-methyl-D-aspartate (NMDA) receptor antagonist [62]. Prescription of this agent early in the morning and midday helps patients with daily and particularly late afternoon fatigue, both physical and cognitive. Dosages after 3 or 4 pm may interfere with sleep, since a common side effect of this agent is insomnia. Other side effects are anticholinergic in nature: dry mouth, constipation, blurred vision, and urinary retention, but in our experience and according to many reports [63], doses of 100 mg early morning and midday or a single 200 mg morning dose should not interfere with sleep hygiene and are well tolerated. A meta-analysis by Asano and

Finlayson [64] concluded that both amantadine and modafinil are beneficial, but not sufficient in isolation, in preventing functional deficits related to fatigue in MS patients. Education regarding fatigue as well as instruction in energy conservation techniques and physical reconditioning were found to be more effective measures than medication alone.

An early report on the use of amantadine [65] found that patients taking amantadine performed better on the Stroop Interference Test, a measure of attention that challenges the patient with distracting and interfering information. In situations of divided attention, risk for falling and injuries resulting from unanticipated balance loss is markedly elevated. Subsequent reports in the many years since the preceding report confirm the positive relation of improved attention and concentration to amantadine and related neurostimulants such as modafinil [66, 67]. In persons with MS, fall reduction and optimizing attention during transfers and gait are among the most important nonpharmacologic interventions to prevent fractures.

Approaches to Treatment

Nonpharmacologic Interventions

General Strategies

During inpatient rehabilitation, the staff must pay careful attention to the daily schedule as well as the personal and work environments of patients with MS. Energy conservation, temperature regulation, sleep hygiene, facilitating attention and concentration, and fall risk reduction are among the most important measures that facilitate meaningful gains in functional activity and mobility, thereby promoting maintenance of bone density. This process begins with organizing and developing an appropriate physical and occupational rehabilitation program. Therapies should be scheduled strategically to optimize the patient's participation and energy level. In acute rehabilitation programs in the United States, patients are required to participate in at least three hours of physical and occupational therapy sessions per day (often in 45 minute increments) as well as additional sessions for speech therapies, nutrition guidance, recreational therapy, group workshops, and rehabilitation psychology sessions. How these sessions are arranged is crucial to the success of the individual patient [68].

Energy conservation is best achieved by pacing activities throughout the day. Some patients also need to separate their physical therapy sessions so that the first happens early in the day and the other later in the day, with a break of several hours in between therapies. Generally patients do better with early morning and midday sessions rather than scheduling all activities later in the afternoon, when fatigue sets in and patients require an assistive device that they did not need in the morning. Therapists and physicians must emphasize safety measures and educate families and patients about anticipating changes in function with late day activities.

Table 4 Recommendations for exercise in patients with MS

Monitor breathing and/or pulse rate
Pace exercise to avoid overdoing
Adapt and modify routines as MS symptoms fluctuate
Time exercise with MS medications
Modify exercises, especially if symptoms cause a difference in strength or ability between one side of the body and the other
Have supervision for protection or stand near a wall or in a corner for balance challenges
Get adequate sleep the night before engaging in sports or taking a class
Schedule physical activity for the time of the day when energy is highest
In warm weather avoid outdoor activities between 10 a.m. and 4 p.m
Dress in layers, in order to add or remove clothing as body temperature changes

Source: National MS Society [2]

For the MS patient, appropriate temperature in the gym provides the proper setting for advancement of physical skills and endurance. Nerve conduction is compromised in warmer temperatures, and thus patients do better functionally and can exercise longer in cooler environments. Temperatures vary based on the individual hospital or therapy center, time of year, number of occupants in the gym, and the needs of the other patients. Arranging to treat a patient in a cooler area of the gym or at a time when fewer people are present allows for more individual tailoring of the environment. Modalities such as cooling vests are helpful in prolonging sessions [68]. Encouraging adequate hydration in the setting of perspiration from activity is important, but careful documentation is recommended due to concerns for patients with neurogenic bladder on an intermittent catheterization program with fluid restrictions. Table fans in the patient room at the bedside can also be helpful for cooling off in between therapy sessions [69].

The MS society has advised the above strategies for patients to minimize symptoms during exercise (Table 4) [2].

Therapy Interventions

Strengthening is a major component of an exercise program for MS patients. Closed chain exercise is ideal to build muscle power as weight-bearing occurs through the lower extremities/spine, promoting bone mineral density formation. This approach is particularly important when an MS patient has osteoporosis as a comorbidity. Closed chain strengthening is also more functional than open chain strengthening because muscular activation occurs in patterns used during mobility and activities of daily living. When implementing strengthening exercises, it is critical to avoid overexertion and provide resistance in a manner which ensures that the patient can maintain proper biomechanics. Core strengthening is integral to an MS exercise program that maximizes proximal stability in order to support distal mobility. A patient with MS who also has osteoporosis can achieve core strengthening through

Table 5 Muscle group with exercise technique/positioning to maximize weight-bearing through bone

Biceps	Stabilization with weight-bearing for contralateral upper extremity reach
Triceps	Repeated bed mobility, chair push-ups
Finger flexors	Functional grip
Abdominals	Posterior pelvic tilt, rhythmic stabilization via proprioceptive neuromuscular reeducation
Back extensors	Quadruped
Hip extensors	Tall kneeling, repeated transfer training, partial single-leg standing for stance stability
Knee extensors	Mini-squats, elliptical machine
Plantar flexors	Toe raises, stair training, speed walking

isometric, pelvic stabilization exercises to address the precaution of trunk flexion. Table 5 demonstrates examples of targeted muscles and a closed chain, functional exercise for various areas of the body.

Balance training can be a challenge in patients with multiple sclerosis and osteoporosis, as an uncompensated loss of balance could result in falls with injury. During skilled therapy sessions, the therapist can design exercise programs to maximize balance challenge while maintaining safety using guarding or support harnesses. Static balance is often challenged by practice conditions characterized by uneven surfaces, decreased base of support, perturbations, and displacement of center of gravity with such functional tasks as reaching. The Berg Balance Score is an example of a fall prediction tool based on challenges to static balance. Patients should be educated to utilize a support surface if carrying out functional tasks when unsupervised. If balance exercises are prescribed as part of the home exercise program, utilizing the corner of a room with a chair anterior to the patient allows for decreased risk of unrecoverable loss of balance.

An efficient method for dynamic balance training is challenging intrinsic and extrinsic conditions during functional mobility. Changes in gait speed, direction, obstacle negotiation, and increasing environmental stimulation are examples of training strategies that promote carryover of gains into function. Standardized testing, such as the Dynamic Gait Index and the Tinetti Performance-Oriented Mobility Assessment, are dynamic balance tests, recognized as reliable and valid in the MS population. An assistive device or a caregiver's supervision may address dynamic balance impairments to meet the MS patient's need to maintain locomotion as long as safely possible [69].

Endurance training is also essential in an MS exercise program. Training that incorporates the principles of closed chain kinetics and forced weight-bearing will encourage good bone health. If the patient is at a high risk of falling, has no available supervision, or has inadequate strength to engage in these exercises, seated therapeutic exercise may be considered, i.e., stationary cycling, treadmill with rails, and chair exercise classes. Endurance training should be preceded by a warm-up period and followed by a cooldown period to minimize dramatic changes in core body temperature and the demands of increased circulation to support blood flow to active muscles [68]. Standardized testing deemed reliable and valid in the MS population includes 12, 6, or 2-minute walk tests, as well as a battery of assessment tools that identify underlying system impairments or target physical and cognition challenges such as the Balance Evaluation Systems Test (BEST) and the Modified Timed Up and Go Test (cognitive or manual).

Gait dysfunction is a prevalent sequela of multiple sclerosis. Common gait characteristics of MS include variable base of support, unequal and shortened step length, and decreased gait velocity [69]. Gait deviations can significantly affect patients with multiple sclerosis because they can lead to joint breakdown from asymmetrical weight-bearing, muscular strain due to poor body mechanics and increased potential of mechanical falls.

Inadequate clearance of the swing limb during gait may result in abnormal gait kinematics, leading to an increased risk of falls. Patients with MS may experience a mechanical fall as a result of tripping due to spasticity of plantar flexors and knee and/or hip extensors. Hip adductor spasticity can result in a narrow base of support or "scissoring" pattern. Spasticity can be addressed by self or manual stretching or the use of an ankle foot orthosis with extended footplate. Spasticity in the stance limb of gait or trunk leads to displacement of the center of gravity during ambulation. Unanticipated spasticity of flexor muscle groups can produce changes in ground reaction forces resulting in joint instability during the stance phase of gait.

Another etiology of inadequate swing limb clearance is weakness of the lower extremity musculature of antigravity muscles including ankle dorsiflexors and hip flexors. Motor fatigue, defined as greater muscular weakness with increased duration of use, results in decreased muscle fiber recruitment during cyclical movement patterns associated with gait [69].

If an MS lesion is identified in the cerebellum, gait deviations may include variable step length, wide base of support (BOS), and decreased coordination [70] with resultant deviation in trajectory of the swing limb. Incoordination of the swing limb contributes to a variable BOS due to deviation in trajectory of the swing limb which, in turn, contributes to fall risks including path deviation, unanticipated lower extremity contact, and inadequate base of support to maintain upright posture. Since patients with MS often experience decreased postural control and inefficient balance reactions, increased falls may occur. Sensory ataxia is also a concern as poor gait kinematics, including postural instability and increased forces at the heel strike phase of gait [69].

Pharmacologic Treatment

For both prevention and treatment of bone loss in multiple sclerosis, pharmacologic options consist of antiresorptive and anabolic medications. Because many MS patients are relatively young and premenopausal, skepticism exists as to the benefit of using bisphosphonates or anabolic agents such as human recombinant N terminal parathyroid hormone (also called PTH I-34 or teriparatide).

Bisphosphonates

No prospective trials of bisphosphonates have been performed exclusively on MS patients, but many exist in similar conditions of muscle disuse, including spinal cord injury and lower limb immobility. Bisphosphonates inhibit bone loss by decreasing the function of the osteoclast through three mechanisms. First, bisphosphonates attach to bone surfaces in the process of active resorption and interfere with the ability of the osteoclasts to form the tight connection at the bony surface necessary for resorption [71, 72]. A second action of bisphosphonates involves decreasing osteoclast progenitor development and recruitment. Third, they are responsible for promoting direct osteoclast apoptosis [73]. Bisphosphonates work by inhibiting a key regulatory enzyme in the osteoclast known as farnesyl diphosphate synthetase. The degree of inhibition of this enzyme varies from one bisphosphonate to another. Zoledronic acid (ZA) is by far the most powerful: 17 times more effective than alendronate and 67 times more powerful than pamidronate.

In a study of ZA use in a small group of 14 patients with acute traumatic SCI and motor complete injuries, Zehnder et al. demonstrated a substantial benefit in preservation of BMD of the total hip, greater trochanter, and lumbar spine [74]. Comparisons of subjects who received ZA and those who received placebo were not significant at the femoral neck. Shapiro et al. examined a similar group of 17 patients and found preservation of bone mineral density at three sites in the proximal femur six months after administration but at only one site by 12 months post administration [75]. The groups tested by the above studies would translate to EDSS scores of 7.5 or worse. Based on the earlier comparison of the relative benefits of exercise for more functional subjects with the suboptimal results seen in less mobile patients, pharmacologic treatment should be strongly considered.

In terms of side effects of bisphosphonates, MS patients may experience gastritis and esophageal burning after the use of oral bisphosphonates such as alendronate or ibandronate. A second concern is the ability to tolerate the acute phase reaction symptoms, common in the 24–48 hours after administration of ZA. In general, the acute neurogenic bladder symptoms are manifest in the form of urgency and increased frequency. However, chronic urinary retention is seen only in late phase MS, without a widespread observation of renal failure or elevated creatinine. MS patients are unlikely to experience renal issues from a single dose of ZA and should be at low risk of the rare elevation in creatinine after administration of ZA. Since they may already be taking a high number of daily medications, compliance in taking all forms of oral forms of bisphosphonates is potentially problematic. The semiannual or annual infusions of selected amino-bisphosphonates greatly reduce noncompliance.

Denosumab

Denosumab is an antiresorptive that inhibits osteoclast activation and interferes with steps involved in osteoclast formation. As a G2 monoclonal antibody that inhibits receptor activator of nuclear factor kappa beta ligand (RANKL), it blocks binding of RANKL to RANK and in doing so interferes or blocks multiple steps in osteoclast formation, activation, function, and longevity [76]. Because it is a human monoclonal antibody, it does not react with other proteins and theoretically should not alter the immune system, although one side effect of its use is increased risk of cellulitis [77]. However, there is no increased risk of development or progression of neoplasia which is a concern with the use of intact PTH (teriparatide). Unlike ZA, denosumab is both safe and clinically effective in persons with renal impairment [78].

In a large cohort investigation (7658 subjects) named the Fracture Reduction Evaluation of Denosumab in Osteoporosis every six Months (FREEDOM) trial [79], Cummings et al. investigated the use of denosumab in postmenopausal but otherwise able-bodied females between ages 60 and 90. They found significant reductions in new fracture rates for women who received denosumab in the vertebral spine by 68 %, in nonvertebral regions by 20 %, and in the hip by 40 %. The above figures represent treatment outcomes after 36 months. Improvement in BMD was noted in a follow-up study to the original FREEDOM trial which extended to eight years. The outcomes from the FREEDOM extension demonstrated a 19.2 % improvement in lumbar spine BMD and an 8.2 % gain in the hip [80] age of subjects in the above trials ranged from 60 to 90, and, other than osteoporosis, no specific mobility deficits were evaluated. Because the majority of MS patients are younger and notably closer to menopause, caution should be used in applying the above outcomes to an MS population.

In terms of side effects and adverse serious events, the original Cummings investigation [79] observed no neutralizing antibodies to the drug and no cases of osteonecrosis of the jaw (ONJ). No increased risk of cancer, infection, cardiovascular events, delayed fracture healing, or hypocalcemia was found in comparison to controls. There was a significantly higher incidence of cellulitis which was categorized as a serious adverse event in the denosumab group, yet no significant increase in overall infection rate was observed. A higher rate of eczema was also seen in those receiving denosumab. Statistically, differences in rates of flatulence were reported among subjects receiving denosumab relative to controls. Neither bowel incontinence nor constipation was reported.

Other investigations of denosumab have produced inconsistent results in terms of side effects. Sugimoto et al. found no increased risk of eczema and skin or respiratory infections but did report one case of ONJ that was treated successfully with oral antibiotics. Another study [81] found no increase in skin infections but did observe a higher incidence of respiratory infections which are of greater concern in hospitalized MS patients or any person with MS in the later stages of their disease, even if in the community.

In terms of eczema exacerbation or skin infections, persons with MS are sensitive to heat and experience sweating during times of over exhaustion or exercise. Toward that end, they are at increased risk of cellulitis in the presence of increased sweating. One strategy to avoid elevated risk of cellulitis is to avoid taking denosumab in the months of elevated temperatures such as June–September. If desired, a schedule of giving the medication between late September and early June would be ideal.

Teriparatide

Teriparatide (recombinant human parathyroid hormone 1–34, brand name Forteo) is a daily 20 mcg subcutaneous administration that increases bone density by direct osteoblastic action. It stimulates bone formation and elevates bone turnover markers, especially during initial months of administration. Discontinuation of the drug will reverse the initial benefit for BMD unless an antiresorptive in the form of a bisphosphonate or comparable agent is initiated immediately.

No prospective clinical trials of teriparatide in MS patients or in acute spinal cord-related disorders resulting in immobilization have been conducted. The primary investigations on teriparatide have been conducted in postmenopausal females or those on steroids. In one of the largest trials demonstrating early efficacy, the European Forteo Observational Study enrolled 1649 postmenopausal females and followed them for 36 months, with 18 months of daily 20 or 40 mg teriparatide dose and then 18 subsequent months without teriparatide as observation. The main objective of the study was to assess fracture incidence rather than BMD values. For those subjects who received the medication, a steady decline in onset of new fractures was noted for each 6-month assessment period. There were 1119 incident fractures in the first six months but only 654 in the last six months of treatment. Moreover, the final six months of the observational period reported an incidence of just 327 fractures. In interpreting the final fracture rates at 30–36 months, it should be noted that over 70 % of study participants were prescribed a bisphosphonate following the first 18 months on teriparatide in order to help maintain any gains in BMD [82]. A summary of nine RCTs evaluating the effect of teriparatide alone versus teriparatide plus alendronate demonstrated positive gains in BMD for the lumbar spine, total hip and, to a lesser extent, the femoral neck for subjects who received only teriparatide.

There is also evidence that teriparatide can assist with symptoms of musculoskeletal back pain [82]; thus, it may have dual utility in patients who have osteoporosis, need for aggressive pharmacologic intervention for osteoporosis, compression fractures, and paraspinal pain resulting from the fractures. Studies examining this precise situation, however, are unavailable. In terms of MS patients, selection of teriparatide as the agent of choice for medical intervention of osteoporosis should be considered only in the context of risk/benefit to the individual patient. There is an increased risk of osteosarcoma with prolonged use of teriparatide, thus the USFDA has limited use of this agent to 24 months per lifetime. The increase in osteosarcoma associated with the drug arose from animal studies, but was concerning enough to warrant the lifetime limit by the FDA [83]. Other common side effects of teriparatide are GI disturbances in the form of nausea and vomiting, leg cramps, and dizziness. No evidence exists regarding increased venous thromboembolism or increased infection rates.

Since no investigations of any antiresorptive drugs or anabolic drugs have been performed in an isolated group of MS patients, clinicians should use their own judgment based on the individual needs of the patient, beginning with the safest agents first. The UK National Institute for Health and Care Excellence provides guidelines for management options in osteoporosis patients in the United Kingdom; in some cases, these recommendations have been applied to patients with MS [11]. This Institute recommends alendronate as the first-line treatment for osteoporosis followed by two other bisphosphonates.

Strategies for Maintaining Bone in Persons with Multiple Sclerosis (MS)

A general strategy for treatment of osteoporosis in MS patients is illustrated in Table 6.

Briefly the philosophy is first and foremost to keep patients active. Every attempt to maintain weight-bearing activity should be pursued, even if this is done with assistive devices. Practitioners should ensure patients have therapeutic serum calcium and vitamin D levels through periodic lab testing. Bone density should be evaluated by DXA screening in those patients who are rapidly or consistently losing motor function or the ability to ambulate, even if manual muscle testing scores remain largely unchanged. Bone markers should also periodically be followed in all MS patients, except those with minimal sensory or motor deficits.

Table 6 Optimizing strategies for bone success in MS

Function /EDSS score	Assessment	Intervention
EDSS 1–4.5	Review diet and exercise, FRAX score, serum calcium, and vitamin D25(OH)	Supplement calcium and vit. D
EDSS 5–6.5	All of the above plus functional assessment, check P1NP, s-CTX, and order screening DXA	All of the above plus order PT/OT, consider changing/stopping problem meds (antiepileptics, PPIs) and osteoporosis meds based on DXA
ESSS 7–9	All of the above plus review functional assessment, order screening DXA annually, and repeat markers based on med treatment	Prescribe adaptive equipment, revise PT/OT plan, and review osteoporosis medications

References

1. Campagnolo DI, Vollmen TL. Multiple sclerosis. In: Kirshblum S, Campagnolo DI, editors. Spinal cord medicine. Philadelphia: Lippincott, Williams and Wilkins; 2011. p. 617–31.
2. National MS Society. http://www.nationalmssociety.org/What-is-MS/Types-of-MS. Accessed 22 Dec 2015.
3. Thomson A. FTY720 in multiple sclerosis: the emerging evidence of its therapeutic value. Core Evid. 2006;1(3):157–67.
4. Gregson CL, Dennison EM, Compston JE, Adami S, Adachi JD, Anderson Jr FA, et al. Disease-specific perception of fracture risk and incident fracture rates: GLOW cohort study. Osteoporos Int. 2014;25(1):85–95.
5. Hughes S, Spelman T, Trojano M, Lugaresi A, Izquierdo G, Grand Maison F, et al. The Kurtzke EDSS rank stability increased 4 years after the onset of multiple sclerosis: results from the MSBase Registry. J Neurol Neurosurg Psychiatry. 2012;83(3):305–10.
6. Kurtzke JF. Rating neurologic impairment in multiple sclerosis: an expanded disability status scale (EDSS). Neurology. 1983;33(11):1444–52.
7. Cosman F, Nieves J, Komar L, Ferrer G, Herbert J, Formica C, et al. Fracture history and bone loss in patients with MS. Neurology. 1998;51(4):1161–5.
8. Weinstock-Guttman B, Gallagher E, Baier M, Green L, Feichter J, Patrick K, et al. Risk of bone loss in mean with multiple sclerosis. Mult Scler. 2004;10(2):170–5.
9. Formica CA, Cosman F, Neives J, Herbert J, Lindsay R. Reduced bone mass and fat-free mass in women with multiple sclerosis: effects of ambulatory status and glucocorticoid use. Calcif Tissue Int. 1997;61(2):129–33.
10. Terzi T, Terzi M, Tander B, Cantürk F, Onar M. Changes in bone mineral density and bone metabolism markers in premenopausal women in multiple sclerosis and the relationship to clinical variables. J Clin Neurosci. 2010;17(10):1260–4.
11. Gupta S, Ahsan I, Mahfooz N, Abdelhamid N, Ramanathan M, Weinstock-Guttman B. Osteoporosis and multiple sclerosis: risk factors, pathophysiology, and therapeutic interventions. CNS Drugs. 2014;28(8):731–42.
12. Vogt MHJ, ten Kate J, Dent RJM, Polman CH, Hupperts R. Increased osteopontin plasma levels in multiple sclerosis patients correlate with bone-specific markers. Mult Scler. 2010;16(4):443–9.
13. Josyula S, Mehta BK, Karmon Y, Teter B, Batista S, Ostroff J, et al. The nervous system's potential role in multiple sclerosis associated bone loss. J Neurol Sci. 2012;319(1–2):8–14.
14. Smolders J, Damoiseaux J, Menheere P, Hupperts R. Vitamin D as an immune modulator in multiple sclerosis, a review. J Neuroimmunol. 2008;194(1–2):7–17.
15. Bikle D, Adams JS, Christakos S. Vitamin D: production, metabolism, mechanism of action, and clinical requirements. In: Rosen CJ, editor. Primer on the metabolic: bone diseases and disorders of mineral metabolism. Ames: Wiley; 2013. p. 235–44.
16. Garcion E, Wion-Barbot N, Montero-Menei CN, Berger F, Wion D. New clues about vitamin D functions in the nervous system. Trends Endocrinol Metab. 2002;13(3):100–5.
17. Chen S, Sims GP, Chen XX, Gu YY, Chen S, Lipsky PE. Modulatory effects of 1,12-dihydrozyvitamin D3 on human B cell differentiation. J Immunol. 2007;179(3):1634–47.
18. Nakashima T, Takayanagi H. Osteoimmunology: crosstalk between the immune and bone systems. J Clin Immunol. 2009;29(5):555–67.
19. Sioka C, Kyritsis AP, Fotopoulos A. Multiple sclerosis, osteoporosis, and vitamin D. J Neurol Sci. 2009;287(1–2):1–6.
20. Zikan V. Bone health in patients with multiple sclerosis. J Osteoporos. 2011;2011:1–9.
21. Mitchell DR, Lyles KW. Glucocorticoid-induced osteoporosis: mechanisms for bone loss; evaluation of strategies for prevention. J Gerontol. 1990;45(5):M153–8.
22. Ziegler R, Kasperk C. Glucocorticoid-induced osteoporosis: prevention and treatment. Steroids. 1998;63(5):344–8.

23. De Vries F, Bracke M, Leufkens HGA, Lammers JWJ, Cooper C, van Staa TP. Fracture risk with intermittent high-dose oral glucocorticoid therapy. Arthritis Rheum. 2007;56(1):208–14.
24. Berris KK, Repp AL, Kleerekoper M. Glucocorticoid-induced osteoporosis. Curr Opin Endocrinol Diabetes Obes. 2007;14(6):446–50.
25. Ozgocmen S, Bulut S, Ilhan N, Gulkesen A, Ardicoglu O, Ozkan Y. Vitamin D deficiency and reduced bone mineral density in multiple sclerosis: effect of ambulatory status and functional capacity. J Bone Miner Metab. 2005;23(4):309–13.
26. Ayatollahi A, Mohajeri-Tehrani MR, Nafissi S. Factors affecting bone mineral density in multiple sclerosis patients. Iran J Neurol. 2013;12(1):19–22.
27. Tüzün Ş, AltWntaş A, Karacan İ, Tangürek S, Saip S, Siva A. Bone status in multiple sclerosis: beyond corticosteroids. Mult Scler. 2003;9(6):600–4.
28. Schwid SR, Goodman AD, Puzas JE, McDermott MP, Mattson DH. Sporadic corticosteroid pulses and osteoporosis in multiple sclerosis. Arch Neurol. 1996;53(8):753–7.
29. Panday K, Gona A, Humphrey MB. Medication-induced osteoporosis: screening and treatment strategies. Ther Adv Musculoskel Disord. 2014;6(5):185–202.
30. Brazelier MT, van Staa TP, Uitdehaag BM, Cooper C, Leufkens H, Vestergaard P, et al. A simple score for estimating the long-term risk of fracture in patients with multiple sclerosis. Neurology. 2012;79(9):922–8.
31. Richards JS, Kogos SC, Ness TJ, Oleson CV. Smoking and neuropathic SCI pain: two case studies. J Spinal Cord Med. 2005;28(4):330–2.
32. Patten SB, Metz LM, Reimer MA. Biopsychosocial correlates of lifetime major depression in a multiple sclerosis population. Mult Scler. 2000;6(2):115–20.
33. Ehde DM, Bombardier CH. Depression in persons with multiple sclerosis. Phys Med Rehabil Clin N Am. 2005;16(2):437–48.
34. Ensrud KE, Blackwell T, Mangione CM, Bowman PJ, Bauer DC, Schwartz A, et al. Central nervous system active medications and risk for fractures in older women. Arch Intern Med. 2003;163(8):949–57.
35. Inose H, Zhou B, Yadav VK, Guo XE, Karsenty G, Ducy P. Efficacy of serotonin inhibition in mouse models of bone loss. J Bone Miner Res. 2011;26(9):2002–11.
36. Karsenty G, Yadav VK. Regulation of bone mass by serotonin molecular biology and therapeutic implications. Annu Rev Med. 2011;62:323–31.
37. Wu Q, Bencaz AF, Hentz JG, Crowell MD. Selective serotonin reuptake inhibitor treatment and risk of fractures: a meta-analysis of cohort and case–control studies. Osteoporos Int. 2012;23(1):365–75.
38. Birnbaum G. Management of multiple sclerosis symptoms. In: Birnbaum G, editor. Multiple sclerosis: clinician's guide to diagnosis and treatment. New York: Oxford University Press; 2009. p. 97–110.
39. Adams AL, Black MH, Zhang JL, Shi JM, Jacobsen SJ. Proton-pump inhibitor use and hip fractures in men: a population-based case-control study. Ann Epidemiol. 2014;24(4):286–90.
40. Yu E, Blackwell T, Ensrud K, Hiller T, Lane N, Orwoll E, et al. Acid-suppressive medications and risk of bone loss and fracture in older adults. Calcif Tissue Int. 2008;83(4):251–9.
41. Vestergaard P, Rejnmark L, Mosekilde L. Proton pump inhibitors, histamine H2 receptor antagonists, and other antacid medications and the risk of fracture. Calcif Tissue Int. 2006;79(2):76–83.
42. Lau YT, Ahmed NN. Fracture risk and bone mineral density reduction associated with proton pump inhibitors. Pharmacotherapy. 2012;32(1):67–79.
43. Pouwels S, Lalmohamed A, Souverein P, Cooper C, Veldt BJ, Leufkens HG. Use of proton pump inhibitors and risk of hip/femur fracture: a population-based case-control study. Osteoporos Int. 2011;22(3):903–10.
44. Ahmad NA, Anderson J, Brenner DM, Chan AT, Chan FK, Chang L, et al. Selected summaries: the final word on proton pump inhibitors and osteoporosis. Gastroenterology. 2013;144:650–3.
45. Consortium for Spinal Cord Medicine. Clinical Practice Guidelines: prevention of thromboembolism in spinal cord injury. 2nd ed. Washington, DC: Paralyzed Veterans Association; 2003.

46. Van Der Kallen J, Giles M, Cooper K, Gill K, Parker V, Tembo A, et al. A fracture prevention service reduces further fractures two years after incident minimal trauma fracture. Int J Rheum Dis. 2014;17(2):195–203.
47. Lee J, Youn K, Choi N, Lee J, Kang D, Song H, et al. A population-based case-control study: proton pump inhibition and risk of hip fracture by bisphosphonate. J Gastroenterol. 2013;48(9):1016–22.
48. Kwok C, Yeong J, Loke Y. Meta-analysis: risk of fractures with acid-suppressing medication. Bone. 2011;48(4):768–76.
49. Yang Y, Lewis J, Epstein S, Metz D. Long-term proton pump inhibitor therapy and risk of hip fracture. JAMA. 2006;296(24):2947–53.
50. Gerson LB. The final word on proton pump inhibitors and osteoporosis? Gastroenterology. 2013;144(3):650–3.
51. Targownik LE, Leslie WD, Davison KS, Goltzman D, Jamal SA, Kreiger N, et al. The relationship between proton pump inhibitor use and longitudinal change in bone mineral density: a population-based from the Canadian Multicentre Osteoporosis Study (CaMos). Am J Gastroenterol. 2012;107(9):1361–9.
52. Corley D, Kubo A, Zhao W, Quesenberry C. Proton pump inhibitors and histamine-2 receptor antagonists are associated with hip fracture among at-risk patients. Gastroenterology. 2010;139(1):93–101.
53. Rajgopal R, Bear M, Butcher M, Shaughnessy S. The effects of heparin and low molecular weight heparins on bone. Thromb Res. 2008;122(3):293–8.
54. Hawkins D, Evans J. Minimising the risk of heparin-induced osteoporosis during pregnancy. Expert Opin Drug Saf. 2005;4(3):583–90.
55. Bilen O, Teruya J. Complications of anticoagulation. Dis Mon. 2012;58(8):440–7.
56. Hirsh J, Bauer KA, Donati MB, Gould M, Samama MM, Weitz JI. Parenteral anticoagulants: American College of Chest Physicians evidence-based clinical practice guidelines. Chest J. 2008;133(6):141S–59.
57. Monreal M, Lafoz E, Olive A, del Rio L, Vedia C. Comparison of subcutaneous unfractionated heparin with a low molecular weight heparin (Fragmin) in patients with venous thromboembolism and contraindications to coumarin. Thromb Haemost. 1994;71(1):7–11.
58. Backos M, Rai R, Thomas E, Murphy M, Dore C, Regan L. Bone density changes in pregnant women treated with heparin: a prospective, longitudinal study. Hum Reprod. 1999;14(11):2876–80.
59. Handschin AE, Trentz OA, Hoerstrup SP, Kock HJ, Wanner GA, Trentz O. Effect of low molecular weight heparin (dalteparin) and fondaparinux (Arixtra ®) on human osteoblasts in vitro. Br J Surg. 2005;92(2):177–83.
60. Carabello PJ, Heit JA, Atkinson EJ, Silverstein MD, O'Fallon WM, Castro MR, et al. Long-term use of oral anticoagulants and the risk of fracture. Arch Intern Med. 1999;159(15):1750–6.
61. Woo C, Chang LL, Ewing SK, Bauer DC. Single-point assessment of warfarin use and risk of osteoporosis in elderly men. JAGS. 2008;56(7):1171–6.
62. PDR Network. Physicians' Desk Reference, 70th ed. Montvale, NJ. 2016.
63. National Multiple Sclerosis Society: Amantadine. www.nationalmssociety.org/Treating-MS/Medications/Amantidine. Accessed 1 Jan 2015.
64. Asano M, Finlayson ML. Meta-analysis of three different types of fatigue management interventions for people with multiple sclerosis: exercise, education, and medication. Mult Scler Int. 2014. doi:10.1155/2014/798285.
65. Cohen RA, Fisher M. Amantadine treatment of fatigue associated with multiple sclerosis. Arch Neurol. 1989;46(6):676–80.
66. Lovera JF, Frohman E, Brown TR, Bandari D, Nguyen L, Yadav V, et al. Memantime for cognitive impairment in multiple sclerosis: a randomized placebo-controlled trial. Mult Scler. 2010;16(6):715–23. doi:10.1177/1352458510367662.
67. Sailer M, Heinze HJ, Schoenfeld MA, Hauser U, Smid HG. Amantadine influences cognitive processing in patients with multiple sclerosis. Pharmacopsychiatry. 2000;33(1):28–37.

68. Sandoval AEG. Exercise in multiple sclerosis. Phys Med Rehabil Clin N Am. 2013;24(4):605–18. doi:10.1016/j.pmr.2013.07.002.
69. Stevens V, Goodman K, Rough K, Kraft GH. Gait impairment and optimizing mobility in multiple sclerosis. Phys Med Rehabil Clin N Am. 2013;24(4):573–92. doi:10.1016/j.pmr.2013.07.002.
70. Sosnoff JJ, Sandroff BM, Pula JH, Morrison SM, Moti RW. Falls and physical activity in persons with multiple sclerosis. Mult Scler Int. 2012;2012:315620. doi:10.1155/2012/315620.
71. Rodman GA, Fleisch HA. Bisphosphonates: mechanisms of action. J Clin Invest. 1996;97(12):2692–6.
72. Fleish HA. Bisphosphonates: mechanisms of action. Endocr Rev. 1998;19(1):80–100.
73. Hughes DE, Wright KR, Uy HL, Sasaki A, Yoneda T, Roodman DG, et al. Bisphosphonates promote apoptosis in murine osteoclasts in vitro and in vivo. J Bone Miner Res. 1995;10(10):1478–87.
74. Zehnder Y, Risi S, Michel D, Knecht H, Perrelet R, Kraenzlin M, et al. Prevention of bone loss in paraplegics over 2 years with alendronate. J Bone Miner Res. 2004;19(7):1067–74.
75. Shapiro J, Smith B, Beck T, Ballard P, Dapthary M, BrintzenhofeSzoc K, et al. Treatment with zoledronic acid ameliorates negative geometric changes in the proximal femur following acute spinal cord injury. Calcif Tissue Int. 2007;80(5):316–22.
76. Bekker PJ, Holloway DL, Rasmussen AS, Murphy R, Martin SW, Leese PT, et al. A single-dose placebo-controlled study of AMG 162, a fully human monoclonal antibody to RANKL, in postmenopausal women. J Bone Miner Res. 2005;20(12):2275–82.
77. Hamdy NA. Targeting the RANK/RANKL/OPG signaling pathway: a novel approach in the management of osteoporosis. Curr Opin Investig Drugs. 2007;8(4):299–303.
78. Jamal SA, Ljunggren Ö, Stehman-Breen C, Cummings SR, McClung MR, Goemaere S, et al. Effects of denosumab on fracture and bone mineral density by level of kidney function. J Bone Miner Res. 2011;26(8):1829–35.
79. Cummings SR, San Martin J, McClung MR, Siris ES, Eastell R, Reid IR, et al. Denosumab for prevention of fractures in postmenopausal women with osteoporosis. N Engl J Med. 2009;361(8):756–65.
80. Papapoulos S, Lippuner K, Roux C, Hall J, Kendler D, Lewiecki EM, et al. Eight years of denosumab treatment in postmenopausal women with osteoporosis: results from the first five years of the FREEDOM extension. J Bone Miner Res. 2013;28 Suppl 1:S503.
81. Reid IR. Efficacy, effectiveness and side effects of medications used to prevent fractures. J Int Med. 2014. doi:10.1111/joim.12339.
82. Fahrleitner-Pammer A, Langdahl BL, Marin F, Jakob F, Karras D, Barrett A, et al. Fracture rate and back pain during and after discontinuation of teriparatide: 36-month data from the European Forsteo Observational Study (EFOS). Osteoporos Int. 2011;22(10):2709–19. doi:10.1007/s00198-010-1498-5.
83. Daddona PE, Matriano JA, Mandema J, Maa YF. Parathyroid hormone (1–34)-coated microneedle patch system: clinical pharmacokinetics for treatment of osteoporosis. Pharm Res. 2011;28(1):159–65.

Chapter 11
Osteoporosis in Patients with Peripheral Neuropathies

Mendel Kupfer and Christina V. Oleson

Peripheral neuropathy, characterized by damage or destruction of neurons that determines how they communicate with each other, affects three types of nerves: sensory, motor, and autonomic (nerves that control involuntary or semi-voluntary function such as heart rate, blood pressure, and digestion) [1]. Damage to only one nerve is termed a mononeuropathy; mononeuritis multiplex neuropathy occurs when two or more isolated nerves in different part of the body are damaged; polyneuropathy implies the involvement of multiple nerves simultaneously. As opposed to hereditary neuropathy, acquired neuropathy has a number of causal factors including systemic diseases, medications and toxins, trauma, infections, autoimmune disorders, and vitamin imbalances. Its symptoms include numbness and tingling in the hands and feet, severe pain or the inability to feel pain at all, loss of coordination and reflexes, and muscle weakness [2, 3]. Diabetes, the primary cause of peripheral neuropathy, will be considered in this chapter together with critical illness polymyopathy and polyneuropathy and their association with immobility and medications. Two autoimmune disorders, Guillain–Barre syndrome and inflammatory demyelinating polyradiculoneuropathy, will also be discussed.

Diabetes Mellitus

Epidemiology

Diabetes mellitus (DM) is a disease of pandemic proportions in both the developed and developing nations. The International Diabetes Foundation reports that, as of 2014, some 387 million people worldwide were living with diabetes, with an estimated increase to 592 million by 2035 [4]. If the current trend persists, diabetes

C.V. Oleson, *Osteoporosis Rehabilitation*, DOI 10.1007/978-3-319-45084-1_11

prevalence in the United States will likely increase from 14 % in 2010 to 21 %, and, possibly, 33 % by 2050, depending upon the health of an aging population, the longevity of diabetic patients, and the survival of increasing numbers of high-risk minority groups [5].

Diabetes is divided into type 1 and type 2 variants, previously known as insulin- and non-insulin-dependent diabetes mellitus; the potential for hyperglycemia is present in both [6]. Type 1 diabetes (T1DM), affecting approximately 5–10 % of all diabetic individuals, is related to a rheumatoid-like autoimmune reaction that destroys the beta cells of the pancreas, leading to decreased production of insulin and, within a short time, total cessation of production. Formerly known as juvenile diabetes, it commonly begins in childhood but can develop in older adults as well. Type 1 diabetes cannot be prevented but can be controlled with daily insulin injections or an insulin pump [6].

In type 2 diabetes (T2DM), occurring in 90–95 % of diabetic patients, the pancreas continues to produce insulin but encounters peripheral receptor resistance/insulin resistance which occurs when fat, muscle, and liver cells fail to respond to insulin, preventing blood sugar from entering these cells as stored energy and leading to a buildup of sugar in the blood, resulting in hyperglycemia. Although the pancreas responds initially by producing more insulin, in time it cannot create a sufficient amount to meet the body's needs. Some 37 % of adults over the age of 20 have early signs of developing insulin resistance (prediabetes) and are at high risk for developing T2DM [7, 8], a condition that particularly targets the overweight and obese population. T2DM can be effectively treated with lifestyle changes including loss of weight, improved diet, and increased levels of physical activity. In addition, metformin, (Glucophage) used alone or with insulin, increases insulin sensitivity and reduces glucose levels without risk of hypoglycemia and weight gain.

Diabetes is associated with a number of health complications including cardiovascular diseases such as heart attack and stroke, kidney disease, blindness and other vision problems, and, the most common complication, peripheral neuropathy. The symptoms of peripheral neuropathy are related to the types of nerves involved, be they sensory, motor, autonomic, or a combination. The longer the duration of diabetes, the greater the risk of diabetic neuropathy. Caused by a number of factors, principally high glucose levels and high lipid levels, diabetic neuropathies are diagnosed on the basis of signs and symptoms including tingling, burning, numbness, and muscle weakness in the extremities as well as problems with coordination, balance, and walking; laboratory tests and electrodiagnostic findings are also employed [9].

The most common diabetic neuropathy, known as chronic distal sensorimotor symmetrical polyneuropathy (DSPN), impacts up to 50 % of diabetes patients; it is commonly manifested by burning and a deep aching pain in the feet and lower limbs and occurs in a relatively symmetrical manner on both sides of the body. DSPN contributes to an increased risk of foot ulceration and Charcot osteoarthropathy, the progressive destruction of bone and joint integrity, and it remains the leading cause of lower leg amputation [10].

Etiology and Pathophysiology of Osteoporosis in Diabetes

Both T1DM and T2DM have serious effects on the skeleton, with bone formation, bone microarchitecture, and bone quality altered in both forms. In terms of bone density, evidence shows a decrease in BMD in T1DM and an increase in T2DM. An increased risk of bone fractures has been found in both but to a lesser degree in T2DM. Given the different pathogenesis of T1DM and T2DM, no uniform entity of diabetic osteopathy exists [11]. Nearly 70 years ago, before the development of dual x-ray absorptiometry, Albright and Reifenstein first demonstrated an association between reduced bone mass and poor glycemic control in childhood diabetes. In the years since, numerous trials have been conducted to examine the nature and extent of bone mineral density and fractures in both types of diabetes; some generalizations have emerged but, to a considerable extent, the results remain inconclusive.

Mechanisms of Diabetic Bone Disease

Diabetes mellitus affects bone through the following mechanisms [12]:

1. Direct metabolic influence of insulin insufficiency on osteoblastic and osteoclastic function
2. Alterations in endocrine secretagogues by pancreatic beta cells, particularly amylin, causing decreased bone integrity (particularly in T1DM)
3. Impact of peripheral neuropathy on proprioception and activity levels
4. Relation between bone loss and both vascular dysfunction and impaired bone microcirculation evident in hyperglycemia
5. Contribution to diabetic retinopathy, resulting in decreased function and disuse osteopenia and osteoporosis from reduced immobility in setting of visual impairment
6. Effect of diabetes medications on bone pathology

Whereas T1DM is widely associated with bone loss and decreased osteoblast activity, T2DM is characterized by preserved-to-increased bone mineral density. As Vestergaard has determined [13], bone mineral density is reduced by 0.2 *Z*- scores in the hip and spine in T1DM, while it is increased by 0.3–0.4 *Z*- scores in T2DM. Yet, in spite of this data, the fracture rate in T2DM is increased over that of the normal population, indicating that the structural strength of bone is impaired.

In this section we will review the mechanisms associated with diabetic bone loss. Given the complex relationship between bone density and fracture risk, it should be emphasized that BMD is only one of the variables responsible for bone strength and quality. Understanding the mechanisms underlying the diabetes–bone relationship and advancing studies of this interaction are critical to the development of new therapies to restore bone loss, particularly as the human life span increases, with a concomitant rise in diabetes complications associated with aging. The following discussion focuses on the effect of diabetes on bone primarily in T1DM with references to T2DM as applicable.

Insulin and Insulin Secretagogues

Historically, as well as in recent years, the majority of studies focusing on the state of bone in T1DM have found decreased BMD in both the spine and hip. Osteopenia is present in about 50–60 % of people with T1DM with osteoporosis occurring in 14–20 % of cases [14]. Both osteopenia and osteoporosis are more prevalent in men than in women. One investigation reported that 14 % of the male patients and none of the females met the criteria for osteoporosis [15]. Similar trends for osteopenia have also been reported for diabetic men versus women [16]. Estrogen may also exert a protective effect on women.

Patients who develop T1DM in childhood and adolescence experience frequent episodes of prolonged bone loss, negatively affecting their ability to attain peak bone mass. Insulin is thought to exert an anabolic effect on bone formation based on data indicating that decreased adolescent growth velocity leads to insulin sufficiency which, in turn, impairs osteoblastic function and produces abnormalities of bone microarchitecture [17]. A 7-year prospective study of BMD in T1DM found that intensive insulin therapy significantly increased body mass index and stabilized BMD at all sites, although patients with retinopathy continued to lose body mass [18].

In addition to insulin, T1DM patients are unable to produce the insulin secretagogue, amylin—a peptide hormone co-secreted with insulin by the beta cells in the pancreas. Amylin enables blood glucose levels to remain relatively stable by slowing digestion, inhibiting secretion of glucagon (a pancreatic hormone that raises blood glucose levels), and enhancing satiety, thereby limiting the possibility of blood glucose "spikes" [19]. In fact, in animal models, supplementation of amylin maintained bone-mass-inhibited biochemical markers of bone reabsorption, and stimulated elevated bone formation [20]. Other secretagogues involved in bone regulation but inhibited in T1DM are glucagon-like polypeptide 2 (GLP2) and gastric inhibitory peptide (GIP). GLP2 receptors have been found on osteoclasts, and their activation is associated with reduced bone reabsorption. GIP receptors are present on osteoblasts, and their activation results in increased secretion of type 1 collagen [21]. It is unclear if the underlying autoimmune process that causes T1DM plays a role in bone metabolism. Table 1 [15, 18, 22–26] describes bone changes in patients with T1DM.

Hyperglycemia

Hyperglycemia exerts adverse effects on both T1DM and T2DM [19]. It leads to nonenzymatic glycosylation of various bone proteins including type 1 collagen, a condition that may impair bone quality [27]. On a cellular level, diabetes is believed to stimulate bone reabsorption by increasing both the number of osteoclasts and their activity through functions involving tumor necrosis factor alpha (TNF-α),

Table 1 Bone changes in patients with type I diabetes mellitus

Sources	*n*	Age (range in years)	Age (mean in years)	Mean duration follow-up (years)	Gender (F/M)	Major findings
Hamilton et al. [22] (2008)	102	20–71	–	Cohort study	52/50	When compared with age-matched control subjects, adult males with T1DM had lower BMD (hip, femoral neck, spine) ($P \leq 0.048$). No significant difference in terms of BMD between females with T1DM versus age-matched control subjects
Lumachi et al. [23] (2009)	18	36–51	–	Cohort study	8/10	~60 % lower BMD was found in patients with T1DM when compared to age-matched control subjects
Rozadilla et al. [24] (2000)	88	–	29	11	43/45	Retinopathy found to be associated with low BMD. Osteoporosis present in 3 %. Decreased lumbar spine BMD. No significant decreased of BMD in the femoral neck of patients with T1DM
Munoz-Torres et al. [25] (1996)	88	–	30	12	49/45	Decreased lumbar spine and femoral neck BMD in patients with T1DM. Osteoporosis present in 19 %. Retinopathy, active smoking, and neuropathy were also associated with decreased BMD
Campos Pastor et al. [18] (2000)	57	–	35	17	30/27	Retinopathy and poor glycemic control were associated with higher rates of osteopenia and osteoporosis (72 % vs. 53 % without retinopathy); benefits of intensive insulin therapy
Kemink et al. [15] (2000)	35	–	38	9	14/21	Decreased lumbar spine and femoral neck BMD in patients with T1DM. Osteopenia associated with decreased serum levels of IGF-1 and bone formation markers
Tuominen et al. [26] (1999)	56	–	61 (F) 62 (M)	18	27/29	Decreased (6.8 in females and 7.6 % in males) femoral neck BMD when compared with age-matched control subjects

macrophage colony-stimulating factor (M-CSF), and the receptor activator of nuclear factor-kB ligand (RANKL). These cytokines activate osteoclast proliferation and differentiation. As described in earlier chapters of this text, hyperglycemia also suppresses osteoblastic function by decreasing runt-related transcription factor 2 (RUNX2), decreasing osteocalcin and osteopontin expression, and reducing osteoblast proliferation. Due to an adverse effect on bone microcirculation, hyperglycemia reduces neurovascularization, thereby decreasing bone formation and impeding bone repair. The cumulative effect of these actions is a net decrease in bone formation.

Indicators of Bone Health

The sympathetic nervous system is thought to have a positive effect on maintenance of bone density but is impaired in the setting of neuropathy, common in both T1DM and T2DM. Research by Rix et al. shows that peripheral neuropathy in T1DM is associated with a greater risk of reduced bone mass in the spine, femur, and distal forearm, indicating that it may be an independent risk factor for reduced BMD not only as a localized process in the affected limbs but in the skeleton more generally [28]. Both diabetic neuropathy and retinopathy may also lower BMD by reducing physical activity needed to build bone and muscle strength as well as by increasing fall risk and resulting fractures.

At the same time, a meta-analysis of studies examining the relation between neuropathy and indicators of bone health in diabetes found no significant association with poor peripheral bone health in seven of the ten studies reviewed [29]. However, four of the ten studies did find an association between poor bone health in patients with neuropathy compared to those without neuropathy. Moreover, the authors acknowledge that methodological limitations in the studies reviewed (e.g., different methods to quantify and classify neuropathy) as well as limitations in the analysis itself (conflation of studies involving both T1DM and T2DM patients and the exclusion of relevant findings from studies that did not meet the review's criteria) point to the need for further investigation.

Adipokines: Leptin and Adiponectin

Adipokines including leptin and adiponectin are strongly associated with T1DM. Serum levels of leptin, a hormone produced by the anterior pituitary, are positively correlated with bone mineral density but are decreased in the setting of T1DM [30, 31]. Leptin increases cortical bone but decreases trabecular bone formation. By acting on the hypothalamus, it works through the sympathetic portion of the central nervous system (CNS) to upregulate bone formation. Whereas diabetic neuropathy exerts its effects on the peripheral nervous system, leptin is more often associated with CNS-related bone metabolism; consequently other mechanisms of leptin may be relevant to DM. Leptin exerts a direct effect on bone through actions on insulin-like growth factor-1 (IGF-I) [32]. Evidence further indicates that leptin may be the key to understanding the link between energy intake and bone metabolism [33].

In contrast, serum levels of adiponectin are negatively correlated with bone mineral density [34]. T1DM is associated with increased adiponectin which is related to insulin sensitivity. Studies indicate that adiponectin is a potent insulin enhancer linking adipose tissue and glucose metabolism throughout the body [35] and that it may influence immune response in T1DM just as leptin affects autoimmune diabetes [36].

To an extent, however, the role of these adipokines remains unclear. Leptin contributes to systemic inflammatory changes and is associated with atherosclerosis, hypertension, and neointimal thickening with vascular disease [35]. Adiponectin, which is present at lower levels in diabetic individuals, has anti-inflammatory properties [37], protects endothelial and vascular smooth muscle cells, and exerts a positive effect in myocardial remodeling [35, 38]. In terms of fractures, the positive effects of adipokines are countered by their negative effect on the cardiovascular system, predisposing diabetes patients to falls and increasing the risk for osteoporosis [19].

Glycation End Products

While the influences on both osteoblast and osteoclast formation and function significantly affect overall BMD, bone quality in individuals with DM is also reduced through several other metabolic processes. The production of advanced glycation end products (AGE) reduces levels of type 1 collagen which, in turn, increases bone flexibility. In stressful circumstances, a less rigid bone is more likely to fracture even under conditions of lower force and lower energy, such as falling or stumbling from a seated or stationary position. Table 2 summarizes the adverse effects of impaired glucose metabolism on bone.

Microvascular Disease

A recent report by Shanbhogue and colleagues considers yet another mechanism [39]. Comparing patients with T1DM against age-matched, healthy controls, they propose that the presence of microvascular disease may be a factor in bone loss for patients with T1DM. Specifically there were no differences between patients *without* microvascular disease and controls. However, T1DM patients *with* microvascular disease demonstrated lower total, trabecular, and cortical volumetric bone mineral density as well as microarchitectural changes in the form of thinner bone cortices at the radius, lower trabecular bone strength, and greater trabecular separation at both radius and tibia which could partially explain the higher level of

Table 2 Adverse effects of impaired glucose metabolism on bone

Factors that decrease BMD	Cause	Solution
Increased urinary calcium excretion	Poor glycemic control	Evaluate and monitor Hg A1c
		Improve dietary control
		Alter antidiabetic medications
Functional hyperparathyroidism	Low bone turnover resulting in decreased osteoblast function (advanced T1DM)	Correct thyroid levels
		Follow thyroid stimulating hormone [TSH] levels
		Optimize vitamin D
		Monitor renal function
Hyperparathyroidism	Excess cortisol seen in early stages of T1DM	Optimize/supplement vitamin D and monitor serum vitamin D 25OH and parathyroid hormone [PTH] levels
Altered vitamin D metabolism	Diabetic nephropathy	Supplement vitamin D possibly with calcitriol rather than cholecalciferol
		Consider renal consultation
Adverse effects of insulin and insulin-like growth factors	Poor glycemic control that may increase need for insulin	Consider endocrine consultation
		Encourage improving glycemic control through nutritional therapy
		Follow growth hormone [GH] levels
		Follow insulin-like growth factor-1 [IGF-1] levels
Estrogen deficiency	Early menopause	Monitor BMD, obtain levels of key pituitary hormones (gonadotropins such as follicle-stimulating hormone [FSH], luteinizing hormone [LH]; as well as growth hormone [GH] and prolactin); in addition, consider pharmacologic interventions during perimenopausal phase

skeletal fragility evident in these subjects. Differences between microvascular positive and negative T1DM remained significant after controlling for age, years of DM, and average glycated hemoglobin over the prior 3-year period. Vitamin D insufficiency and celiac disease are still other causal factors in diabetes-induced osteoporosis.

Fracture Risk

Type 1 Diabetes

Vestergaard et al. have reported a trend toward an increased fracture risk at most skeletal sites in type 1 diabetes as well as a marked trend toward higher fracture risk in the presence of complications; most of the studies examined in his analysis focused on hip fracture [13]. For example, Nicodemus et al. [40] reported that postmenopausal women were 12.25 times more likely to experience a hip fracture—a finding confirmed by subsequent studies of diabetic men and women in the relevant age groups [41] and in a different study, specifically in women ages 34–59 [42]. A recent study by Weber et al. [43] was the first to report that an increase in fracture risk begins in childhood and adolescence and extends over the life span of T1DM patients. Men ages 60–69 and women ages 40–49 have double the fracture risk of those without diabetes. Moreover, people with retinopathy and neuropathy have a higher fracture risk in the lower extremities with falls being a major contributing factor.

Type 2 Diabetes

In recent years, increased fracture risk, formerly associated primarily with T1DM, has become a growing concern in T2DM patients, although they are still affected to a lesser degree. In terms of hip fractures, Nicodemus et al. found a 1.7-fold increased risk of hip fractures in postmenopausal women with T2DM than in those without diabetes [40]. An association between higher fracture incidence and such factors as longer disease duration, decreased bone quality, diabetic complications, inadequate glycemic control, the use of insulin or oral diabetes medications, and increased fall risk has also been identified and reported. Despite the paradox of higher bone density coexistent with increased fracture risk in T2DM, Schwartz et al. determined [44] that women ages 65 and older were at greater risk of developing hip, proximal humerus, and foot fractures than nondiabetic women, in part because of associated comorbidities including decreased bone quality and impaired balance and gait due to neuropathy, and visual impairment resulting from diabetic retinopathy and cataracts.

The recognition that diabetes compromises bone health, particularly in an aging population, strengthens the need to incorporate bone assessment together with possible treatment options as an integral part of long-term diabetes care. A 2015 International Osteoporosis Foundation review of bone fragility in T1DM [45] strongly recommends early and regular evaluation of fracture risk in T1DM coupled with the implementation of fracture prevention strategies; in addition, it advocates intensified efforts to evaluate the efficacy of anti-osteoporotic agents in the context of diabetes.

Complications of Diabetes Mellitus Related to Bone and Physical Function

Charcot Osteoarthropathy

Diabetes mellitus and its neuropathies are regarded as the most common cause of Charcot osteoarthropathy (COA), also known as Charcot foot. A chronic, progressive, potentially limb-threatening disease, it is relatively rare, occurring in an estimated 0.08–7.5 % of patients with both T1DM and T2DM [46]. Characterized by destruction of bone and joint integrity, it initially presents with redness, swelling, and increased warmth, progressing to severe deformities including collapse of the midfoot and ulcers that could predispose to amputation.

COA is associated with vascular calcification which includes abnormal calcified deposits in the smooth muscle of blood vessels of all sizes and with atherosclerosis that results in vascular stiffness and increases systolic blood pressure [47]. The primary underlying etiology of the disease is thought to be increased trauma resulting from impaired sensory feedback of the joint under conditions of both peripheral and autonomic neuropathy. This trauma, often minimal in nature, causes excess production of pro-inflammatory cytokines including TNF-α which, in turn, leads to an increase in RANKL-mediated osteoclast activation, causing bone fracture and destruction [47, 48].

The first step in treating COA is to control the heat and swelling and stabilize the foot to prevent disease progression and minimize deformity. Nonoperative treatment generally includes the use of a total contact cast or a bivalved cast (Aircast walker) followed by bracing and the use of footwear designed to accommodate preexisting deformities, relieve pressure, and ensure joint stability [48]. Surgical treatment, reserved for patients with recurrent joint instability and ulceration, may entail removal of a bony prominence, midfoot fusion, and realignment osteotomy. Pharmacological therapies including bisphosphonates and calcitonin as well as anabolic agents such as human parathyroid hormones are being investigated as treatment options with some early success [49].

Diabetes Medications Detrimental to Bone

The link between fracture risk and diabetes medication is most clearly established in the class of drugs called thiazolidinediones (rosiglitazone/Avandia and pioglitazone/Actos). Although their efficacy in controlling diabetic hyperglycemia has been demonstrated, their prolonged use negatively impacts osteoblastogenesis by decreasing activity of both osteoblast transcription factors (e.g., RUNX2) and osteoblast signaling pathways (e.g., ICF-1) [50]. As a result, thiazolidinediones decrease bone formation and bone mineral density while increasing bone reabsorption, leading to greater fracture risk. A large, population-based case–control analysis demonstrated that the use of rosiglitazone and pioglitazone in men and women with T2DM for 12 or more months may be linked to a two to threefold increased risk of hip and nonvertebral osteoporotic fractures [51]. Both drugs are now in limited use as a result of FDA warnings about the adverse heart-related side effects of rosiglitazone and the heightened risk of bladder cancer of pioglitazone [52].

Recently, canagliflozin (Invokana, Invokamet), a sodium–glucose cotransporter-2 (SGLT2), has been used in combination with a sulfoylurea, pioglitazone, or short acting insulins to lower blood sugar in T2DM by stimulating the kidneys to remove sugar through the urine. In 2015 the FDA issued two warnings regarding the use of canagliflozin, one dealing with bone fracture risk and decreased BMD [53] and the other with the presence of too much acid in the blood (acidosis) due to the production of high levels of ketones [54]. Drawing on the results of several clinical trials, the first warning was based on findings that fractures occur more frequently with canagliflozin than with placebos and within a time span of 12 weeks after initiating treatment. It is not FDA approved for patients with T1DM.

Antiepileptic medications such as gabapentin and pregabalin are commonly used as therapy for the pain associated with diabetic peripheral polyneuropathy. As a class, they affect balance and coordination, increasing fall and fracture risk; moreover, they also lead to vitamin D25(OH) insufficiency and deficiency [55]. Large-scale RCTs as well as long-term follow-ups are needed to elucidate the efficacy of antiepileptic drugs in neuropathic pain [56]. Patients with diabetic polyneuropathy may also receive selective serotonin–norepinephrine reuptake inhibitors (SNRIs), a class of antidepressant medications that is associated with decreased bone mineral density, increased falls, and a greater risk of nonspine fracture including hip fractures [57].

Prevention and Treatment of Diabetes Mellitus-Related Bone Disease

Treatment of bone disease in diabetes requires a multipronged approach. Several of the following therapies apply to osteoporosis in general. Others are related to conditions specific to diabetes.

Nonpharmacologic Interventions

The first step is to minimize any inciting events that adversely affect bone demineralization and increase fracture risk including poor glycemic control, harmful medications, and falls. Patients with T1DM are at particularly high risk of osteoporotic fractures, with T2DM patients affected to a lesser degree; however, both groups of patients should be made aware of the principal causes of osteoporosis in diabetes, particularly insulin deficiency and the impact of peripheral neuropathy and retinopathy. As Brown et al. emphasize, no osteoporosis screening recommendations have been adopted for patients with diabetes, but it is deemed prudent to provide screening for both men and women (particularly thin women), with T1DM complications [58]. In T2DM, conventional dual-emission x-ray absorptiometry scans may be misleading given that, in this condition, higher BMD coexists with increased fracture risk due primarily to falls [19].

Poor nutrition and a compromised lifestyle are factors contributing to the development of osteoporosis in diabetes. Diets with adequate amounts of calcium and vitamin D or supplements if needed should be maintained in order to help ensure

Table 3 Factors that increase falls in diabetic patients

Factor	Cause	Solution
Diabetic neuropathy	Altered sensation and proprioception and balance Foot ulcers that alter weight-bearing	Proper footwear PT evaluation Use of assistive devices (cane, walker) if appropriate Improve glucose control
Diabetic retinopathy and cataracts	Retinal vascular changes that impair visual acuity caused by years of poor glucose control	Routine optical evaluation
Orthostatic hypotension	New medications, excessive doses of antihypertensive medications, or dehydration	Educate patient on getting up from seated position Avoid drastic dose alternations in antihypertensive medications
Hypoglycemia	May cause syncope or dizziness	Close monitoring of glucose levels throughout day

bone health and optimal glucose control. Smoking and excessive alcohol intake should be avoided. Weight management is an issue for both excessively thin women with T1DM and obese and overweight women with T2DM. Risk factors for falls including advanced age, household hazards, and impaired balance should also be minimized (Table 3).

The next factor in both prevention of further decline and ongoing treatment is regular physical therapy to develop proprioceptive and balance skills and to increase and maintain bone and muscle strength. With the assistance of a physical therapist, if needed, diabetic patients should be encouraged to walk, jog, dance as well as practice yoga and engage in weight-bearing and resistance exercises. As predicated in Wolff's law (bone adapts to the loads placed upon it), bone strength is directly correlated with use. Given painful peripheral polyneuropathy, retinopathy, and poor proprioception as well as possible cardiac deconditioning and a propensity for coronary vascular accidents, diabetic patients experience a decline in activity. In contrast, maintaining appropriate activity levels not only contributes to healthy bone remodeling as well as muscle coordination and balance, but it also exerts beneficial effects on glycemic control, atherosclerosis risk, and weight control [58].

Pharmacologic Treatment

A number of medications that positively alter the bone formation and reabsorption balance have proved effective in treating diabetic osteoporosis. In the first instance, recombinant insulin therapy, acting through its osteoblast receptors, exerts an osteogenic effect on osteoblasts [12]. As Gopalakrishnan et al. [59] have shown, insulin in combination with estradiol counters the deleterious effect of high concentrations of glucose on osteoblast proliferation and function.

The antidiabetic drug, metformin, positively influences bone turnover and is associated with a decrease in risk fracture. It not only has a direct osteogenic effect at all glucose concentrations [60] but in animal studies, it has been shown to exert a positive impact on osteoblast differentiation and function both in vivo and in vitro [61]. Long used in T2DM, metformin has recently assumed new importance as the focus of a proposed study examining its efficacy in treating several age-related ailments including cardiovascular disease, cancer, and cognitive impairment—a significant departure from studies addressing treatments for only a single disease [62].

A study of ovariectomized and non-ovariectomized rats demonstrates that glimepiride, a first-line drug in the treatment of T2DM, inhibits the deleterious bone changes caused by estrogen deficiency in ovariectomized rats and heightens bone formation, indicating that it may reduce the risk of osteoporosis, particularly in postmenopausal women [63].

In terms of prescription agents for osteoporosis, the bisphosphonates—specifically alendronate, risedronate, and pamidronate—have become a significant addition to the therapeutic armamentarium for osteoporosis. By reducing osteoclast activity, they inhibit bone resorption, thereby preventing bone loss and inducing increased BMD. Interestingly, recent studies have indicated a possible correlation between the use of alendronate and both a decrease in daily insulin requirements as well as a possible decrease in T2DM itself. As a treatment for senile T1DM alendronate produced an increase in BMD accompanied by a reduction in the required daily consumption of insulin, perhaps because it alleviated some of the pain, rigidity, and restricted movement in osteoporosis, enabling patients to improve their physical activity [64].

An examination of the use of alendronate in patients with T2DM revealed a reduced risk of T2DM in users of alendronate as opposed to a 21 % increased risk of developing the disease in those not receiving the drug. Increased physical activity may also be a factor in this analysis [65]. Similarly, a British study found that the long-term use of bisphosphonates reduced the chance of developing T2DM by one-half with a greater risk reduction in women (51 %) than in men (23 %); a slight increase in risk occurred in the period from 1 to 2.5 years of exposure, followed by a sustained decrease thereafter [66]. These findings await confirmation. Few if any bisphosphonate treatments have been studied in patients with both diabetes and osteoporosis, although small studies have shown the efficacy of pamidronate in COA [58].

Compared with bisphosphonates, the selective estrogen receptor modulator, raloxifene, exhibits relatively modest BMD gains but causes reductions in vertebral fractures similar to those of bisphosphonates. A randomized clinical trial involving 40 postmenopausal women with T2DM found that raloxifene did not affect either glycemic control or insulin sensitivity [67]. Although approved by the FDA for treatment of postmenopausal women with osteoporosis, the androgynous peptide, calcitonin, is regarded as a second-tier therapy because of the availability of more effective drugs, the lack of definitive evidence on calcitonin's efficacy in preventing fracture, and recent studies indicating a possible causal relationship with cancer [68].

Also approved by the FDA but with a 2-year limitation, parathyroid hormone (PTH) is generally reserved for patients at greatest risk of fracture, not only because of its cost but also because of its possible relation to increased risk of osteosarcoma [58]. This risk has only been observed in laboratory animals, but individuals with high-risk conditions such as Paget's disease of the bone or prior radiation should avoid PTH [69].

Future Treatments

The protein PPAR-γ, currently the focus of efforts to develop insulin sensitivity in T2DM, shows highly preliminary but promising results as a new therapeutic approach to bone formation. PPAR-γ is known to inhibit the production of stem cells in bone marrow, preventing the cells from developing into bone, cartilage, and connective tissue. In a laboratory trial involving mice and human tissue, Marciano et al. found that when stem cells were treated with a compound that represses PPAR-γ activity, a statistically significant increase occurred in osteoclast formation leading to increased bone formation. The next step is to test the compound in animal models of bone loss, aging, obesity, and diabetes [70]. These and other investigations related to PPAR-γ, together with the development of new medications, are forthcoming.

Critical Illness Polyneuropathy and Polymyopathy

Critical illness polyneuropathy (CIP), particularly when associated with sepsis and systematic inflammatory response syndrome (SIRS), is one of the most common neuromuscular complications of critical illness. An axonal degenerative polyneuropathy presenting as both limb and respiratory muscle weakness, CIP affects primarily distal motor fibers as opposed to proximal ones [71]. It is often cited as an underlying factor in a patient's difficulty in weaning from a mechanical ventilator, thereby increasing the risk of intensive care morbidity; greater susceptibility to infection and organ failure are also likely to result [72]. CIP and an overlapping syndrome, critical illness myopathy (CIM), are thought to occur in approximately 25–50 % of patients admitted to the intensive care unit with SIRS or sepsis [73].

The etiology of critical illness polyneuropathy is unclear. Observations of its clinical course have led to speculation that it may be caused by a defect in the transportation of nutrients through the axon—a process that requires significant energy expenditure which may be deficient due to the sepsis and various interleukins and cytokines that affect cellular respiration. Further, microcirculation to peripheral nerves may be impaired by sepsis and its cardiovascular consequences as well as by elevated glucose levels associated with diabetic polyneuropathy [74].

In terms of diagnosis, the following criteria for critical illness polyneuropathy have been put forward by Latronico and Bolton [75]:

1. Patient is critically ill with multi-organ dysfunction.
2. Patient has limb weakness or difficulty in weaning after non-neuromuscular etiologies have been ruled out.
3. Electrophysiological evidence of axonal motor and sensory polyneuropathy exists.
4. Detrimental response on repetitive nerve stimulation is absent, thus excluding neuromuscular junction pathology.

A diagnosis of CIP is established if all four of these criteria are met. In the absence of limb weakness or difficulty in weaning from a ventilator but in the presence of other criteria, critical illness polyneuropathy is considered probable but cannot be confirmed.

Medical care for CIP emphasizes intensive insulin treatment (IIT), early mobilization through physiotherapy, and electrical muscle stimulation. Studies indicate that CIP and its accompanying hyperglycemia may be mitigated with strict glucose control [76]. A 2001 RCT enrolling 1,548 surgical ICU patients demonstrated that IIT to maintain blood glucose level at or below 110 mg per deciliters reduced overall in-hospital mortality by 34 % and CIP by 44 %, with patients less likely to require prolonged mechanical ventilation and intensive care [76]. On the basis of these results, IIT was widely prescribed. However, a subsequent 2009 trial involving 3,054 patients on IIT and 3,054 on conventional glucose control reported that IIT increased the absolute risk of death at 90 days by 2.6 % and recommended that a blood glucose level of 180 mg or less per deciliter be adopted. IIT is also known to increase the risk of hypoglycemia [77].

Early treatment with immunoglobulin M-enriched intravenous immunoglobulin (IVIG) initially seemed promising but ultimately has not been efficacious in the prevention and treatment of critical illness polyneuropathy in patients with multiple organ failure and sepsis/SIRS nor does it influence the length of ICU stay or mortality in these patients [78]. Early mobilization combined with physiotherapy in the ICU shows limited but promising results in terms of improved functional independence as well as reduced inflammation and disability. A progressive four-step mobility and walking program, conducted by a multidisciplinary team, is among the potential interventions designed to reduce the duration of mechanical ventilation and the length of hospital stays [79].

It should be noted, however, that two recent systematic reviews—one dealing with the effect of physical rehabilitation on activities of daily living and quality of life [80] and the other with the impact of exercised-based intervention following ICU discharge [81]—produced inconclusive results, largely attributable to marked differences between studies, variability in the way they were performed and presented, failure to meet inclusion criteria, and insufficient methodological rigor. Further research is needed to elucidate the benefits of physical therapy in various critical illnesses as well as the intensity and frequency of physical activity required to produce optimal results [82].

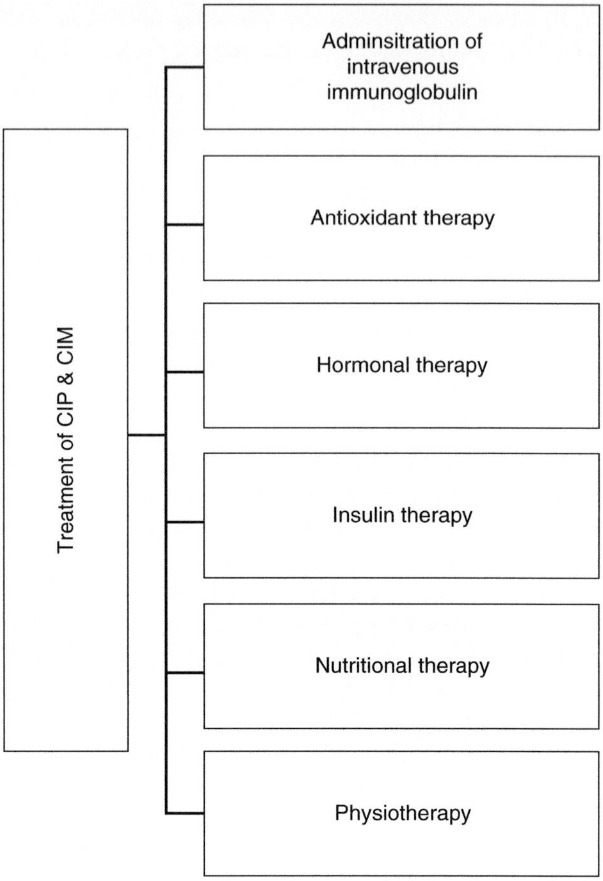

Fig. 1 Approaches to treatment of CIP and CIM. The figure illustrates many approaches to treatment with the more aggressive treatments at the top and less aggressive approaches below. While initial studies on IVIG indicated it might be a possible treatment, later, more robust investigations found it conferred substantially less benefit. The figure is not meant to imply a stepwise progression of treatment; in fact, nutritional therapy and physiotherapy should be done in all patients with CIP and CIM (*Source*: Zhou et al. [72]. Adapted with permission)

As an alternative to active exercise, electrical muscle stimulation (ESTIM) is emerging as a safe and effective therapy for ICU patients, particularly those with heart failure and chronic obstructive pulmonary disease (COPD). In their study of the effects of ESTIM on muscle strength, Karatzanos et al. indicated that ESTIM had a beneficial effect on the muscle strength of ICU patients primarily in terms of the muscle groups stimulated but also in those not involved, indicating its potential ability to improve overall muscle strength and to promote early mobilization [83]. Approaches to treatment for CIM and CIP are illustrated in Fig. 1 [72].

Complications Related to Bone

Critical illness and ICU care may be associated with decreased bone mineralization in part because of the immobility associated with this condition. Immobilization is a long-established but seldom-recognized cause of recurrent hypercalcemia which, in turn, can lead to multiple organ dysfunction, impaired renal function, gastrointestinal disorders, and neurological symptoms including weakness and depression [84]. In the presence of sepsis, hypercalcemia of immobility may be worsened due to pro-inflammatory cytokines such as IL1, IL6, and TNF-α that accelerate osteoclastic resorption.

Medications for Treatment of Hypercalcemia

Treatment options for hypercalcemia exist, principally in the form of bisphosphonates, specifically pamidronate and zoledronic acid, and in the form of and the human monoclonal antibody, denosumab.

Gallacher et al. demonstrated that pamidronate at doses as low as 10 mg is safe and effective in immobilization-related hypercalcemia and proposed that sepsis be added to the list of risk factors for developing the disorder [85]. In cases of severe renal insufficiency, bisphosphonates may cause renal toxicity; thus denosumab, which is not excreted by the kidneys, has been introduced as an alternative medication to reduce serum calcium concentration, with demonstrated success [86]. Unlike an IV infusion of bisphosphonates, denosumab is given as a two-yearly subcutaneous injection, meaning that it can be easily administered in a skilled nursing facility without monitoring; it remains in the blood stream for months and could eventually have wider applicability for those with immobilization hypercalcemia [87]. Both bisphosphonates and the monoclonal antibody denusomab are also given for treatment of osteoporosis.

Like bisphosphonates, denosumab has been associated with atypical femur fractures [88]; however, such fractures are uncommon and both medications are likely to prevent more fractures than they cause [89]. In its primary use as an FDA-approved medication for postmenopausal osteoporosis, denosumab treatment, sustained over a period of six years, remained well tolerated, reduced bone turnover, increased bone mineral density, and reduced the risk of vertebral and nonvertebral fractures while maintaining a low fracture rate, even below that projected for a virtual placebo group [90].

Medications Causing Bone Loss

In addition to immobility, medications commonly administered to critically ill patients affect bone mineral density and fracture risk. The benefits and risk of prescribing these drugs, particularly for the long term, should be considered in the context of the severity of the disease and its complications as well as the evidence supporting the drug's efficacy.

Proton Pump Inhibitors

Proton pump inhibitors (PPIs) are regarded as the leading therapy for gastroesophageal reflux disease. In contrast to their less potent counterpart, histamine-2 receptor antagonists (H2RAs) which work by inhibiting histamine action in the parietal cells of the stomach, PPIs including omeprazole, pantoprazole, esomeprazole, and lansoprazole block the site of acid production in these cells, while H2RAs such as famotidine and ranitidine inhibit the action of histamine on parietal cells in the stomach, reducing the secretion of stomach acid. Numerous studies on the possible effect of PPIs on fracture risk have been undertaken with conflicting results; no association or a small decrease in fracture risk has been detected with H2RAs.

Whereas the PPI, omeprazole, has been found to decrease bone resorption in vitro [91], proton pump inhibition has been associated with the reduction in calcium absorption [92]. It has been postulated that a decrease in gastric pH inhibits calcium absorption since patients who have undergone gastrectomy (surgical removal of all or part of the stomach) and those with hypochlorhydria (inability of the stomach to produce hydrochloric acid) evidence decreased calcium absorption. Countering these results is the finding that patients with vagotomy (surgical severance of part of, or a resection of, the vagus nerve) but without gastrectomy do not experience bone density loss [93].

A trial involving postmenopausal women indicated that 30 days of continuous PPI therapy did not alter functional calcium absorption [94]. In addition, a recent study using the Manitoba Bone Mineral Density Database [95, 96] found no association between PPIs and either osteoporosis or accelerated BMD loss, independent of a link with fracture risk. The Manitoba study matched 2,193 subjects evidencing osteoporosis of the hip with 5,527 normal controls and 3,596 subjects with osteoporosis of the lumbar spine with 10,257 normal controls. Proton pump inhibitor use was defined as greater than 1,500 standard proton pump inhibitor doses over a 5-year period of time. In both a cross-sectional and a longitudinal analysis, results indicated that chronic use of PPIs inhibition was not associated with increased likelihood of BMD loss or osteoporosis (as determined by bone mineral densitometry), at either the hip or lumbar spine. The majority of patients with CIP do not require long-term GI prophylaxis but rather use these agents to get through the current hospital course and potentially a short duration after hospitalization to protect against stress ulcers, particularly in a setting where blood thinners for deep vein thrombosis prophylaxis are prescribed. This situation lies in contrast to that experienced by patients with more chronic conditions of severe gastrointestinal reflux, or valvular heart disease where high dose anticoagulation is required for the patient's remaining life.

Just as the studies relating to BMD loss are contradictory, so too are studies examining the link between PPIs and fracture risk. Two large trials published in 2006 reported evidence of an association between the two. Vestergaard et al. [97] demonstrated that PPIs produce a limited increase in fracture risk for use within one year in contrast to H2RAs that appeared to produce a small decrease fracture risk over the same period. In a nested case–control study, Yang et al. corroborated the Vestergaard et al. results by determining that PPIs, when taken for more than one year, led to increased fracture risk and that the risk was significantly greater with PPI use than with H2RAs; moreover the adjusted rate of fractures was significantly higher in patients taking a long-term high dose of PPIs [98].

At a time when PPI use was still relatively low, a trial examining its relationship to hip fracture found no increase in fracture risk in patients in the absence of other medical risk factors, such as alcohol dependence and neurologic disease.

A subsequent study of more than 130,000 postmenopausal women enrolled in the Women's Health Initiative revealed no connection between PPIs and hip fracture at a 7-year follow-up but did identify a 47 % increased risk for spine fracture and a 26 % increased risk for forearm/wrist fracture. A marginal effect on 3-year BMD change was present at the hip but not at other sites [99].

On the basis of these and other epidemiological studies, in 2010, the FDA instituted a product label change on both prescription and over-the-counter PPIs including a warning that "PPI therapy may be associated with an increased risk for osteoporosis-related fracture of the hip, wrist or spine with the risk of fracture increased in patients who received high-dose, long–term PPI therapy for a year or longer." A year later, the FDA rescinded the ruling on over-the-counter PPIs, citing the unlikelihood of fracture risk based on their lower doses and recommended short-term use [100].

In the years since the FDA ruling, researchers have continued to indicate a link between PPIs and fracture risk, but the magnitude of the risk still remains uncertain. In contrast to earlier studies, the newer trials indicate a lower risk of osteoporosis at the lumbar spine and hip as well as a more modest increase in spine, forearm/wrist, and total fractures [101]. Yet findings remain contradictory. A Canadian study found no correlation between PPI use over 10 years and accelerated bone mineral density loss [102]. However, a large American trial involving nearly 80,000 postmenopausal women [103] reported that, compared with nonusers, women who took PPIs regularly for at least two years evidenced a 35 % higher risk of hip fracture, with longer use associated with greater risk. The relationship was sustained after adjusting for body mass index, physical activity, calcium intake, and the use of drugs (bisphosphonates, corticosteroids) that affect fracture risk. After other factors contributing to hip fractures were taken into account, only one, smoking, was found to independently contribute to the association: in current and former smokers, the risk of hip fracture increased to greater than 50 %.

While postmenopausal women remain a focus of PPI studies, men and younger adults have also been studied. In a trial involving men taking omeprazole and pantoprazole, PPI consumption was associated with an increasing risk of fractures in long-term PPI users, in the most adherent users, and in most recent users [104]. This association, together with a dose-responsive effect, is also evident in young adults but not in children [105].

Thus far, some 35 studies of PPIs and fractures involving two million participants [106] have been conducted. In assessing the results, several analyses have pointed out that these are nearly all retrospective, observational studies which have a greater potential for bias and produce less accurate estimates [107]. Nonetheless, given the marked increase in PPI use—an estimated 113 million prescriptions, excluding over-the-counter medications, are filled globally each year [108]— concerns over PPI use appear to be warranted. Again the risks and benefits of therapy should be taken into account, especially at a time when PPIs are considered to be overprescribed. In general, PPIs are indicated in cases of severe acid peptic disorders including gastroesophageal reflux disease (GERD), peptic ulcers, and dyspepsia with an indication that they not be used in higher doses or for a longer period than needed [101]. High-risk patients such as postmenopausal women, the elderly, the nutritionally deficient, and those with osteoporosis who are at a high risk of falling should be monitored regularly. Most patients with upper GI symptoms can be treated with the lowest effective dose or with far less expensive H2RAs which have little or no association with increased fracture risk.

Large prospective RCTs are needed to confirm or refute the results of past observational studies on PPIs as well as to determine causality and magnitude of risk. The most widely "assumed" mechanism [92] underlying the relation between PPIs and bone fractures involves long-term use leading to increased calcium absorption which, in turn, results in a negative calcium balance and increased risk of osteoporosis, bone loss, and fractures. However, a clearly defined, noncontroversial mechanism awaits further investigation.

Loop Diuretics

Although not directly associated with sepsis, loop diuretics are another class of medications commonly used in the ICU environment to manage congestive heart disease and anasarca (extreme generalized edema). In a 2006 trial with postmenopausal women, Rejnmark et al. reported that the loop diuretic, bumetanide, inhibits sodium and chloride reabsorption, thereby blocking calcium reabsorption, increasing renal excretion and bone turnover, and significantly decreasing bone mineral density by 2 % at the total hip and forearm [109].

By contrast, a large, prospective study of postmenopausal women enrolled in the Women's Health Initiative [110] found no significant association between ever-use of loop diuretics and changes in BMD, fall occurrence, and total and clinical vertebral fractures. The study did confirm a link between prolonged use (over three years) and increased fracture risk. Whether it was sufficiently empowered to address the relation between loop diuretics and bone fracture has been questioned on the basis that the data documented only long-term use [111].

Conflicting findings emerge from two other studies of hip bone loss in older women and men. Lim et al. reported a small but significantly higher rate of bone loss in female loop diuretic users compared with nonusers after a mean duration of 4.4 years [112]. In men, the adjusted rates of loss were twofold greater among intermittent loop diuretic users and 2.5-fold greater among continuous users. These inconclusive results may be attributable, in part, to potential bias, heterogeneity, residual confounding, lack of relevant data, and other methodological issues, leaving open the question of whether and to what extent the association can be confirmed. A 2015 meta-analysis of 113 studies indicates that users of loop diuretics had a significant positive association with overall risk of total and hip fractures [113].

Anticoagulants

Deep vein thrombosis (DVT) prophylaxis is often administered to patients in the form of unfractionated or low-molecular-weight heparin, both of which are associated with impaired bone metabolism. Intravenous heparin has been found to not only decrease cancellous bone volume in a dose and time-dependent manner but also to produce a dose-dependent decrease in alkaline phosphatase, a marker of bone formation, and a dose-dependent increase in urinary type 1 collagen cross-linked pyridinoline (PYD), a marker of bone resorption. It is also postulated that effects of heparin upon bone are long lasting with deficits seen for many years after intense heparin therapy [114].

A derivative of heparin, low-molecular-weight heparin, is a commonly used alternative to unfractionated heparin and is linked with fewer hematologic side effects. Whereas standard heparin is known to cause spontaneous fracture of the rib and vertebrae, studies have borne out the fact that low-molecular-weight heparin is linked to decreased risk for developing osteoporosis [115]. Monreal et al. found that 15 % of nonpregnant women treated with unfractionated heparin reported vertebral fractures within six months of initiating therapy, while only 2.5 % treated with the low-molecular-weight heparin, dalteparin, reported similar fractures [116]. Fondaparinux, a synthetically produced anticoagulant used in similar fashion to low-molecular-weight heparin but often reserved for those with heparin-induced thrombocytopenia, has not been associated with changes in bone metabolism or integrity [114].

Guillain–Barre Syndrome (GBS)/Chronic Inflammatory Demyelinating Polyradiculoneuropathy (CIDP)

Epidemiology

Guillain–Barre syndrome (GBS) is defined as an acute inflammatory disease of the peripheral nerves caused by damage to the myelin, the insulation surrounding sensory, motor, or autonomic nerve fibers. It is also termed acute demyelinating polyneuropathy (AIDP). Symptoms, including numbness, weakness and cramping in the limbs, and difficulty breathing, develop rapidly and progress within a 2–4-week period, followed by a plateau and eventual improvement in the majority of cases; there is no recurrence and little if any further deterioration. Because of its acute onset and rapid decline, GBS can be confused with critical illness polyneuropathy. Table 4 compares features of CIP and Guillain–Barre [72].

Chronic inflammatory demyelinating polyneuropathy (CIDP) is regarded as the chronic form of GBS (AIDP). While both AIDP and CIDP are caused by an attack on myelin, they differ in terms of onset and progression. Unlike GBS, CIDP develops more slowly and may progress for as long as eight weeks with a possibility of recurrence; without treatment, some 30 % of CIDP patients mobilize predominantly by wheelchair [117]. Although CIDP exists in several different phenotypic variants, it is primarily characterized by loss of sensation or abnormal sensation such as tingling and pain and weakness associated with loss of reflexes and manifested by difficulty in walking. Just as recognition of different types of GBS has led to advances in treatment, so greater understanding of

Table 4 Comparison of critical illness polyneuropathy (CIP) and Guillain–Barre syndrome (GBS)

	CIP	GBS
Prodromal indications	Sepsis and multiple organ failure	Respiratory or gastrointestinal infection
Clinical presentation	Typically the onset follows an intensive care unit admission	Typically the onset precedes an intensive care unit admission
Electrophysiology	Axonal motor and sensory polyneuropathy	Unresponsive nerves or demyelinating polyneuropathy; spontaneous neuronal activity; Axonal motor and sensory polyneuropathy
Cerebrospinal fluid	Typically normal	Albuminocytologic dissociation
Magnetic resonance imaging	Absent of any significant findings	On occasion, there will be indications involving the enhancement of spinal nerve roots
Biopsy	Primarily axonal degeneration of the distal peripheral nerves without inflammation	Primarily demyelinating process with inflammation, or motor axonal degeneration only, or motor and sensory axonal degeneration
Treatment	Typically antiseptic treatment is appropriate, but no specific therapy is indicated	Plasmapheresis, intravenous immunoglobulin
Outcome	Patient may have spontaneous recovery with variable timing; 50 % of patients with full recovery	Usually more than 75 % of patients with full recovery

Source: Zhou et al. [72]. Used with permission

these phenotypes should help guide diagnostic and treatment strategies for CIDP [118]. Table 5 illustrates the comparison of CIDP and GBS [117, 119–121].

Treatment of GBS

Distinguishing between GBS and CIDP is important in terms of determining optimal therapies. To hasten improvement, Guillain–Barre is generally treated with either plasma exchange or high-dose intravenous immunoglobulin (IVIG), both of which are equally effective. Because it is easier to administer, IVIG is the treatment of choice beginning as soon as possible after diagnosis. Accelerated recovery occurs in some patients but others experience residual deficits [122]. In a Cochrane review of the use of corticosteroids in GBS, moderate quality evidence revealed that, when given alone, corticosteroids do not significantly

Table 5 Differentiation between CIDP and GBS

	CIDP	GBS
What is it?	A neurological disorder characterized by progressive weakness and impaired sensory function in the legs and arms. Considered the chronic counterpart of Guillain–Barre	An acute inflammatory disease of the peripheral nerves that causes an autoimmune attack on the myelin leading to a loss of myelin
How to differentiate	Considered when a patient thought to have Guillain–Barre syndrome deteriorates again after eight weeks from onset or when deterioration occurs three times or more	Symptoms include paresthesia in toes and fingers on both sides of the body, loss of reflexes (such as knee jerk), slowed nerve conduction velocity, high protein in cerebrospinal fluid
Likelihood of osteoporosis	Unlikely; risk increases with intake of steroids; more likely in elder patients	Unlikely; fracture risk increases with pain treatment
Likelihood of neuropathy	More likely; polyneuropathy	Less likely; may develop in some cases

Sources:
National Institute of Neurological Disorders and Stroke [119]
National Institute of Neurological Disorders and Stroke [120]
Center for Peripheral Neuropathy [121]
John Hopkins Medicine. Guillain–Barre and CIDP. http://www.hopkinsmedicine.org/neurology_neurosurgery/centers_clinics/peripheral_nerve/conditions/guillain_barre_and_cidp.html. Accessed 17 Jan 2016

hasten recovery or affect the long-term outcome [123]. New clinical trials are underway to test the hypothesis that complement inhibitors such as eculizumab may control inflammation, reduce nerve injury, and prevent progression of weakness in GBS [124].

Patients with GBS often need aggressive rehabilitation to maintain body functioning during recovery. Mechanical ventilation is required by 20–30 % of those with the disorder, and other machines may be needed to assist body function. Manual manipulation of patient's limbs is employed as a first step, followed by physical therapy including training in safe transfers and balance, passive range of motion exercises, the use of partial body weight support systems, airway clearance techniques, and hydrotherapy [125].

Like GBS, CIDP responds to IVIG, to plasma exchange, and, to a limited extent, to corticosteroids, all administered on a short-term basis with similar effectiveness. IVIG improves disability for at least 2–6 weeks and up to 48 and possibly even 48 weeks, a similar efficacy to plasma exchange and oral prednisone; however, long-term benefits are unknown [126]. Moderate to high-quality evidence indicates that plasma exchange leads to short-term improvements in disability, but rapid deterioration occurs shortly after treatment cessation [127]. Corticosteroids are commonly used in practice with one study showing no significant difference between monthly dexamethasone and daily prednisone.

As Gorson has observed, IVIG is time-consuming and expensive; plasma exchange is invasive and can be administered only by highly trained personnel in specialized centers with hematologic testing imperative throughout the infusion process; corticosteroids have several serious side effects and are poorly tolerated in the long term [128]. There is no consensus on the best long-term strategy for CIDP. In considering new medications, the benefits of the relatively safe IVIG/ plasma exchange therapies must be balanced against as yet undetermined risks of drugs currently under investigation [129].

GBS/CIDP Complications Related to Bone

Vitamin D deficiency has been associated with autoimmune-related neurologic diseases including both Guillain–Barre and CIDP. Although impaired serum levels of vitamin D deficiency may cause an abnormally regulated immune response, the link to bone involvement is unclear because the active form of vitamin D, specifically vitamin 1,25 $(OH)_2D_3$, may not fluctuate in autoimmune disease. A study by Elf et al. found that patients with primary immune-mediated peripheral neuropathies were deficient in vitamin D and had significantly lower serum vitamin D25-OH levels values than healthy controls [130], suggesting the need to monitor vitamin D status, ensuring that immune cells respond to the ameliorative effect of vitamin D. As previously indicated, corticosteroid use is ineffective and possibly deleterious in the treatment of GBS but is employed in CIDP, independently reducing already diminished levels of vitamin D25-OH to severe levels [131].

Glucocorticoid-induced osteoporosis, the most common form of secondary osteoporosis, occurs in 50 % of patients taking glucocorticoid medications and has a profound effect on bone formation by impairing osteoblastic differentiation and function and increasing bone resorption even in the early treatment phase [132]. Thus far, glucocorticoids appear to affect bone regardless of their dosage [133]. Fractures seen in patients with glucocorticoid-induced osteoporosis occur at a higher BMD level than in postmenopausal osteoporosis [134]. As a consequence, guidelines for treatment of postmenopausal osteoporosis should not be applied to patients taking glucocorticoid steroids. Instead, vitamin D and calcium, along with bisphosphonates, are administered to patients who anticipate exposure to glucocorticoids for 3–6 months [133]. The combination of all three agents has been shown to increase BMD by as much as twice the increase produced by vitamin D alone. Moreover, the efficacy of bisphosphonates is further enhanced with concomitant use of vitamin D [135].

GBS, in itself, evidences no independent association with any fracture risk. The only exception occurs in patients undergoing pain treatment which doubles the risk of fracture—a finding also apparent in controls being treated for pain [136]. Patients with GBS that later presents as CIDP may suffer from prolonged periods of immobilization which increases bone resorption and results in hypercalcemia [87]. The proposed mechanism is an increase in osteoclast-driven reabsorption manifested in reduced bone formation and decreased osteoblastic activity, offsetting the balance of bone metabolism toward reabsorption. The most direct treatment of hypercalcemic immobility consists of ambulation, passive and active range of motion exercises, and other forms of physical therapy. In situations where mobilization of the patient is not feasible, bisphosphonates, as well as denosumab, are the preferred pharmacologic treatment. However, caution must be exercised in those with renal insufficiency if selecting a bisphosphonate [86].

There are over 100 different types of peripheral neuropathy, each with its own set of causes, symptoms, and therapies. The prognosis depends on the underlying causes and the extent of the nerve damage; the earlier the diagnosis, the greater the chance of slowing or reversing the process. In some cases, nerve damage is permanent, and pain can persist for a lifetime. Research is focusing on a broad spectrum of contributing factors ranging from the biological mechanisms involved and the role of genetic mutations to the impact of neurotropic factors and new strategies for relieving neuropathic pain.

References

1. National Institute of Diabetes and Digestive and Kidney Diseases. Diabetic neuropathies: the nerve damage of diabetes. U.S. Department of Health and Human Services, National Institutes of Health, 2013. http://www.niddk.nih.gov/health-information/health-topics/Diabetes/diabetic-neuropathies-nerve-damage-diabetes/Pages/diabetic-neuropathies-nerve-damage.aspx. Accessed 5 Dec 2015.
2. National Institute of Neurological Disorders and Stroke. Peripheral neuropathy fact sheet. 2016. http://www.ninds.nih.gov/disorders/peripheralneuropathy/detail_peripheralneuropathy.htm. Accessed 15 Jan 2016.
3. Cleveland Clinic. Diseases and conditions: neuropathy. http://my.clevelandclinic.org/services/neurological_institute_neuromuscular-center/diseases-conditions/peripheral-neuropathies. Accessed 15 Jan 2016.
4. International Diabetes Foundation. IDF Diabetes Atlas. Brussels, Belgium. http://www.idf.org/sites/default/files/Atlas-poster-2014_EN.pdf. Accessed 5 Dec 2015.
5. Boyle JP, Thompson TJ, Gregg EW, Barker LE, Williamson DF. Projection of the year 2050 burden of diabetes in the US adult population: dynamic modeling of incidence, mortality, and prediabetes prevalence. Popul Health Metrics. 2010. doi:10.1186/1478-7954-8-29.
6. Alberti KG, Zimmet PZ. Definition, diagnosis and classification of mellitus and its complications. Part 1: diagnosis and classification of diabetes mellitus provisional report of a WHO consultation. Diabet Med. 1998;156(87):539–53.
7. Center for Disease Control and Prevention. National diabetes statistics report. 2014. http://www.cdc.gov/diabetes/pubs/statsreport14/national-diabetes-report-web.pdf. Accessed 5 Dec 2015.
8. Tabak AG, Herder C, Rathmann W, Brunner EJ, Kivimaki M. Prediabetes: a high-risk state for diabetes development. Lancet. 2012;379(9833):2279–90. doi:10.1016/S0140-6736(12)60283-9.
9. Boulton AJM, Vinik AI, Arezzo JC, Brit V, Feldman EL, Freeman R. Diabetic neuropathies: a statement by the American Diabetes Association. Diabetes Care. 2005;28(4):956–62.
10. Tesfaye S, Boulton AJM, Dickerson AH. Mechanisms and management of diabetic painful distal symmetrical polyneuropathy. Diabetes Care. 2013;36(9):2456–65.

11. Leidig-Bruchner G, Ziegler R. Diabetes mellitus a risk for osteoporosis? Exp Clin Endocrinol Diabetes. 2001;109 Suppl 2:S493–514.
12. Wongdee K, Charoenphandhu N. Osteoporosis in diabetes mellitus: possible cellular and molecular mechanisms. World J Diabetes. 2011;2:41–8.
13. Vestergaard P. Discrepancies in bone mineral density and fracture risk in patients with type 1 and type 2 diabetes—a meta-analysis. Osteoporos Int. 2007;18(4):427–44.
14. Rakel A, Sheehy O, Rahme E, LeLorier J. Osteoporosis among patients with type 1 and type 2 diabetes. Diabetes Metab. 2007;34:193–205. doi:10.1016/j.diabet.2007.10.008.
15. Ingberg CM, Palmer M, Aman J, Arvidsson B, Schvarez E, Berne C. Body composition and bone mineral density in long-standing type 1 diabetes. J Intern Med. 2004;255(3):392–8.
16. Kemink SA, Hermus AR, Swinkels LM, Lutterman JA. Smais. Osteopenia in insulin-dependent diabetes mellitus; prevalence and aspects of pathophysiology. J Endocrinol Invest. 2000;23(5):295–303.
17. Thrailkill KM, Lumpkin CK, Bunn RC, Kemp SF, Fowlkes JL. Is insulin an anabolic agent in bone? Dissecting the diabetic bone for clues. Am J Physiol Endocrinol Metab. 2005;289(5):E735–45.
18. Campos Pastor MM, Lopez-Ibarra PJ, Escobar-Imenez F, Serrano Pardo MD, Garcia-Cervigon AG. Intensive insulin therapy and bone mineral intensity in Type 1 diabetes mellitus: a prospective study. Osteoporos Int. 2000;11(5):455–9.
19. Hofbauer LC, Brueck CC, Singh SK, Dibnig H. Review: osteoporosis in patients with diabetes mellitus. J Bone Mineral Res. 2007;22(9):1317–28.
20. Horcajada-Molteni MN, Chanteranne B, Lebecque P, Davicco MJ, Young A, Barlet JP. Amylin and bone metabolism in streptozotocin-induced diabetic rats. J Bone Miner Res. 2001;16(5):958–65.
21. Clowes JA, Khosla S, Eastell R. Potential role of pancreatic and enteric hormones in regulating bone turnover. J Bone Miner Res. 2005;20(9):1497–506.
22. Hamilton EJ, Rakic V, Davis WA, Chubb SA, Kamber N, Prince RL, et al. Prevalence and predictors of osteopenia and osteoporosis in adults with type 1 diabetes. Diabet Med. 2009;26:45–52. doi:10.1111/j.1464-5491.2008.02608.x.
23. Lumachi F, Camozzi V, Tombolan V, Luisetto G. Bone mineral density, osteocalcin, and bone-specific alkaline phosphatase in patients with insulin-dependent diabetes mellitus. Ann N Y Acad Sci. 2009;1173 Suppl 1:E64–7. doi:10.1111/j.1749-6632.2009.04955.x.
24. Rozadilla A, Nolla JM, Montana E, Fiter J, Gomez-Vaquero C, Soler J. Bone mineral density in patients with type 1 diabetes mellitus. Joint Bone Spine. 2000;67:215–8.
25. Munoz-Torres M, Jodar E, Escobar-Jimenez F, Lopez-Ibarra PJ, Luna JD. Bone mineral density measured by dual X-ray absorptiometry in Spanish patients with insulin-dependent diabetes mellitus. Calcif Tissue Int. 1996;58:316–9.
26. Tuominen JT, Impivaara O, Puukka P, Ronnemaa T. Bone mineral density in patients with type 1 and type 2 diabetes. Diabetes Care. 1999;22:1196–200.
27. Vashishth D, Gilson GJ, Khoury JI, Schaffler MB, Kimura J, Fyhrue DP. Influence of nonenzymatic glycation on biomechanical properties of cortical bone. Bone. 2001;28(2):195–201.
28. Rix M, Andreassen H, Eskildsen P. Impact of peripheral neuropathy on bone density in patients with type I diabetes. Diabetes Care. 1999;22(5):827–31.
29. Barwick AL, de Jonge XAKJ, Tessier JW, Ho A, Chuter VH. The effect of diabetic neuropathy on foot bones: a systematic review and meta-analysis. Diabet Med. 2014;31(2):136–47.
30. Thomas T, Gori, Spelsberg TC, Khosla S, Riggs BL, Conover CA. Response of bipotential human marrow stromal cells to insulin-like growth factors: effect of binding protein production, proliferation, and commitment to osteoblasts and adipocytes. Endocrinology. 1999;140(11):5036–44.
31. Holloway WR, Collier FM, Aitken CJ, Myers DE, Hodge JM, Malakellis M, et al. Leptin inhibits osteoclast generation. J Bone Miner Res. 2002;17(2):200–9.
32. Martin A, David V, Malaval L, Lafarge-Proust MH, Vico L, Thomas T. Opposite effects of leptin on bone metabolism: a dose-dependent balance related to energy intake and insulin-like growth factor –1 pathway. Endocrinology. 2007;148(7):3419–25.

33. Khosla S. Leptin—central or peripheral to the regulation of bone metabolism. Endocrinology. 2002;143(11):4161–4.
34. Kanazawa I. Adiponectin in metabolic bone disease. Curr Med Chem. 2012;19(32):5481–92.
35. Berg AH, Scherer PE. Adipose tissue, inflammation, and cardiovascular disease. Circ Res. 2005;96(6):939–49.
36. Imagawa A, Funahashi T, Nakamura T, Moriwaki M, Tanaka S, Nishizawa K, et al. Elevated serum concentration of adipose-derived factors, adiponectin, in patients with type 1 diabetes. Diabetes Care. 2002;25(9):1665–6.
37. Ouchi N, Walsh K. Adiponectin as an anti-inflammatory factor. Clin Chim Acta. 2007;380(1–2):24–30.
38. Shibata R, Sato K, Pimentel DR, Takemura Y, Kihara S, Ohashi K, et al. Adiponectin protects again myocardial ischemia-reperfusion injury through AMPK-and COX-2-dependent mechanisms. Nat Med. 2005;11(10):1096–103.
39. Shanbhogue VV, Hansen S, Frost M, Jorgensen NR, Hermann AP, Henriksen JE. Bone geometry, volumetric density, microarchitecture, and estimated bone strength assessed by HR-pQCT in adult patients with type 1 diabetes mellitus. J Bone Miner Res. 2015;30(12):2188–99.
40. Nicodemus KK, Folsom AR. Type 1 and type 2 diabetes and incident hip fractures in postmenopausal women. Diabetes Care. 2001;24(7):1192–7.
41. Miao J, Brossard K, Noreen O, Ugarph-Morawski A, Ye W. Elevated hip fracture risk in type 1 diabetic patients: a population-based cohort study in Sweden. Diabetes Care. 2005;28(12):2850–5.
42. Janghorbani M, Feskanich D, Willett WC, Hu F. Prospective study of diabetes and risk of hip fractures: the Nurses' Health Study. Diabetes Care. 2006;29(7):1573–8.
43. Weber DR, Haynes K, Leonard MR, Willi SM, Denburg MR. Type 1 diabetes is associated with an increased risk of fracture across the life span: a population-based cohort study using the Health Improvement Network (THIN). Diabetes Care. 2015;38(120):19113–20.
44. Schwartz AV, Selimeyer DE, Ensrud KE, Cauley JA, Tabor HK, Schreiner PJ, et al. Older women with diabetes have an increased risk of fracture: a prospective study. J Clin Endocrinol Metab. 2001;86(1):32–8.
45. International Osteoporosis Foundation. IOF urges early evaluation of fracture risk in diabetes. 2015. http://www.iofbonehealth.org/news/iof-urges-early-evaluation-fracture-risk-diabetes. Accessed 8 Feb 2016.
46. Kaynak G, Birsel O, Guven MF, Ogut T. An overview of the Charcot foot pathophysiology. Diabet Foot Ankle. 2013. doi:10.3402/dfa.v410.2117.
47. Petrova NL, Shanahan CM. Neuropathy and the vascular-bone axis in diabetes: lessons from Charcot osteoarthropathy. Osteoporos Int. 2014;25(4):1197–207.
48. Gouveri E, Papanas N. Charcot osteoarthropathy in diabetes: a brief review with an emphasis on clinical practice. World J Diabetes. 2011;2(5):59–65.
49. Petrova NL, Edmonds ME. Acute Charcot neuro-osteoarthropathy. Diabetes Metab Res Rev. 2016;32(Suppl S1):281–6.
50. Meier C, Schwartz AV, Egger A, Lecka-Czernik B. Effects of diabetes drugs on the skeleton. Bone. 2016;82:93–100. doi:10.1016/jbone.2015.04.026.
51. Meier C, Kraenzlinm ME, Bodmer M, Jick SS, Jick H, Meier CR. Use of thiazolidinediones and fracture risk. Arch Intern Med. 2008;168(8):820–5.
52. Lecka-Czernik B. Safety of anti-diabetic therapies on bone. Clin Rev Bone Miner Metab. 2013;11(1):49–58.
53. U.S. Food and Drug Administration. FDA drug safety communication: FDA revises label of diabetes drug canagliflozin (invokana, invokamet) to include updates on bone fracture risk and new information on decreased bone mineral density. 2015. http://www.fda.gov/Drugs/DrugSafety/ucm461449. Accessed 2 Feb 2016.
54. U.S. Food and Drug Administration. FDA drug safety communication: FDA warns that SGLT2 inhibitors for diabetes may result in a serious condition of too much acid in the blood. 2015. http://www.fda.gov/Drugs/DrugSafety/ucm446845. Accessed 2 Feb 2016.

55. Menon B, Harinarayan CV. The effect of anti-epileptic drug therapy on serum 25-hydroxyvitamin D and parameters of calcium and bone metabolism – a longitudinal study. Seizure. 2010;19(3):153–8.
56. Eisenberg E, River Y, Shifrin A, Krivoy N. Antiepileptic drugs in the treatment of neuropathic pain. Drugs. 2007;67(9):1265–89.
57. Ensrud KE, Blackwell T, Mangione CM, Bowman PJ, Bauer DC, Schwartz A, et al. Central nervous system-active medications and risk for fracture in older women. Arch Intern Med. 2003;163(8):949–57.
58. Brown SA, Sharpless JL. Osteoporosis: an under-appreciated complication of diabetes. Clin Diabetes. 2004;22(1):10–20.
59. Gopalakrishnan V, Vignesh RC, Arunakaran J, Aruldhas MM, Srinivasan N. Effects of glucose and its modulation by insulin and estradiol on BMSC differentiation into osteoblastic lineages. Biochem Cell Biol. 2006;84(1):93–101.
60. Zhen D, Chen Y, Tang X. Metformin reverses the deleterious effects of high glucose on osteoblast function. J Diabetes Complicat. 2010;24(5):334–44.
61. Molinuevo MS, Schurman L, McCarthy AD, Cortizo AM, Tolosa MJ, Gangoiti G, et al. Effects of metformin on bone marrow progenitor cell differentiation: in vivo and in vitro studies. J Bone Miner Res. 2010;25(2):211–21.
62. Novelle MG, Ali A, Dieguez C, Bernier M, de Cabo R. Metformin: a hopeful approach in the aging research. In: Olshansky SJ, Martin GM, Kirkland JL, editors. Aging: the longevity dividend. New York: Cold Spring Harbor Laboratory Press; 2016. p. 179–90.
63. Fronczek-Sokol J, Pytlik M. Effect of glimepiride on the skeletal system of ovariectomized and non-ovariectomized rats. Pharmacol Rep. 2014;66(3):412–7.
64. Maugeri D, Panebianco P, Rosso D, Calanna A, Speciale S, Santangelo A, et al. Alendronate reduced the daily consumption of insulin (DCI) in patients with senile type 1 diabetes and osteoporosis. Arch Gerontol Geriatr. 2002;34(2):117–22.
65. Chan DC, Yang RS, Ho CH, Tsai YS, Wang JJ, Tsai KT. The use of alendronate is associated with decreased incidence of type 2 diabetes mellitus—a population-based cohort study in Taiwan. PLoS ONE. 2015;10(4), e0123279.
66. Toulis KA, Nirantharakumar K, Ryan R, Marshall T, Hemming K. Bisphosphonates and glucose homeostasis: a population-based, retrospective cohort study. J Clin Endocrinol Metab. 2015;100:1933–40. doi:10.1210/jc.2014-3481.
67. Andersson B, Johannsson G, Holm G, Bengtsson BA, Sashegyi A, Pavo I, et al. Raloxifene does not affect insulin sensitivity or glycemic control in postmenopausal women with type 2 diabetes mellitus: a randomized clinical trial. J Clin Endocrinol Metab. 2002; 87(1):122–8.
68. U.S. Food and Drug Administration. Changes to the indicated population for miacalcin (calcitonin-salmon). http://www.fda.Drugs/DrugSafety/PostmarketDrugSafetyInformationfor PatientsandProviders/ucm 388641.htm. Accessed 7 Feb 2016.
69. Eli Lilly Company. Safety information and updates to prescribing information for Forteo. http://uspl.lilly.com/forteo/forteo.html#pi. Accessed 26 Feb 2016.
70. Marciano DP, Kuruvilla DS, Boregowda SV, Asteian A, Hughes TS, Garcia-Ordonez R, et al. Pharmacological repression of PPARγ promotes osteogenesis. Nat Commun. 2015;6:7443. http://www.nature.com/ncomms/2015/150612/ncomms8443/full/ncoomms 8443./html. Accessed 7 Feb 2016.
71. Bolton CF, Bryan GY, Zochodne DW. The neurological complications of sepsis. Ann Neurol. 1993;33:94–100.
72. Zhou C, Wu L, Ni F, Ji W, Wu J, Zhang H. Critical illness polyneuropathy and myopathy; a systemic review. Neural Regen Res. 2014;9(1):101–10.
73. Lacomis D. Neuromuscular disorders in critically ill patients: review and update. J Clin Neuromuscul Dis. 2011;12(4):197–218.
74. Osias J, Manno E. Neuromuscular complications of critical illness. Crit Care Clin. 2014;30(4):785–94. doi:10.1016/j.ccc.2014.06.008.
75. Latronico N, Bolton CF. Critical illness polyneuropathy and myopathy: a major cause of muscle weakness and paralysis. Lancet Neurol. 2011;10(10):931–41.

76. Van den Berghe G, Wouters P, Weekers F, Verwaest C, Bruyninckx F, Schetz M, et al. Intensive insulin therapy in critically ill patients. N Engl J Med. 2001;345(19):1359–67.
77. Finfer S, Chittock DR, Su SY, Blair D, Foster D, Dhingra V, et al. Intensive versus conventional glucose control in critically ill patients. N Engl J Med. 2009;360(13):1283–97.
78. Brunner R, Rinner W, Haberler C, Kitzberger R, Sycha T, Herkner H, et al. Early treatment with IgM-enriched intravenous immunoglobulin does not mitigate critical illness polyneuropathy and/or myopathy in patients with multiple organ failure and SIRS/sepsis: a prospective, randomized, placebo-controlled, double-blinded trial. Crit Care. 2013;17(5):R213.
79. Perme C, Chandrasekhar R. Early mobility and walking program for patients in intensive care units: creating a standard of care. Am J Crit Care. 2009;18(3):212–21.
80. Mehrholz J, Pohl M, Kugler J, Burridge J, Muckel S, Eisner B. Physical rehabilitation for critical illness myopathy and neuropathy. Cochrane Database Syst Rev. 2015;3, CD010942. doi:10.1002/14651858.CD010942.pub2.
81. Connolly B, Salisbury L, O'Neill B, Geneen L, Douiri A, Grocott MP, et al. Exercise rehabilitation following intensive care unit discharge for recovery from critical illness. Cochrane Database Syst Rev. 2015. doi:10.1002/14651858.CD008632.pub2.
82. Adler J, Malone D. Early mobilization in the intensive care unit: a systematic review. Cardiopulm Phys Ther J. 2012;23(1):5–13.
83. Karatzanos E, Gerovasli V, Zervakis D, Tripodski ES, Apostoiou K, Vasileiadis I, et al. Electrical muscle stimulation: an effective form of exercise and early mobilization to preserve muscle strength in critically ill patients. Crit Care Res Pract. 2012. doi:10.1155/2012/432752.
84. Cheng CJ, Chou CH, Lin S. An unrecognized cause of recurrent hypercalcemia: immobilization. South Med J. 2006;99(4):371–4.
85. Gallacher SJ, Ralston SH, Dryburgh FJ, Logue FC, Allam BF, Boyce BF, et al. Immobilization-related hypercalcaemia—a possible novel mechanism and response to pamidronate. Postgrad Med J. 1990;66(781):918–22.
86. De Beus E, Boer WH. Denosumab for treatment of immobilization-related hypercalcaemia in a patient with advanced renal failure. Clin Kidney J. 2012;5(6):566–71.
87. Booth KA, Hays CI. Using denosumab to treat immobilization hypercalcemia in a post-acute care patient. J Clin Endocrinol Metab. 2014;99(10):3531–5. doi:10.1210/js.2013-4205.
88. Thompson RN, Armstrong CL, Heyburn G. Bilateral atypical femoral fractures in a patient prescribed denosumab–a case report. Bone. 2014;61:44–7. doi:10.1016/j.bone2013.12.027.014.
89. Aspenberg P. Denosumab and atypical femoral fractures. Acta Orthop. 2014;85(1):1. doi:10.3109/17453674.2013.859423.
90. Bone HG, Chapuriat R, Brandi ML, Brown JP, Czerwinski E, Krieg MA, et al. The effect of three or six years of denosumab exposure in women with postmenopausal osteoporosis: results from the FREEDOM extension. J Clin Endocrinol Metab. 2013;98:4483–92. doi:10.1210/jc.2013-1597.
91. Tuukkanen J, Vaananen HK. Omeprazole, a specific inhibitor of H+K+ATPase inhibits bone resorption in vitro. Calcif Tissue Int. 1986;38(2):123–5.
92. Ito T, Jensen RT. Association of long-term proton pump inhibitor therapy with bone fractures and effects on absorption of calcium, vitamin B12, iron, and magnesium. Curr Gastroenterol Rep. 2010;12(6):448–57.
93. Marcinowska-Suchowierska EB, Talalaz MY, Wlodarcyzk AW, Bielecki K, Zawadzski JJ, Brzozzowski R. Calcium/phosphate/vitamin D homeostasis and bone mass in patients after gastrectomy, vagotomy, and cholecystectomy. World J Surg. 1995;19(4):597–601.
94. Hansen KE, Jones AN, Lindstrom MJ, Davis LA, Ziegler TE, Penniston KL, et al. Do proton pump inhibitors decrease calcium absorption? J Bone Miner Res. 2010;25(12):2786–95.
95. Targownik LE, Lix LM, Leung G, Leslie WD. Proton-pump inhibitor use is not associated with osteoporosis or accelerated bone mineral density loss. Gastroenterology. 2010;138(3):896–904.
96. Jung HK. Is there any association of osteoporosis with proton pump inhibitor use? (Gastroenterology 2010;138:896–904). J Neurogastroenterol Motil. 2010;16(3):35–6.
97. Vestergaard P, Ejnmark L, Mosekilde L. Proton pump inhibitors, histamine H2 receptor antagonists, and other antacid medications and the risk of fracture. Calcif Tissue Int. 2006;7(9):76–83.

98. Yang YX, Lewis JD, Epstein S, Metz DC. Long-term proton-pump inhibitor therapy and risk of hip fracture. JAMA. 2006;296(24):2947–53.
99. Gray SL, LaCroix AZ, Larson J, Robbins J, Cauley JA, Manson JAE. Proton pump inhibitor use, hip fracture, and change in bone mineral density in postmenopausal women: results from the Women's Health Initiative. Arch Intern Med. 2010;170(9):765–71.
100. FDA Drug Safety Communication: possible increased risk of fractures at the hip, wrist, and spine with the use of proton pump inhibitors. U.S. Food and Drug Administration. 2010–2011. http://www.fda.gov/Drugs/DrugSafety/PostmarketDrugSafetyInformationforPatientsandProviders/ucm213206.htm. Accessed 12 Jan 2016.
101. Heidelbaugh JJ. PPI therapy: when to worry about fracture risk. J Fam Pract. 2011;60(5):255–60.
102. Targownik LE, Leslie WD, Davison KS, Goltzman D, Jamal SA, Kreiger N, et al. The relationship between proton pump inhibitor use and longitudinal change in bone mineral density: a population based [study] based [on] the Canadian Multicentre Osteoporosis Study (CaMos). Am J Gastroenterol. 2012;107:1361–9. 10/10038/ajg.2012.200.
103. Khalili H, Huang ES, Jacobson BC, Camargo Jr CA, Fiskanich D, Chan AT. Use of proton pump inhibitors and risk of hip fracture in relation to dietary and lifestyle factors: a prospective cohort study. BMD. 2012;344:e372. doi: http://dx.doi.org/10.1136/bmj.e372.
104. Adams AL, Black MH, Zhang JL, Shi JM, Jacobsen SJ. Proton-pump inhibitor use and hip fractures in men: a population-based case-control study. Ann Epidemiol. 2014;24(4):286–98.
105. Freedberg DE, Haynes K, Denburg MR, Zemel BS, Leonard MB, Abrams KJA, et al. Use of proton pump inhibitors is associated with fractures in young adults: a population-based study. Osteoporos Int. 2015;26(10):2501–7.
106. Leontiadis GI, Moayyedi P. Proton pump inhibitors and risk of bone fractures. Curr Treat Options Gastroenterol. 2014;12(4):414–23.
107. Johnson DA, Oldfield IV EC. Reported side effects and complications of long-term proton pump inhibitor use. Clin Gastroenterol Hepatol. 2013;11(5):458–64.
108. Shah NH, LePendu P, Bauer-Mehren A, Ghebremariam YT, Iyer SV, Marcus J, et al. Proton pump inhibitor usage and risk of myocardial infarction in the general population. PLoS ONE. 2015. 10.11371/journal.pone.0124653.
109. Rejnmark L, Vestergaard P, Heickendorff L, Andreasen F, Mosekilde L. Loop diuretics increase bone turnover and decrease BMD in osteopenic menopausal women, results from a randomized controlled study with bumetanide. J Bone Miner Res. 2006;21(1):163–70.
110. Carbone LD, Johnson KC, Bush AJ, Robbins J, Larson J, Thomas A, et al. Loop diuretic use and fracture in postmenopausal women: findings from the Women's Health Initiative. Arch Intern Med. 2009;169(2):132–40.
111. Bergman DA. Perspective. In: Prolonged use of loop diuretics, fracture risk in postmenopausal women. Endocrine Today. 2009. http://www.healio.com/endocrinology/bone-mineral-metabolism/news/print/endocrine-today. Accessed 10 Feb 2016.
112. Lim LS, Fink HA, Blackwell T, Taylor BC, Ensud KE. Loop diuretics use and rates of hip bone loss, and risk of falls and fractures in older women. J Am Geriatr Soc. 2009;57(5):855–62.
113. Xiao F, Qu X, Zhai Z, Jiang C, Li H, Liu X, et al. Association between loop diuretic use and fracture risk. Osteoporos Int. 2015;26:775–84. doi:10.1007/s00198-014-2979-8.
114. Rajgopal R, Bear M, Butcher MK, Shaughnessy SG. The effects of heparin and low molecular weight heparins on bone. Thromb Res. 2008;122(3):293–8.
115. Pettila V, Kaaja R, Leinonen P, Ekblad U, Kataza M, Ikkala E. Thromboprophylaxis with low-molecular weight heparin in pregnancy. Thromb Res. 1999;96:275–82.
116. Monreal M, Lafoz E, Olive A, del Rio L, Vedia C. Comparison of subcutaneous unfractionated heparin with a low molecular weight heparin (Fragmin) in patients with venous thromboembolism and contraindications to coumadin. Thromb Haemost. 1994;71(1):7–11.
117. John Hopkins Medicine. Guillain-barre and CIDP. http://www.hopkinsmedicine.org/neurology_neurosurgery/centers_clinics/peripheral_nerve/conditions/guillain_barre_and_cidp.html. Accessed 17 Jan 2016.

118. Mathey EK, Park SB, Hughes RAC, Pollard JD, Armati PJ, Barnett MH, et al. Chronic inflammatory demyelinating polyradiculoneuropathy: from pathology to phenotype. J Neurol Neurosurg Psychiatry. 2014;86:973–85. doi:10.1136/jnnp-2014-309697.
119. National Institute of Neurological Disorders and Stroke. NINDS chronic inflammatory demyelinating polyneuropathy (CIDP). http://www.ninds.nih.gov/disorders/cidp/cidp.html. Accessed 17 Jan 2016.
120. National Institute of Neurological Disorders and Stroke. Guillain-barré syndrome fact sheet. http://www.ninds.nih.gov/disorders/gbs/detail_gbs.htm#3139_3. Accessed 17 Jan 2016.
121. Center for Peripheral Neuropathy. Guillain-barré syndrome/acute demyelinating polyneuropathy.http://peripheralneuropathycenter.uchicago.edu/learnaboutpn/typesofpn/inflammatory/guillainbarre.shtml. Accessed 17 Jan 2016.
122. van den Berg B, Waigaard C, Drenthen J, Fokke C, Jacobs BC, van Doorm P. Guillain-Barre syndrome: pathogenesis, diagnosis, treatment and prognosis. Nat Rev Neurol. 2014;10:469–82. doi:10.1038/nrneurol.2014.121.
123. Hughes RA, Swan AV, van Koningsveld R, van Doorn PA. Corticosteroids for Guillain-Barre syndrome. Cochrane Database Syst Rev. 2006;19(2), CD001446.
124. Inhibition of complement activation (Eculizumab) in Guillain-Barre Syndrome (ICA-GBS). National Health Service Great Glasgow and Clyde, University of Glasgow. 2014. https://clinicaltrials.gov/ct2/show/NCT02029378. Accessed 30 Oct 2015.
125. Orsini M, de Freitas MRG, Presto B, Mello MP, Reis CHM, Silveira V, et al. Guideline for neuromuscular rehabilitation in Guillain-Barre Syndrome: what can we do? Rev Neurocience. 2010;18(4):572–80.
126. Eftimov F, Winer JB, Vermeulen M, de Haan R, van Schaik. Intravenous immunoglobin for chronic inflammatory demyelinating polyradiculoneuropathy. Cochrane Database Syst Rev. 2013;12, CD001797. doi:10.1002/14681858.CD001797.pub3.
127. Mehndiratta MM, Hughes RA, Agarwal P. Plasma exchange for chronic inflammatory demyelinating polyradiculoneuropathy. Cochrane Database Syst Rev. 2015;(8):CD003906. doi:10.1002/14651858.CD003906.pub4.
128. Gorson KC. An update on the management of chronic inflammatory demyelinating polyneuropathy. Ther Adv Neurol Disord. 2012;5(6):359–73.
129. Mathey EK, Pollard JD. New treatment for chronic inflammatory demyelinating polyneuropathy. Eur Neurol Rev. 2013;8(1):51–6.
130. Elf K, Ashmark H, Nygren I, Punga AR. Vitamin D deficiency in patients with primary immune-mediated peripheral neuropathies. J Neurol Sci. 2014;345(1–2):184–8.
131. Skversky AL, Jumar J, Abramowitz MK, Kaskel FJ, Melamed ML. Association of glucocorticoid use and low 25-hyroxyvitamin D levels: results from the National Health and Nutrition Examination Survey (NHANES): 2001–2006. J Clin Endocrinol Metab. 2011;96(12):3838–45.
132. Canalis E, Mazziotti G, Glustina A, Bilezikian JP. Glucocorticoid- induced osteoporosis: pathophysiology and therapy. Osteoporos Int. 2007;18:1319–28.
133. Mazziotti G, Canalis E, Giustina A. Drug-induced osteoporosis: mechanisms and clinical implications. Am J Med. 2010;123(10):877–84.
134. Van Staa TP, Laan RF, Barton JP, Cohen S, Reid DM, Cooper G. Bone density thresholds and other predictors of vertebral fracture in patients receiving oral glucocorticoid therapy. Arthritis Rheum. 2003;48(11):3224–9.
135. Amin S, Lavalley MP, Simms RW, Felson DT. The comparative efficacy of drug therapies used for the management of corticosteroid-induced osteoporosis: a meta-regression. J Bone Miner Res. 2002;17(8):1512–26.
136. Pouwels S, de Boer A, Leufkens HGM, Weber WEJ, Cooper C, van Staa TP, et al. Risk of fracture in patients with Guillain-Barre syndrome. Osteoporos Int. 2014;25(7):1845–51.

Chapter 12
Osteoporosis in Rheumatologic Conditions and Inflammatory Disorders

Christina V. Oleson

The concept of inflammation-induced bone loss among patients with rheumatic diseases has gained increasing attention in the medical community in recent years. Osteoporosis may begin with inflammation, but joint pain, relative immobilization, with increasing loss of function, and glucocorticoid therapy also contribute substantially to evolving bone loss. A number of rheumatologic conditions including systemic sclerosis are considered noninflammatory, yet individuals with this condition and others of a similar nature are also at increased risk of osteoporosis. In this chapter, the pathogenesis, diagnosis, and epidemiology of inflammatory and noninflammatory-induced osteoporosis will be discussed with respect to several rheumatologic disorders: rheumatoid arthritis (RA), systemic lupus erythematosus (SLE), and ankylosing spondylitis (AS). Management approaches, both pharmacologic and nonpharmacologic, will be considered.

Rheumatoid Arthritis (RA)

Etiology and Pathogenesis

The hallmark of rheumatoid arthritis is chronic joint inflammation, which can lead to erosive destruction of joints. Locally, this destruction occurs along the subchondral bone at the margins of joints and at the boundary between articular cartilage and bone. However, bone loss can also be more generalized throughout the skeleton, a process that leads to clinically significant osteoporosis. The severity of disease activity, as indicated by inflammatory markers, is an independent risk factor for development of osteoporosis.

C.V. Oleson, *Osteoporosis Rehabilitation*, DOI 10.1007/978-3-319-45084-1_12

Predictive Factors and Models

In a landmark study to determine which patients with RA should be tested for osteoporosis, Haugenberg and colleagues [1] proposed five criteria—age, weight, inflammation, immobility, and ever-use of corticosteroids.

More recently, Hauser et al. developed a clinical prediction model to assess the most influential factors in osteoporosis development in RA subjects [2]. Termed the osteoporosis prediction in RA tool (OPRA), it enables clinicians to use a point allocation according to the two factors with the strongest predictive qualities for osteoporosis development. While the authors of this report evaluated erythrocyte sedimentation rate (ESR), Larsen score, and years since menopause (in females), only older age and lower BMI were found to be independent predictive measures [2].

Epidemiology of Osteoporosis in RA

In the United States, an estimated 1.5 million individuals are affected by rheumatoid arthritis, a condition involving chronic joint inflammation with potential consequences of joint erosions and destruction. Women are two to three times more likely to develop RA than men, with the most common onset of the condition between ages 30 and 60. Although osteoporosis is among the more common extra-articular manifestations of RA, epidemiologic studies have been highly variable. Older investigations may overestimate prevalence because many of these were conducted at large rheumatology clinics that served the most severely impaired RA patients. In 2000, a study examining 925 women with RA, most of whom were postmenopausal, found that frequency of osteoporosis as measured by DXA was 28.8 % at the lumbar spine and 36.2 % at the femoral neck [3, 4]. Despite the large sample size of this study, the prevalence estimates are likely elevated, due to the selection of patients from 21 rheumatology centers who were referred to a specialist for advanced management of RA. Among the more recent literature, efforts have been made to give more accurate estimates of osteoporosis with RA. Population-based studies are more representative of actual disease prevalence. A study of 394 patients drawn from a county registry of RA patients in Oslo, Norway, found that the overall prevalence of osteoporosis was increased by a factor of two, compared with an age-matched population of non-RA subjects living in the same region [5]. Using the standard definition of osteoporosis as determined by DXA, the prevalence of osteoporosis for the population as a whole was 16.8 % in the lumbar spine (L2-4) and 14.7 % for both the femoral neck and the total hip, among all subjects in the population, but a stepwise increase occurred in each succeeding decade, with the 60–70 year old group having the highest percentage of osteoporosis at each of the three locations and the greatest percentage of BMD reduction at individual bone sites. Predictors of low BMD were older age, glucocorticoid use, and physical disability.

Since the report of Haugenberg and colleagues in 2000 [5], earlier and more aggressive treatment with stronger, disease-modifying antirheumatic drugs (DMARDs) has been initiated. This change in the approach to patient care may reduce osteoporosis or delay its onset. Other, more recent investigations have also been undertaken. In the trial by Hauser et al. [2] nearly all patients had received DMARDs and over half were also on oral or intramuscular glucocorticoids or had taken them in the past. The researchers found that 29.9 % of RA patients had osteoporosis compared with 17.4 % age and gender-matched non-RA patients. Female gender, age, years since menopause, erythrocyte sedimentation rate (ESR), and body mass index (BMI) were the strongest risk factors for osteoporosis development.

Many of the larger studies dealt predominantly or solely with women, but some, centering on men with RA, indicated a prevalence of osteoporosis from 10 % to 29 %. Most of the studies were small and focused on different age groups, accounting for this varied prevalence [6–9]. They found a higher prevalence of osteoporosis in their study group of 50 men, but the age of subjects was 67. Femoral osteoporosis was seen in 29 % of the subjects, while lumbar spine osteoporosis was observed in 19 %. Interestingly, reduced BMD was independent of testosterone levels, distinguishing these findings from those seen in men with senile osteoporosis unrelated to rheumatic disorders [6].

Fractures in RA Patients

A number of investigations have explored the circumstances leading specifically to fractures, with and without osteoporosis, in the RA population. A large investigation of 110 patients, prospectively followed for 8.4 years, revealed that years of prednisone use, high disability index, older age, and limited physical activity, as well as prior diagnosis of osteoporosis, were predictive of incidence for fracture. Regarding vertebral fractures specifically, evidence of vertebral deformity on imaging, corticosteroid use greater than one year, and diagnosis of low BMD at the hip could predict fractures in lumbar spine. Both fear of falling and history of prior falls were significant associations with fractures primarily in the hip. Kaz Kaz and colleagues [10] showed that tender joints and prior level of disability were predictive for falls, but they did not specifically investigate if falls directly translated to fractures. Women who were unable to do stand-ups and demonstrated inability or limited ability to perform heel–toe walking also carried higher ESRs, worse outcomes on the Health Assessment Questionnaire (one of the first patient-reported outcomes) [11], and a greater number of tender joints.

Another investigation [12] examining correlates of falls and fear of falling found similar results but focused more directly on pain control. In this study by Jamison et al., increased pain intensity, in addition to a greater number of comorbid medical conditions and lower functional walking status, was seen in RA patients with fear of falling but were less prevalent in healthy control subjects. Amin and colleagues [13] have shown that in contrast to prior investigations, fracture rates were considerably higher in younger RA patients relative to older ones (odds ratio 4.3 for subjects under age 50 yet 1.7 among those age 51 or older). Reasons for this finding may be a greater level of activity and participation in higher fall risk actions in younger individuals.

Treatment of Osteoporosis in RA

Pharmacologic Intervention

Based on the dose and duration of glucocorticoids used for treatment of RA, patients may experience a negative calcium balance and, in turn, vitamin D levels below serum levels of 30 ng/ml—the desired level for bone protection of skeletal stores [14]. Given the minimal cost, the low risk of vitamin D toxicity, and potential benefit in reduction of fracture risk, a 2000 Cochrane review concluded that all patients requiring glucocorticoids should be started on calcium and vitamin D supplementation [15]. An individual's dietary calcium intake should be evaluated to determine the optimal dose. Serum vitamin D 25OH levels are the best measure of vitamin D physiologic status. A minimum desirable level would be 30 ng/ml, but aiming for 40–60 ng/ml is ideal in patients taking steroids. Increases in serum levels to this extent are best accomplished with supplemental oral vitamin D ranging from 1,000 to 2,000 IU in most cases, although selected individuals with levels under 30 ng/ml will require higher doses [16]. In addition, evidence suggests that active vitamin D analogs may be more effective in fracture reduction in patients receiving high-dose glucocorticoids, regardless of the medical condition for which they are prescribed [17].

Anti-TNF therapeutic agents have shown promise in arresting the synthesis of antiresorptive factors responsible for bone loss in several rheumatic conditions, including RA. Their effectiveness has been demonstrated over short-term prospective studies [18] as well as longer-term evaluations of up to two years [19]. More recently, Korczowska and colleagues found that infliximab is active as early as two weeks into treatment [20]. By examining levels of a number of inflammatory cytokines including TNF-α, IL-6, IL-17, and IL-23, as well as markers of bone formation (osteocalcin) and two markers of bone resorption (deoxypyridinoline and N-telopeptide), they determined that all cytokines and metabolic indexes evidenced reduced levels at follow-up times of two weeks, 14 weeks, six months, and one year. Adalimumab, another anti-TNF-α agent, has also demonstrated the ability to preserve but not increase BMD in the lumbar spine and femoral neck. This group investigated 50 patients with RA followed prospectively over a year for changes in BMD. While no increase was seen in the overall study sample, an association was found between the decrease in serum CRP at 16 weeks and an increase in BMD in the femoral neck at one year [21].

To date, bisphosphonates have been the primary mode of treatment for glucocorticoid-induced osteoporosis. Alendronate, risedronate, and zoledronic acid have all received FDA approval for treatment of glucocorticoid-induced osteoporosis (GIO), but osteoporosis due to RA is not caused solely by steroids. Medications that address a variety of physiologic abnormalities in rheumatoid patients are best suited to this population. Studies on both alendronate and risedronate indicate that they reduce future fracture risk [22, 23]. Eastell et al. showed that risedronate prevented further bone loss in patients with RA who were taking glucocorticoids [24] and Lems et al. reported that alendronate had a protective effect on markers of bone loss as well as BMD in RA patients taking chronic low-dose steroids [25]. Ebina and colleagues [26] investigated the effect of switching from weekly or daily risedronate or alendronate to a once monthly oral regimen of minodronate, an agent thought to have superior effects in inhibiting farnesyl diphosphate synthase, an enzyme that which induces an apoptosis of osteoclasts and thereby compromises their antiresorptive properties of bone. This agent is approved for use in Japan but currently not in the United States. The additional benefit gleaned from the study was that compliance with a monthly agent was potentially superior to that with a daily or weekly pill.

Limited data exists on the effect of once annual zoledronic acid (ZA) for the treatment of osteoporosis in RA. While ZA has been approved for the prevention and treatment of GIO, its use is just now gaining acceptance in the RA population. One major clinical trial demonstrated that ZA was superior to risedronate in increasing lumbar spine BMD over a prospective time of one year [27]. Subjects involved in the treatment evaluation arm had all received at least three months of glucocorticoids. A summary of therapies to date is given in Table 1 [19–21, 27–30].

To date, no studies on PTH (also called teriparatide, brand name Forteo) have been conducted with a specific focus on osteoporosis treatment for RA patients. In two reports [28, 29], Saag et al. illustrated the benefit of PTH in patients with GIO by demonstrating that it was superior to alendronate in terms of changes in BMD and in prevention of morphometric vertebral fractures. In a recent commentary by Gennari and Bilezekian [31] the idea that teriparatide may be a superior treatment for RA-associated osteoporosis has emerged, based on its direct action on osteoblasts and osteocytes (Fig. 1) [31].

Nonpharmacologic Intervention

Due to increased inflammation, restricted movement, and tight, painful joints, patients with RA have 30–75 % the muscle strength of able-bodied, similarly aged adults and one-half the endurance of age-matched adults. Reduced muscle strength in combination with the above factors leads to an overall lower level of physical activity and fitness [32]. Lack of fitness and an increased sedentary lifestyle contribute to the 50–60 % increased incidence of cardiovascular-related mortality observed in individuals with RA [33]. Exercise can help reduce these rates if a physical training program is appropriately tailored to increase muscle strength in a way that will prevent further joint trauma and educate patients about safe forms of exercise in cardiovascular disease. A 2009 Cochrane review examined eight clinical trials [34]

Table 1 Medication study outcomes

Drug	Recommendations	Notes/references
Zoledronic acid	A single 5 mg IV infusion	One major clinical trial demonstrated that ZA was superior to risedronate in increasing lumbar spine BMD over a prospective time of one year [27]
PTH teriparatide	20 mcg injection subq/day into thigh or abdominal wall	Demonstrated benefits of PTH in patients with GIO; indicated PTH was superior to alendronate in terms of changes in BMD and prevention of morphometric vertebral fractures [28, 29]
Calcium	1,000–1,500 mg/day	Caution in patients with renal disease or history of kidney stones [30]
Vitamin D (in setting of glucocorticoids)	1,000–1,500 IU/day	Give amount necessary to maintain serum vitamin D25OH at 30 ng/ml or higher [30]
Anti-TNF		
Infliximab	3 mg/kg IV infusion at baseline, two weeks, six weeks, then every eight weeks	Increases BMD [20]; improves bone metabolism and BMD in patients with RA and AS [19]
Adalimumab	40 mg subq per 14 days	Maintains but does not increase BMD in lumbar spine and femoral neck [21]

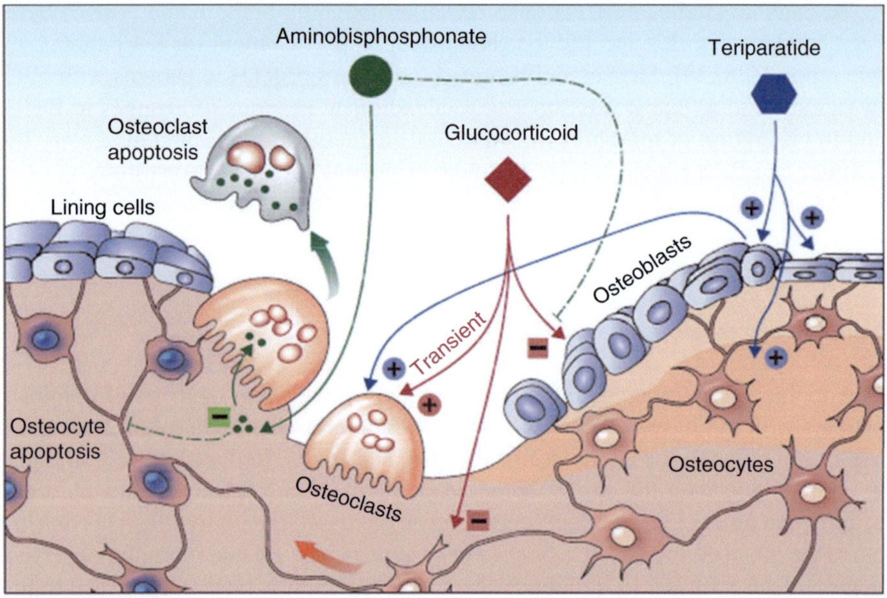

Fig. 1 Effects of glucocorticoids, bisphosphonates, and teriparatide on bone cells. *Dashed lines* indicate potential effects of bisphosphonates (*Source*: Gennari and Bilezekian [31]. Reprinted with permission)

Table 2 Criteria for functional status classification in rheumatoid arthritis

Class I	Full functional ability to perform activities of daily living, including self-care, vocational, and avocational
Class II	Limited functional ability to perform avocational activities. Relatively normal ability to perform typical vocational and self-care activities
Class III	Limited functional ability to perform both vocational and avocational activities. Relatively normal ability to perform typical self-care activities
Class IV	Limited functional ability to perform vocational, avocational, and typical self-care activities

Source: Hochberg et al. [35]

related to exercise in patients with RA and concluded that both overall fitness and more specific strength training are required to improve functional outcome. Moreover, if dynamic activity is carried out properly, no increased disease activity or pain should ensue.

The preceding recommendations are largely based on the less involved patients with RA. The American College of Rheumatology has published guidelines on the four levels of functional capacity of patients with RA as given in Table 2 and the majority of studies to date have focused on patients at the less severe Class I or II level of the disease [35].

In a study conducted by de Jong et al., subjects who underwent a 75 min, twice weekly exercise session involving bike training, circuit training, volleyball, basketball, or other ball sports, experienced increased physical well-being and functional status [36]. The majority of subjects saw no radiologic progression of joint appearance, but a subset of those with baseline severe radiologic damage did see a progression of disease. In general, aerobic and resistance exercise conditioning has been shown to improve functional capacity, muscle strength [32, 37], and cardiovascular conditioning, particularly in terms of blood pressure and lipid profiles [38]. However, caution is required in subjects with Class III or IV RA since patients with more severe disease at baseline remain at high risk of disease exacerbation and increased joint damage [36].

Systemic Lupus Erythematosus (SLE)

Etiology and Pathogenesis

Systemic lupus erythematosus (SLE) is a chronic autoimmune condition involving inflammation in multiple body parts including the skin, joints, heart, lung, blood, kidney, and brain. The increased antibody production that precipitates the chronic inflammation leads to pain as well as adverse effects on the joints, with both problems contributing to generalized immobility of patients with SLE. Survival and morbidity rates have improved drastically over recent years, and evidence is emerging that long-term health conditions, including osteoporosis, are receiving appropriate attention in management of persons with lupus. The etiology of bone loss in SLE represents the combined effects of traditional risk factors of osteoporosis (advanced age, postmenopausal status in women, low body weight, dietary deficiencies) as well as those inherent in rheumatoid conditions, including inflammation, metabolic factors, hormonal factors, serologic titers, and adverse effects of medication [39].

Chronic systemic inflammation leads to increased levels of tumor necrosis factor (TNF). It also increases oxidized low-density lipoproteins (oLDLs), which, in turn, induce elevated production of receptor activator of nuclear factor-kB ligand (RANKL) and further increase levels of TNF. Because both RANKL and TNF activate osteoclasts, increased bone resorption occurs. At the same time, oLDLs decrease bone formation by reducing osteoblast maturation. The combined effects result in lower BMD [39]. Additional evidence of decreased osteoblast activity stems from observations of decreased osteocalcin titers, indicating low bone formation, as supported by a study of premenopausal women with untreated SLE [40].

Hormonal factors have been shown to predispose SLE patients to bone loss as is the case in other populations. Specifically SLE patients experience more frequent episodes of months of amenorrhea, earlier (premature) menopause, and hyperprolactinemia. Males may experience low plasma androgen levels. Decreased vitamin D levels are another contributor to low BMD. Patients with SLE are consistently counseled to avoid sunlight, and others may be prescribed drugs such as hydroxychloroquine that directly blocks conversion of inactive to active forms of vitamin D [39, 41]. In addition, foods rich in vitamin D may add to GI distress given the prevalence of GI inflammation in SLE.

Serologically, the presence of anti-Ro antibodies is associated with a lower femoral BMD. This finding may be due to serologic adverse effects or it may be an indirect consequence of avoidance of sunlight. According to Mok et al. [42], anti-Ro antibodies are more commonly present in Chinese relative to Caucasian patients, perhaps because Chinese practice guidelines advise against sun exposure in SLE patients with anti-Ro antibodies. Ordinarily, a substantial percentage of vitamin D is absorbed from sunlight in certain seasons. Thus lack of exposure to sun may contribute to vitamin D deficiency as one factor in osteoporosis development. The presence of anti-Smith antibodies (a highly specific marker of SLE) and the absence of anti-Ro antibodies were found to correlate with improved femoral neck BMD [42].

In terms of medications that contribute to osteoporosis in SLE, Jardinet et al. reported a loss of lumbar spine bone in premenopausal SLE patients given corticosteroid therapy over a prolonged period of time [43, 44] but exactly how long is uncertain. Studies are divided as to whether corticosteroids confer an overall positive effect on BMD by reducing inflammation and enabling patients to be more active while allowing inflammatory markers to remain at lower levels. In their review of 16 articles focusing on the effect of corticosteroid use on osteoporosis in SLE, Garcia-Carrasco et al. [41] reported that seven studies found no association, but nine others demonstrated an adverse effect of steroids. In general, prolonged use

Table 3 Summary of studies of BMD in SLE patients

Source	Design	No. of patients	BMD lumbar region	BMD hip
Bultink et al. (2005) [48]	Transversal	107	39 % osteopenia and 4 % osteoporosis in any location	74 % osteopenia, 3 % osteoporosis
Mok et al. (2005) [42]	Cross-sectional	34	33 % osteopenia, 42 % osteoporosis	74 % osteopenia, 3 % osteoporosis
Becker et al. (2001) [45]	Cross-sectional	67	11 % osteopenia, 6 % osteoporosis	13 % osteopenia, 3 % osteoporosis
Lakshminarayanan et al. 2001 [47]	Cross-sectional	92	32 % osteopenia, 15 % osteoporosis	35 % osteopenia, 12 % osteoporosis
Sinigaglia et al. (2000) [3]	Cross-sectional	84	23 % osteoporosis in any location	
Pons et al. (1995) [49]	Cross-sectional and longitudinal	43	18 % osteoporosis in patients with corticosteroids	
Formiga et al. (1995) [55]	Cross-sectional	74	12.1 % osteoporosis in any location	

of higher doses of steroids appears to have a deleterious effect on BMD in either hip, lumbar spine, or both [41], whereas pulsed steroids given for short-term exacerbations or complications have a decreased long-term effect [41, 44].

In addition to corticosteroids, cyclophosphamide, typically used to address life-threatening organ involvement, is associated with premature menopause and osteoporosis. Cyclosporine reduces new bone formation by activating osteoclasts and suppressing osteoblasts. High-dose methotrexate, also associated with bone loss and fractures, is occasionally given to patients with advanced SLE [46]. In contrast to other agents used to treat SLE symptoms, use of hydroxychloroquine is noted to have a positive effect on BMD at the spine [42, 47] as well as the hip [47]. Table 3 [3, 42, 45, 47–50] summarizes risks of low BMD in lumbar spine and separately in the hip, based on the results of individual investigations.

Fractures in SLE Patients

The prevalence of fractures in SLE patients ranges from 6 % to 26 %, with symptomatic fractures occurring in only 6–12.5 % of these patients [51]. Despite this elevated occurrence, only a few high-quality studies on fracture prevalence, prevention, and treatment, as described below, have been conducted Ramsey-Goldman [51] and coauthors determined that fracture risk was related to duration of treatment with glucocorticoids, whereas Zonana-Nacach et al. [52] examined the cumulative exposure to corticosteroids in terms of overall dose, finding that for every 36.5 g of corticosteroid consumed, the risk of fracture nearly doubled.

Subsequently, Lee et al. [46], along with Ramsey-Goldman and colleagues [51], considered the frequency of fractures in a cohort study of 304 women with established SLE who were followed for six years. Overall 12.3 % experienced fractures and among those BMD *Z*-scores at the hip but not at the spine were significantly lower in the group of SLE patients with fractures compared to those without fractures. Borba et al. [53] investigated the presence of vertebral fractures in a cross-sectional study of 70 patients having established SLE and 22 controls. Although the mean age of subjects was only age 32, fracture deformity in image screening was found in 21 % of subjects with SLE but in none of the aged-matched healthy controls.

Focusing on risk factors for vertebral fractures, Mendoza-Pinto and colleagues [54] studied 210 subjects with a mean age 48 in which osteopenia was present in 50.3 % of subjects with vertebral body fracture and osteoporosis in 17.4 %. At least one vertebral fracture was detected in 26.1 %. Patients with vertebral fractures had a higher mean age (50 ± 14 vs. 41 ± 13.2 years, $p=0.001$), higher disease damage (57.1 % vs. 34.4 %, $p=0.001$), lower BMD at the total hip (0.902 ± 0.160 vs. 982 ± 0.137 g/cm^2, $p=0.002$), and postmenopausal status (61.9 % vs. 45.3 %, $p=0.048$). Stepwise logistic regression analysis revealed that only age ($p=0.001$) and low BMD at the total hip ($p=0.007$) remained as significant factors for the presence of vertebral fracture [54]. A summary of risk factors for fractures is given in Table 4 [51, 55].

Evidence suggests that fractures in SLE are not necessarily a function of low BMD. A study of Dutch patients found that 20 % of subjects had vertebral fracture, defined as greater than 20 % reduction of vertebral body height—a criterion developed by Genant et al. [56]. Using this measure, the threshold for identifying a fracture by radiographs is lower than that in other studies, potentially accounting for the higher fracture occurrence. Nevertheless, it should be noted that of the 107 participants, 73 % of those with fractures by the Genant et al. semiquantitative identification tool had height reductions of 20–25 % in at least one vertebra, 23 % of subjects had 25–40 % vertebral body height reduction, and 4 % had vertebral body height reduction greater than 40 %. Yet among the entire sample, only 4 % of subjects had a DXA scan with *T*-scores below 2.5, the threshold for meeting the definition of osteoporosis. In this investigation, males had a higher fracture rate than did females. Moreover, findings reported that 11 % of subjects had a prior nonvertebral fracture. This study also identified a number of conditions commonly seen among rehabilitation patients that further increase risk of fractures (Table 4).

Treatment

Initial Measures

Prior to considering pharmacologic treatment, the traditional first steps are optimizing overall nutrition, limiting alcohol, and eliminating smoking, if applicable. Beyond these measures, optimizing calcium and vitamin D stores is advised [57].

Table 4 Risk factors for fractures in SLE

Risk factor	Frequency or relative risk based on chosen study outcome	Notes
Age at diagnosis	RR not calculated	Older age is more likely to cause fracture
Cumulative glucocorticoid exposure	RR 1.17–1.3	Prolonged use is worse
Use of oral contraceptives	RR not calculated	Lower use associated with higher fracture risk
Timing of menopause	RR not calculated	Early menopause more likely to be associated with fracture
Dementia	RR 1.67	
Seizures	RR 2.01	
History of one or more cerebrovascular events	RR 1.49	
Prior osteoporotic low velocity fracture	RR 4.26	
Use of oral diabetic agents	RR 1.39	
Concurrent malignancy	RR 1.23	

Sources: Adapted from Ramsey-Goldman et al. [51], Bultink et al. [55]
RR Relative Risk

Calcitriol has been found to reduce bone loss in subjects with SLE who were on corticosteroids. Lambrinoudaki and colleagues found improvement of BMD at the lumbar spine in premenopausal women with SLE who took 0.5 mcg calcitriol daily for two years, compared with controls [58]. Conversely in a study of hypogonadal amenorrheic women, hormone replacement therapy but not calcitriol led to improvements in BMD of the lumbar spine. No increase in BMD in either the hip or radius was noted.

Estrogens and Androgens

No specific studies on selective estrogen receptor modulators exist, but recent interest has emerged in exploring the use of dehydroepiandrosterone (DHEA) for treatment of disease activity and osteoporosis due to SLE [57]. Along with its metabolite dehydroepiandrosterone sulfate (DHEAS), DHEA is the most abundant circulating adrenal steroid in humans [59]. Normal human levels of DHEA are 1–50 nM, but levels of DHEA, DHEAS, and androgens decline in states of chronic inflammation including RA and SLE and are reduced even further by steroids [60]. In a number of clinical trials described in the review by Sawalha and Kovats [59], the average daily use of corticosteroids was significantly reduced in the months following initiation of a daily dose of DHEA, but studies differed on the effectiveness of trial doses of DHEA in improving the Systemic Lupus Erythematosus Activity Index.

In terms of whether DHEA and DHEAS exert direct effects on bone, studies demonstrate conflicting results. In a small study of 19 SLE patients [61], the nine subjects who received DHEA showed no change in BMD at six months, whereas the ten placebo subjects experienced significant reduction in BMD. The subjects in this study all had advanced forms of active, systemic lupus affecting multiple organ systems. A second study of 37 subjects by Formiga et al. [62] found a positive correlation between DHEAS levels and BMD in the lumbar spine and femoral neck. The same study demonstrated a negative correlation in DHEAS and serum PTH, which may explain the potential role that DHEA may play in protecting bone. However, other studies have shown less of a benefit from DHEA, particularly one investigation looking at subjects with quiescent SLE [63]. Researchers are now attempting to determine (1) which groups of SLE patients may benefit from DHEA and (2) at what stage of the disease, in terms of duration and severity, are DHEA and its metabolite DHEAS most likely to make a significant difference in function and bone health [59].

Bisphosphonates

Although a number of investigations have examined the benefits of bisphosphonates on BMD in subjects receiving corticosteroids for rheumatoid conditions, no single study focuses solely on those with SLE. However, patients with SLE represent 5–15 % of subjects in several investigations. The majority of these analyses did not separate groups of patients but instead, often combined men, premenopausal, and postmenopausal women, and in doing so, complicated the ability to draw conclusions. Overall, positive effects on BMD were seen in most subsets of patients [22, 27, 64]. However, no conclusions could be drawn regarding the effectiveness of bisphosphonates for fracture prevention due to the absence of fractures in both the control and treatment groups, reported in the prevention studies on GIO. To date, no dedicated studies on the value of PTH, growth hormone, or insulin-like growth factor have been undertaken in SLE patients or in patients with GIO that include a notable percentage of participants with SLE. However, interest in exploring the potential for agents that work on the osteoblast continues to grow.

Ankylosing Spondylitis

Ankylosing spondylitis (AS) is an inflammatory, arthritic condition involving the axial skeleton and traditionally affecting males, often starting before age 40 [65]. Inflammation is both erosive leading to osteopenia and proliferative, with abnormal bony overgrowth and bridging syndesmophytes that fuse the vertebrae to create the appearance of a "bamboo spine." [65]. The result is rigid kyphotic posture as well as mid back and shoulder pain, limiting spinal flexibility and functional mobility. The structural changes may also affect the ribs and can compromise breathing mechanics. Patients may be subject to atelectasis and pneumonia, and, in severe cases, the architectural changes actually predispose the spine to spinal cord injury [66]. Perhaps even more frustrating for patients is that AS is often diagnosed late, in its advanced stages. The most effective treatment agents, TNF-α blockers, have limited impact if given late but are fairly successful if administered early in the disease process [65]. Although AS only affects 0.5 % of the US population, it results in work disability, eventual withdrawal from the workforce, substantial health costs, and a reduced quality of life [67].

The causes of AS are a mix of genetic and environmental factors, influenced by both autoimmune and autoinflammatory factors. Genetic evidence points to specific immune pathways, namely, interleukins 17 and 23 upregulation, activation of nuclear factor kappa B, and genes controlling CD8 and CD4 T-cell subsets. Autoreactive T cells and autoantibodies denote an autoimmune process, while autoinflammatory processes are characterized by mutations in single immunomodulatory genes and accelerated cytokine production [65]. In terms of environmental factors that contribute to the disease or accelerate an already established case, certain microbes can trigger a disease flare. Internal and external mechanical stress can promote inflammation throughout the body, particularly in the axial spine and fibrocartilaginous enthuses and enhance production of interleukin IL-23R$^+$ T cells. In addition animal studies suggest that weight-bearing and biomechanical stress contribute to the inflammatory component of AS [68].

Diagnosis of Osteoporosis in AS

Although osteoporosis is common in AS, it is often diagnosed late due to visual confounding by syndesmophytes and ankyloses. Consequently, BMD measurements may be artificially high and the extent of osteopenia or osteoporosis may not be appreciated [69].

Because spinal hyperostosis in AS is often positioned around the zygapophyseal joints, the vertebral endplates of disks, and the annulus fibrosus, with relative sparing of the lateral sides, lateral DXA scans may be more useful than anteroposterior (AP) views in terms of evaluating possible osteoporosis. Moreover lateral scanning permits exclusive examination of the vertebral body, comprised of 80 % trabecular bone [70]. In Klingberg et al.'s [70] study of 87 AS women and 117 men using both lateral and AP lumbar BMDs, the lateral view revealed significantly more cases of osteoporosis in men with AS than did the AP view. At the same time, the AP view revealed high rates of osteoporosis in women, whereas the lateral view did not, indicating that certain modalities of imaging are better suited to males versus females in making an early diagnosis. In a number of senses, both the lateral and AP view may be needed since the combination will allow a three-dimensional volumetric BMD which is a superior measure to a two-dimensional area BMD.

Emohare and coauthors [71] went a step further and tested computerized tomography (CT) attenuation models in lieu of DXA as a tool to assess osteoporosis and fractures in AS patients. In a group of 17 patients, they diagnosed 82–88 % of subjects with osteoporosis based on the threshold sensitivity of the machine selected. Pickhardt et al. [72] has proposed the novel concept that data from abdominal CT images, which included the L1 vertebra but were obtained for other purposes, can be used to identify patients with osteoporosis without additional radiation exposure or expense: If the L1 vertebra was not fractured, an estimate of lumbar bone density can be made without having the patient undergo another scan.

Challenges exist not only in the diagnosis of osteoporosis but, also, at times in the identification of fractures. A number of cases illustrate the challenges that syndesmophytes and the spinous overgrowth create. In the cervical spine, new fractures may be missed in the immediate hours after an injury such as a fall. Pain may be present, but radiographs may not reveal a fracture until 24 hour later, and then, often only by MRI or CT [73]. In the case described by Fatemi et al., a nondisplaced fracture was missed by plain imaging and CT; not until 20 hour later, when the fracture had become displaced and the patient had returned to the hospital with new neurologic symptoms, was an MRI performed. Harrop et al. [74] have also described a case of a missed surgical fracture but only a high-definition multidetector CT revealed the deformity; standard CT, plain radiographs, and MRI all failed to diagnose the fracture. The question of whether MRIs should be done after any injury to the neck or lower spine in AS patients is raised in the literature. While the cost of an MRI is not insignificant, it bears no comparison to the potential cost to patients and society of a spinal cord injury arising from an undiagnosed fracture. Figures 2 and 3 demonstrate cervical spine fracture as well as extensive ankylosing spondylitis in thoracic and lumbar portions of this patient's spine. This question warrants further analysis in future investigations.

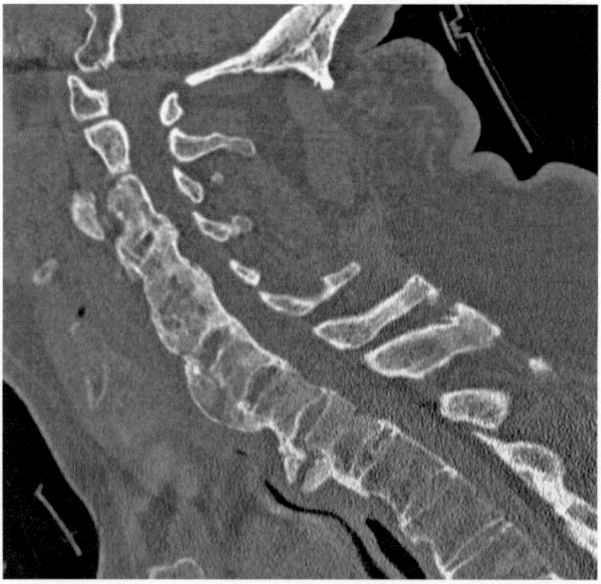

Fig. 2 CT scan of cervical spine demonstrating ankylosing spondylitis. In a 75-year-old male with longstanding disease. Image demonstrates an age-indeterminate fracture of C5 anterior osteophyte with upper thoracic ankylotic changes (*Source*: Thomas Jefferson University Department of Radiology, Philadelphia, PA. Used with permission)

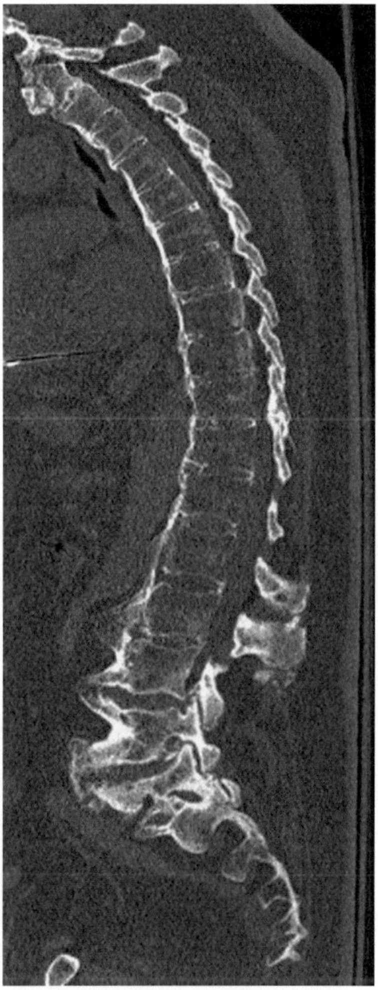

Fig. 3 CT of thoracolumbar spine in a patient with ankylosing spondylitis. Image illustrates the middle and lower thoracic as well as the lumbosacral spine demonstrating ankylosing spondylitis throughout multiple areas, along with superimposed multi-level degenerative changes (*Source*: Thomas Jefferson University Department of Radiology, Philadelphia, PA. Used with permission)

Etiology and Pathophysiology of Osteoporosis in AS

The study by Klingberg et al. [70] found that low BMD in AS patients was associated with female sex, older age, low body mass index, heredity for fractures, scores on the physical activity at home and work index [75], and the number of years since menopause. Additional factors relate to function and medications: disease duration, high Bath Ankylosing Spondylitis Metrology Index (BASMI), high modified Stoke Ankylosing Spondylitis Spine Score (mSASSS), elevated inflammatory parameters (ESR, CRP), and low hemoglobin. Factors that influenced osteoporosis in AS, as well as others that were examined and not relevant to AS, are summarized in Table 5 [69, 70, 76–78].

Table 5 Factors associated with osteoporosis in patients with AS

Source	*n*	Outcome of study
Franck et al. [69]	504	OPG levels are typically low, possibly contributing to the immune response and relative state of osteoclastogenesis seen in these patients
Klingberg et al. [70]	204	Low BMD was associated with female sex, older age, low body mass index, heredity for fractures, scores on the physical activity at home and work index, and number of years since menopause in the case of female patients
Gratacos et al. [76]	34	Only subjects with persistent active disease experienced significant bone loss early on; 5 % loss was seen in the lumbar spine and 3 % in the femoral neck over 19 months; of note, no significant bone loss was found in those with inactive disease; the group with active disease also showed elevated IL-6, but other factors including physical activity or medications for treatment impacted BMD
Maillefert et al. [77]	54	No significant change in lumbar BMD in the 34 subjects on average in the 2-year assessment but did observe a decline in femoral neck BMD of 1.6 %. The levels of ESR and CRP were only significantly elevated in the group with bone loss in the femoral neck
Cai et al. [78]	1001	Serum vitamin D levels and disease activity were tightly correlated (SMD = 0.71, $p < 0.001$), more so for the value of ESR than for CRP or BASDAI. Calcium and PTH levels were not related to disease activity

Among these factors, a number of researchers give greater weight to the degree of inflammation in fostering and advancing the extent of bone loss in AS. A prospective study of 34 patients with AS by Gratacos and colleagues [76] found that only subjects with persistent active disease experienced significant bone loss early in the disease course. Loss was seen in the lumbar spine (5 %) and in the femoral neck (3 %) over 19 months for those with active disease, whereas no significant bone loss was found in those with inactive disease. Moreover, the group with active disease had significantly higher levels of IL-6, but other factors including physical activity or medications for treatment impacted BMD.

A subsequent study by Maillefert et al. examined changes in bone density in patients with AS over a prospective 2-year period [77]. The questions posed were whether change in BMD in the lumbar spine and in the femoral neck were related to any of the three factors: physical impairment, persistent systemic inflammation as defined by ESR ≥28 mm/h, or mean C-Reactive Protein (CRP) ≥15 mm/l. The authors found no change in lumbar BMD in the 34 subjects on average in the 2-year assessment but did observe a decline in femoral neck BMD of 1.6 %. The levels of ESR and CRP were only significantly elevated in the group with bone loss in the femoral neck.

Biochemical markers of bone metabolism are altered in patients with AS. Franck and colleagues [69] examined how osteoprotegerin (OPG) levels might relate to inflammation and osteoporosis in AS patients. As a decoy protein receptor for the receptor activator of nuclear factor kappa B ligand (RANKL), OPG can bind to RANKL and, in doing so, prevent RANK-mediated nuclear factor kappa B activation, a step that is essential to transcription of immune-related genes and a regulator of innate immunity [79]. The researchers found that OPG levels in AS patients are low, possibly contributing to their immune response. Another function of OPG is to reduce the production of osteoclasts by inhibiting their differentiation. This step is essential to preventing excess bone resorption; if OPG levels are low, a relative state of osteoclastogenesis ensues [80].

The role of vitamin D in osteoporosis prevention in AS patients remains uncertain. A study by Cai et al. in 2015 examined a series of eight case–control studies with a total of 533 AS patients and 478 matching controls [78]. They explored the correlation between ESR, CRP, Bath Ankylosing Spondylitis Disease Activity Index (BASDAI) and levels of both serum calcium, PTH, and serum vitamin D25OH. Results found that serum vitamin D levels and disease activity were tightly correlated (standard mean difference (SMD) = −0.71, $p<0.001$), more so for the value of ESR than for CRP or BASDAI. Calcium and PTH levels were not related to disease activity. Additional studies on the role of vitamin D are indicated, but there is little harm in ensuring that patients have at least a serum vitamin D level of 30–35 mg/dl, which is the low end of the therapeutic range.

Epidemiology of Osteoporosis and AS

A number of studies have examined the prevalence of osteoporosis, measured under varying modalities, in patients with AS. The best recent estimate sets the overall prevalence of osteoporosis at 25 % and vertebral fractures at 10 %, noting that these figures are challenged by falsely elevated BMD and by lack of presentation by many patients, due to the absence of symptoms in advance of any fracture and often even following a vertebral fracture [81]. In general, osteoporosis is routinely underdiagnosed and undertreated due to diagnostic challenges, so prevalence estimates in early studies have been low, particularly in investigations that preceded recommendations to use CT or lateral DXA. In a review article by van der Weidjen et al. [82], seven investigations are considered with findings of low BMD in 51–54 % of subjects; however, a BMD level low enough to meet the WHO diagnosis of osteoporosis was only present in 13–16 % of patients. While this review focused on patients within 10 years of diagnosis, symptom onset of AS may precede its diagnosis and can be interpreted as neck or back pain. In many cases, AS is diagnosed late and screening for osteoporosis does not occur until it has reached more advanced stage [81].

In the report by Klingberg et al. [70] examining 204 patients with AS, 34 % of patients under age 50 had a BMD *Z*-score of <−1.0 at the hip and/or lumbar spine, and 4.9 % had BMD below the expected range for age, *Z*-score <2.0. However, for patients over 50, osteoporosis was far more prevalent: 43.6 % were osteopenic and 20.8 % met the definition of osteoporosis by World Health Organization standards. For both male and female patients combined, the spine was the most common location of osteopenia or osteoporosis, followed by the radius and then the femoral neck.

Ghozlani et al. examined the prevalence of both osteoporosis and vertebral fractures in persons with AS [83]. Osteoporosis was present in 25 % of their sample of 80 subjects, and 18.8 % had vertebral fractures. The group did not report rates of osteopenia. Relevant factors for low BMD were disease duration, elevated Bath Ankylosing Spondylitis Disease Activity Index, longer disease duration, and lower BMI. Wang et al. studied 504 subjects with more advanced AS than the other authors and found a much greater prevalence of osteoporosis in AS patients (9.7 % vs. 0 %) as well as osteopenia (57.5 % vs. 34.9 %), when compared with 106 age- and gender-matched controls [84]. At the lumbar spine, risk factors for bone loss were juvenile onset of disease, morning stiffness lasting more than 30 minutes, and elevated ESR, whereas at the femur, risk factors were male gender, older age, ankylosis of the hip and lack of regular AS treatment. Interestingly, the use of glucocorticoids did not correlate with bone loss in either the spine or hip.

Fractures in AS

The reported prevalence of vertebral fractures in AS patients ranges from 12 % to 32.4 %. One large investigation of 66,000 patients gave an estimate below 1 %, but this was based on patient questionnaires. Often patients may not realize they have a vertebral body collapse consistent with fracture unless pain or weakness results. Notably, 47 % of those completing questionnaires reported fractures that were significant enough to cause neurological damage [85]. The advantage of this study is that it was a population-based study and not drawn from a rheumatology clinic where cases tend to be more complex.

In the study by Ghozlani [83], fractures in lumbar vertebrae were seen in 18.8 % of patients, with the strongest risk factors being disease duration and mSASSS. This group only looked at vertebral fractures of grade 2 (reduction of 26–40 % loss of height) and grade 3 (reduction of >40 % loss of height). A summary of prior studies on prevalence of osteoporosis and vertebral fractures is given in Table 6 [70, 81–83, 85, 86].

Pharmacologic Treatment

Vitamins and Hormones

Although there are no formalized treatment guidelines for osteoporosis in AS endorsed by relevant European or North American organizations, AS screening for osteoporosis should occur in the first several years of diagnosis. The initial step in management consists of appropriate preventative measures, including review of dietary intake of calcium and vitamin D, screening baseline levels of serum calcium PTH and serum vitamin D25OH, and evaluation of endocrine abnormalities in

Table 6 Prevalence of osteoporosis and vertebral fractures in patients with ankylosing spondylitis

Source	*n*	Age	Sex (M/F)	AS disease duration, yrs	Modality	Results OP (%), VF (%)	Comments
Van der Weidjen et al. [82]	482	35	419/63	8	DXA (*T*-score)	OP 13–16 %	Systematic review
Klingberg et al. [70]	204	50	117/87	15	DXA (*T*-score)	OP 21 %	Based on lateral DXA scans, which showed low BMD in comparison to the AP projection
Ghozlani et al. [83]	80	39	67/13	11	DXA (*T*-score)	OP 25 %	Some vertebrae from the T4–L4 region were not adequately visualized
Vosse et al. [85]	59	57	44/13	25	Patient questionnaire	VF 0.4 %	Subjects completed questionnaires regarding CVFs

Sources: Adapted from Davey-Ranasinghe [81] and El Maghraoui A. [86]
AP anterioposterior, *DXA* dual-energy x-ray absorptiometry, *OP* osteoporosis, *VFs* vertebral fractures, *CVFs* clinically confirmed vertebral fractures

estrogen, testosterone, growth hormone, and thyroid function. However, there are no controlled trials of osteoporosis prevention or treatment with vitamin D, calcium, anabolic steroids, or other forms of hormone replacement.

Bisphosphonates

Two trials of pamidronate given to reduce inflammation rather than treat osteoporosis revealed a reduction in bone turnover markers [87, 88]. However no improvement in BMD was observed over the study evaluation period of 3–6 months. Both investigations took place 15–20 years ago and additional trials of alternative bisphosphonates may ultimately demonstrate greater potential.

Two published trials of zoledronic acid (ZA) for inflammation secondary to AS should be noted [89, 90]. In one investigation by Sargin and Senturk [89], ZA was well tolerated, and, after three months, reduced disease activity, less spine pain, and lower inflammatory markers (ESR and CRP) were found. The mechanism of bisphosphonates involves inhibition of osteoclastic activity and modulation of pro-inflammatory cytokines. Measures of bone turnover and bone density such as telopeptides, P1NP, or DXA scans were not examined. To date, no controlled studies of other bisphosphonates have been published that focus on improvement of BMD in AS patients.

TNF-α Inhibitors

As the reports of Gratacos [76] and Maillefert [77] have shown, disease duration and elevated ESR as well as CRP correlate with bone loss, and thus the role of TNF-α inhibitors may offer promise for treatment and further prevention of osteoporosis. Because TNF-α is a cytokine that increases bone resorption in states of estrogen deficiency and erosive arthritis affecting periarticular regions, blocking the action of TNF-α should theoretically result in a net gain of bone content.

Infliximab is a human neutralizing monoclonal antibody used successfully to decrease inflammation in rheumatoid conditions and spondyloarthropathies. Allali et al. [91] focused on 29 patients with various forms of spondyloarthropathy, most receiving 5 mg/kg at weeks 0, 2, and 6. Significant gains were seen in BMD of spine, total hip, and greater trochanter. Only four patients received corticosteroids during the study; notably, no increase in BMD was seen at any site in the four subjects. Values of ESR and CRP for the group as a whole demonstrated significant decreases between baseline and week number six and between baseline and final visit at approximately six months posttreatment.

A recent phase III clinical trial of 279 subjects taking infliximab for AS-related osteoporosis demonstrated a 2.5 % increase in spinal BMD and 0.5 % gain in hip BMD relative to control subjects who, in comparison, achieved BMD gains of 0.5 % in the spine and 0.2 % in the hip [92]. Subjects received either the study drug or placebo every two weeks. Early response to infliximab was seen in the form of elevated bone alkaline phosphatase (BAP) and/or increased osteocalcin, two alternative markers of bone formation. Subjects with high BAP early in the study and those with elevated osteocalcin levels just two weeks into the trial demonstrated significant gains in BMD at the end of the study, two years after the first dose of the drug.

Nonpharmacologic Treatment

Deficits in postural stability, coordination, proprioception, and balance are inherent in AS [73]. Pompeu et al. has described the consequences of altered posture with AS, specifically the combination of increased thoracolumbar kyphosis and hip flexion that displace the body's center of gravity anteriorly, resulting in horizontal gaze and a compensatory increase in knee flexion and ankle plantar flexion [93]. In a study of 12 AS subjects matched with 12 healthy age-equivalent controls, those with AS demonstrated significant reductions in range of motion for hip and knee extension, markedly decreased heel strike and plantar flexion in the initial contact phase of gait, and notable deficits in dynamic and static balance [94]. Physical therapists should focus on correction of these deficits as early as possible to maximize remaining function.

Impairments in proprioception and vestibular function have been reported in patients with AS. How much of a role nonsteroidal anti-inflammatory agents (NSAIDs) may play in this observation is unclear. This class of drugs has been known to cause ototoxicity, and, given the high use in populations with rheumatic diseases, the effect of NSAIDs on balance and proprioception is potentially detrimental [73]. Spinal enthesopathy may intensify deficits further.

When vision (via kyphosis) is impaired along with sensation and proprioception, the risk of falls is increased significantly. This concern, combined with motor weakness, endurance deficits, and adverse medication effects, only increases the need for structured physical therapy to educate patients on protective fall techniques and anticipatory safety measures. No studies on AS patients have focused on an exercise program specific to osteoporosis, but the risk of spinal fractures is substantial at all phases of disease. Many therapy centers incorporate structured home exercise programs to meet functional deficits and offer long-term guidance for safe mobility in the home and community.

References

1. Haugenberg G, Orstovik RE, Uhlig T, Falch JA, Halse JI, Kvien TK. Clinical decision rule in rheumatoid arthritis: do they identify patients at high risk for osteoporosis? Testing clinical criteria in a population based cohort of patients with rheumatoid arthritis recruited from the Oslo Rheumatoid Arthritis Register. Ann Rheum Dis. 2002;61:12085–9.
2. Hauser B, Riches PL, Wilson JF, Horne AE, Ralston SH. Prevalence and clinical prediction of osteoporosis in a contemporary cohort of patients with rheumatoid arthritis. Rheumatology. 2014;53(10):1759–66.
3. Sinigaglia L, Nervetti A, Mela Q, Bianchi G, Del Puente A, Di Munno O, et al. A multicenter cross sectional study on bone mineral density in rheumatoid arthritis. Italian Study Group on Bone Mass in Rheumatoid Arthritis. J Rheumatol. 2000;27(11):2582–9.
4. Reid DM, Kennedy NS, Nicoll J, Smith MA, Tothill P, Nuki G. Total and peripheral bone mass in patients with psoriatic arthritis and rheumatoid arthritis. Clin Rheumatol. 1986;5:372–8.
5. Haugenberg G, Uhlig T, Falch JA, Halse JI, Kvien TK. Bone mineral density and frequency of osteoporosis in female patients with rheumatoid arthritis. Arthritis Rheum. 2000;43:522–30.
6. Stafford L, Bleasel J, Giles A, Handelsman D. Androgen deficiency and bone mineral density in men with rheumatoid arthritis. J Rheumatol. 2000;27:2786–90.
7. Tengstrand B, Hafstrom I. Bone mineral density in men with rheumatoid arthritis is associated with erosive disease and sulfasalazine treatment but not with sex hormones. J Rheumatol. 2002;29:2299–305.
8. Haugeberg G, Uhlig T, Falch JA, Halse JI, Kvien TK. Reduced bone mineral density in male rheumatoid arthritis patients: frequencies and associations with demographic and disease variables in ninety-four patients in the Oslo County Rheumatoid Arthritis Register. Arthritis Rheum. 2000;43:2776–84.
9. Sinigaglia L, Varenna M, Girasole G, Bianchi G. Epidemiology of osteoporosis in rheumatic diseases. Rheum Dis Clin N Am. 2006;32:631–58.
10. Kaz Kaz H, Johnson D, Kerry S, Chinappen U, Tweed K, Patel S. Fall-related risk factors and osteoporosis in women with rheumatoid arthritis. Rheumatology (Oxford). 2004;43(10):1267–71.
11. Bruce B, Fries JF. The Health Assessment Questionnaire (HAQ). Clin Exp Rheumatol. 2005;23 Suppl 39:14–8.
12. Jamison M, Neuberger GB, Miller PA. Correlates of falls and fear of falling among adults with rheumatoid arthritis. Arthritis Rheum. 2003;49:673–80.
13. Amin S, Gabriel S, Achenbach S, Atkinson E, Melton LJ. Fracture risk is increased in young women with rheumatoid arthritis. J Bone Miner Res. 2011;26(Suppl 1):669–76.

14. Rodrigues Pereira RM, Freire de Carvalho J, Canalis E. Glucocorticoid-induced osteoporosis in rheumatic diseases. Clinics (San Paolo). 2010;65(11):1197–205.
15. Homik JJ, Suarez-Almazor ME, Shea B, Cranney A, Wells G, Tugwell P. Calcium and vitamin D for corticosteroid-induced osteoporosis. Cochrane Database Syst Rev. 2000;2, CD000952.
16. Heaney RP. The vitamin D requirement in health and disease. J Steroid Biochem Mol Biol. 2005;97:13–9.
17. Richy F, Schact E, Bruyere O, Ethgen O, Gourlay M, Reginster JY. Vitamin D analogs versus native vitamin D in preventing bone loss and osteoporosis-related fractures. Calcif Tissue Int. 2005;76:176–86.
18. Lange U, Teichmann J, Muller-Ladner U, Strunk J. Increase in bone mineral density of patients with rheumatoid arthritis treated with anti-TNF alpha antibody: a prospective open-label pilot study. Rheumatology. 2005;44:1546–8.
19. Dischereit G, Tarner IH, Muller-Ladner U, Lange U. Infliximab improves bone metabolism and bone mineral density in rheumatoid arthritis and ankylosing spondylitis: a prospective 2-year study. Clin Rheumatol. 2013;32:377–81.
20. Korczowska I, Lackl JK, Hrycaj P. Influence of infliximab on cytokines network and markers of bone remodeling in rheumatoid arthritis patients. Yonsei Med J. 2013;54(1):183–8.
21. Wijbrandts CA, Klaasen R, Dijkgraaf MGW, Gerlag DM, van Eck-Smit BLF, Tak PP. Bone mineral density in rheumatoid arthritis patients 1 year after adalimumab therapy: arrest of bone loss. Ann Rheum Dis. 2009;68:373–6.
22. Saag KG, Emkey R, Schnitzer TJ, Brown JP, Hawkins F, Goemaere S, et al. Alendronate for the prevention and treatment of glucocorticoid-induced osteoporosis. N Engl J Med. 1998;339:292–9.
23. Feng Z, Zeng S, Wang Y, Zheng Z, Chen Z. Bisphosphonates for the prevention and treatment of osteoporosis in patients with rheumatic diseases: a systemic review and meta-analysis. PLoS ONE. 2013;8(12), e80890. doi:10.1371/journal.pone.0080890.
24. Eastell R, Devogelaer JP, Peel NF, Chines AA, Bax DE, Sacco-Gibson N, et al. Prevention of bone loss with risedronate in glucocorticoid-treated rheumatoid arthritis patients. Osteoporos Int. 2000;11:331–7.
25. Lems WF, Lodder MC, Lips P, Bijlsma JW, Geusens P, Schrameijer N, et al. Positive effect of alendronate on bone mineral density and markers of bone turnover in patients with rheumatoid arthritis on chronic treatment with low-dose prednisone: a randomized, double-blind, placebo-controlled trial. Osteoporos Int. 2006;17:716–23.
26. Ebina K, Noguchi T, Hirao M, Hashimoto J, Kaneshiro S, Yukioka M, et al. Effects of switching weekly alendronate or risedronate to monthly minodronate in patients with rheumatoid arthritis: a 12-month prospective study. Osteoporos Int. 2016;27(1):351–9.
27. Reid DM, Devogelaer JP, Saag K, Roux C, Lau CS, Reginster JY, et al. Zoledronic acid and risedronate in the prevention and treatment of glucocorticoid-induced osteoporosis (HORIZON): a multicenter double-blind, double-dummy, randomized controlled trial. Lancet. 2009;373(9671):1253–63.
28. Saag KG, Shane E, Boonen S, Marin F, Donley DW, Taylor KA, et al. Teriparatide or alendronate in glucocorticoid-induced osteoporosis. N Engl J Med. 2007;357(20):2028–39.
29. Saag KG, Zanchetta JR, Devogelaer JP, Adler RA, Eastell R, See K, et al. Effects of teriparatide versus alendronate for treating glucocorticoid-induced osteoporosis: thirty-six month results of a randomized double-blind controlled trial. Arthritis Rheum. 2009;60(11):3346–55.
30. National Osteoporosis Foundation. Clinician's guide to prevention and treatment of osteoporosis. Washington, DC: National Osteoporosis Foundation; 2013. p. 14–23.
31. Gennari L, Bilezekian JP. Glucocorticoid-induced osteoporosis: hope is on the HORIZON. Lancet. 2009;373(9671):1225–6.
32. Pedersen BK, Saltin B. Exercise as medicine-evidence for prescribing exercise as therapy in 26 different chronic diseases. Scand J Med Sci Sports. 2015;25 Suppl 3:1–72.
33. Lindhardsen J, Gislason GH, Ahlehoff O, Madsen OR, Hansen PR. Excess mortality from cardiovascular disease in patients with rheumatoid arthritis. Ugeskr Laeger. 2011;173:343–6.

34. Hurkmans E, van der Giesen FJ, Vliet Vlieland TPM, Schoones J, Van den Ende ECHM. Dynamic exercise programs (aerobic capacity and/or muscle strength training) in patients with rheumatoid arthritis (review). Cochrane Database Syst Rev. 2009;4, CD006853.
35. Hochberg MC, Chang RW, Dwosh I, Lindsey S, Pincus T, Wolfe F. The American College of Rheumatology 1991 revised criteria for the classification of global functional status in rheumatoid arthritis. Arthritis Rheum. 1992;35(5):498–502.
36. de Jong Z, Munneke M, Lems WF, Zwinderman AH, Kroon HM, Jansen A, et al. Is a long term high-intensity exercise program effective and safe in patients with rheumatoid arthritis: results of a randomized controlled trial. Arthritis Rheum. 2003;48:2415–24.
37. Strasser B, Leeb G, Strehblow C, Schobersberger W, Haber P, Cauza E. The effects of strength and endurance training in patients with rheumatoid arthritis. Clin Rheumatol. 2011;30:623–32.
38. Stavropoulos-Kalinoglou A, Metsios GS, Veldhuijzen van Zanten JJ, Nightingale P, Kitas GD, Koutedakis Y. Individualized aerobic and resistance exercise training improves cardiorespiratory fitness and reduces cardiovascular risk in patients with rheumatoid arthritis. Ann Rheum Dis. 2013;72:1819–25.
39. Bultink IEM, Vis M, van der Horst-Bruinsma IE, Lems WF. Inflammatory rheumatic disorders and bone. Curr Rheumatol Rep. 2012;14:224–30.
40. Teichmann J, Lange U, Stracke H, Federlin K, Bretzel RG. Bone metabolism and bone mineral density of systemic lupus erythematosus at the time of diagnosis. Rheumatol Int. 1999;18:137–40.
41. Garcia-Carrasco M, Mendoza-Pinto C, Escárcega RO, Jiménez-Hernández M, Etchegaray Morales I, Munguia Realpozo P, et al. Osteoporosis in patients with systemic lupus erythematosus. Isr Med Assoc J. 2009;11:486–91.
42. Mok CC, Mak A, Ma KM. Bone mineral density in postmenopausal Chinese patients with systemic lupus erythematosus. Lupus. 2005;14:106–12.
43. Jardinet D, Lefebvre C, Depresseux G, Lambert M, Devogelaer J-P, Houssiau FA. Longitudinal analysis of bone mineral density in pre-menopausal female systematic lupus erythematosus patients: deleterious role of glucocorticoid therapy at the lumbar spine. Rheumatology. 2000;39:389–92.
44. Kipen Y, Briganti E, Strauss B, Will R, Littlejohn G, Morand E. Three year followup on bone mineral density change in premenopausal women with systemic lupus erythematosus. J Rheumatol. 1999;26:310–7.
45. Becker A, Fischer R, Scherbaum WA, Schneider M. Osteoporosis screening in systemic lupus erythematosus: impact of disease duration and organ damage. Lupus. 2001;10:809–14.
46. Lee C, Manzi S, Ramsey-Goldman R. Bone loss and fractures in systemic lupus erythematosus. In: Maricic M, Gluck OS, editors. Bone disease in rheumatology. Philadelphia: Lippincott; 2005. p. 79–86.
47. Lakshminarayanan S, Walsh S, Mohanraj M, Rothfield N. Factors associated with low bone mineral density in female patients with systemic lupus erythematosus. J Rheumatol. 2001;28:102–8.
48. Bultink IEM, Lems WF, Kostense PJ, Dijkmans BAC, Voskuyl AE. Prevalence of and risk factors for low bone mineral density and vertebral fractures in patients with systemic lupus erythematosus. Arthritis Rheum. 2005;54:2044–50.
49. Pons F, Peris P, Guañabens N, Font J, Huguet M, Espinosa G, Ingelmo M, Muñoz-Gomez J, Setoain J. The effect of systemic lupus erythematosus and long-term steroid therapy on bone mass in pre-menopausal women. Br J Rheumatol. 1995;34(8):742–6.
50. Formiga F, Moga I, Nolla JM, Pac M, Mitjavila F, Roig-Escofet D. Loss of bone mineral density in premenopausal women with systemic lupus erythematosus. Ann Rheum Dis. 1995;54(4):274–6.
51. Ramsey-Goldman R, Dunn JE, Huang CF, Dunlop D, Rairie JE, Fitzgerald S, et al. Frequency of fractures in women with systemic lupus erythematosus: comparison with United States population data. Arthritis Rheum. 1999;42:882–90.
52. Zonana-Nacach A, Barr S, Magder LS, Petri M. Damage in systematic lupus erythematosus and its association with corticosteroids. Arthritis Rheum. 1999;42:1801–8.

53. Borba VZ, Matos PG, da Silva Viana PR, Fernandes A, Sato EI, Lazaretti-Castro M. High prevalence of vertebral deformity in premenopausal systemic lupus erythematosus patients. Lupus. 2005;14:529–33.
54. Mendoza-Pinto C, García-Carrasco M, Sandoval-Cruz H, Muñoz-Guarneros M, Escárcega RO, Jiménez-Hernández M, et al. Risk factors of vertebral fractures in women with systemic lupus erythematosus. Clin Rheumatol. 2009;28(5):579–85.
55. Bultink IE, Harvey NC, Lalmohamed A, Cooper C, Lems WF, van Staa TP, et al. Elevated risk of clinical fractures and associated risk factors in patients with systemic lupus erythematosus versus matched controls: a population-based study in the United Kingdom. Osteoporos Int. 2014;25(4):1275–83.
56. Genant HK, Wu CY, van Kujik C, Nevitt MC. Vertebral fracture assessment using a semiquantitative technique. J Bone Miner Res. 1993;8:1137–48.
57. Sen D, Keen RW. Osteoporosis in systemic lupus erythematosus: prevention and treatment. Lupus. 2001;10:227–32.
58. Lambrinoudaki I, Chan DT, Lau CS, Wong RW, Yeung SS, Kung AW. Effect of calcitriol on bone mineral density in premenopausal Chinese women taking chronic steroid therapy. A randomized, double blind, placebo controlled study. J Rheumatol. 2000;27:1759–65.
59. Sawalha AH, Kovats S. Dehydroepiandrosterone in systemic lupus erythematosus. Curr Rheumatol Rep. 2008;10(4):286–91.
60. van Vollenhaven RF. Dehydroepiandrosterone in systemic lupus erythematosus. Rheum Dis Clin N Am. 2000;26:349–62.
61. van Vollenhoven RF, Park JL, Genovese MC, West JP, McGuire JL. A double-blind, placebo-controlled trial of dehydroepiandrosterone in severe systemic lupus erythematosus. Lupus. 1999;8(3):181–7.
62. Formiga F, Moga I, Nolla JM, Navarro MA, Bonnin R, Roig-Escofet D. The association of dehydroepiandrosterone sulfate levels with bone mineral density in systemic lupus erythematosus. Clin Exp Rheumatol. 1997;15(4):387–92.
63. Hartkamp A, Geenen R, Godaert GL, Bijl M, Bijlsma JW, Derksen RH. The effect of dehydroepiandrosterone on lumbar spine bone mineral density in patients with quiescent systemic lupus erythematosus. Arthritis Rheum. 2004;50(11):3591–5.
64. Cohen S, Levy RM, Keller M, Boling E, Emkey RD, Greenwald M, et al. Risedronate therapy prevents corticosteroid-induced bone loss: a twelve-month, multicenter, randomized, double-blind, placebo-controlled parallel-group study. Arthritis Rheum. 1999;42(11):2309–18.
65. Smith JA. Update on ankylosing spondylitis: current concepts in pathogenesis. Curr Allergy Asthma Rep. 2015;15:489–98.
66. Mayo Clinic. Ankylosing spondylitis: symptoms and causes. http://www.mayoclinic.org/diseases-conditions/ankylosing-spondylitis/basics/definition/con-20019766. Accessed 10 Oct 2015.
67. Boonen A, Severens JL. Ankylosing spondylitis: what is the cost to society, and can it be reduced? Best Pract Res Clin Rheumatol. 2002;16:691–705.
68. Sherlock JP, Joyce-Shaikh B, Turner SP, Chao CC, Sathe M, Grein J, et al. IL-23R induces spondyloarthropathy by acting on ROR-gamma+ CD3+CD4-CD8- entheseal resident T cells. Nat Med. 2012;18:1069–76.
69. Franck H, Meurer T, Hofbauer LC. Evaluation of bone mineral density, hormones, biochemical markers of bone metabolism, and osteoprotegerin serum levels in patients with ankylosing spondylitis. J Rheumatol. 2004;31(11):2236–41.
70. Klingberg E, Lorentzon M, Geijer M, Gothlin J, Hilme E, Hedberg M, et al. Osteoporosis in ankylosing spondylitis-prevalence, risk factors, and methods of assessment. Arthritis Res Ther. 2012;14(R108):1–12.
71. Emohare O, Cagan A, Polly DW, Gertner E. Opportunistic computed tomography screening shows a high incidence of osteoporosis in ankylosing spondylitis patients with acute vertebral fractures. J Clin Densitom. 2015;18(1):17–21.
72. Pickhardt PJ, Pooler BD, Lauder T, del Rio AM, Bruce RJ, Binkley N. Opportunistic screening for osteoporosis using abdominal computer tomography scans obtained for other indications. Ann Intern Med. 2013;158(8):588–95.

73. Fatemi G, Gensler LS, Learch TJ, Weisman MH. Spine fractures in ankylosing spondylitis: a case report and review of imaging as well as predisposing factors to falls and fractures. Semin Arthritis Rheum. 2014;44(1):20–4.
74. Harrop JS, Sharan A, Anderson G, Hillibrand AS, Albert TJ, Flanders A, et al. Failure of standard imaging to detect a cervical fracture in a patient with ankylosing spondylitis. Spine. 2005;30(14):E417–9.
75. Mannerkorpi K, Hernelid C. Leisure time physical activity instrument and physical activity at home and work instrument. Development, face validity, construct validity, and test-retest reliability for subjects with fibromyalgia. Disabil Rehabil. 2005;27:695–701.
76. Gratacos J, Collado A, Pons F, Osaba M, Sammarti R, Roque M, et al. Significant bone mass in patients with early, active ankylosing spondylitis. Arthritis Rheum. 1999;42:2319–24.
77. Maillefert JF, Aho LS, El Maghraoui A, Dougados M, Roux C. Changes in bone density in patients with ankylosing spondylitis: a two-year follow-up study. Osteoporos Int. 2001;12:605–9.
78. Cai G, Wang L, Fan D, Xin L, Liu L, Hy Y, et al. Vitamin D in ankylosing spondylitis: review and meta-analysis. Clin Chim Acta. 2015;438:316–22.
79. Krakauer T. Nuclear factor-kappaB: fine-tuning a central integrator of diverse biologic stimuli. Int Rev Immunol. 2008;27(5):286–92. doi:10.1080/08830180802317957.
80. Luis Neyro J, Jesus Cancelo M, Palacios S. Inhibition of RANKL in the pathophysiology of osteoporosis. Clinical evidences of its use. Ginecol Obstet Mex. 2013;81(3):146–57.
81. Davey-Ranasinghe N, Deodhar A. Osteoporosis and vertebral fractures in ankylosing spondylitis. Curr Opin Rheumatol. 2013;25(4):509–16.
82. van der Weidjen MA, Claushuis TA, Nazari T, Lems WF, Dijkmans BA, Van der Horst-Bruinsma IE. High prevalence of low bone mineral density in patients within 10 years of onset of ankylosing spondylitis: a systematic review. Clin Rheumatol. 2012;31:1529–35.
83. Ghozlani I, Ghazi M, Nouijall A, Mounach A, Rezqi A, Achemlal L, et al. Prevalence and risk factors of osteoporosis and vertebral fractures. Bone. 2009;43:772–6.
84. Wang D, Zeng Q, Chen S, Gong Y, Hou Z, Xiao Z. Prevalence and risk factors of osteoporosis in patients with ankylosing spondylitis: a 5-year follow-up study of 504 cases. Clin Exp Rheum. 2015;33(4):465–70.
85. Vosse D, Feldkeller E, Erlendsson J, Guesens P, vander Linden S. Clinical vertebral fractures in patients with ankylosing spondylitis. J Rheumatol. 2004;31(10):1981–5.
86. El Maghraoui A. Osteoporosis and ankylosing spondylitis. Joint Bone Spine. 2004;71:291–5.
87. Maksymowych WP, Jhangri GS, Leclercq S, Skeith K, Yan A, Russell AS. An open study of pamidronate in the treatment of refractory ankylosing spondylitis. J Rheumatol. 1998;25:714–7.
88. Maksymowych WP, Lambert R, Jhangri GS, Leclercq S, Chiu P, Wong B, et al. Clinical and radiological amelioration of refractory peripheral spondyloarthritis by pulse intravenous pamidronate therapy. J Rheumatol. 2001;28:144–55.
89. Sargin G, Senturk T. Zoledronic acid effective as rescue treatment for ankylosing spondylitis refractory to TNF inhibition. Ann Pharmacother. 2015;49(3):368–9.
90. Clunie GR, Ginawi A, O'Conner P, Bearcroft W, Garber S, Bhagat S, Grainger A, Gaston JS. An open-label study of zoledronic acid (Aclasta 5 mg iv) in the treatment of ankylosing spondylitis. Ann Rheum Dis. 2014;73(6):1273–4.
91. Allali F, Brebon M, Porcher R, Maillefert JF, Dougados M, Roux C. Increase in bone mineral density of patients with spondyloarthropathy treated with anti TNF-α. Ann Rheum Dis. 2003;62:347–9.
92. Visvanathan S, van der Heijke D. Effects of infliximab on markers of inflammation and bone turnover and associations with bone mineral density in patients with ankylosing spondylitis. Ann Rheum Dis. 2009;68(2):175–82.
93. Pompeu JE, Romano RS, Pompeu SM, Lima SM. Static and dynamic balance in subjects with ankylosing spondylitis: literature review. Rev Bras Reumatol. 2012;52(3):409–16.
94. Del Din S, Carraro E, Sawacha Z, Guitto A, Bonaldo L, Masiero S, et al. Impaired gait in ankylosing spondylitis. Med Biol Eng Comput. 2011;49:801–9.

Chapter 13
Osteoporosis in Gastrointestinal Diseases of Malabsorption and Inflammation

Christina V. Oleson

Chronic conditions affecting the gastrointestinal tract and its functions can have profound long-term effects on bone. Pathological conditions resulting in malabsorption of key vitamins and minerals, as well as altered metabolism of essential components of bone, can have lasting effects on bone health. Individuals with Crohn's disease, ulcerative colitis, pancreatic insufficiency, celiac disease, and restrictive forms of bariatric surgery, as well as gastric bypass or partial small bowel resection, are at significant risk for osteoporosis. This chapter will cover the above topics and offer strategies for clinician awareness and monitoring, diagnosis, and treatment approaches, both nonpharmacologic and pharmacologic in nature.

Inflammatory Malabsorption Disorders

Inflammatory Bowel Disease

Definition and Pathophysiology

Inflammatory bowel disease (IBD) is an umbrella term that combines both Crohn's disease and ulcerative colitis. Both disorders are characterized by fatigue, abdominal pain, diarrhea, GI bleeding, and structural tissue damage to the intestine [1]. Crohn's disease involves periodic or unremitting inflammation of the gastrointestinal tract anywhere along the alimentary pathway (esophagus to anus), whereas ulcerative colitis affects primarily the large bowel which is less involved in nutrient absorption. Fever, nutrient malabsorption, and anemia are common among persons with Crohn's disease [2]. Frequently, those with Crohn's experience reduced levels of vitamin B12, vitamin D, and folate, as well as low prealbumin. If the disease is mild to moderate, medical management of the condition includes antibiotics such as

C.V. Oleson, *Osteoporosis Rehabilitation*, DOI 10.1007/978-3-319-45084-1_13

metronidazole or fluoroquinolone. However for those with severe disease, emergent hospitalization and initiation of corticosteroids or agents that act against tumor necrosis factor alpha (TNF-α), such as infliximab or adalimumab, are the standard of care.

Osteoporosis and IBD

Osteoporosis has been associated with IBD particularly in the advanced stages. It has also been linked to an increased risk of fragility (low trauma) fractures, but the cause and effect of this is less well known. The pathophysiology of bone loss in IBD is secondary to inflammatory processes and their consequences; inappropriate absorption of nutrients, calcium, vitamin D and trace minerals, and ongoing use of osteotoxic medications that may harm bone yet benefit the overall management of IBD. The process of bone loss begins when increased T-cell activity accelerates cytokine production which, in turn, stimulates osteoclasts [3]. These cytokines include IL-1α, IL-1β, IL-6, IL-11, IL-17, TNF-α, and prostaglandin E-2 [4]. Upregulation of IL-6 is particularly problematic because it reduces levels of male and female sex hormones which support osteoblastic activity [5].

Additional bone loss occurs through a receptor ligand pathway identified on osteoblast and osteoclast precursor cells. A surface ligand known as the receptor activator of nuclear factor kappa B ligand (RANKL) can bind to either an osteoclast precursor, called the receptor activator of nuclear factor kappa (RANK), or to a decoy receptor known as osteoprotegerin (OPG). The osteoblast cell produces the soluble decoy receptor OPG. The process of RANKL binding to RANK promotes a cascade of events that matures osteoclasts and causes osteoporosis. The decoy receptor is the key to blocking this process of bone loss by attempting to have RANKL bind to OPG instead; unfortunately the activity of OPG is inadequate to balance the bone loss of the RANKL-mediated osteoclastogenesis. In the setting of prolonged inflammation, OPG levels continue to remain elevated so there is an ongoing attempt by the body to limit further bone loss [6]. In an investigation by Moschen et al. [7], levels of OPG were 2.4 times normal in Crohn's and 1.9 times greater than normal levels in ulcerative colitis. Despite this counter attempt, a negative bone balance results.

Corticosteroids (also known as glucocorticoids) are traditionally utilized in the treatment of IBD, particularly in the more advanced forms of the disease. Not only do glucocorticoids promote osteoblastic apoptosis, but they also impair calcium absorption and promote renal excretion of calcium [4]. They are associated with increased fracture risk, with the greatest detriment in the initial months of treatment, but adverse effects are reduced in the long term if steroids are discontinued [8]. Another encouraging development in recent years is the introduction of budesonide for the treatment of IBD. This corticosteroid has low systemic bioavailability and does not lead to bone loss associated with traditional steroids [4].

Bone Density and Fracture Risk with IBD

The prevalence of osteoporosis and IBD is estimated to range from 42 to 70 %. These estimates are derived from studies generated by tertiary care centers rather than from population-based studies. A more accurate estimate of 5–6 % can be found by looking at a reasonable cross section of the population [1, 9]. Vestergaard found that 32–38 % of persons with Crohn's and 23–25 % of those with ulcerative colitis experience osteopenia [10]. However the relative risk (RR) of fractures is only modestly increased: RR of 1.2 for any fracture and 2.2 for spine fractures for those with Crohn's; 1.1 for any fracture and 1.5 for spine fractures for those with ulcerative colitis.

The American Gastroenterological Association (AGA) has developed a position statement on guidelines for osteoporosis management in a number of gastrointestinal diseases, including IBD [11]. According to this report, IBD has a modest effect on BMD, with a *Z*-score of −0.5. The prevalence of patients with osteoporosis and IBD is 15 %, but increasing age significantly influences results in terms of both prevalence of osteoporosis and fracture incidence, estimated at one per 100 patient years. According to the committee's findings, corticosteroid use was the variable most likely responsible for osteoporosis, but use was difficult to calculate in terms of magnitude of effect due to variability of the disease itself. Also unlike other studies which demonstrated males are more likely than females to be affected by Crohn's disease-related osteoporosis, the AGA stated that the risk of developing osteoporosis in males and females was equivalent. In addition, while other reports [10] found the risk of bone loss to be higher in Crohn's than in ulcerative colitis, the AGA maintained that the risks were comparable.

In terms of prevention of osteoporosis for those with IBD, the AGA recommends the vitamin and calcium supplementation, noted below, as well as periodic assessment by DXA for any patient with IBD who has more than one additional risk factor for osteoporosis including chronic corticosteroid use (defined as three months or longer [1]), hypogonadism, male gender, postmenopausal status if female gender, age greater than 50, or prior history of fracture. Moreover it advises that DXA scans be repeated every 2–3 years for patients with established osteoporosis (*T*-score <2.5) [12].

As described in the early chapters of this text, peak bone mass varies by sex and skeletal site. The degree of bone mineralization increases gradually to a maximum level in the third decade for both genders [13]. The inability to achieve peak bone density by age 25–30 and maintain it until ages 30–40 for women and 40–50 for men places individuals at risk for developing osteoporosis. Since Crohn's disease affects children and teenagers, early efforts to attain maximal BMD by participating in weight-bearing exercise during early life and by optimizing vitamin D and calcium intake should be undertaken. Despite relatively inactive inflammation and disease activity, Laakso et al. found that over a prospective 5-year period, when pre- and postpubertal children should be increasing BMD, children with IBD either maintained their current bone density or, even worse, lost bone over the observation period [14]. This same study found that 25 % of subjects were deficient in vitamin D. Wingate et al. [15] compared the effects of supplemental vitamin D3 in dosages of 400 IU versus 2000 IU in 83 subjects from ages 8–18 with mean BMD of 24 ng/ml. Both groups were able to increase BMD to a mid-range threshold of 20 ng/ml over a duration of six months. However, the desired serum vitamin D25OH level of 30 ng/ml was achieved by only 35 % of subjects receiving supplementation of 400 IU cholecalciferol daily, compared with 79 % of the group that received 2000 IU daily.

Irritable Bowel Syndrome

Irritable bowel disease or syndrome (IBS) is a condition involving chronic abdominal pain and altered bowel habits in the absence of a defined pathology of the GI tract [16]. It is a functional bowel disorder characterized by alternating bouts of constipation and diarrhea, painful defecation, and increased levels of inflammatory cytokines [17]. This condition, highly prevalent in the US population with estimates now at 10–20 %, is more common in young adult or middle-aged females. An early epidemiologic study by Whitehead et al. [18] examined a number of comorbid conditions among IBS patients and noted an increased incidence of osteoporosis among IBS subjects relative to control subjects.

Using the National Emergency Department Sample (NEDS) database, which is comprised of emergency room visit data from 20 % of the hospitals in the United States, Stobaugh et al. [19] found that of 317,857 visits, 752 or 5.6 % carried a simultaneous diagnosis of osteoporosis, with 0.6 % also having a diagnosis of either a pathologic or traumatic fracture of spine or extremities. The odds ratio (OR) was 4.28 for a concurrent diagnosis of osteoporosis and 2.36 for diagnosis of an osteoporosis-related fracture. The authors carefully controlled for common comorbidities that would lead to false elevations in prevalence, including family history of osteoporosis, vitamin D deficiency, various forms of cancer, renal disease, thyroid disease, and eating disorders.

Authors compared prevalence of osteoporosis and osteoporosis-related fractures in IBS with Crohn's disease, ulcerative colitis, and celiac disease. The OR for fractures was greater for IBS than either Crohn's (1.98) or UC (1.72) but was not as high as that of celiac disease (OR of 3.21). The increased risk of osteoporosis in IBS is unclear, but several experts believe it may be linked to elevated levels of serotonin found among IBS patients [20]. In addition, the elevated serotonin levels are associated with heightened states of IBS and its ongoing pathogenesis [21]. Additional causes of osteoporosis may be related to a reduced intake of milk and other calcium products since patients with IBS frequently report intolerance to such food sources [19]. Studies on treatment for bone disease in IBS are lacking. Of note, steroids can decrease the intensity of bouts of IBS, but their use may have adverse effects on bone if prescribed for over three months [16].

Treatment for Inflammatory Malabsorptive Disorders (IBD and IBS)

Pharmacologic Interventions

The strategies for pharmacologic intervention involve a reduction in medications causing bone loss and an initiation of those that build or maintain bone. Corticosteroids and immunomodulating agents have been significant factors in furthering bone loss in IBD and related conditions. If an individual's inflammatory level permits, reducing corticosteroids in the form of prednisone or methylprednisolone should be considered. Frequently, this is not possible. Vestergaard et al. [22] found that doses as small as 6.7 mg daily increase fracture risk in a dose-dependent manner. However, other steroids, specifically hydrocortisone and oral budesonide, did not increase overall fracture risk. Several years prior to the Vestergaard study, a similarly favorable outcome on preservation of bone mass was published by Schoon et al. [23]. Even though a 3.35 % loss of BMD for the group treated with methylprednisolone seems unsubstantial compared with budesonide loss of 0.9 %, the findings are significant ($p=0.002$). For a follow-up time of six months, a 3.35 % bone loss is concerning.

Azathioprine-treated patients as well as those with anti TNF-α therapy may experience benefits in terms of maintaining or increasing BMD [4]. The theory behind treatment with an agent directed against TNF-α is based on the upregulation of osteoclastic function by cytokines including TNF. Reducing the inflammation component of IBD would help maintain bone but may not actually increase BMD. However, one retrospective study of subjects, conducted at an outpatient Crohn's disease clinic, examined the use of infliximab with simultaneous use of alendronate or risedronate and compared BMD findings to those with infliximab alone. This investigation revealed improved overall BMD with a combination of infliximab and bisphosphonate relative to infliximab alone. However, the use of infliximab alone did result in a preservation of existing BMD but not an increase in density [24].

The British Society of Gastroenterology (BSG) advises that all patients over age 65 with IBD receive bisphosphonates at the start of steroid treatment [25]. The FDA has approved bisphosphonates for patients with known osteoporosis, history of traumatic fractures, or use of steroids for more than three months due to a high risk of developing osteoporosis. Because bisphosphonates are not without their own set of side effects, particularly in the elderly, the BSG advises obtaining a DXA before starting a patient on a bisphosphonate and deferring start of medication unless the DXA has a *T*-score of <1.5.

In terms of clinical trials focused on subjects with IBD, one double-blind trial involving 61 patients, each of whom received either 12 months of 5 mg risedronate plus 600 mg calcium or placebo and calcium, yielded a 2.0 % increase in BMD in the spine and 1.9 % at the hip for those on risedronate [26]. Favorable

BMD outcomes at one, two, and three years at the spine, trochanter, and femoral neck were seen in a second study of risedronate [27]. Studies on the benefits of alendronate, ibandronate, and zoledronic acid have also been conducted [28]. A meta-analysis of five large clinical trials involving 423 participants found that, as a class of drugs, bisphosphonates improved hip BMD but not spine BMD at 12 months. No differences between subjects receiving bisphosphonates and those taking placebo were found at 24 months for either spine or hip BMD, and no differences were found for rates of new vertebral fractures or incidence of side effects. Nevertheless, individual trials have found some positive trends for BMD outcomes for focused groups of patients.

A small trial of 32 subjects using low-dose alendronate 10 mg daily was published by Haderslav et al. in 2000, prior to the widespread acceptance of IV bisphosphonates for management of chronic osteoporosis. Authors found a 4.6 % increase in lumbar spine BMD among patients who received alendronate in comparison to a 0.9 % decline in control subjects [29]. The study was not powered sufficiently to detect a fracture rate difference, and with a follow-up time of only 12 months, large differences would be unlikely. No significant differences in GI adverse effects were seen. Since a weekly dosage of alendronate at 70 mg has become available, dosages of 10 mg daily have gone out of favor due to patient choice and low compliance. However, symptoms of GI burning, pain, and nausea, to which patients with Crohn's disease are predisposed, are less likely to occur with a 10 mg tablet as opposed to a 70 mg tablet.

Other investigations of subjects with postmenopausal osteoporosis have suggested that compliance with oral regimens is limited by GI intolerance and lifestyle inconveniences [30]. A recent soluble formulation of alendronate may be better tolerated in persons prone to GI symptoms. Coaccioli et al. [31] found that after one year of use of a 70 mg soluble weekly alendronate, 92.4 % of subjects were still taking the soluble form, but only 65.4 % of those using the tablets were still adhering to their medication. No subjects after three months and only 5 % after six months had chosen to discontinue treatment with soluble alendronate in comparison to 5 % at three months and 23 % at six months for those using traditional oral alendronate, risedronate, or ibandronate tablets.

Siffledeen and colleagues explored the use of etidronate 400 mg on BMD in patients with Crohn's disease [32]. All subjects received daily calcium of 500 mg and vitamin D3 of 400 IU but only half received etidronate, with the remaining 50 % receiving placebo. Based on BMD outcomes at both 12 and 24 months, both groups demonstrated improved BMD values of similar degrees. No benefit was realized by the addition of etidronate to calcium and vitamin D.

Bartram et al. conducted the first clinical trial examining the effects of an IV bisphosphonate in patients with Crohn's disease. The group receiving both calcium and IV pamidronate increased BMD significantly more than the subjects receiving calcium alone [33]. Their comparison of IV ibandronate versus sodium fluoride on 66 patients with Crohn's disease showed both groups had improved BMD at the spine but not the femur [34].

Nonpharmacologic Interventions

Individually tailored rehab programs should be initiated for patients with IBD and other malabsorptive disorders including celiac disease and conditions involving ileal dysfunction, due to malnutrition and potentially to proprioceptive and sensory deficits involving low levels of key vitamins. Those with critically low levels of pyridoxine (vitamin B6) may experience proprioceptive deficits. In addition individual case reports of neuropathic sensory changes in the form of absent or impaired light touch, vibration, and pinprick have been reported for patients who have undergone gastric bypass and have experienced critically low vitamin D levels as a result [35]. In the case described by Guanche and Oleson, the patient experienced no clinical symptoms for several months after surgery. Rather, symptoms appeared at the end of winter when vitamin D levels are typically at their nadir and followed a gastrointestinal virus involving intractable nausea and vomiting. Therapists need to focus not only on strengthening management and fall prevention but also on compensatory techniques for patients who lack sensory feedback. These patients must learn to rely on vision or other means of adaptation to compensate for sensory proprioceptive deficits.

Bariatric Surgery and Related Procedures

Patients who have undergone gastric bypass or partial small bowel resection for cancers, volvulus, or ischemia are at increased risk of osteoporosis. Any area that is resected or dysfunctional and involves the proximal small bowel will necessarily compromise the absorption of vitamin D and other key nutrients [11]. Postgastrectomy is a general term that would describe any resection of the GI tract, but specific portions that are resected or circumvented are more harmful than others in terms of malabsorption states. Resection may occur for a deliberate purpose such as weight loss through one of several types of bariatric surgery. Alternatively, resection of a portion of the GI tract may be performed to remove a mass with the purpose of debulking a malignant tumor, thereby limiting further metastases or preventing obstruction. In this chapter, we will focus on resections for the purpose of weight loss, since oncologic resections have considerable variation and individual patient responses are unique.

Surgical Options and Definitions

In 2011, over 340,000 bariatric surgeries were performed worldwide. Currently, these procedures are indicated for those with a BMI greater than 40 without obesity-related health issues or greater than 35 with specific obesity-related health

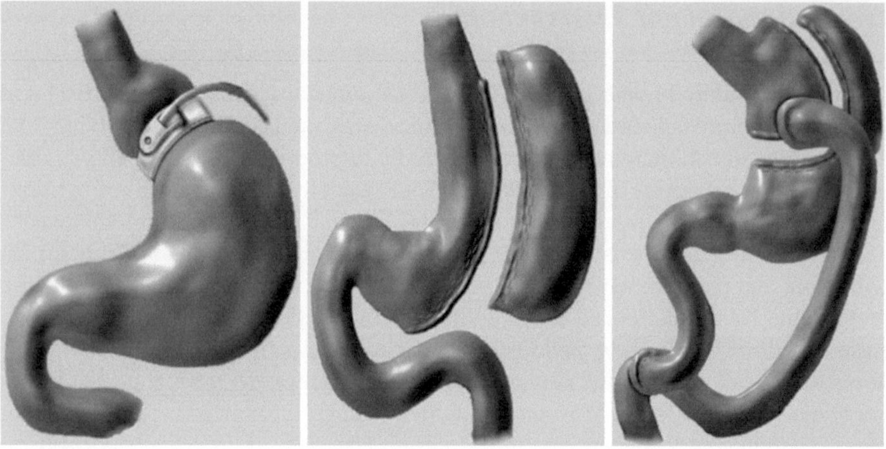

Fig. 1 A comparison of laparoscopic adjustable gastric banding (LAGB), sleeve gastrectomy (SG), Roux-en-Y gastric bypass (RYGB). From *left* to *right*: LAGB, SG, and RYGB (*Source*: Smith et al. [41]. Reprinted with permission)

conditions of diabetes mellitus, hypertension, and obstructive sleep apnea [36]. Several common procedures have been used to generate weight loss. They can be divided into those that induce weight loss by mechanical restriction of food passage through the digestive tract and those that induce more substantial weight loss through malabsorption in combination with some elements of restriction. There are also newer theories concerning neurohormonal pathways that appear to contribute to weight loss [37]. The laparoscopic adjustable gastric band (LAGB) and Roux-en-Y gastric bypass (RYGB) were the most common procedures undertaken in 2008, but by 2011, the number of patients undergoing RYGB had declined, and a less aggressive procedure known as the sleeve gastrectomy (SG) had increased [38, 39]. Numbers issued by the American Society for Metabolic and Bariatric Surgery in 2014 indicate that of the 179,000 surgeries performed the previous year, 34.2 % were RYGB as opposed to 37.5 % in 2012, while SG surgeries increased from 33 % in 2012 to 42.1 % in 2013 [40]. (The specifics of each procedure are illustrated in Fig. 1 [41].)

Restrictive Bariatric Procedures

The LAGB constricts the initial portion of the stomach, slowing down the transit of food and thereby inducing a feeling of early satiety [37]. In this fully reversible procedure, a saline-filled band is inserted around the proximal stomach and reduces the stomach cavity to 10–20 ml [42]. While the LAGB can result in 30–50 % excess body weight reduction, proximal slippage of the band necessitates revision surgery within 5–7 years of the initial operation for 25–50 % of patients. This complication, in combination with recently developed, equally effective alternatives, has made LAGB a less popular option in recent years [43, 44].

A newer surgical option known as the gastric sleeve or sleeve gastrectomy (GS) involves resection of a large section of the lateral stomach, with the remainder stapled shut. The mechanism of weight loss is primarily through reduction of gastric capacity to approximately 120 ml [45] and decreased appetite. Weight loss is gradual over 12–18 months, and significant nutrient malabsorption does not occur because there is no involvement of the small intestine. Appetite attenuation is closely related to the elimination of a portion of the abdomen responsible for the secretion of ghrelin, an anti-satiety hormone which signals the desire to continue eating.

Although initially developed as the first stage of the combined restrictive and malabsorption procedure, SG alone has successfully resulted in a 55–60 % weight loss in some studies and is now offered as a primary procedure [46]. The elimination of ghrelin and other neurohormones including glucagon-like peptide-1 may contribute to the success of GS through continued dietary compliance of patients. One benefit of all restrictive bariatric surgeries is the sparing of the proximal small bowel where many essential vitamins and nutrients are absorbed [47]. The absence of this portion of the small intestine may lead to osteoporosis in part because of lack of vitamin D. Despite the above benefits, postoperative development of gastric reflux or exacerbation of preexisting reflux after SG can be as high as 40 %. Many patients require a surgical solution to the reflux because medications, including proton pump inhibitors, are helpful yet insufficient to overcome the functional problem created by the surgery [48].

Malabsorptive Bariatric Surgeries

In contrast to the adjustable gastric band and GS interventions, the RYGB and duodenal switch circumvent moderate to large portions of the small intestine. Weight loss occurs by redirecting digested food from the stomach to distal gut, bypassing proximal portions of the small intestine that function in key nutrient absorption. Both procedures result in a "common channel" that is shared by both digested food and pancreatic enzymes; their combined action is required for nutrient absorption. The pancreatic enzymes travel through an independent pathway and link up with the food channel further along the path. Not until they come together in the common channel is any food (particularly protein) absorbed [37]. The shorter the channel, the greater the likelihood of insufficient absorption, especially if the length is less than 120 cm from the start of the channel to the ileocecal valve [47]. Certain procedures carry a higher risk of side effects than others. A summary of the complications with the three most common types of procedures is given in Table 1 [49].

RYGB is synonymous with the term "gastric bypass" and results in as much as a 65 % excess body weight loss. The sleeve gastrectomy–duodenal switch combined procedure offers the greatest loss, up to 80 % of excess body weight. This is a modification of earlier versions of the biliopancreatic diversion [50–53]. Even in revised form, patients can become severely malnourished, particularly in vitamin

Table 1 Complications associated with bariatric surgery procedures

Procedure	Complications
Laparoscopic Roux-en-Y gastric bypass	Leaks
	Anastomotic narrowing and strictures
	Marginal ulcers
	Jejunal ischemia
	Small bowel obstruction
	Internal hernias
	Intussusception
	Recurrent weight gain
	Gastrogastric fistula
Laparoscopic adjustable gastric banding	Stomal stenosis
	Malpositioned band
	Pouch dilation
	Distal band slippage
	Perforation
	Gastric volvulus
	Intraluminal band erosion
	Port-related and band-related complications
Laparoscopic sleeve gastrectomy	Gastric leaks
	Gastric strictures and gastric outlet obstruction
	Gastric dilation
	Gastroesophageal reflux

Source: Levine and Carucci [49]

B12 levels, and must be closely followed with blood tests of fat- and water-soluble vitamins and trace elements like zinc and copper [54].

Many considerations go into the decision for surgery. The desired amount of weight to be lost for medical reasons, the risks of a given procedure to the individual patient, and the patient's prior history with weight loss attempts must all be carefully balanced. The patient's own commitment to preparing for the surgery medically and psychologically and their commitment to follow-up care and ongoing nutrition are as important if not more important than the actual surgical procedure chosen. Table 2 describes important selection criteria [55].

Nutritional Deficiencies After Surgery

Malabsorption arises in both macro- and micronutrients following bariatric surgeries. Deficits in many of the key nutrients serving to support bone structures serve as major contributing factors to the development of postsurgical osteoporosis [47]. The major macronutrient affected is protein. When reduced length of the small intestine results in inadequate time for pancreatic enzymes to act on ingested dietary protein, insufficient protein absorption occurs. Anemia and hypoalbuminemia are observed

Table 2 Selection criteria for bariatric surgery

Factor	Criteria
Weight: adults	Body mass index ≥35 kg/m² and obesity-associated comorbidity
	Body mass index ≥40 kg/m²
Weight: children	Severe comorbidity and >95th percentile of weight for age
Weight loss history	Failed attempts of nonsurgical weight loss, including profit-making commercial programs
Commitment	Expectation that patient will adhere to postoperative care including follow-up visits, recommended medical management, and recommended tests or procedures
Exclusion	Current drug or alcohol abuse
	Severe, uncontrolled psychiatric illness
	Reversible endocrine disorders that may lead to obesity
	Inability to comprehend bariatric surgery details (benefits, risks, expected outcomes, alternatives, lifestyle changes, etc.)

Source: Mechanick et al. [55]

in gastric bypass and duodenal switch [47]. Generalized edema that leads to mobility deficits and severe muscle wasting may require physical therapy, in addition to nutritional correction measures such as liquid protein supplementation, to aid functional recovery. As muscle wasting progresses, patients shift stress from their muscles to their bones for ambulation and transfers. In addition, profoundly weak proximal muscles may make activities such as sit to stand transfers more challenging and an increased fall rate is predictable. If BMD is low, falls and altered stress on bones during weight-bearing activities may lead to fractures.

Micronutrients include water-soluble B and C vitamins; fat-soluble vitamins A, D, E, and K; and trace minerals such as copper and zinc. Another key mineral of concern is calcium. In assessing risk of developing bone disease, any nutrient that results in weakness, alters proprioception, causes myalgias, compromises awareness, or results in functional deficits that increase fall risk or reduce mobility warrants discussion. Vitamin B12 deficiency occurs in patients who have undergone procedures that bypass the lower stomach [37] with findings indicating inadequate B12 in 40% of patients after the first year following traditional RYGB [56, 57]. Vitamin B12 deficiency results in pernicious anemia, affecting both the dorsal tracts of the spinal cord responsible for proprioception and vibration as well as the corticospinal tracts responsible for motor function. A severe form of Vitamin B12 deficiency compromises safety in cases of weight-bearing, ambulation, and transfers, leading to self-care deficits and an increased risk of falls.

Vitamin B1 (thiamine) deficiency arises from bypass of the jejunum where absorption occurs or from recurrent emesis, caused by reduced gastric size or stomal stenosis. Loss of thiamine can present after either gastric banding or gastric bypass [36]. Seen in 49% of patients after RYGB [58], thiamine deficiency induces Wernicke's encephalopathy involving nystagmus, ophthalmoplegia, confusion, and ataxia [59]. Polyneuropathy has been reported after gastric bypass [59–61]. Nakamura et al. [60] emphasize that a single dose of supplemental thiamine may correct a lab reading for serum levels of vitamin B1, but if neurological deficits have occurred because the patient has gone untreated in previous months, functional deficits in the form of ataxia and gait dysfunction will remain. Electrodiagnostic studies often confirm a distal axonal sensory polyneuropathy and support the need for physical therapy to educate patients in compensatory measures that improve safety during ambulation and prevent falls [60].

Both calcium and vitamin D are absorbed from portions of the gastrointestinal tract that are bypassed in RYGB and similar malabsorptive bariatric procedures. Due to vitamin D malabsorption, calcium metabolism is compromised through a physiologic mechanism apart from the absence of absorption from the missing region of gastrointestinal tissue. A hypocalcemic state ensues and secondary hyperparathyroidism follows [47]. After gastric bypass, calcium deficiency is seen in 10–25 % of patients after one year and 25–48 % after two years. Vitamin D deficiency one year after a malabsorptive surgery ranges from 17 % to 52 % and becomes significantly worse as years pass unless treatment is initiated. In a series of investigations by Brolin, vitamin D deficiency was seen in 50 % of patients five years after surgery if they had a short common channel 75 cm from the ileocecal valve [56]. Although aggressive supplementation will be helpful in preventing further metabolic disease, this alone may be insufficient in patients with malabsorptive procedures, and dosages of 50,000 IU ergocalciferol weekly may be needed.

Although vitamin D and calcium deficiency are far more common after malabsorptive procedures than after restrictive GI surgeries, deficits in both bone density and individual nutrient deficiencies may occur nonetheless. A study of 73 adolescent patients found that four subjects (5.5 %) had vitamin D deficiency. Restrictive food intake may play a role, but because this study involved teenagers, dietary compliance may be challenging, although physician follow-up in this study was 90 %, far exceeding statistics in most adult bariatric follow-up clinics. Aarts et al. found that in a study of 60 patients who were consuming a daily multivitamin containing 400 IU vitamin D, 39 % were deficient following SG procedures [62]. In this same study, 5 % of patients had vitamin B12 deficiency and 15 % had folic acid deficiency, but what is more remarkable are the chronically *elevated* levels of vitamin A, B1, and B6. Findings highlight the need for comprehensive and frequent postoperative metabolic monitoring coupled with a more aggressive nutritional approach, similar to that offered to restrictive surgery patients. A simple multivitamin is far from adequate and may have an inappropriate mixture of too little vitamin D and too much vitamin A or B6. Table 3 gives suggestive preoperative nutritional assessment measures which should be reviewed with each patient prior to planning surgery [63].

Epidemiology of Osteoporosis After Bariatric Surgery

Scibora et al. [37] have conducted comprehensive reviews of retrospective and prospective studies of osteoporosis and bone density changes related to bariatric surgeries. Because bone loss is a well-established outcome of gastrectomy for

Table 3 Suggested preoperative nutrition assessment

General	Specific
Weight history	Recent weight loss attempts
	Weight gain and loss trends
	Personal weight loss goals
Medical history	Comorbidities
	Medications and supplements
	Food allergies and intolerances
	Body fat distribution
	Available lab values
	Dentition problems
	Eyesight problems
Psychiatric history	Eating disorder history
	Psychiatric diagnoses
	Alcohol, tobacco, drug use
Nutrition and food	Food, mood, and activity log
	Eating patterns
	Restaurant meal intake
	Food cravings
	Cultural and religious dietary considerations
Physical activity	Current activity level
	Physical conditions that limit activity
	Previous enjoyment of physical activities
	Time spent sedentary daily
Psychosocial	Confidence in ability to maintain weight loss
	Support system, family dynamics
	Motivations and reasons for wanting surgery
	Willingness to comply with protocol
	Emotional connection with food
	Stress level and coping mechanisms
Education	Literacy level
	Language barrier

Source: Allied Health Sciences Section Ad Hoc Nutrition Committee, Aills L et al. [63]

non-weight loss purposes, clinicians have long been aware of the risk of osteoporosis following bariatric surgeries [64]. Data from cross-sectional and retrospective studies of BMD in the hip, radius, and lumbar spine have been difficult to interpret due to a number of confounding issues. Obese patients typically have higher BMD than normal weight controls due to the presence of estrogen content in fat cells; thus, comparing postoperative yet still overweight gastric bypass patients to normal weight controls may present challenges. Moreover, many of the cross-sectional studies were unable to separate pre- and postmenopausal women, resulting in a heterogeneous population and compromising any conclusions for specific groups.

Prospective studies examining changes in BMD within the same individual at preoperative and postoperative time points have proven to be more valuable. Overall these investigations support decreases in BMD following malabsorptive as opposed to restrictive surgeries, with the greatest reduction seen in BMD at the hip relative to the lumbar spine or radius [37]. After restrictive surgeries in which the weight loss is less than that achieved from malabsorptive procedures, bone loss at the hip is found to vary by site and is inconsistent among studies. The femoral neck BMD declined by approximately 2.3 % one year after LAGB in a study of premenopausal women [65]. In restrictive procedures where weight loss is accomplished through constriction-forced dieting due to limited abdominal size, weight loss and bone loss continue into the second and subsequent years after surgery. A two-year study demonstrated that femoral neck BMD declined 3.5 % [65, 66]. Although vertical gastric banding is a restrictive procedure done far less frequently today, studies did find that it results in greater bone loss at the proximal hip of 10–14 % [65]. Patients now have other options which may be more favorable from a number of medical perspectives. Bone turnover markers were elevated following SG in one small-scale investigation of 15 patients indicating ongoing effects of bone loss [67].

Greater bone loss is consistently observed with malabsorptive procedures. A number of reports estimate that total bone loss at the femoral neck following either RYGB or the more aggressive biliopancreatic diversion (also now rarely performed) ranges from 9–10.9 % at the femoral neck and 8–10.5 % at the total hip. Postoperative care in the majority of bariatric surgical centers includes vitamin supplementation with vitamin D. But teams caring for patients in a postoperative setting lack a standard protocol, and the amounts that each patient receives vary by institution. In the setting of 800 IU vitamin D3 and 1200 mg daily calcium supplementation [68], femoral neck BMD one year after surgery declined by 10.9 %; in another investigation with even greater supplementation of vitamin D and calcium, BMD of the femoral neck declined by 9.2 % while the total hip saw an 8 % decrease. Since most of the weight loss occurs in the first year following RYGB, findings of stability of BMD in the second and third years following surgery are conceivable [65].

Fleischer et al. [69] assert that the degree of bone loss following restrictive procedures parallels the degree of weight loss. Their prospective study of 23 patients one year following RYGB demonstrates bone loss at the total hip of 8 % and at the femoral neck of 9.2 %. In addition, elevated markers of bone loss in the form of N-telopeptide confirm an active bone loss process. This finding is further supported by a simultaneous increase in PTH and a reduction of urinary calcium, even in patients who increased calcium and vitamin D intake postoperatively to 2400 mg and 1600 IU, respectively. This study is only one of a number of investigations [70, 71] demonstrating increases in markers of bone loss and of PTH. Bruno et al. [70] did show that supplementing patients with 1200 IU vitamin D, more than the Fleisher investigation that prescribed 600 IU for subjects under 50 and 800 IU for those over age 50, prevented development of postoperative vitamin D deficiency. However, even 1200 IU was insufficient to prevent elevation of bone turnover markers.

Bone loss in the lumbar spine is again seen more commonly in patients undergoing malabsorptive rather than restrictive bariatric procedures. After LAGB surgery, one study [66] showed a 3.5 % and 1.6 % increase in BMD, respectively. Several other investigations [72–74] demonstrated either no change or a small increase that was not statistically significant. In SG, Hsin et al. [74] found no change in lumbar spine BMD between L1 and L4 after one year. In contrast, RYGB and similar malabsorptive procedures result in a reduction of lumbar BMD by 3.6–8 % in premenopausal patients, even in those who are supplemented proactively with calcium and vitamin D, the amounts of which vary by study [37, 68, 75]. More aggressive supplementation is unable to help preserve BMD in more aggressive malabsorptive procedures. Tsiftsis et al. [75] noted a 7–8 % decline in lumbar BMD after biliopancreatic diversion in 26 premenopausal women who were given 2 g of calcium daily. This group was also supplemented with vitamin D.

Quite often, bone loss and fractures can occur in nontraditional osteoporotic sites following bariatric surgery, but many of the fractures are not observed until years after surgery. In a large prospective study of 258 subjects, representing 2286 person-years, 79 individuals experienced 132 fractures. Conducted between 1989 and 2004, this investigation has one of the longest follow-up periods of published works to date. In total, 56 % of subjects experienced only one fracture, while 26.5 % reported two or more fractures. The cumulative incidence of fracture after 15 years was 58 %, with the most common mechanism of injury being a fall. However, many fractures occurred in nontraditional osteoporotic sites: 22 % in the feet or toes, 7.6 % in the ribs, and 15 % in hands or fingers [76].

Treatment for Bariatric Surgery Patients

Pharmacologic Interventions

Nutrition Supplementation

The Endocrine Society has developed specific recommendations for treatment of deficiencies anticipated after bariatric surgery, especially after malabsorption procedures, with the expectation of preventing major instances of malnutrition if supplementation is done at the beginning of postoperative care. These recommendations include taking two multivitamin tablets daily, preferably separated in time, as well as consuming 1200–2000 mg of elemental calcium and at least 1000 IU of cholecalciferol (Vitamin D3), if the individual is replete in vitamin D25OH at the time of surgery. Those with greater deficiencies would understandably need higher doses of vitamin D3 or a 50,000 IU capsule of vitamin D2 (ergocalciferol) [36]. These clinical practice guidelines further advise that if aggressive supplementation of nutrients is attempted and fails, revision surgery may be needed to avert severe malnutrition [36].

As illustrated in the prior section, supplementation with various nutrients is helpful but not sufficient in the more aggressive forms of bariatric surgery, particularly in malabsorptive procedures but also in some restrictive procedures such as SG involving the rapid and substantial loss of ghrelin. Gjessing et al. [77] found substantially elevated PTH levels and hypocalcemia one year after SG. The resultant malabsorption of calcium, in conjunction with ongoing hyperparathyroidism, contributes to osteoporosis. Through the above mechanism, supplementation with additional calcium and vitamin D appears unlikely to help. Reduction in PTH and downregulation of osteoclasts or upregulation of osteoblasts may need to be approached from a different direction. Interestingly, Hsin et al. [74] used the guidelines developed by the AGA in his study, and with the exception of the lumbar spine BMD, many regions of the skeleton nonetheless experienced extensive bone loss following bariatric procedures.

Emerging Concept of Bariatric Osteomalacia

A number of studies looking at postmenopausal osteoporosis rarely find that vitamin D or calcium alone can have a singular impact on the development of osteoporosis. However, the situation is very different for those who have experienced malabsorptive bariatric procedures, with results demonstrating the positive impact of aggressive supplementation with calcium citrate and cholecalciferol. Williams [78] describes a case of one female who originally had low BMD in her radius but after eight months of aggressive supplementation achieved a 55 % improvement of BMD. Following treatment, she experienced no further development of calcium oxalate stones and reported less muscle and bone pain together with better endurancc and strength.

The pattern of bariatric osteomalacia can be so profound that myopathy as well as peripheral neuropathy can develop. A number of case reports describe these events, which can have a devastating effect on a patient's level of independence. Such cases require astonishingly large doses of vitamin D (in one case 1200 IU orally daily plus 400,000 IU intramuscularly every month) to realize improvement in lab values following SG and RYGB [79–81].

Medications

Because oral bisphosphonates carry a high risk of gastrointestinal reflux, these agents are largely contraindicated after bariatric procedures. In fact, reflux is one of the most common adverse effects following SG and a number of malabsorptive procedures. Bisphosphonates and NSAIDs are two classes of drugs that have been specifically reported to worsen symptoms [78]. Intravenous bisphosphonates, subcutaneous denosumab, or other oral medications without side effects of gastric reflux are worth discussing, but few reports examining these alternatives have been published outside of limited case studies. Oral alendronate was used successfully in one small investigation of 13 patients who had undergone one of several types of gastrectomy for gastric cancer, one being RYGB with the others being Billroth I and II and partial as well as total gastrectomy [82]. No reports exist for treatment with intravenous zoledronic acid, but one article does describe two cases of pamidronate used effectively for treating immobilization hypercalcemia in the postoperative period following RYGB [83]. The two subjects described by Alborzi and Leibowitz required direct ICU admission from home following RYGB for dangerously elevated serum calcium levels which were attributed to a combination of inactivity postoperatively, specifically reduced weight-bearing on a skeleton which had been used to carrying significant amounts of weight, and disruption of the calcium homeostatic axis which indirectly elevates osteoclastic activity. In the above cases, pamidronate was found to be safe and effective for hypercalcemia. Although its benefit for osteoporosis prevention has not been investigated, the initial safety data from the above case reports are encouraging.

In addition to considering medications to reduce fracture risk and optimizing nutritional stores, physicians should carefully investigate the long-term consequences of certain common medications given in the postoperative period, many of which can be continued long term. Cholestyramine is often used for diarrhea in patients who have developed a partial short gut syndrome, particularly common after RYGB in patients with a longer Roux limb and relatively shorter common channel. Cholestyramine reduces adverse effects of diarrhea by sequestering bile acids; however, it also reduces calcium absorption resulting in impaired vitamin D absorption and osteomalacia [78]. Because cholestyramine can cause bowel obstruction over time, many clinicians do not prescribe it for long-term use; however, evidence suggests that bone complications are avoided in persons using the medication simply for temporary relief of diarrhea.

Nonpharmacologic Treatment

As the findings of Alborzi and Leibowitz [83] illustrate, early mobilization following bariatric procedures is essential not only from the standpoint of conditioning but to prevent adverse postoperative complications of hypercalcemia, urinary calcium wasting, potential kidney stones, and ultimately osteoporosis. Even if some of the postoperative activity involves movement with reduced lower extremity weight-bearing such as pedaling a stationary bike, calcium exodus from the bones may be partially curtailed. The most important goal is to get patients up and moving through their daily routine, while incorporating exercise into that routine. Nakamura's long-term follow-up study [76] further demonstrates that exercise in the perioperative period is protective against fractures long term, particularly if weight-bearing exercise is maintained in the years following surgery. Activities such as walking, light aerobics, and treadmill may be a safe place to begin. A physical therapist or athletic trainer well educated in the precautions needed following bariatric surgery should be an essential participant in the rehabilitation plan.

Thiamine deficiency results in neuropsychiatric challenges including hallucinations if severe, confusion, and ataxia, ultimately making gait unsafe [47]. Speech therapists focus on attention and concentration, especially in busy or loud environments when patients become easily distracted or their attention is divided. Unplanned awakening in the middle of the night may increase confusion and can predispose patients to falls. Such events have resulted in a variety of injuries, including fracture to hips, spine, and forearms. Therapists focus on family education for those at home, while low beds, seizure pads on the floor, additional side rails to prevent climbing out without assistance, and bed alarms are used in the inpatient setting. In cardiac abnormalities including bradycardia and tachycardia, endurance can be altered through progressive muscle strengthening and activities that increase oxygen demand, especially stair climbing. Progressive strengthening and close attention to cardiac parameters are needed in initial therapy sessions. Numbness and weakness are other physical manifestations of both thiamine and pyridoxine deficiency. Vestibular training can help with both conditions.

Mononeuropathy, polyneuropathy, and radiculopathy have all been reported after various forms of bariatric surgery [84]. For patients who have experienced bariatric osteomalacia with adverse consequences of neuropathy or myopathy, case reports highlight the need for a comprehensive physical and occupational therapy program to correct functional deficits in the months immediately following surgery. Outcomes for these patients vary, with some improving fully and others partially. All reports indicate that recovery involves learning compensatory techniques and improving endurance and strength to address profound proximal muscle weakness, altered sensation, and proprioception. Georgoulas et al. [81] describes a patient with profound myopathy and waddling gait, needing to push off the chair with her hands due to quadriceps and gluteal weakness. In this case, profound vitamin D deficiency was treated with an extended period of intramuscular ergocalciferol and oral cholecalciferol. Moderate recovery in muscle strength was observed but not until months later, and laboratory studies indicated that alkaline phosphatase and serum phosphate did remain mildly elevated through vitamin supplementation.

In the case with osteomalacia illustrated by Panda [79], functional improvement was significant, but it remained unclear when initial electrodiagnostic findings might resolve. In his patient, evidence of acute denervation in the form of positive sharp waves and fibrillations was seen in the vastus lateralis, while high-amplitude, long-duration motor unit action potentials with decreased recruitment in proximal and distal muscles were found in bilateral lower extremities. From the initial EMG report, diagnosis was clear but prognosis was not straightforward and limited similar case reports are available to guide clinicians. Patients with neuropathy due to severe malnutrition and vitamin deficiencies progress in a manner different from those with traumatic or metabolic causes of denervation. In this instance, every patient is unique due to the amount of weight loss, the particular details of the surgery even among those with the same procedure, the physical condition of the patient preoperatively, and their nutritional reserve. It remains unclear if a comprehensive physical therapy program, combined with aggressive nutritional repletion, will translate to full functional recovery and, if so, how long that process will take. This remains a major challenge for the rehabilitation physician attempting to provide guidance to patients and caregivers of those experiencing functional deficits after surgery.

Final Thoughts

For patients with inflammatory conditions of malabsorption including Crohn's disease and ulcerative colitis, management of the primary condition seems to be the key to success. The less the inflammation, the lower the upregulation of cytokines and other secondary compounds that leach calcium from bone. When such efforts fail, medications to treat osteoporosis can be utilized along with a comprehensive nutritional plan that addresses current deficiencies and emphasizes long-term prevention.

For those who have undergone bariatric surgery, careful presurgical screening should be carried out, including examination of levels of serum calcium, vitamin D 25OH, and PTH. Unfortunately, DXA scans often cannot be done preoperatively due to the usual 300 lb weight capacity of DXA scanners but, if possible, should be obtained before and within six months of surgery. Pre- and postoperative laboratory values should also be followed in the pre- and postoperative period including markers of bone formation, bone loss, PTH, and serum vitamin D25OH along with calcium. Deficits seen prior to surgery including low vitamin D should be addressed at that time.

Secondly, nutritional support with macro- and micronutrients is needed from the very start of the postoperative period and cannot end at a 1-year surgical follow-up. These patients need a lifetime plan. The same bone markers and electrolytes evaluated prior to surgery should be followed postoperatively, with the addition of alkaline phosphatase and serum phosphate to ensure that osteomalacia is not developing. The importance of initiating a comprehensive physical activity program preoperatively and a more intensive program after surgery cannot be underestimated. Prevention of immobilization hypercalcemia and functional mobility deficits is essential. Finally, an entire team of medical providers is needed from the planning stage of bariatric surgery, through the peri- and postoperative time, and for selected providers, throughout the life of the patient. Essential members of this team include the bariatric surgeons, physiatrists, endocrinologists, nutritionists, physical therapists, occupational therapists, and in many cases psychologists. All of these individuals play a critical role in ensuring the long-term health and success of individuals following bariatric surgery.

References

1. Targownik LE, Bernstein CN, Leslie WD. Inflammatory bowel disease and the risk of osteoporosis and fracture. Maturitas. 2013;76(4):315–9. doi:10.1016/j.maturitas.2013.09.009.
2. Wilkins T, Jarvis K, Patel J. Diagnosis and management of Crohn's disease. Am Fam Physician. 2011;84(12):1365–75.
3. Abraham C, Cho JH. Inflammatory bowel disease. N Engl J Med. 2009;361(21):2066–76. doi:10.1056/NEJMra0804647.
4. Ali T, Lam D, Bronze MS, Humphrey MB. Osteoporosis in inflammatory bowel disease. Am J Med. 2009;122(7):599–604. doi:10.1016/j.amjmed.2009.01.022.
5. Manolagas SC. The role of IL-6 type cytokines and their receptors in bone. Ann N Y Acad Sci. 1998;840:194–204.
6. Bernstein CN, Sargent M, Leslie WD. Serum osteoprotegerin is increased in Crohn's disease: a population-based case control study. Inflamm Bowel Dis. 2005;11(4):325–30.
7. Moschen AR, Kaser A, Enrich B, Ludwiczek O, Gabriel M, Obrist P, et al. The RANKL/OPG system is activated in inflammatory bowel disease and relates to the state of bone loss. Gut. 2005;54(4):479–87.
8. van Staa TP, Leufkens HG, Cooper C. The epidemiology of corticosteroid-induced osteoporosis: a meta-analysis. Osteoporos Int. 2002;13(10):777–87.
9. Wada Y, Hisamatsu T, Naganuma M, Matsuoka K, Okamoto S, Inoue N, et al. Risk factors for decreased bone mineral density in inflammatory bowel disease: a cross-sectional study. Clin Nutr. 2015;34(6):1202–9. doi:10.1016/j.cinu.2015.01.003.
10. Vestergaard P. Prevalence and pathogenesis of osteoporosis in patients with inflammatory bowel disease. Minerva Med. 2004;95(6):469–80.
11. American Gastroenterological Association. Medical position statement: guidelines on osteoporosis in gastrointestinal diseases. Gastroenterol. 2003;124(3):791–4.
12. Bernstein CN, Leslie WD, Leboff MS. AGA technical review on osteoporosis in gastrointestinal diseases. Gastroenterology. 2003;124(3):795–841.
13. Watkins J. Structure and function of the musculoskeletal system. 2nd ed. eBook: Human Kinetics; 2010.
14. Laakso S, Valta H, Verkasalo M, Toiviainen-Salo S, Mäkitie O. Compromised peak bone mass in patients with inflammatory bowel disease–a prospective study. J Pediatr. 2014;164(6):1436–43. doi:10.1016/j.jpeds.2014.01.073.
15. Wingate KE, Jacobson K, Issenman R, Carroll M, Barker C, Israel D, et al. 25-Hydroxyvitamin D concentrations in children with Crohn's disease supplemented with either 2000 or 400 IU daily for 6 months: a randomized controlled study. J Pediatr. 2014;164(4):860–5. doi:10.1016/j.jpeds.2013.11.071.
16. Torii A, Toda G. Management of irritable bowel syndrome. Intern Med. 2004;43(5):353–9.
17. Liebregts T, Adam B, Bredack C, Röth A, Heinzel S, Lester S, et al. Immune activation in patients with irritable bowel syndrome. Gastroenterology. 2007;132(3):913–20.
18. Whitehead WE, Palsson OS, Levy RR, Feld AD, Turner M, Von Korff M. Comorbidity in irritable bowel syndrome. Am J Gastroenterol. 2007;102(12):2767–76.
19. Stobaugh DJ, Deepak P, Ehrenpreis ED. Increased risk of osteoporosis-related fractures in patients with irritable bowel syndrome. Osteoporos Int. 2013;24(4):1169–75. doi:10.1007/s00198-012-2141-4.
20. Cremon C, Carini G, Wang B, Vasina V, Cogliandro RF, De Giorgio R, et al. Intestinal serotonin release, sensory neuron activation, and abdominal pain in irritable bowel syndrome. Am J Gastroenterol. 2011;106(7):1290–8. doi:10.1038/ajg.2011.86.
21. Gershon MD, Tack J. The serotonin signaling system: from basic understanding to drug development for functional GI disorders. Gastroenterology. 2007;132(1):397–414.
22. Vestergaard P, Rejnmark L, Mosekilde L. Fracture risk associated with different types of oral corticosteroids and effect of termination of corticosteroids on the risk of fractures. Calcif Tissue Int. 2008;82(4):249–57. doi:10.1007/s00223-008-9124-7.

23. Schoon EJ, Bollani S, Mills PR, Israeli E, Felsenberg D, Ljunghall S, et al. Bone mineral density in relation to efficacy and side effects of budesonide and prednisolone in Crohn's disease. Clin Gastroenterol Hepatol. 2005;3(2):113–21.
24. Pazianas M, Rhim AD, Weinberg AM, Su C, Lichtenstein GR. The effect of anti-TNF-alpha therapy on spinal bone mineral density in patients with Crohn's disease. Ann N Y Acad Sci. 2006;1068:543–56.
25. Lewis NR, Scott BB. Guidelines for osteoporosis in inflammatory bowel disease and coeliac disease. British Society of Gastroenterology. 2007. http://bsg.org.uk.
26. Henderson S, Hoffman N, Prince R. A double-blind placebo-controlled study of the effects of the bisphosphonate risedronate on bone mass in patients with inflammatory bowel disease. Am J Gastroenterol. 2006;101:119–23.
27. Palomba S, Manguso F, Orio Jr F, Russo T, Oppedisano R, Sacchinelli A, et al. Effectiveness of risedronate in osteoporotic postmenopausal women with inflammatory bowel disease: a prospective, parallel, open-label, two-year extension study. Menopause. 2008;15(4 Pt 1):730–6. doi:10.1097/gme.0b013e318159f190.
28. Guo Z, Wu R, Gong J, Zhu W, Li Y, Li N, et al. The efficacy and safety of bisphosphonates for osteoporosis or osteopenia in Crohn's disease: a meta-analysis. Dig Dis Sci. 2013;58(4):915–22. doi:10.1007/s10620-012-2465-0.
29. Haderslev KV, Tjellesen L, Sorensen HA, Staun M. Alendronate increases lumbar spine bone mineral density in patients with Crohn's disease. Gastroenterology. 2000;119(3):639–46.
30. Claxton AJ, Cramer J, Pierce C. A systematic review of the associations between dose regimens and medication compliance. Clin Ther. 2001;23(8):1296–310.
31. Coaccioli S, Celi G, Crapa ME, Masia F, Brandi ML. Alendronate soluble solution: a higher adherence rate in the treatment of osteoporosis. Clin Cases Miner Bone Metab. 2014;11(2):123–5.
32. Siffledeen JS, Fedorak RN, Siminoski K, Jen H, Vaudan E, Abraham N, et al. Randomized trial of etidronate plus calcium and vitamin D for treatment of low bone mineral density in Crohn's disease. Clin Gastroenterol Hepatol. 2005;3(2):122–32.
33. Bartram SA, Peaston RT, Rawlings DJ, Francis RM, Thompson NP. A randomized controlled trial of calcium with vitamin D, alone or in combination with intravenous pamidronate, for the treatment of low bone mineral density associated with Crohn's disease. Aliment Pharmacol Ther. 2003;18(11-12):1121–7.
34. Klaus J, Reinshagen M, Herdt K, Adler G, von Boyen GB, von Tirpitz C. Intravenous ibandronate or sodium-fluoride–a 3.5 years study on bone density and fractures in Crohn's disease patients with osteoporosis. J Gastrointestin Liver Dis. 2011;20(2):141–8.
35. Guanche MM, Oleson CV. Poster 288 Rehabilitation of severe vitamin D deficiency secondary to gastric bypass surgery. PM&R. 2011;3(10):S271. doi:10.1016/j.pmrj.2011.08.315.
36. Heber D, Greenway FL, Kaplan LM, Livingston E, Salvador J, Still C, Endocrine Society. Endocrine and nutritional management of the post-bariatric surgery patient: an Endocrine Society clinical practice guideline. J Clin Endocrinol Metab. 2010;95(11):4823–43. doi:10.1210/jc.2009-2128.
37. Scibora LM, Ikramuddin S, Buchwald H, Petit MA. Examining the link between bariatric surgery, bone loss, and osteoporosis: a review of bone density studies. Obes Surg. 2012;22(4):654–67. doi:10.1007/s11695-012-0596-1.
38. Buchwald H, Oien DM. Metabolic/bariatric surgery worldwide 2008. Obes Surg. 2009;19(12):1605–11. doi:10.1007/s11695-009-0014-5.
39. Buchwald H, Oien DM. Metabolic/bariatric surgery worldwide 2011. Obes Surg. 2013;23(4):427–36. doi:10.1007/s11695-012-0864-0.
40. American Society for Metabolic and Bariatric Surgery. Estimate of bariatric surgery numbers 2014. http://asmbs.org/resources/estimate-of-bariatric-surgery-numbers. Accessed 2015.
41. Smith BR, Schauer P, Nguyen NT. Surgical approaches to the treatment of obesity: bariatric surgery. Endocrinol Metab Clin N Am. 2008;37(4):943–64.
42. Brolin RE. Bariatric surgery and long-term control of morbid obesity. JAMA. 2002;288(22):2793–6.

43. Himpens J, Cadière GB, Bazi M, Vouche M, Cadière B, Dapri G. Long-term outcomes of laparoscopic adjustable gastric banding. Arch Surg. 2011;146(7):802–7. doi:10.1001/archsurg.2011.45.
44. DeMaria EJ, Sugerman HJ, Meador JG, Doty JM, Kellum JM, Wolfe L, et al. High failure rate after laparoscopic adjustable silicone gastric banding for treatment of morbid obesity. Ann Surg. 2001;233(6):809–18.
45. Braghetto I, Korn O, Valladares H, Gutiérrez L, Csendes A, Debandi A, et al. Laparoscopic sleeve gastrectomy: surgical technique, indications and clinical results. Obes Surg. 2007;17(11):1442–50.
46. D'Hondt M, Vanneste S, Pottel H, Devriendt D, Van Rooy F, Vansteenkiste F. Laparoscopic sleeve gastrectomy as a single-stage procedure for the treatment of morbid obesity and the resulting quality of life, resolution of comorbidities, food tolerance, and 6-year weight loss. Surg Endosc. 2011;25(8):2498–504. doi:10.1007/s00464-011-1572-x.
47. Bal BS, Finelli FC, Shope TR, Koch TR. Nutritional deficiencies after bariatric surgery. Nat Rev Endocrinol. 2012;8(9):544–56. doi:10.1038/nrendo.2012.48.
48. Carter PR, LeBlanc KA, Hausmann MG, Kleinpeter KP, de Barros SN, Jones SM. Association between gastroesophageal reflux disease and laparoscopic sleeve gastrectomy. Surg Obes Relat Dis. 2011;7(5):569–72. doi:10.1016/j.soard.2011.01.040.
49. Levine MS, Carucci LR. Imaging of bariatric surgery: normal anatomy and postoperative complications. Radiology. 2014;270(2):327–41.
50. Scopinaro N, Gianetta E, Friedman D. Biliopancreatic diversion for obesity. Probl Gen Surg. 1992;9:362–9.
51. DeMeester TR, Fuchs KH, Ball CS, Albertucci M, Smyrk TC, Marcus JN. Experimental and clinical results with proximal end-to-end duodenojejunostomy for pathologic duodenogastric reflux. Ann Surg. 1987;206(4):414–26.
52. Lagace M, Marceau P, Marceau S, Hould FS, Potvin M, Bourque RA, et al. Biliopancreatic diversion with a new type of gastrectomy: some previous conclusions revisited. Obes Surg. 1995;5(4):411–6.
53. Hess DS, Hess DW. Biliopancreatic diversion with duodenal switch. Obes Surg. 1998;8(3):262–82.
54. Aasheim ET, Björkman S, Søvik TT, Engström M, Hanvold SE, Mala T, et al. Vitamin status after bariatric surgery: a randomized study of gastric bypass and duodenal switch. Am J Clin Nutr. 2009;90(1):15–22. doi:10.3945/ajcn.2009.27583.
55. Mechanick JI, Kushner RF, Sugerman HJ, Gonzalez-Campoy JM, Collazo-Clavel ML, Guven S, et al. Executive summary of the recommendations of the American Association of Clinical Endocrinologists, the Obesity Society, and American Society for Metabolic & Bariatric Surgery medical guidelines for clinical practice for the perioperative nutritional, metabolic, and nonsurgical support of the bariatric surgery patient. Endocr Pract. 2008;14(3):318–36.
56. Brolin RE, LaMarca LB, Kenler HA, Cody RP. Malabsorptive gastric bypass in patients with superobesity. J Gastrointest Surg. 2002;6(2):195–203.
57. Bloomberg RD, Fleishman A, Nalle JE, Herron DM, Kini S. Nutritional deficiencies following bariatric surgery: what have we learned? Obes Surg. 2005;15(2):145–54.
58. Lakhani SV, Shah HN, Alexander K, Finelli FC, Kirkpatrick JR, Koch TR. Small intestinal bacterial overgrowth and thiamine deficiency after Roux-en-Y gastric bypass surgery in obese patients. Nutr Res. 2008;28(5):293–8. doi:10.1016/j.nutres.2008.03.002.
59. Teitleman M, Katzka DA. A case of polyneuropathy after gastric bypass surgery. MedGenMed. 2005;7(2):21.
60. Nakamura K, Roberson ED, Reilly LG, Tsao JW. Polyneuropathy following gastric bypass surgery. Am J Med. 2003;115:679–80.
61. Maryniak O. Severe peripheral neuropathy following gastric bypass surgery for morbid obesity. Can Med Assoc J. 1984;131(2):119–20.

62. Aarts EO, Janssen IM, Berends FJ. The gastric sleeve: losing weight as fast as micronutrients? Obes Surg. 2011;21(2):207–11. doi:10.1007/s11695-010-0316-7.
63. Aills L, Blankenship J, Buffington C, Furtado M, Parrott J. American Society for Metabolic and Bariatric Surgery allied nutritional guidelines for the surgical weight loss patient. Surg Obes Relat Dis. 2008;4(5 Suppl):S73–108. doi:10.1016/j.soard.2008.03.002.
64. Zittel TT, Zeeb B, Maier GW, Kaiser GW, Zwirner M, Liebich H, et al. High prevalence of bone disorders after gastrectomy. Am J Surg. 1997;174(4):431–8.
65. Giusti V, Gasteyger C, Suter M, Heraief E, Gaillard RC, Burckhardt P. Gastric banding induces negative bone remodelling in the absence of secondary hyperparathyroidism: potential role of serum C telopeptides for follow-up. Int J Obes (Lond). 2005;29:1429–35.
66. Cundy T, Evans MC, Kay RG, Dowman M, Wattie D, Reid IR. Effects of vertical-banded gastroplasty on bone and mineral metabolism in obese patients. Br J Surg. 1996;83(10):1468–72.
67. Serra Aracil X, Bombardó Juncá J, Mora López L, Alcantara Moral M, Ayguavives Garnica I, Darnell Marti A, et al. Site of local surgery in adenocarcinoma of the rectum T2N0M0. Cir Esp. 2009;85(2):103–9. doi:10.1016/j.ciresp.2008.09.007.
68. Vilarrasa N, Gómez JM, Elio I, Gómez-Vaquero C, Masdevall C, Pujol J, et al. Evaluation of bone disease in morbidly obese women after gastric bypass and risk factors implicated in bone loss. Obes Surg. 2009;19(7):860–6. doi:10.1007/s11695-009-9843-5.
69. Fleischer J, Stein EM, Bessler M, Della Badia M, Restuccia N, Olivero-Rivera L, et al. The decline in hip bone density after gastric bypass surgery is associated with extent of weight loss. J Clin Endocrinol Metab. 2008;93(10):3735–40. doi:10.1210/jc.2008-0481.
70. Bruno C, Fulford AD, Potts JR, McClintock R, Jones R, Cacucci BM, et al. Serum markers of bone turnover are increased at six and 18 months after Roux-en-Y bariatric surgery: correlation with the reduction in leptin. J Clin Endocrinol Metab. 2010;95(1):159–66. doi:10.1210/jc.2009-0265.
71. Coates PS, Fernstrom JD, Fernstrom MH, Schauer PR, Greenspan SL. Gastric bypass surgery for morbid obesity leads to an increase in bone turnover and a decrease in bone mass. J Clin Endocrinol Metab. 2004;89(3):1061–5.
72. Pugnale N, Giusti V, Suter M, Zysset E, Héraïef E, Gaillard RC, et al. Bone metabolism and risk of secondary hyperparathyroidism 12 months after gastric banding in obese pre-menopausal women. Int J Obes Relat Metab Disord. 2003;27(1):110–6.
73. von Mach MA, Stoeckli R, Bilz S, Kraenzlin M, Langer I, Keller U. Changes in bone mineral content after surgical treatment of morbid obesity. Metabolism. 2004;53(7):918–21.
74. Hsin MC, Huang CK, Tai CM, Yeh LR, Kuo HC, Garg A. A case-matched study of the differences in bone mineral density 1 year after 3 different bariatric procedures. Surg Obes Relat Dis. 2015;11(1):181–5. doi:10.1016/j.soard.2014.07.008.
75. Tsiftsis DD, Mylonas P, Mead N, Kalfarentzos F, Alexandrides TK. Bone mass decreases in morbidly obese women after long limb-biliopancreatic diversion and marked weight loss without secondary hyperparathyroidism. A physiological adaptation to weight loss? Obes Surg. 2009;19(11):1497–503. doi:10.1007/s11695-009-9938-z.
76. Nakamura KM, Haglind EG, Clowes JA, Achenbach SJ, Atkinson EJ, Melton 3rd LJ, et al. Fracture risk following bariatric surgery: a population-based study. Osteoporos Int. 2014;25(1):151–8. doi:10.1007/s00198-013-2463-x.
77. Gjessing HR, Nielsen HJ, Mellgren G, Gudbrandsen OA. Energy intake, nutritional status and weight reduction in patients one year after laparoscopic sleeve gastrectomy. SpringerPlus. 2013;2:352–7.
78. Williams SE. Metabolic bone disease in the bariatric surgery patient. J Obes. 2011;2011:634614. doi:10.1155/2011/634614.
79. Panda S, Sharma K. Osteomalacia induced peripheral neuropathy after obesity reduction surgery. Ann Indian Acad Neurol. 2013;16(4):690–2. doi:10.4103/0972-2327.120466.

80. Irani PF. Electromyography in nutritional osteomalacic myopathy. J Neurol Neurosurg Psychiatry. 1976;39(7):686–93.
81. Georgoulas TI, Tournis S, Lyritis GP. Development of osteomalacic myopathy in a morbidly obese woman following bariatric surgery. J Musculoskelet Neuronal Interact. 2010;10(4): 287–9.
82. Suzuki Y, Ishibashi Y, Omura N, Kawasaki N, Kashiwagi H, Yanaga K, et al. Alendronate improves vitamin D-resistant osteopenia triggered by gastrectomy in patients with gastric cancer followed long term. J Gastrointest Surg. 2005;9(7):955–60.
83. Alborzi F, Leibowitz AB. Immobilization hypercalcemia in critical illness following bariatric surgery. Obes Surg. 2002;12(6):871–3.
84. Thaisetthawatkul P, Collazo-Clavell ML, Sarr MG, Norell JE, Dyck PJ. A controlled study of peripheral neuropathy after bariatric surgery. Neurology. 2004;63(8):1462–70.

Chapter 14
Osteoporosis in Cardiopulmonary, Kidney and Liver Disorders

Christina V. Oleson

Osteoporosis coexists with other chronic diseases to provide what Colon-Emeric et al. [1] termed "multimorbidity" interactions, often leading to significant deterioration in either or both conditions. This chapter focuses on four chronic diseases—cardiovascular and pulmonary conditions as well as kidney and liver disorders. As with osteoporosis, these conditions are associated with aging, even if aging, as in the case of cystic fibrosis, begins as early as adolescence. In each case, either the condition itself or its treatment may lead to new-onset osteoporosis, exacerbate existing osteoporosis, or increase fracture risk even when an individual's BMD would not suggest a risk. For example, low bone mineral bone density and vitamin D deficiency are associated with chronic obstructive pulmonary disease (COPD), while its treatment including prolonged use of oral corticosteroids can induce osteoporosis. In aspects of liver failure, fractures can occur even with moderate declines in BMD, generally not in the range when fractures would otherwise occur. In the diseases selected, we will examine the prevalence of one condition in consort with the other, the impact of the interaction of these conditions, and the drug–disease interactions.

Cardiovascular Conditions

Despite advances in treatment, cardiovascular disease (congestive heart failure, heart attack, coronary artery disease, abnormal heart rhythms, and other heart conditions) and osteoporosis remain the most common health problems in the world, accounting for the largest share of morbidity and mortality in an aging population [2]. Over 20 million persons worldwide suffer from congestive heart failure, and another 75 million carry a diagnosis of osteoporosis [3]. Of those in the United States, two million experience osteoporosis-related fractures annually [4]. Numerous investigations have found a high correlation between the degree of heart failure, its duration in a given patient, and loss of BMD. Moreover, reports have indicated an inverse relationship between heart failure and BMD in the total hip, femoral neck,

C.V. Oleson, *Osteoporosis Rehabilitation*, DOI 10.1007/978-3-319-45084-1_14

and lumbar spine [5]. This section will discuss the epidemiology of the relationship of heart disease to osteoporosis, explore possible mechanisms of association, and offer suggestions for treatment.

Etiology and Pathogenesis of Bone Loss in Cardiac Conditions

Congestive Heart Failure (CHF)

It has long been known that renal and hepatic failure result in altered bone metabolism, but only recently has evidence emerged of a relationship between heart failure and increased bone turnover. In a 2003 study, Nishio et al. explored the rate of bone loss in spinal BMD in patients with CHF, based upon polymorphisms of the vitamin D receptor (VDR) [6]. One particular receptor genotype, FF VDR, was associated with a higher rate of bone loss, leading this group to propose that patients with this genotype may benefit from higher calcium intake to compensate for suboptimal metabolic processing of vitamin D.

Both the pathophysiology and therapy for CHF may adversely alter mineral homeostasis and the balance of calcitropic hormones. Although some studies found such imbalances only after heart transplantation, accumulating evidence suggests the imbalance between bone formation and resorption started in the advanced stage of cardiac failure, not subsequent to the transplant. Shane et al. [7] found that among patients with severe CHF {Class III or IV, left ventricular ejection fraction average 19 % or lower, New York Heart Association (NYHA)} [8], 35 % were deficient in Vitamin D25(OH) with levels less than 16 ng/ml, and 69 % had hyperparathyroidism (PTH levels above 65 picograms/ml). Moreover, bone resorption markers including hydroxyproline, pyridinoline, and deoxypyridinoline were elevated, although both men and women had normal levels of serum osteocalcin, a marker of bone formation. Overall, participants demonstrated osteoporosis rates of 7 % in the lumbar spine, 6 % at the total hip, and 19 % at the femoral neck, while osteopenia was present in 43 % of subjects at the lumbar spine, 47 % at the total hip, and 42 % at the femoral neck. In addition, all were receiving loop diuretics, digoxin, or angiotensin-converting enzyme inhibitors.

Similar outcomes were noted in a study 13 years later by Zotos et al. [9]. Osteoporosis in heart failure is associated with secondary hyperparathyroidism and has adverse prognostic implications [10]. Bone mass loss in chronic heart failure is associated with secondary hyperparathyroidism and has prognostic significance. Compared with healthy subjects, men with CHF had significant reductions in BMD in the total body and total femur, and had evidence of hyperparathyroidism given the presence of elevated PTH values. In addition, all four levels of NYHA classes were included in the study, but changes were more severe in subjects with Class III and IV heart disease. So, is the bone loss observed physiologic, possibly related to oxidative stress and reduced cardiac output; activity based, due to low amounts of exercise; or secondary to medications?

Coronary Artery Disease (CAD) and Valvular Disease

Although age, gender, age-related renal insufficiency, low calcium intake, and vitamin D deficiency are seen in both coronary artery disease and valvular disease, recent research points to additional factors related to heart disease that contribute to bone loss and predispose patients to a formal diagnosis of osteoporosis. Animal studies suggest apolipoprotein E (Apo-E) may play a protective role. Specifically, mice deficient in Apo-E had increased rates of both arterial and aortic valve calcifications—findings that correlated directly with the extent of BMD loss [11]. An earlier study in humans by Aksoy et al. [12] found a relationship between aortic valve calcifications and low BMD but did not suggest Apo-E as a possible mechanism and alluded instead to a possible mechanism involving parathyroid hormone abnormalities in association with aging.

In terms of a relationship between CAD and osteoporosis, both conditions were initially thought to follow an independent, parallel progression. However, evidence from recent studies focused on aging supports a direct relationship between the two. Very early roentgenographic studies indicated an association between calcification of the abdominal aorta and osteoporosis in the lumbar spine [13]; 20 years later, these findings were supported by molecular biology studies demonstrating that arterial calcification was regulated by mechanisms similar to bone formation, rather than by passive precipitation of calcium phosphate [14]. An association with vitamin D deficiency has also been identified. As Stojnovic et al. have observed [2], insufficient vitamin D linked with low BMD increases fracture risk, resulting in secondary hyperparathyroidism, calcification of coronary arteries, and increases in cardiovascular disease. Low BMD of the hip represents a high risk of cardiovascular disease in both men and women, whereas aortic calcification is a strong predictor of low BMD and fragility fractures [15].

Data regarding the association of atherosclerosis and osteoporosis have been confounded by evaluations of varying patient populations with different technologies: earlier studies used lateral spine x-rays; later ones employed electron beam computerized tomography (ECBT), and only a few used both DXA and EBCT [16]. Barengolts and colleagues [17] have suggested that estrogen may play a role in protecting against coronary atherosclerosis as well as osteoporosis and that relative estrogen deficiency may contribute to temporal onset of both conditions. They also found that 31 % of the group with osteopenia and 76 % of participants with osteoporosis had elevated coronary calcium scores, with calcium deposits located primarily in the left anterior descending artery measured by ECBT. These findings highlight reasons to address the presence of CAD in the osteoporotic population and heighten the need for prevention of both disorders.

Until recently, there has been no evidence that the association between osteoporosis and heart failure acts both ways. However, a study by Pfister et al. [18] has found for the first time that lower BMD predicts the development of heart failure after 9.3 years of follow-up, following adjustment for age, sex, cardiovascular risk factors, and sociodemographic status. Although yet to be confirmed, this finding raises such questions as to whether increasing BMD in childhood or young adulthood could reduce subsequent heart failure and whether increased BMD resulting from antiresorptive therapies could affect heart failure risk [19].

The Influence of Medications

As in other conditions involving immobility and compromised circulation, patients with CHF have an increased risk of thromboembolic events. To avoid vascular complications, anticoagulation is often prescribed for many months and potentially a lifetime. The risk of heparin and low molecular weight heparin-induced osteoporosis increases with time, but in the long term, many patients are prescribed either warfarin or newer oral anticoagulants that improve compliance [20]. As described in other chapters, these medications, both oral and subcutaneous, appear to have a lower adverse effect on bone than do traditional heparins. Newer anticoagulants involve no daily monitoring but are difficult to reverse. These agents, also known as direct oral anticoagulants, are more expensive than warfarin and frequently not covered by insurance; if funded by insurance in part, patients are often unable to afford the remaining cost of copayments, specifically in the United States. Traditionally, warfarin has been used, and although it requires monitoring with blood tests, cost remains comparably lower. Data indicates that warfarin is less problematic in terms of preserving skeletal integrity than are other agents [21].

Statins are commonly prescribed as secondary prophylaxis for those with CAD and may be appropriate in patients with CHF as well. Many patients are prescribed statins for a number of years before developing heart failure severe enough to be associated with bone loss. A number of reports have suggested a benefit in terms of BMD improvement or fracture reduction with use of hydroxymethylglutaryl coenzyme A (HMG-CoA) reductase inhibitors, including such popular agents as atorvastatin (Lipitor), lovastatin (Mevacor), rosuvastatin (Crestor), and simvastatin (Zocor). Chang et al. [22] found that statins increased BMD in type 2 diabetes, and Edwards et al. [23] demonstrated that BMD was increased in a larger cross-sectional study of postmenopausal women. The rationale behind the possible benefit of HMG-CoA reductase inhibitors lies in its ability to decrease levels of mevalonate which indirectly enhances osteoblastic differentiation.

At the same time, studies of the relation of statins to bone loss have produced conflicting results. At the turn of the century, several trials [24–29] postulated that use of statins over extended periods of time and with different comorbidities could lead to fracture reduction. Since this group of patients may have impaired sensation, their risk of fractures is, by definition, elevated. However, in 2002, a large prospective 10-year investigation by Sirola et al. found no significant benefit in extended use of statins—not among those with existing hypercholesterolemia nor in those with normal cholesterol levels [30]. No significant difference in BMD of the lumbar spine or femoral neck was identified among those who reported occasional statin use, those who followed the protocol and took statins regularly, and control subjects who did not use statins (some who had high cholesterol and others who had normal blood cholesterol). Subsequent evidence from a Women's Health Initiative Observational Study revealed no statistically significant difference in bone mineral density nor in fracture rates among statin users and nonusers [31]. An analysis of the effect of rosuvastatin, the first randomized control data ($n = 17{,}802$ men and women), confirmed that statin therapy did not reduce fracture risk [32].

Diuretics may have a positive or negative effect on bone balance, depending on the individual agent. Thiazide diuretics such as hydrochlorothiazide and potassium-sparing agents such as spironolactone decrease excretion of renal calcium, thus promoting bone building. In contrast, loop diuretics favor bone resorption, since they assist in renal calcium excretion. Although beta blockers may positively impact bone, the data is again conflicting. A study examining a newer beta blocker, nebivolol, demonstrated that it induces nitrous oxide release, which may be protective in bone preservation and prevention of osteoporosis [5, 33]. While one trial linked beta blockers with increased fracture risk [34], a large cohort study ($n = 39{,}938$) found that beta blockers resulted in a reduced risk of hip fractures, with an attributable effect percentage of negative 3.5 % and a standard incidence rate (SIR) of 0.7 [35].

These findings were in agreement with two recent meta-analyses and one epidemiological investigation. In the meta-analyses, Yang et al. [36] observed a reduction in fracture risk by 17 % (RR 0.83), while Toulis et al. [37] found a reduction of 14 % in women and 20 % in men.

The epidemiological investigation by Rejnmark et al. [38] found that not only beta blockers but also calcium channel blockers and ACE inhibitors are related to a small but significant reduction in fracture risk. Large epidemiological studies have demonstrated the association between calcium channel blockers and reduced fracture risk. While some in vitro investigations suggest that this class of drugs inhibits osteoclastic function, definitive human studies confirming such a mechanism are lacking. In the population-based study by Ruths et al. [35], hip fractures were reduced among subjects using calcium channel blockers with SIR of 0.8, not significantly different from the 7 % reduction in fracture risk found in the Rejnmark et al. [38] investigation.

Although ACE inhibitors appear to increase risk of fractures in a number of studies, other trials demonstrate a neutral effect. Their action on bone remains unclear, largely because of conflicting results due to different ages of the populations studied, mixed genders versus all female or all male, and use of other cardiac medications, in addition to angiotensin receptor antagonists [35]. In terms of mechanism of action, angiotensin I stimulates bone resorption in osteoblast and osteoclast cultures, whereas angiotensin II accelerates bone resorption by activating osteoclasts. Agents that block angiotensin I or II would, in theory, inhibit the resorptive process [39]. A summary of the effects that different classes of cardiac medications have on bone is given in Table 1.

Epidemiology of Bone Loss in Persons with Cardiac Disease

The risk factors and prevalence of bone loss in persons with advanced heart disease are difficult to estimate, since risks are closely dependent on the extent of disease, age of the individual patient or groups of patients, medications, comorbidities, and lifestyle. A similar statement could apply to risk of fractures, since syncopal events

Table 1 Commonly prescribed cardiac medications and their relative effects on bone

Drug class	Mechanism of action	Effect on bone	Medication concerns
Anticoagulants			
Heparin	Both standard and low MW heparin increase bone resorption by reducing osteoprogenetin and favoring RANKL-induced osteoclast differentiation, as well as inhibiting osteoblast differentiation. The result is decreased bone formation	Significant decrease	A newer oral anticoagulant, fondaparinux, has rapid onset; reversibility is not a concern
Low MW heparin		Moderate decrease	
Warfarin	Decreases the γ-carboxylation of and calcium-binding properties of osteocalcin, which is involved in bone formation	Mild-moderate decrease	
HMG-CoA reductase inhibitors			
Atorvastatin, lovastatin, rosuvastatin, simvastatin	Decreases mevalonate, which indirectly increases osteoblast differentiations	Suggested BMD increases and fractures decrease	N/A
Diuretics			
Thiazides (hydrochlorothiazide, chlorthalidone)	Decreases renal Ca excretion	Promote bone building	Thiazides and K+ sparing preferred over loop diuretics if clinically acceptable for patient
Potassium sparing agents (spironolactone, Aldactone)	Decreases renal Ca excretion, Increases K stores, Decreases aldosterone-mediated bone loss	Increases bone building	
Loop diuretics	Increases renal Ca excretion	Increases bone resorption	
Beta blockers			
Nebivolol	B-Adrenergic receptor inhibition Induces NO release which may be protective in bone preservation and prevention of osteoporosis	Likely a positive effect on bone	Evidence insufficient to warrant any specific agent over another
Atenolol	No specific action on bone cells delineated	Majority of larger studies indicate a positive effect on bone	
Metoprolol			

(continued)

Table 1 (continued)

Drug class	Mechanism of action	Effect on bone	Medication concerns
Nitrates	NO stimulation of osteoblastic activation	Likely a positive effect on bone	N/A
Calcium channel blockers	Studies suggest decreases osteoclast function	Decreases risk of fractures	N/A
ACE inhibitors	Angiotensin action on osteoblasts or calcium metabolism	Appear to increase fractures; neutral effect on bone	Consider other antihypertensive if clinically acceptable for patient
Angiotensin receptor blockers	Possible action at the angiotensin receptor	May inhibit bone resorption	N/A

Sources:
Aluoch et al. [5]
Ruths et al. [35]

and hypotension as well as new medications or changes in doses of existing medications can substantially increase the risk of falls. Table 2 summarizes the findings of a cross section of studies in the last 15 years, looking at a variety of populations.

In patients with advanced degrees of heart failure who are awaiting a transplant, evidence suggests a correlation between trabecular bone loss and time of evolution of the disease prior to transplant [40]. Garcia-Delgado et al. identified an increase in markers of bone resorption as well as decreased bone mass at lumbar and hip sites among patients before cardiac transplantation. Waiting time for the transplant was the most important predictive factor in bone loss at the lumbar spine, and as the next chapter will discuss, patients with recent organ transplants experience an even greater degrees of bone loss.

Treatment of Bone Loss in Cardiac Conditions

Given that osteoporosis occurs in 23 % of patients with heart failure pretransplant [41] and that medications given posttransplant (corticosteroids, immunosuppressants) contribute to further bone loss, preventative efforts and early treatment should be initiated prior to reaching the stage of organ transplantation [42].

For patients with heart failure on cardiac medications, particularly antihypertensive agents, selection of a non-loop diuretic such as spironolactone or one of the thiazides is favored over agents such as furosemide. In terms of effect on bone, data on ACE inhibitors is mixed, but if other equally suitable options for treatment of hypertension exist, then such agents should be considered. As with many other conditions, optimizing calcium and vitamin D stores is advisable in high-risk patients. Shane et al. [7] found that in two groups of heart failure patients, those with more

Table 2 Presence of osteoporosis in patients with cardiac conditions

Population studied/source	N control subjects	N experimental subjects	Outcome in control subjects	Osteopenia or osteoporosis in experimental subjects	Special notes
Aortic valve calcification (AVC) subjects (Aksoy et al. [12])	65 (AVC–)	49 (AVC+)	60 % with osteopenia or osteoporosis by BMD in L spine L1–4	82 % osteopenia or osteoporosis, by BMD in L spine L1–4	Presence of hypertension and age in AVC+ subjects
Postmenopausal sample of population-based females being screened for osteoporosis, with/without CAD (Barengolts et al. [17])	11 with normal BMD	20 with osteopenia and 14 with osteoporosis by DXA	Coronary calcium score in all arteries 41.9 ± 83.1, in LAD 30.2 ± 69.1	Coronary calcium score in all arteries for osteopenia 115.1 ± 182, in LAD 68,9 ± 115 and for osteoporosis was 221.7 ± 54.3 for all arteries and 166.6 ± 243.6 for LAD	Osteoporosis based on BMD at L spine, total hip FN, or Ward's triangle. Overall prevalence OP 31 %, calcium deposits 76 %
Men and women with NYHA Class III or IV CHF (Shane et al. [7])	Study sample with unknown bone disease but known CHF	N 101 total with 79 men and 22 women,	N/A	Osteopenia in 43 % at L spine, 47 % at total hip, and 42 % at FN. Osteoporosis in 7 % L spine, 6 % total hip, and 19 % FN	Osteopenia and osteoporosis present in approximately 50 % sample in either spine hip or both locations
Men with and without CHF screened for presence of osteoporosis (Terrovitis et al. [10])	13 male patients without CHF	60 male patients with CHF	Absence of osteopenia or osteoporosis on average in control group	*T*-score BMD in femur for Class I/II-1.1 and for Class II/IV patients was −1.9	Both classes had significant differences in BMD from controls

L spine lumbar spine, *FN* femoral neck

severe conditions, requiring ongoing hospitalization for intravenous inotropic agents or a management of left ventricular assistive device (LVAD), had significantly lower stores of serum vitamin D25-OH and notably reduced levels of the active form of vitamin D 1,25-$(OH)_2$. In contrast, the comparison group of heart failure outpatients had modestly deficient levels of vitamin D titers. Oral supplementation and, if possible, brief outdoor exposure to sunlight are advised if patients can tolerate these interventions.

More severely involved heart failure patients would have reduced exercise tolerance and limited community mobility, further contributing to osteoporosis. For patients with advanced CHF, including those with LVADs, lower extremity strengthening, weight-bearing exercises such as walking, and aerobic conditioning are all acceptable forms of exercise after VAD implantation [43]. Moreover, they lessen the severity of proximal muscles and osteoporosis which often occur in the transplant population.

Pulmonary Conditions and Osteoporosis

Advanced pulmonary disease most commonly occurs in the form of chronic obstructive pulmonary disease (COPD) including emphysema and chronic bronchitis and cystic fibrosis (CF). While other forms of restrictive pulmonary disease lead to organ failure, this section will focus primarily on the effects of COPD and cystic fibrosis on osteoporosis. Given their high prevalence in the elderly population coupled with the frequency of osteoporosis in the same age group, it is not surprising that more than 60 % of COPD patients in a recent study had osteopenia and 29 % met the criteria for osteoporosis [44]. For CF, a prevalence study of 103 patients aged 16–53 indicated that 10 % had osteoporosis and another 36 % had osteopenia [45]. Because the last three decades have seen CF life expectancies rise to a median age of nearly 40 years, those treating patients with the disease are just now seeing how bone health is affected by years of compromised pulmonary function, multiple infections, and malabsorption of nutrients [46].

Epidemiology of Osteoporosis and COPD

The prevalence of osteoporosis in COPD generally varies between 21 % and 59 % depending upon the diagnostic methods used, the age and gender of the sample, and the duration and severity of COPD in a study group [47, 48]. The few studies that demonstrated prevalence under 20 % used either quantitative ultrasound in part for the diagnosis, which is not the standard of care, or included subjects with obstructive airflow disease who had not met the definition of "chronic" in terms of disease duration. Although COPD is the third leading cause of death in the United States [49], it is not considered a risk factor for osteoporosis by the American College of Physicians, nor is smoking, despite its close association with COPD [50]. In contrast, the FRAX tool for prediction of fractures includes COPD but not smoking. Selected pulmonary parameters, inactivity, steroids, and other medications are among the risk factors for osteoporosis in those with COPD.

In their 2011 review of a number of studies involving samples of 40 to over 100 subjects, Lehouck et al. [47] found that osteoporosis occurred to a greater degree in subjects with lower forced expiatory volume in 1 second (FEV_1) scores and in those with advanced disease who are awaiting organ transplant [51]. In a study by Silva et al. [52] in which 42 % of subjects with COPD were osteoporotic and another 42 % were osteopenic, a significant correlation was found between femoral neck *T*-score and body mass index (BMI), with a significant inverse relationship between femoral neck *T*-score and BODE, a combined value including body mass index, air flow obstruction, dyspnea, and exercise capacity. In addition, correlations were found between a DXA *T*-score and $FEV_{1,}$ forced vital capacity (FVC), and percent of predicted diffusing capacity of the lung for carbon monoxide. The severity and rate of progression of COPD would have a marked influence on maintaining BMD.

By contrast, a 2011 study by Graat-Verboom et al. [53] examining 255 outpatients with stable COPD revealed an astonishing 51 % had osteoporosis defined by a combination of spinal x-rays and DXA. A summary of recent studies on prevalence rates is given in Table 3.

The Global Initiative for Chronic Obstructive Lung Disease (GOLD) has defined four levels of COPD severity, ranked I–IV, the end stage [64]. GOLD rankings take into account extrapulmonary manifestations of COPD, one of which is osteoporosis.

Among the most consistent risk factors for osteoporosis in the COPD population is the prolonged use of oral corticosteroids or glucocorticoids (GCs). An extensive review by van Staa et al. [65] demonstrates that the total cumulative dose of corticosteroids is inversely related to BMD. Although this study was not specifically focused on COPD patients, it does illustrate the substantial risk that COPD patients face in terms of maintaining bone health with cumulative years of GCs use.

The risk of developing osteoporosis with inhaled corticosteroids (ICS), as opposed to oral or intravenous corticosteroids (ICS), appears to be low based on a meta-analysis by Drummond et al. [66] who observed no significant difference in BMD among those COPD subjects using and not using ICS. Similarly, the TORCH trial (Towards a Revolution in COPD Health) [55], involving 658 patients with COPD, found minimal decreases in BMD (1.7–3.2 %) with use of ICS therapy in the first three years. However, the risk for fractures with ICS is increased, according to a number of investigations described in the following section.

Table 3 Prevalence of osteoporosis and vertebral compression fracture in COPD

Condition Author/source	Patient group	Subjects	BMD measure ments	Prevalence of osteoporosis, %	RX diagnosis of VCF	Prevalence of VCF, %
Osteoporosis						
Graat-Verboom et al. [54]	COPD patients (GOLD I–IV) referred for PR	554	Whole-body BMD (DXA)	21	…	…
Ferguson et al. [55]	COPD patients (GOLD II–IV)	658	BMD LS and hip (DXA)	24	…	…
Sin et al. [56]	COPD patients (GOLD I–IV)	5215	BMD total femur (DXA)	4–33	…	…
Førli et al. [51]	COPD patients awaiting LTX	40	BMD LS and FM (DXA)	59	…	…
Iqbal et al. [57]	Patients with chronic lung disease	130	BMD LS and hip (DXA)	36	…	…
Sabit et al. [58]	COPD patients (GOLD I–IV)	75	BMD LS and hip (DXA)	24	…	…
Bolton et al. [59]	Respiratory outpatients referred for PR	81	BMD total body, LS, and hip (DXA)	32	…	…
Compression fractures						
Jørgensen et al. [60]	Ambulatory COPD outpatients (GOLD III–IV)	62	…	…	Thoracic and lumbar spine radiographs	24
Nuti et al. [61]	Ambulatory COPD outpatients (GOLD I–IV)	2981	…	…	Lateral chest radiograph	41

(continued)

Table 3 (continued)

Condition Author/source	Patient group	Subjects	BMD measure ments	Prevalence of osteoporosis, %	RX diagnosis of VCF	Prevalence of VCF, %
Papaioannou et al. [62]	COPD patients (GOLD not reported)	127	…	…	Lateral chest radiograph	27
McEvoy et al. [63]	Male COPD patients (GOLD not reported)	312	…	…	Lateral lumbar and thoracic radiograph	49–63
Graat-Verboom et al. [53]	Ambulatory COPD outpatients (GOLD I–IV)	255	BMD LS, and hip (DXA)	51.4	Lumbar, lateral chest, and thoracic radiograph	36.5

GOLD Global Initiative for Chronic Obstructive Lung Disease, *LS* lumbar spine, *LTX* lung transplant, *PR* pulmonary rehabilitation, *RX* radiograph, *VCF* vertebral compression fractures. (*Source*: Lehouck et al. [47]. Used with permission)

Epidemiology of Fractures in COPD

As some investigations on COPD patients demonstrate, BMD assessed by DXA measures only bone density, not bone microarchitecture and bone quality. However, the use of DXA as a measure of BMD to determine fracture risk may not be ideal in some settings. Quantitative CT (QCT), an alternative method of assessment, was employed in a large study ($n=3317$) dealing with the effect of smoking on both osteoporosis and vertebral fracture risks in patients, with and without COPD [66]. In a smaller companion sample of 111 subjects taken from this larger group, Jaramillo et al. [67] applied both QCT and standard DXA tests, finding that QCT identified more subjects as osteopenic or osteoporotic than did DXA and that these subjects had a greater number of fractures. In this sample, 6 % of the QCT-classified osteopenic subjects and 37 % of those classified as osteoporotic had vertebral fractures. More broadly, the trial concluded that COPD was independently associated with not only low volumetric bone density, after adjusting for race, BMI, smoking, steroid use, and age, but also with an increased prevalence of vertebral fractures, with the highest number of fractures between T6-12, a region that is perhaps better evaluated by quantitative CT than DXA.

In a further analysis of ICS in COPD, Loke et al. [68] evaluated 16 randomized controlled trials (RCTs) and 14 observational studies relating to the use of two different ICS, fluticasone or budesonide, for at least 90 weeks. Findings demonstrated an increased odds ratio (OR) for fractures of 1.27 for all studies and 1.19 for the four trials of greatest duration (three years). The preceding meta-analysis evaluated risks of vertebral and nonvertebral fractures, with evidence demonstrating ICS were associated with both types of fractures. However, no comparison of likelihood of one

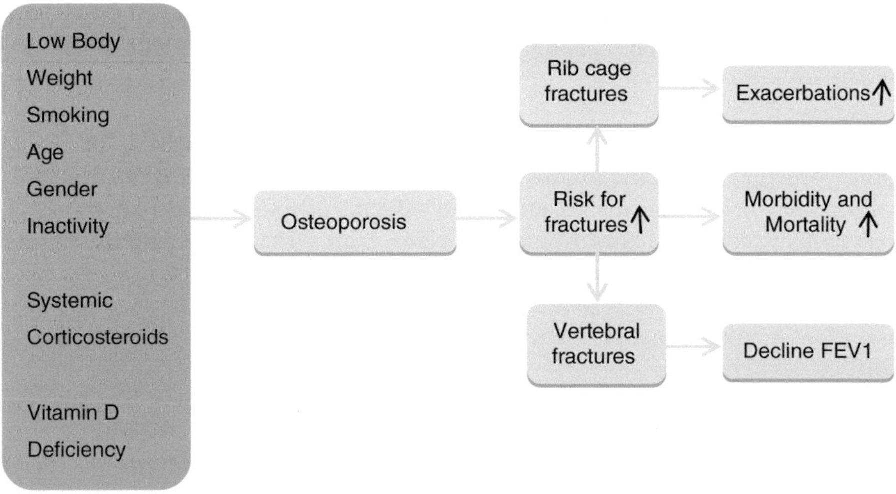

Fig. 1 Risk factors for osteoporosis in COPD and functional consequences (*Source*: Lehouck et al. [47]. Used with permission)

type of fracture versus another was possible, since the studies used different combinations of ICS or different solo agents.

Clinicians often balance the benefits of steroids for prevention and management of COPD exacerbations against the deleterious effects on other organ systems including bone health. Yet even very low daily doses can have deleterious effects: 2.5 mg/day presents a modest increased risk of fractures, while amounts greater than 7.5 mg/day confer a fivefold increased fracture risk [65, 69]. However, the risk of fractures does dissipate with discontinuation of steroids.

Etiology and Pathogenesis

Many different elements—physiologic, environmental, and pharmacological—contribute to osteoporosis in those with COPD and emphysema. Chronic hypoxemia, chronic inflammation, hypogonadism, dietary deficiencies in vitamin D and calcium, chronic use of corticosteroids, and other disease-modifying agents reduced physical activity and contributed to a sedentary lifestyle [70]. Figure 1 illustrates the risk factors for osteoporosis and functional consequences [47].

Liang and Feng [44] have demonstrated a relationship between systemic inflammation of low to moderate grades and low BMD in relatively stable COPD patients. It is known that the inflammatory cytokines, IL-6 and TNF alpha, induce expression of RANKL and RANKL-mediated bone resorption. Chronically elevated stores of these cytokines were found to be associated significantly with low BMD ($p=0.023$ and 0.010, respectively) as was the level of C-reactive protein (CRP), falling just short of statistical significance ($p=0.062$). These findings held true after adjustment for age, gender, use of inhaled corticosteroids, and severity of airway obstruction. States of chronic inflammation also suppress the WNT/β-catenin signaling pathway that stimulates osteoblasts, thereby contributing to the development of osteoporosis [71].

As in other conditions of inflammation including rheumatic disorders, the use of glucocorticoids (aka corticosteroids) increases expression of RANKL and decreases osteoprotegerin (OPG) [72]. In addition to reducing apoptosis of osteoclasts which resorb bone, enhanced bone resorption occurs, with subsequent inhibition of production and maturation of osteoblasts. These combined effects result in a net loss of bone with ongoing resorption and prolonged inhibition of bone formation. Initial use of GCs adversely alters trabecular bone but prolonged inflammation can also affect cortical bone.

Low vitamin D also compromises optimal absorption of calcium from the gut and influences immature osteoblastic cells to stimulate RANKL which, in turn, stimulates osteoclasts to promote bone resorption. In addition to exerting a direct influence on cells involved in bone metabolism, adequate serum levels vitamin D help to maintain muscle strength, thereby reducing the risk of falls [73–75]. An estimated 20–30 % of patients with COPD have reduced limb muscle strength relative to healthy controls [76].

Finally a mechanical abnormality related to altered lung structure and involving air trapping and parenchymal destruction may account for a substantial portion of bone loss, based on evidence that lung volume reduction surgery in advanced emphysematous patients significantly improves BMD in patients one year after undergoing this procedure [77].

Nonpharmacologic Treatment of COPD and Osteoporosis

Optimizing Function Prior to Formal Exercise

As stated above, evidence suggests lung volume reduction surgery has a positive effect on BMD as opposed to other surgical interventions which confer no direct, osteoporotic benefit with COPD. Optimizing pulmonary function prior to pulmonary rehabilitation can be valuable. Blocking or decreasing exacerbations of COPD with inhaled anticholinergics, such as ipratropium or tiotropium as well as short acting beta-2 agonists such as albuterol, helps with dyspneic symptoms and can indirectly improve pulmonary endurance for participation in aerobic exercise including weight-bearing activities. If any component of airway hyperactivity and bronchospasm exists, mast-cell stabilizers such as cromolyn sodium can alleviate airway inflammation which limits exercise tolerance [78].

Supplemental oxygen can improve endurance during physical therapy and aerobic activities by reducing shortness of breath. Perceived exertional activity during aerobic conditioning improves cognitive function, which is critical in settings where fall risk exists and attention to safety is imperative. Unless there is documented

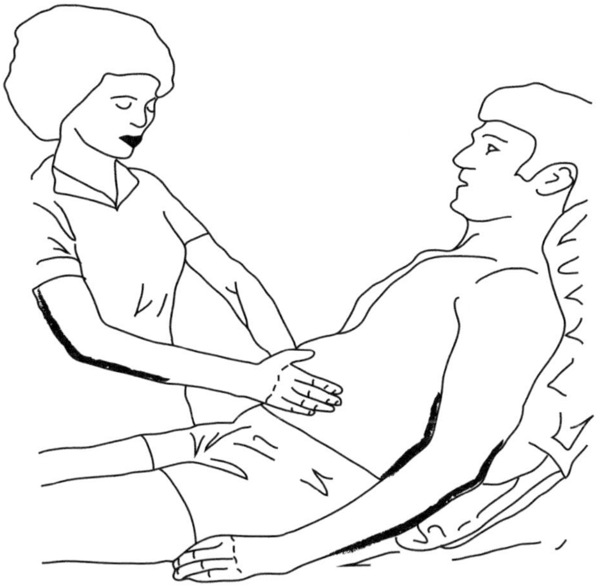

Fig. 2 Illustration of diaphragmatic breathing. Diaphragmatic breathing is appropriate for COPD patients who demonstrate predominantly upper thoracic expansion but limited abdominal movement or with inward movement of the lower rib cage during inspiration. This technique may be difficult to learn and is most easily performed, at least initially, in the semi-Fowler or side-lying position. Once mastered, the therapist should progress to the sitting position, followed by standing, and finally walking and stair climbing (*Source*: http://www.slideshare.net/sharminsusiwala22/a-detailed-description-on-breathing-exercises)

reduction in oxygen saturations with exercise, supplemental oxygen is unlikely to ameliorate function. Improving breathing with diaphragmatic and segmental breathing techniques can increase tidal volume and maximize oxygen uptake with reduced effort (Figs. 2 and 3) [79]. Pursed lip breathing prevents air trapping and small airway collapse, improving gas exchange, while it also reduces dyspnea and the work of breathing [80]. The combination of diaphragmatic and pursed lip breathing leads to higher arterial blood gas numbers, signifying improved oxygen supply to muscles and key organs. In this manner, exercise endurance is enhanced, and overall sense of fatigue is lessened.

Optimizing Nutrition: Vitamin D and Calcium

Because most patients with COPD tend to be older and many have comorbidities, standard supplementation with oral vitamin D3 on the order of 800 IU daily is advised for all those with normal to near normal serum vitamin D25OH levels [47]. Many will have difficulty simply maintaining therapeutic levels of vitamin D without a daily dose of a supplement. At the same time, several researchers advise the administration

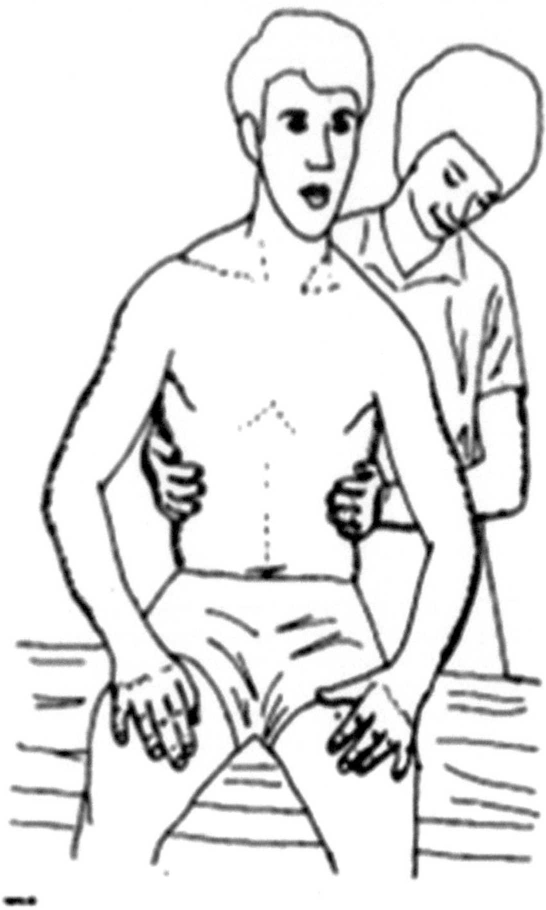

Fig. 3 Illustration of segmental breathing. Segmental breathing involves localized expansion exercises used to direct airflow to specific regions. This technique is often used in hypoventilation states as with painful conditions and muscle guarding in which patients self-limit their thoracic expansion. This type of scenario may occur following vertebral compression fractures; spine surgery for traumatic or insufficiency fractures (which have less pain than traumatic fractures); kyphoplasty; post thoracotomy, trauma to the chest wall, post-chest radiation fibrosis, pneumonia, and postmastectomy scars (*Sources*: For illustration and text above, see http://www.slideshare.net/sharminsusiwala22/a-detailed-description-on-breathing-exercises. See also Garritan [80])

of high potency vitamin D to any COPD patient with levels <10 ng/ml, because inadequate levels of the active form of vitamin D 1,25 (OH)2 D can adversely affect inflammation, thus exacerbating other comorbidities found in COPD [81]. Ensuring a diet adequate in calcium intake is also essential. For those patients who are lactose intolerant or who consume few products rich in calcium, oral supplementation is recommended.

Physical and Occupational Therapy in COPD

Formalized therapy in those with COPD and osteoporosis must be tempered by continual recognition of the need to improve ventilation and reduce the work of breathing [82]. Ideally, patients should start with 5 minutes sessions but work up to 15 minutes of resistive training pulmonary exercises daily. Focusing on activities of daily living, they generally begin with reconditioning exercises which encompass upper extremity range of motion and gentle resistance exercises with arm elevation as well as pool or bicycle routines [83]. Although none of these workouts involve weight-bearing through the spine or lower extremities, less intense exercise may initially be required to build adequate core strength before the more challenging activities of walking or stair climbing can be undertaken safely. Alternating walking with unsupported upper extremity exercise produces a safe combination of weight-bearing and non-weight-bearing exercise in keeping with the standard pulmonary rehabilitation protocol.

An individually prescribed exercise program, incorporating devices such as inspiratory orifices, should include a warm-up, followed by a time of gradually increasing physical exercise, and then a cooldown. Ideally, a pulmonary rehabilitation therapist working in conjunction with a patient's pulmonologist or internist should be involved in the design and initial intensity of a given patient's program. To maximize blood flow to lungs and avoid splanchnic diversion of oxyhemoglobin, exercise should not be initiated for at least 90–120 minutes after eating. In addition, nutritional selection, especially prior to therapy sessions, is important, since high carbohydrate meals produce the most carbon dioxide for the amount of oxygen used, whereas metabolism of fat produces the least carbon dioxide expenditure [84].

All programs should include a daily 12 minutes walk, with the distance recorded in order to monitor progress and estimate future exercise tolerance. Rest breaks are essential in the early and, depending on the severity of COPD, the later phases of pulmonary rehabilitation. Overexertion and pulmonary fatigue can compromise gas exchange and lead to hypercapnia. Arterial blood gases may need to be monitored. Ideally heart rate should not increase more than 20 % from baseline in initial phases of pulmonary rehabilitation reconditioning, and no more than 30 % in patients who are well advanced in the therapy program. Warning signals to discontinue or suspend therapy temporarily include heart rate >125, oxygen saturations below 91 %, or greater than 13 on the Borg perceived exertion scale (Table 4) [85]. If oxygen saturations do not improve despite supplemental oxygen or if any EKG changes involving premature ventricular contractions (PVCs) appear, therapy for the day should be suspended, and physicians should alter the plan of care to lessen intensity.

Pharmacologic Intervention

Antiresorptive Agents

In terms of medications that directly address osteoporosis, bisphosphonates have the longest follow-up evidence, demonstrating their ability to protect against postmenopausal and glucocorticoid-induced osteoporosis. The monoclonal antibody, denosumab, is effective in these conditions as well but has not been specifically

Table 4 Borg perceived exertional scale

How you might describe your exertion	Borg rating of your exertion	Examples (for most adults <65 years old)
None	6	Reading a book, watching television
Very, very light	7–8	Tying shoes
Very light	9–10	Chores like folding clothes that seem to take little effort
Fairly light	11–12	Walking through the grocery store or other activities that require some effort but not enough to speed up your breathing
Somewhat hard	13–14	Brisk walking or other activities that require moderate effort and speed your heart rate and breathing but don't make you out of breath
Hard	15–16	Bicycling, swimming, or other activities that take vigorous effort and get the heart pounding and make breathing very fast
Very hard	17–18	The highest level of activity you can sustain
Very, very hard	19–20	A finishing kick in a race or other burst of activity that you can't maintain for long

Source: Borg [85]

studied in COPD. In a major clinical trial examining the effect of alendronate (a once weekly oral bisphosphonate) on BMD, Smith et al. [86] used a daily 10 mg oral dose of the drug with 600 mg oral calcium supplementation for 12 months in subjects with established osteoporosis (*T*-score, –2.5 by DXA). Compared to controls who received a placebo with 600 mg daily elemental calcium, subjects given alendronate with calcium demonstrated significant improvement in BMD of the lumbar spine segments L2-4 but no improvement in the femoral neck or total hip.

Given the risks of osteoporosis in persons with COPD, the American College of Rheumatology has recommended that patients whose DXA scans are in the osteopenic range (*T*-score below –1) and who regularly use glucocorticoids be offered treatment in the form of antiresorptive agents, even in the absence of initial fractures. These recommendations published in 2001 predate the release of PTH and so do not address how its use might fit into the guidelines, now over a decade old [87]. Newer recommendations in 2010 place an emphasis on dosing of glucocorticoids and selection of bisphosphonate and in some cases teriparatide, although the latter agent receives a lower level of support than bisphosphonates, mainly based on the evidence published up to that time (2010, when evidence was just building regarding this medication) [88]. Imaging via DXA is incorporated in other tools of determination such as the FRAX score, which is used in the revised model. The guidelines suggest a number of limitations with reliance on FRAX, since it uses only the BMD at the hip rather than the spine, where many glucocorticoid-induced fractures are seen.

Additional guidance on approaches to treatment in high-risk patients such as those with COPD, and the timing of monitoring clinical response to treatment is needed in light of recent pharmacologic advances, radiographic imaging, and biological markers of response to interventions.

Cystic Fibrosis

Epidemiology of Cystic Fibrosis, Osteoporosis, and Fracture

Cystic fibrosis (CF) is an autosomal recessive disorder that affects approximately 30,000 people in the United States and a somewhat higher number throughout the rest of the world [89]. The most common lethal genetic disease in the Caucasian population, it affects the protein known as cystic fibrosis transmembrane conductance regulator (CFTR) which controls the movement of sodium, chloride, and water in and out of cells, predominantly in the lungs but also in the pancreas, digestive system, and liver. With too little or abnormal CFTR, the mucus secreted in these areas becomes thickened, causing obstructions, infection, and loss of function [90].

Generally diagnosed by age two, half of patients with CF recorded in 2014 were, for the first time, over the age of 18, with a survival rate of 39.3 years compared with 29.2 years in 1986. Many patients live well into their 40s and 50s [91]. Advancements in newborn screening programs, leading-edge therapeutic options, and improved management have all contributed to rising life expectancy; however, that lengthened life span has led to an increased occurrence of age-related comorbidities, including CF-associated osteoporosis [92].

As Gore et al. have observed [93], decreased BMD and higher fracture rates occur at a young age, 30 years earlier than in a non-CF population; they increase with age, the severity of the disease, and the use of corticosteroids. Beginning with the 1979 Mischler study [94], subsequent trials have corroborated the finding that CF patients have a demonstrated low BMD. Whereas Mischler used direct photon absorptiometry to find that 44 % of 27 patients (ages 5–24) had significant bone deficiency, Conway et al. [95] employed densitometry and multiple indices of disease severity to determine that, in a sample of 114 adolescents and adults, 79 % of 53 men and 56 % of 61 women had osteopenia or osteoporosis at one or more sites. They further documented a clear relationship between low BMD and disease severity as well as between reduced BMD and corticosteroid use. In terms of bone mineralization, 26 % of 66 patients singled out for this complication had pronounced anterior vertebral collapse, resulting in rib and thoracic compression fractures that restrict both coughing efficiency and the ability to undertake chest physiotherapy.

Further research confirms the marked prevalence of osteoporosis and fractures in patients with CF. In a study involving 50 clinically stable CF adults with 53 controls, Aris et al. [96] demonstrated that the CF cohort experienced accelerated bone breakdown without a compensatory increase in bone formation, suggesting that such factors as inflammatory cytokines and PTH increase osteoclast activity and play a role in CF bone disease [96]. In comparison with age-matched controls, patients with both CF and osteoporosis have a 100-fold increased risk of vertebral fractures and a tenfold increased risk of rib fractures [97]. In a 2010 meta-analysis of young adults with CF (mean age = 18.5–32 years), the prevalence of vertebral fractures varied between 5.0 % and 31.0 %, and the prevalence of nonvertebral fractures was as high as 20–40 %, but it could not be determined whether these fractures were truly osteoporotic [98]. As Goalski and Aris [99] have observed, no association between BMD and fractures has been specifically proved in CF studies. However, the link is so strong outside of CF that it dictates treatment.

Finally, a recent study of areal bone density comparing a cohort of CF adults (ages 18–50) who were evaluated in 1995–1999 (historic) with a comparable cohort examined in 2011–2013 (current) has produced unanticipated, disturbing results [100]. Despite advances in care management and heightened life expectancy, areal BMD was no better in the current cohort than it was 15 years ago. However, the present-day cohort did evidence improvements in pulmonary function, vitamin D deficiency, and secondary hyperparathyroidism. The underlying factors contributing to this static state include difficulty achieving nutritional goals, greater intake of systematic and inhaled glucocorticoids, delayed puberty, and CFTR dysfunction.

Pathogenesis of CF

As the occurrence of CF-related bone disease continues to rise with increased life expectancy, the number of age-related risk factors increases concomitantly, including those directly related to osteoporosis as well as those unique to CF, specifically the role of the CF transmembrane conductance regulator. The interaction of these factors leads to an uncoupling of the dynamic status of bone turnover, resulting in decreased bone formation and increased bone resorption [101].

Factors contributing to osteoporosis in CF originate in childhood. In comparison with healthy subjects, those with CF during childhood and adolescence fail to achieve adequate bone mass because of the interaction of delayed puberty, chronic infections, and hormonal imbalance [93]; in addition, the BMD in an age group of 4.9–17.8 years was found to decline at a rapid rate of approximately 1 SD every 6–8 years [102]. A high proportion of CF patients—85–90 %—evidence endocrine pancreatic insufficiency leading to digestive problems and malabsorption of vitamins A, E, K, and D. Both vitamin K and vitamin D levels, so critical to bone formation, are significantly reduced in cystic fibrosis. Whereas vitamin K deficiency is linked to low levels of carboxylated osteocalcin, vitamin D deficiency impairs the ability to achieve peak bone mass and limits calcium absorption by increasing bone turnover through PTH stimulation [103].

In severe CF, acute pulmonary exacerbations are associated with higher levels of cytokines (e.g., tumor necrosis factor-alpha (TNF-α), interleukin (IL)-1, and IL-6) that stimulate osteoclastic bone resorption and cause bone loss [93]. Corticosteroids employed to improve respiratory function in CF are known to adversely affect bone, with oral corticosteroids decreasing BMD in the lumbar spine and femoral neck and inhaled corticosteroids resulting in low total body BMD [95, 104]. High-dose corticosteroid therapy is particularly important following lung transplantation, but it contributes to a rapid decline in BMD associated with increased fracture risk. In contrast to an earlier prevailing belief that osteoporosis with fractures contraindicates lung transplants, most transplant centers now regard osteoporosis as a "remediable comorbidity," with only uncontrolled pain related to fractures considered to be a contraindication [105, 106].

Specific to osteoporosis in CF, dysfunction of the CFTR has recently been implicated as another factor leading to bone disease. In trials with knockout mice, the existence of an abnormal CFTR protein called delta F509 was linked with osteopenia, reduced cortical bone, and thinning of the trabecular bone [107], while a study of CF adults revealed that delta 509 mutation is an independent risk factor for osteoporosis [108, 109]. In addition, Shead et al. [110] have demonstrated the presence of CFTR in human osteoblasts, osteocytes, and osteoclasts. Implications of these findings require further research.

Diagnosis and Treatment

In accordance with guidelines established by the Cystic Fibrosis Foundation [111], screening for CF-related bone disease should begin in childhood in order to determine the extent of bone density loss and to implement preventative and treatment measures. A baseline BMD determined by standard dual-energy x-ray absorptiometry (DEXA) of the lumbar spine and hip is recommended for all patients at age 18; children ages eight and over should be tested if they evidence risk factors such as previous history of fractures, delayed FEV_1 <50 % predicted, and glucocorticoids 5 mg/day or more for a minimum of 90 days/year.

Vitamin Supplementation

Vitamin D and K supplementation as well as supplemental doses of calcium at 1300–1500 mg daily is a first step in both prevention and treatment. To maintain a target level of serum vitamin D25(OH) of 30 mg/mL and optimize calcium metabolism in CF patients, updated guidelines for vitamin D [112] stipulate giving 400–500 IU/day for children 12 months and younger, 800–1000 IU/day for ages 1–10, and 800–2000 IU/day for those 11 years and older. An age-specific intake of 0.3–0.5 mg/day of vitamin K is recommended, based on recent research demonstrating its positive impact on the posttranslational activation of osteocalcin which promotes bone formation and mineralization [113].

Physical Therapy

In CF, physical activity must be tailored to the needs and capabilities of the individual patient. Observational studies of CF children and adults have shown a positive relationship between regular aerobic weight-bearing exercise and BMD, as well as a complementary role in chest physiotherapy. However, controlled intervention trials examining the effect of exercise on bone mass accrual are lacking.

Consequently existing evidence is limited to indications that patients with mild to moderate CF are physically able to participate in regular exercise that benefit muscle strength as well as bone and lean mass—if they have sufficient dietary energy intake and motivation [114].

Pharmacologic Intervention

Bisphosphonates, including oral alendronate and risedronate or intravenous pamidronate and zoledronic acid, have been shown to be effective in CF. These agents are recommended in patients with a *T/Z* scores less than −2.0 and in those with *T/Z* scores between −1.0 and −2.0 who have a history of fractures, are awaiting a lung transplant or are losing BMD at the rate of >3–5.0 annually [111]. In a Cochrane review of seven small trials, bisphosphonates consistently increased BMD but did not demonstrate fracture reduction or survival benefits [115]. A recent trial involving CF patients aged 5–30 found that BMD increased by 16.3 % in patients receiving alendronate for one year as opposed to 3.1 % for patients on placebo; moreover the patients on alendronate achieved a normal-for-age BMD Z-score after one year. Adverse effects included nonsevere gastrointestinal, muscle, and bone pain [116]. Given their efficacy in cystic fibrosis and their greater degree of tolerance, oral bisphosphonates remain the first-line therapy for the disease.

Denosumab, teriparatide, and growth hormone are among the promising therapies for osteoporosis in cystic fibrosis, but further tests are needed to determine their potential in the specific context of CF. As an antiresorptive agent in bone disease, denosumab improves bone density in lumbar spine and hip and, unlike bisphosphonates, increases cortical bone density [101]. Although its long-term effects are yet to be assessed, its short-term benefits, coupled with relatively few side effects and twice-yearly dosing, strengthen the likelihood that it will become an effective intervention in CF-related bone disease. The parathyroid hormone, teriparatide, known to increase osteoblast formation and bone growth, may prove useful in CF patients experiencing severe osteoporosis or previous fractures [117]. A study of children and young adults up to age 25 has demonstrated that recombinant growth hormone improves intermediate outcomes in height, weight, and lean tissue mass as well as improvements in exercise tolerance; however, long-term RCMs are needed before it can be administered on a routine basis [118].

The promise of increased survival rates and advanced treatments for CF and its related diseases is enhanced by the existence of more than 120 care centers and 55 affiliated programs, including 96 for adult treatment, at teaching and community hospitals across the country. Initiated in 1960 and accredited by the CF Foundation, this network of multidisciplinary facilities sets and maintains standards for care, research, and education; provides data on health outcomes to the CF Patient Registry; designs CF clinical trials; and identifies the most promising therapies; thereby serving as a model of effective healthcare for other chronic diseases [119, 120].

Renal Osteodystrophy and Disorders of Mineral Metabolism

Abnormalities of bone in the spectrum of chronic kidney disease–mineral and bone disorders (CKD–MBD, also called renal osteodystrophy) can result in a number of serious consequences for long-term bone health including the formation of heterotopic bone, excessive vascular calcification, and abnormalities of bone formation. Irregularities in the metabolism of both calcium and phosphate occur, even in the early stages of renal disease, and moderately impaired glomerular filtration rates (GFR) are evidenced by elevated levels of fibroblast growth factor 23 (FGF23) and hyperparathyroidism. This section will explain the pathophysiology of renal disease and its effect on bones and offer approaches to treatment [121]. Before focusing on the skeletal pathology component of CKD, it is necessary to describe the broader context of metabolic bone changes and related organ pathology involved in CKD.

Pathophysiology of CKD–MBD

In the course of renal disease, a number of circulating inhibitors and promoters work in negative ways to decrease bone formation and bone mineralization (Fig. 4). Fibroblast growth factor FGF23 is increased along with sclerostin, both of which promote bone resorption and bone remodeling, although FGF23 does so only indirectly through mechanisms involving PTH and vitamin D. Produced by osteocytes and osteoblasts, FGF23 exerts a direct action on renal tubules and parathyroid glands. As kidney disease progresses, the number of working nephrons in the kidney continually declines. Hence, more phosphate is excreted by each of the remaining nephrons, a mechanism that is only possible through increased activity of FGF23 and parathyroid hormone (PTH) [122]. The constant elevated production of PTH resulting from hyperplasia of the parathyroid glands results in increased RANKL production. The consequences of increased RANKL in this setting are significant: high turnover renal osteodystrophy, desensitization of the PTH receptor, and excessive bone resorption [121].

Additional effects of actions of FGF23 include inhibition of the enzyme 25-hydroxyvitamin D 1-α hydroxylase that produces calcitriol, resulting in decreased intestinal calcium absorption and ultimately hypocalcemia. This cascade of events also reduces the number of active vitamin D receptors on cells in the parathyroid contributing to more definitive adverse changes in CKD–MBD of those with advanced renal disease [123]. High serum phosphorous, low serum calcium, and low calcitriol levels collectively contribute to persisting and worsening hyperparathyroidism. By controlling the levels of calcium and phosphorous early in the course of CKD, practitioners can help to prevent one of the most severe complications of renal osteodystrophy, i.e., hyperparathyroidism [124].

There are three different types of metabolic disorders in CKD: high bone turnover states, low bone turnover states, and mixed disorders. If hyperparathyroidism

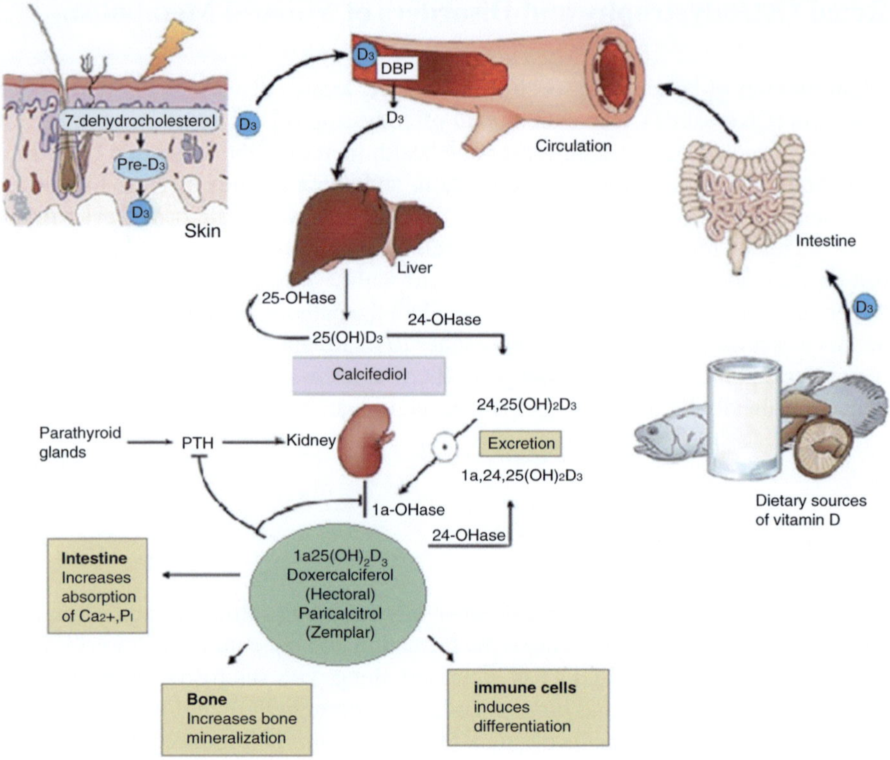

Fig. 4 The metabolism of vitamin D and location of actions of vitamin D analogs. Vitamin D analogs doxercalciferol and paricalcitol act similarly to 1α-25OH (calcitriol) but may have less effect on the intestine and bone compared with calcitriol (See page 303)

is present, a high bone turnover state develops which is characterized by irregular collagen production known as woven bone. In comparison to mineralized bone, woven bone lacks strength because of haphazard orientation of the type I collagen fibers that form osteoid. Furthermore, due to enhanced resorption as compared with formation, bone mass is decreased. In contrast, if the prevailing PTH level is insufficient to overcome PTH resistance characteristic of severe CKD, the result is a low bone turnover state, a condition classified as either adynamic bone or osteomalacia. Adynamic bone is characterized by complete lack of osteoid production and new bone formation, whereas osteomalacia results from normal osteoid production but impaired ability to mineralize the osteoid. In CKD, osteomalacia most frequently occurs from aluminum toxicity. In mixed uremic osteodystrophy, both a mineralization defect and high bone turnover state exist [121]. All three disorders are influenced by the extent of vitamin D metabolic irregularities, any immunosuppressive treatment adversely affecting bone maintenance, dietary restrictions, and associated health problems including diabetes. Table 5 compares the various types of bone turnover pathology seen in CKD [121].

Table 5 Pathology and diagnosis of bone turnover in CKD

Predominant hyperparathyroidism	Low bone turnover	Mixed uremic osteodystrophy	Undefined
Intact PTH >500 pg/ml	Adynamic bone disorder (AMD) 1. Intact PTH <100 pg/ml 2. Normal alkaline phosphatase or bone-specific alkaline phosphatase	PTH >300 pg/ml	PTH >100 pg/ml <500 pg/ml
Elevated alkaline phosphatase or bone-specific alkaline phosphatase	Osteomalacia 1. Intact PTH <100 pg/ml 2. Normal alkaline phosphatase or bone-specific alkaline phosphatase 3. Low osteocalcin 4. Elevated aluminum	Elevated aluminum	

Source: Hruska and Seifert [121]

The intact PTH level varies depending on the severity of CKD. Elevated levels of intact PTH are often desired in later stages of CKD (3–5D) in order to have optimal bone health due to the known skeletal resistance to PTH with uremia. Therapy should be aimed at improving calcium, phosphorous, and vitamin D levels, as well as focusing on PTH levels [124]. If intact PTH falls outside the desired range of 2–9 times, the upper limit of normal in a patient with CKD stage 5D, management plans must be further individualized in conjunction with close coordination with the patient's nephrologist. Nearly all of the laboratory studies and medical treatments desired at this stage of evaluation can be performed in an inpatient rehabilitation setting. Only in cases of severe CKD (stages 3–5D), which are consistently unresponsive to medical interventions including both dialysis adjustments and pharmacologic agents, would a parathyroidectomy need to be considered.

Diagnostic Evaluation

Serum calcium (or ionized calcium if albumin levels are low), phosphorous, intact PTH, and bone-specific alkaline phosphatase should be measured at baseline when GFR falls below 60 ml/min. Serum vitamin D 25OH should be monitored at least twice annually, especially at the end of winter when levels reach their nadir. Due to diurnal, postprandial, and dialysis (pre and post) variability, it is helpful to pick a consistent time for patients to be analyzed and compare those values over months. In addition, titers used by laboratories differ, particularly for vitamin D and alkaline phosphatase. Although P1NP is an alternative marker of bone formation to bone-specific alkaline phosphatase, it is not widely available, takes longer to process and obtain results (often sent out of a clinic to a specialized lab), and is between three and four times the cost of bone-specific alkaline phosphatase [125]. In reality, the most important measures used for day-to-day management of CKD–MBS remain calcium, phosphorous, vitamin D, and PTH.

Bone alterations are most accurately diagnosed by bone biopsy with histomorphometric analysis. While performing a biopsy has utility at any stage of renal disease, it is most important to undertake histomorphometric analysis in CKD stages 3–5D. In the setting of advanced CKD, bone biopsy should also be considered with any of the following conditions [124]:

- Fractures or bone pain with no trauma or apparent cause
- Suspected aluminum associated bone disease (aluminum deposits in the bone)
- Possible osteomalacia
- Unexplained hypercalcemia or hypophosphatemia
- Prior to initiating treatment with bisphosphonates
- Before parathyroidectomy

Regarding DXA scans to assess bone density, these studies are useful in early CKD, although the guidelines described in the report by Bellorin-Font [124] suggest that they are minimally effective in advanced CKD (stages 3–5D). DXA remains the preferred means of assessing BMD due to high precision, short scanning time, and low radiation dose [126]. Quantitative ultrasound (QUS) may have potential as an alternative to DXA. Taal et al. [127] examined patients with various stages of CKD and found that the two diagnostic tools were significantly correlated. However, while the high negative predictive value of QUS allowed physicians to rule out osteoporosis in those patients less likely to have the condition, the low positive predictive value meant that patients at higher risk and tested in the osteoporotic range required further confirmation with DXA, quantitative CT, or another modality.

In the absence of bone biopsy, quantitative CT and micro MRI are more useful than DXA to differentiate the percentage of bone loss due to osteoporosis and the percentage due to CKD–MBD. If treatment for osteoporosis is recommended, a bone biopsy will ultimately have to be done to rule out adynamic bone disease before selecting pharmaceutical agents for intervention [128].

Osteoporosis and Fractures in CKD

The prevalence of osteoporosis in the CKD population is higher than that in the general population. Estimates however are highly varied because bone changes in CKD encompass abnormalities in bone mineral density (measured by DXA), bone microarchitecture (cortical and trabecular bone balance), bone geometry (shape and size of bone, which is related to bone fragility and fracture risk), and molecular elements (component parts such as collagen type and linkages). Taal et al. [127] found that among 88 patients with CKD of mixed severities, 48.9 % had reduced BMD and 19.3 % had BMD values low enough to fall within the fracture threshold. Both femoral neck and lumbar spine were evaluated in this report [127].

Among CKD stage 5 patients, Stehman-Breen et al. [129] found osteopenia prevalence at the femoral neck to be 60 % among African-Americans and 86 % among Caucasians, while the prevalence of osteoporosis in the same two groups was 22 and 59 %, respectively. Hip fracture is increased by a factor of 4 over the risk in the normal population [129, 130]. Even more impressive is the 99-fold increase in hip fracture prevalence among men under age 45 with CKD and women over 85, although with the latter category, it is more difficult to understand how CKD may affect a number of other risk factors among older women. In contrast, Coco and Rush found that low PTH was associated with increased risk of hip fracture [131].

Although many patients with osteoporosis experience greater bone loss in the trabecular region than in cortical areas, those with end-stage renal disease (ESRD) or CKD demonstrate loss of cortical bone specifically [132]. Microarchitectural changes are among the essential components of renal osteodystrophy within a broader spectrum of CKD. In fact, osteoporosis can be observed in four different yet related situations in patients with CKD. For those individuals who experience bone resorption that exceeds formation, hyperphosphatemia and hypercalcemia occur in the absence of additional skeletal deposition of bone, resulting in heterotopic mineralization within the vasculature [121]. The latter situation directly links the bone pathology of CKD–MBD to cardiovascular disease and increased mortality [133]. In summary, four different scenarios of osteoporosis can be seen in CKD–MBD:

High bone turnover renal osteodystrophy
Low turnover renal osteodystrophy
Preexisting osteoporosis, now worsened by onset of renal disease
New onset gonadal hormone deficiency related to CKD, now causing osteoporosis

Bellorin-Font et al. [124] present several tables describing studies with patients who have experienced hip or spine fractures. The studies span a 45-year period, some confined to one gender or the other and vary widely in participant numbers. The reader is referred to their review of additional findings on selected groups of CKD 5D patients.

Pain Associated with Osteoporosis from CKD

Severe bone pain is common in those with renal osteodystrophy and advanced CKD, regardless of the particular etiology that caused bone loss. Of the four subtypes, low bone turnover osteodystrophy and aluminum-based bone disease have the highest reports of bone pain. In addition, these two etiologies carry the greatest risk of bone fractures. While bone pain more commonly occurs with an insidious onset that progresses slowly, an isolated joint in the lower extremities or chest can suddenly cause increased pain. If such an instance occurs, clinicians should rule out a low-trauma fracture, because insufficiency fractures have been known to occur spontaneously in the lower extremities and vertebral bodies [121].

Treatment of CKD–MBD

Unlike many other medical and neurological degenerative conditions that combine treatment of the underlying condition with aggressive management to alter the balance of bone resorption and formation, initial treatment of CKD–MBD is heavily focused on regulating calcium, phosphorous, vitamin D, and innate parathyroid hormone-metabolic interactions. Two agencies have created guidelines for management of metabolic bone disease in CKD stages 3–5D (National Kidney Foundation, Kidney Disease Outcomes Quality Initiative (KDOQI), developed in 2003 and the Kidney Disease: Improving Global Outcomes (KDIGO) in 2009) [134]. While the earlier recommendations proposed keeping calcium levels in the mid-to-low end of normal and phosphate levels at 3.5–5.5 mg/dl, the 2009 guidelines relax these stipulations. KDIGO permits calcium and phosphate levels in the normal range except for phosphorous values for CKD stage 5D which should ideally be "toward" the normal range [135]. The newer guidelines further recommend up to 2–9 times the upper limit of normal for PTH, in order to optimize blood levels of other nutrients in CKD stage 5D, whereas for stages 3–5, they believe that optimal levels are unknown and that specific limits on values are hard to achieve. The goals of treatment are [135]:

1. To achieve neutral phosphate balance without causing other electrolyte abnormalities (specifically in calcium) or creating protein malnutrition.
2. To limit hyperparathyroidism and control PTH levels, thereby avoiding progression of secondary hyperparathyroidism to tertiary hyperparathyroidism, a condition in which only surgical removal of 3.5 of 4 parathyroid glands can restore normal PTH levels.
3. To optimize vitamin D25-OH levels to the extent that they can prevent the non-CKD adverse aspects of vitamin D deficiency, thereby protecting other bodily functions.
4. To achieve the objectives, cinacalcet may be needed in addition to active vitamin D analogs such as calcitriol, paricalcitol, and doxercalciferol. Compared with conventional therapy, this combination has had greater success in controlling PTH while also preventing hyperphosphatemia escalation [136].

Controlling Phosphate Levels

Although controlling dietary phosphorus is widely recommended for management of renal disease, evidence exists that reduction of dietary phosphorous through restriction of oral protein intake can worsen bone density. In a study examining the effects of a low-protein, phosphorus-restricted diet in subjects with advanced kidney disease, Lafage et al. found that a number of patients experienced a decrease in bone remodeling that may promote adynamic bone disease. This process fosters subsequent bone loss from oversuppression of bone remodeling [137]. In a subsequent 5-year study of a similar cohort, patients exhibited low BMD associated with sustained osteoclastic activity and more than half developed moderate to severe osteoporosis [138].

Reduction of serum phosphate can also be accomplished with the use of phosphate binders such as calcium acetate or sevelamer. Calcium-based binders have the added benefit of improving osteoporosis protection. However, these agents should not be combined with other forms of calcium supplementation to avoid the possibility of hypercalcemia.

Recent studies point to disturbing prospects for those with elevated phosphate levels including increased risk of cardiovascular events and premature mortality even in patients with early renal disease [128]. What is not clear is whether reduction in dietary phosphorous in particular will help change the outcome. Theoretically, prevention of secondary hyperparathyroidism brought about by reduction of phosphorous in the diet should alleviate high turnover bone loss, but studies have shown that patients with advanced renal disease still experience high percentages of osteoporosis in the absence of secondary hyperparathyroidism.

Vitamin D Management

The emphasis in vitamin D management is consistently focused upon prevention of hyperparathyroidism, in particular, secondary hyperparathyroidism that falls outside the desired range for a given individual's state of renal function. As stated previously, in advanced renal disease, permissive secondary hyperparathyroidism is ideally in the range of 2–9 times normal, but not beyond that. The level of acceptable PTH values depends on the severity of CKD. A finding of low vitamin D beyond what can be anticipated by dysfunctional metabolism of the kidney has been recognized as a significant health risk. Low vitamin D should be treated initially with either cholecalciferol or weekly ergocalciferol. Other forms of vitamin D (e.g., calcitriol) which act after renal processing carry a greater risk of hypercalcemia. While practitioners may ultimately need to treat with calcitriol, initial attempts with less potent agents should be trialed [124, 128]. If less potent measures work to enhance levels of serum D25 and maintain serum calcium and phosphate at normal levels, then more aggressive intervention is unnecessary. Follow-up testing should be done 4–6 weeks after treatment begins.

Should the above approach fail, two new alternatives for vitamin D supplementation in renal disease patients are now available. Vitamin D analogs such as doxercalciferol and paricalcitol act similarly to calcitriol but may have lower tendency to cause problematic hypercalcemia and hyperphosphatemia compared with calcitriol. Table 6 compares the new vitamin D analogs in terms of mechanism and sites of action as well as benefits and drawbacks of the individual agents [139–144]. Figure 4 (page 298) illustrates their respective sites of action in the metabolic pathway of vitamin D.

Table 6 Alternative vitamin D analogs in end-stage renal or liver disease

Name of drug	Location of action	Benefits	Concerns	Mode of delivery	Price for 30 capsules*
Calcitriol	Bone	Lower cost	Increasing intestinal calcium absorption with the resultant of hypercalcemia	IV injection or oral	0.25 mg: $ 43.55
	Intestine	The mechanism and risks of it are fully understood	Hyperphosphatemia		0.5 mg: $45.30
	Kidney	May be indicated to treat hypocalcemia	Increased risk of extraskeletal calcification		
Paricalcitol (trade name Zemplar)	Bone	Effective in achieving suppression of elevated levels of PTH	High cost	IV injection or oral	1 mcg: $541.10
	Intestine	Minimal hypercalcemia and hyperphosphatemia	No published direct comparison to calcitriol to assess differences in efficacy and safety		2 mcg: $1122.15
	Kidney		The mechanism is not fully understood		
Doxercalciferol (trade name Hectorol)	Bone	It is already hydroxylated at the 1-α-position, and requires only hydroxylation at the 25 position, accomplished in the liver	High cost	IV injection or oral	0.5 mcg: $424.85
	Intestine	By avoiding the need for activation in the kidney, patients with little or no kidney function can use this agent	Limited use to treat hypocalcemia		2.5 mcg: $1452.20
	Kidney	Oral administration was shown to be safe and highly effective for the treatment of SHPT	It has not been directly compared to calcitriol to assess difference in efficacy and safety		
		Minimal hypercalcemia and hyperphosphatemia			

Sources * 2016 prices
Lindberg [139]
Slatopolsky et al. [140]
Martin et al. [141]
Coburn et al. [142]
Frazao et al. [143]
Tan et al. [144]

Traditional Osteoporosis Medications

Limited studies in persons with CKD have been conducted on use of the more common agents for treatment of osteoporosis: estrogen, selective estrogen receptor modulators (SERMs), calcitonin, bisphosphonates, and monoclonal antibodies such as denosumab.

Estrogen and Selective Estrogen Reuptake Modulators (SERMs)

Several studies in women are worth noting. In an investigation involving premenopausal women with CKD stage 5 undergoing hemodialysis, hormone replacement therapy (HRT) was used to counter estrogen deficiency but was not randomized. After one year of treatment and subsequent DXA measurement, lumbar spine BMD increased markedly in the treatment group but decreased in the controls [145]. The concern is that some researchers report an association between estrogen and increased cardiovascular events and that this 1999 study predated much of the newer research on the subject.

A randomized, placebo controlled examination of raloxifene (a SERM) on BMD in lumbar spine and femoral neck was conducted in 50 postmenopausal women on hemodialysis [146]. Compared with those on placebo, women who received raloxifene experienced improvement in lumbar BMD but not in femoral neck BMD. In a second study of postmenopausal women on hemodialysis with existing diagnosis of either advanced osteopenia or osteoporosis, a significant increase in lumbar BMD with reduction of bone markers of resorption was noted [147]. Although those on hemodialysis are at risk of venous thromboembolism, pulmonary embolism, and clotting difficulties with dialysis catheters, none of these complications were found in this investigation. There has been evidence that raloxifene levels are higher, and renal clearance of the medication lower, in men with reduced renal function, compared to men with normal renal function [148].

Bisphosphonates

In considering the use of bisphosphonates in CKD–MBD, a number of concerns have been raised including oversuppression of bone in patients who already have adynamic bone disease. Vitamin D levels should be evaluated and optimized prior to initiation of treatment to prevent hypocalcemia and maximize potential benefit of a bisphosphonate. Hypocalcemia post administration underlies the need to ensure that calcium levels are adequate prior to initiation, particularly in terms of administering the more potent intravenous agents such as zoledronic acid.

A number of safety measures have been instituted for those with renal insufficiency and renal failure desiring to take bisphosphonates. In such cases, intestinal bisphosphanate absorption is less than 1 % with only 40–50 % absorbed by the bone [149]. The remaining 40–60 % of the small portion that is absorbed is excreted unchanged in the urine, potentially damaging renal tubules in a patient who is either dehydrated or at risk of nephrotoxicity from other drugs. For those with renal disease, the glomerular filtration rate (GFR) needs to be above 30 ml/min for bisphosphonates to be used safely.

In those with borderline renal functions, some bisphosphonates such as zoledronic acid need to be given with caution, but many options exist to allow patients to benefit from these agents with adjustment of administration. Ways to improve safety and avoid any damage to the kidney include optimizing hydration with IV fluid prior to or during administration of the drug, using a lower dose, and extending the infusion time to over one or more hours as opposed to 15–30 minutes. Some reports suggest pamidronate may represent a greater risk than zoledronic acid among IV bisphosphonates, while intravenous ibandronate may have the lowest risk of the three agents [128, 150]. Although pamidronate is not as widely used for osteoporosis treatment, it is still commonly administered for hypercalcemia of malignancy. For those with borderline GFR (30–35 ml/min), transient elevation in serum creatinine, which can be seen post infusion with ibandronate or zoledronic acid [151, 152], resolves with time and can be more quickly corrected with oral or IV hydration post infusion. The use of oral bisphosphonates in CKD–MBD stages 2–4 suggests that nephrotoxicity is not a concern and that positive results in terms of decreased fracture risk and improvement of BMD have been found with both alendronate [150, 153] and risedronate [154].

Liver Disease and Osteoporosis

Osteoporosis is a frequent complication of liver disease, particularly in the end stage (ESLD) and in cases of chronic cholestasis when substances normally excreted in bile are retained. Liver disorder begins with inflammation of the bile ducts, ultimately leading to scarring and cirrhosis—the end point in patients with chronic progressive liver disease. Patients who develop ascites (abnormal accumulation of excessive fluid in the abdominal cavity), variceal hemorrhage, hepatic encephalopathy, or renal impairment are said to have ESLD [155]. Its occurrence is primarily attributable to long-standing alcohol abuse, hepatitis B/C, and fatty liver disease occurring in those with obesity and diabetes.

In such cases, transplantation has become an increasingly viable option; however, patients encounter a long waiting list. Whereas some 6730 liver transplants were performed in the United States in 2014, more than 12,000 patients remained on an active waiting list [156].

Osteoporosis is the primary metabolic bone disease found in patients with chronic liver disease. Many factors including altered metabolism of vitamin D, poor diet, reduced mobility, limited physical activity, and medications given to prevent pain, edema, or thromboembolism contribute to bone loss. This section will examine the epidemiology and causes of osteoporosis in liver disease and discuss treatment options at both the pre- and posttransplant stages.

Epidemiology and Causes of Osteoporosis in Liver Disease: Pretransplant Phase

In preparation for liver transplantation, a process which decreases bone density, patients undergo routine screening laboratory studies focusing on baseline levels of serum vitamin D25OH, PTH, and imaging to determine the presence of osteoporosis or osteopenia. Investigations carried out in this pretransplant phase have gained increasing attention, because of high rates of bone fractures generally following transplant, and concern is now being raised that much of the predisposition to fractures arises from processes that are already significantly advanced before transplantation occurs. Declining functional mobility with a corresponding increase in fluid retention shifts the weight distribution and compromises balance; nutrition declines as patients lose appetite from a sense of abdominal fullness, and vitamin D metabolism is compromised by poor liver function.

Based on five separate investigations, Krol et al. [157] found that either osteopenia or osteoporosis was present in one-half of the population with ESLD. Vertebral fractures were also prevalent but there was no association between BMD and fracture occurrence [157].

As in other conditions, BMD in ESLD patients is defined by DXA scanning. However, patients with cirrhosis and ascites may have falsely elevated BMD values prior to paracentesis, with more accurate levels immediately following evacuation of excess fluid, particularly when the amount drained exceeds 4 l. This disparity is most problematic when measuring the lumbar spine or the hip, with minimal impact observed at the femoral neck [158].

Alcalde-Vargas et al. [159] conducted a retrospective study of BMD findings among cirrhotic patients undergoing evaluation for future liver transplant. Their population, consisting of 350 subjects, included a mix of patients with alcoholic cirrhosis, hepatitis B and C, and primary and secondary biliary cirrhosis. Overall, 72 % of participants had either osteoporosis or osteopenia in the hip or spine: more specifically, the global hip showed 22 % of patients with osteopenia and 4 % with osteoporosis, femoral neck had 43 % with osteopenia and 5 % with osteoporosis, and lumbar spine had 40 % with osteopenia and 23 % with osteoporosis. In addition to liver disease, other risk factors that increased the odds ratio of low bone mass included female gender, lower body mass index, and tobacco use. Of the large number of investigations of osteoporosis in association with ESLD, the majority focus on the very late stages of ESLD, in preparation for liver transplantation.

In a prospective study of non-cholestatic (non-impairment of bile flow) liver disease, Mahmoudi et al. examined patients with alcoholic cirrhosis as well as with hepatitis B and C [160]. As with prior investigations, the lumbar spine demonstrated a higher percentage of osteoporosis relative to the femoral neck: 11 % versus 4 %. In addition, since the lumbar spine has a higher degree of trabecular bone than the hip, it is not surprising that rates of osteoporosis are greater in the lumbar spine. Throughout this study, the observed percentages of both osteopenia and osteoporosis were much lower than in many other studies, due to a focus on the viral etiology of liver disease and a population of less severe liver disease patients. Among the three etiologies studied (hepatitis B, hepatitis C, and alcohol-related liver disease), no statistical differences in rates of osteoporosis of the lumbar spine were found, but significant differences were observed between hepatitis B and C in the femoral neck, with hepatitis C patients having lower BMD. Participants in the study were evaluated much earlier in the process of their liver disease, classified as Child-Pugh Category A (mildest form), whereas the participants in studies described previously were primarily class B or C (the most severe form) or a mix of all three severities. Studies that focus on more heterogeneous liver disease patients, those with ESLD, cholestatic liver disease (chronic cholestasis), and primary biliary cirrhosis have all typically shown higher rates of bone loss.

A number of reasons exist for the onset of osteoporosis in this population. Physiologically, although a number of osteoclastogenic proteins that promote bone loss are made in the liver, it appears their decline in both number and relative function as liver disease progresses is inadequate to offset decreased activity of bone-building osteoblasts. In liver disease, chronic use of alcohol, cholestasis, and decreased level of insulin growth factor 1 (IFG-1), which stimulates osteoblast function [160], has negative effects on bone that far outweigh any loss of osteoclastogenic cells. Hepatic osteodystrophy, an abnormal mineralization of the bony matrix, is similarly seen in advanced liver disease due primarily to prolonged vitamin D deficiency or cholestasis. However, osteodystrophy is far more common in renal than in hepatic disease.

Vitamin Deficiencies

Vitamins A, D, E, K are processed through the liver, so those with ESLD are likely to experience vitamin deficiencies, with prevalent vitamin D deficiency—up to 92.4 % in patients with chronic liver disease [161]—directly linked to osteoporosis. Overall, malnutrition is seen in up to 80 % of subjects with ESLD, making supplementation by means of dietary measures unlikely [162]. Prior research has demonstrated an inverse relationship between levels of serum vitamin D25OH and nonalcoholic fatty liver disease or nonalcoholic steatohepatitis [163, 164].

Poor nutritional intake, hepatic dysfunction, malabsorption, or a combination of all three conditions can potentially contribute. In those with cirrhosis and chronic cholestasis, inadequate delivery of bile slats due to liver disease contributes to inadequate absorption of fat soluble vitamins A, D, and others. In an effort to separate the factors responsible for vitamin D deficiency, Venu et al. [165] examined possible associations with Child-Pugh score, bilirubin levels, etiology of cirrhosis, and body mass index (BMI). While none of these factors were related to vitamin D deficiency, Child-Pugh class, bilirubin level, and elevated BMI correlated with vitamin A deficiency. Although the latter is not directly related to osteoporosis, it is associated with night blindness, thereby posing a hazard for fall risk in certain situations. Like any group of patients with osteoporosis, those with liver disease who fall unexpectedly are at increased risk of fractures.

Fractures and their Relation to BMD and to Liver Disease

In a meta-analysis by Bang et al. [166], articles reviewed demonstrated that alcoholic liver disease (ALD) conferred a relative risk (RR) of 1.944 for the development of bone fractures but only 0.849 for the development of osteoporosis. No significant difference in ALD patients and controls was found in terms of BMD, demonstrating that while there is a definite increased risk of fractures, the elevated fracture rate is potentially independent of BMD. Although RR for fractures in ALD patients was elevated regardless of whether the control group was a healthy age-matched population or an age-matched chronic nonalcoholic liver disease population, RR of osteoporosis was elevated only in comparison with healthy individuals but not with nonalcoholic liver disease patients.

The Krol et al. trial [157], discussed above, found that, at time of screening for transplantation, vertebral fractures were evident in 56 % of their study population, independent of the severity of bone loss. At the same time, they did identify large numbers of patients with bone loss: 19 % were osteoporotic at the lumbar spine and 10 % at the femoral neck, while 38 % were osteopenic at the lumbar spine and 42 % at the femoral neck. Based on their evidence, they conclude that the lack of association between BMD and fracture prevalence may be related to bone quality, as opposed to solely bone quantity, suggesting that routine spinal radiographs should be performed in advance of transplant. These steps are necessary to identify skeletal fragility as a baseline for evaluating if fracture risk persists, worsens, or improves after transplant.

Nonpharmacologic Treatment

Physical Therapy

Early mobilization with appropriate cardiopulmonary monitoring (including possible telemetry, spot checking oxygen saturations) is advised as part of the transition home following hospitalization for complications of ESLD, including pulmonary compromise from massive ascites, difficulties with fluid mobilization from the legs in conjunction with ascites, and increased fall risk. The goals are to optimize aerobic capacity and to increase musculoskeletal strength and endurance [167]. Therapists focus on basic skills including sit-to-stand transfers to alleviate swelling in the abdominal and pelvic region, short distance ambulation with the use of assistive devices as needed, and energy conservation techniques including paced breathing. If the patient had a borderline need for oxygen in the past (used only during upper respiratory infections or during activities of high energy demand), this need should be re-evaluated for potential increased oxygen demand.

Physical and occupational therapy, whether in acute care or in an inpatient rehab setting, should offer patients and families anticipatory guidance in the form of techniques to adjust mobility strategies relevant to fluid management, which will vary with diet and disease progression and remission. In the pretransplant phase, knowledge of such strategies is essential because patients need to make this adjustment just during the many months of waiting until a liver becomes available.

Vitamin D Supplementation

As discussed in the earlier renal section, paricalcitol (which is similar to calcitriol in that it acts subsequent to liver hydroxylation and provides the step otherwise responsible from the liver and kidney) or calcidio1 (25-hydroxy vitamin D) provides vitamin D in active forms without needing hydroxylation in the liver. Calcidiol lasts a long time in the body and is just one step short of the most active form of vitamin D [139]. A blood test to determine baseline vitamin D levels, in fact, measures 25-hydoxy vitamin D, the action of which is illustrated in Fig. 4.

Surgical Intervention in the Case of Fractures

Surgical intervention for multiple compression fractures has been proposed by Karatoprak et al. [168]. These authors described favorable outcomes in two patients who underwent vertebroplasty at 12 different levels overall, done in several stages. Although no 12-month follow-up complications were seen in these patients, this approach to treatment is one of last resort. As clinicians, it is hoped that we can address the issue of osteoporosis in ESLD prior to reaching this point in the disease.

Pharmacologic Treatment

Few studies on the use of pharmacologic treatment in patients with ESLD at the pre transplant stage have been conducted, with a small number of publications on estrogen and bisphosphonates. One trial of bisphosphonates via parenteral delivery offers an alternative to oral GI side effects or IV administration. Several of these studies have involved patients with primary biliary cirrhosis (PBC), a chronic disease that causes the small bile ducts in the liver to become inflamed and damaged, often leading to cirrhosis. It generally occurs between the ages of 30 and 65 with women more affected than men [169].

Estrogens

Given a 20–44 % prevalence of osteoporosis in patients with PBC [170], oral and transdermal estrogens have been used to prevent further bone loss. In an investigation by Menon et al. [171], the authors determined that estrogen replacement therapy, in a matched sample of 46 postmenopausal women, was safe and effective. The group of PBC subjects who received estrogen therapy had significantly better retention of BMD over a 4.8 year follow-up, relative to a control group of PBC patients not receiving estrogen.

Ormarsdottir and colleagues examined use of transdermal hormone replacement therapy (HRT) in postmenopausal women with PBC [172]. Although their sample size was small ($n = 18$, eight experimental and ten controls), they found few serious side effects to the liver. HRT with transdermal estrogen twice weekly in combination with daily vitamin D and calcium supplementation resulted in significantly higher BMD (3 %) at the lumbar spine L2–4 relative to a control group receiving only vitamin D and calcium. In the femoral neck, BMD declined by 0.6 % in the control group but increased by 1.7 in those receiving PRT.

Bisphosphonates

Although alendronate, etidronate, and raloxifene have been studied in PBC patients, few investigations exist for other agents in this class. Several trials involving oral alendronate alone and another comparing alendronate to etidronate have been conducted. Musialik and colleagues [173] studied the effect of alendronate on bone mass in patients with both PBC and established osteoporosis. After 12 months of 70 mg of alendronate weekly, they reported a 5 % increase in BMD at L2–4 of the lumbar spine, without biochemical evidence of downregulation of bone-building cells given normal osteocalcin. In what is reported to be the first randomized placebo controlled study of alendronate (70 mg weekly) in patients with PBC and *T*-scores less than −1.5, Zein et al. [174] demonstrated that, after one year, BMD increased significantly at both lumbar spine (10.5 %) and proximal femur (1.4 %), whereas the placebo groups showed a decline at both sites. In addition the study found no difference between the rates of compression fractures in the alendronate compared with placebo group, leading the authors to conclude that, given the BMD findings, a similar anti-fracture effect would be found with alendronate.

In a small investigation ($N = 32$ women) comparing the efficacy of alendronate versus etidronate on osteoporosis and fractures in patients with PBC [175]. Guanabens et al. [175] reported that both agents increased BMD at the spine and proximal femur but the magnitude of the improvement was significantly greater in those receiving alendronate. No significant differences occurred in fracture rates in the two groups; those on alendronate had no fractures in the spine and only two peripheral fractures. Neither liver function nor cholestasis was impaired in either treatment.

A somewhat larger study ($n = 42$) comparing alendronate to ibandronate produced more encouraging results [176]. Patients randomized to receive ibandronate showed a 5.7 % increase in BMD in the spine, compared with a 4.5 % increase in those on alendronate. Compliance with once-monthly dosing of ibandronate (150 mg) was greater than with weekly dosing of alendronate (70 mg). Ibandronate is known to have insignificant efficacy at the hip, a finding that was confirmed by this investigation: 2.0 % increase in hip BMD for alendronate versus 1.2 % for ibandronate. While the difference in increase from one agent to the other was not significant, the baseline and two-year follow-up for BMD in alendronate was statistically significant ($p=0.04$), as opposed to an insignificant difference for ibandronate. After two years, both groups demonstrated reduction of markers of bone resorption. As Angelo [177] observed in a commentary on this study, the duration of treatment and the follow-up was too short to permit an assessment of the efficacy of these bisphosphonates in reducing the number of fractures in PBC despite the fact that an increase in BMD should theoretically reduce fracture risk.

A recent report examined benefits of zoledronic acid, pamidronate, and ibandronate delivered parenterally, with nine of the 34 participants having a history of liver transplant [178]. Of the 34 subjects, the 17 who received pharmacologic intervention were divided into two groups with one group receiving ibandronate and pamidronate and the other receiving zoledronic acid; however, data did not permit analysis of one bisphosphonate versus another. In the 17 receiving treatment, eight patients (47 %) improved in lumbar spine BMD by 8.7 % and in proximal femur BMD by 0.8 %, but nine participants became slightly worse.

Other Agents

The selective estrogen reuptake inhibitor, raloxifene, has been used in a single pilot study of postmenopausal women with PBC. The seven subjects completing the 1-year trial of 60 mg/raloxifene/daily showed significant BMD increases of 2.7 % in lumbar spine density but not in the femoral neck [179]. Calcitonin inhibits bone resorption with subcutaneous, parenteral, or more convenient intranasal delivery. However in a 6-month trial of calcitonin given parenterally to patients with PBC, no statistical improvement was seen in the study group [180].

Future Considerations for Treatment

A 2011 Cochrane review [181] evaluated six large investigations involving agents for treatment of osteoporosis in primary biliary cirrhosis. While individual studies showed some promise for prevention and early treatment, bisphosphonates, in general, had no significant effect on BMD. The review cited the need for large-scale, randomized clinical trials on a number of agents used in pilot studies and specifically advised investigation of other agents not previously studied, such as denosumab, an alternative to bisphosphonate therapy. Used in patients undergoing dialysis or with chronic renal insufficiency, denosumab has the advantage of demonstrated safety in patients with hepatorenal syndrome.

The authors of the Cochrane review also addressed the need for additional studies of one of the most potent bisphosphonates, zoledronic acid, as well as anabolic agents such as teriparatide and strontium ranelate, although the latter carries a high risk of venous thromboembolism. As with many chronic and serious conditions associated with bone loss, there is inadequate time for patients to risk becoming a placebo in a clinical trial of two arms, with one receiving an actual drug for treatment and the other effectively receiving no medical intervention. Finally, additional studies need to examine outcome measures of fractures rather than BMD as a result of pharmacologic intervention. If the BMD is improved by any of the agents discussed above but the fracture rate remains the same, recommendations for their use will not be widely accepted.

References

1. Colon-Emeric C, O'Connell MB, Haney E. Osteoporosis piece of multi-morbidity puzzle in geriatric care. Mt Sinai J Med. 2011;78(4):515–26. doi:10.1002/msj.20269.
2. Stojanovic OI, Lazovic M, Lazovic M, Vuceljic M. Association between atherosclerosis and osteoporosis, the role of vitamin D. Arch Med Sci. 2011;7(2):179–88. doi:10.5114/aoms.2011.22066.
3. Brüggenjürgen B, Israel CW, Klesius AA, Ezzat N, Willich SN. Health services research in heart failure patients treated with a remote monitoring device in Germany—a retrospective database analysis in evaluating resource use. J Med Econ. 2012;15(4):737–45.
4. Schuiling KD, Robinia K, Nye R. Osteoporosis update. J Midwifery Womens Health. 2011;56(6):515–27. doi:10.1111/j.1542-2011.2011.00135.x.
5. Aluoch AO, Jessee R, Habal H, Garcia-Rosell M, Shah R, Reed G, et al. Heart failure as a risk factor for osteoporosis and fractures. Curr Osteoporos Rep. 2012;10(4):258–69. doi:10.1007/s11914-012-0115-2.
6. Nishio K, Mukae S, Aoki S, Itoh S, Konno N, Ozawa K, et al. Congestive heart failure is associated with the rate of bone loss. J Intern Med. 2003;253(4):439–46.
7. Shane E, Mancini D, Aaronson K, Silverberg SJ, Seibel MJ, Addesso V, et al. Bone mass, vitamin D deficiency, and hyperparathyroidism in congestive heart failure. Am J Med. 1997;103(3):197–207.
8. Dolgin M. Nomenclature and criteria for diagnosis of diseases of the heart and great vessels. Criteria Committee of the New York Heart Association. 9th ed. Boston: Little, Brown; 1994.
9. Zotos P, Terrovitis J, Karga E, Nanas S, Kaldara E, Chalazonitis A, et al. Osteoporosis in heart failure is associated with secondary hyperparathyroidism and has adverse prognostic implications. Circulation. 2010;21[Suppl Abstract] 13703.
10. Terrovitis J, Zotos P, Kaldara E, Diakos N, Tseliou E, Vakrou S, et al. Bone mass loss in chronic heart failure is associated with secondary hyperparathyroidism and has prognostic significance. Eur J Heart Fail. 2012;14(3):326–32. doi:10.1093/eurjhf/hfs002.
11. Hjortnaes J, Butcher J, Figueiredo JL, Riccio M, Kohler RH, Kozloff KM, et al. Arterial and aortic valve calcification inversely correlates with osteoporotic bone remodeling: a role for inflammation. Eur Heart J. 2010;31(16):1975–84.
12. Aksoy Y, Yagmur C, Tekin GO, Yagmur J, Topal E, Kekilli E, et al. Aortic valve calcification: association with bone mineral density and cardiovascular risk factors. Coron Artery Dis. 2005;16(6):379–83.
13. Boukhris R, Becker KL. Calcification of the aorta and osteoporosis. Aroentgenographic study. JAMA. 1972;219(10):1307–11.
14. Watson KE, Bostrom K, Ravindranath R, Lam T, Norton B, Demer L. TGF-beta 1 and 25-hydroxycholesterol stimulate osteoblast-like vascular cells to calcify. J Clin Invest. 1994;93(5):2106–13.
15. Schulz E, Arfai K, Liu X, Sayre J, Gilsanz V. Aortic calcification and the risk of osteoporosis and fractures. J Clin Endocrinol Metab. 2004;89(9):4246–52.

16. Bakhireva LN, Barrett-Connor EL, Laughlin GA, Kritz-Silverstein D. Differences in association of bone mineral density with coronary artery calcification in men and women: the Rancho Bernardo study. Menopause. 2005;12(6):691–8.
17. Barengolts EI, Berman M, Kukreja SC, Kousnetsova T, Lin C, Chomka EV. Osteoporosis and coronary atherosclerosis in asymptomatic postmenopausal women. Calcif Tissue Int. 1998;62(3):209–13.
18. Pfister R, Michaels G, Sharp SJ, Luben B, Wareham NJ, Khaw KT. Low bone mineral density predicts incident heart failure in men and women: the EPIC (European Prospective Investigation into Cancer and Nutrition)-Norfolk prospective study. JACC Heart Fail. 2014;2(4):380–9. doi:10.1016/j.jchf.2014.03.010.
19. Lyles KW, Colon-Emeric CS. Does low bone mineral density cause a broken heart? J Clin Heart Fail. 2014;2(4):390–1. doi:10.1016/j.jchf.2014.04.002.
20. Wawrzynska L, Tomkowski WZ, Przedlackl J, Hajduk B, Torbicki A. Changes in bone density during long-term administration of low molecular weight heparins or acenocoumarol for secondary prophylaxis of venous thromboembolism. Pathophysiol Haemost Thromb. 2003;33(2):64–7.
21. Jamal SA, Browner WS, Bauer DC, Cummings SR. Warfarin use and risk for osteoporosis in elderly. Study of osteoporotic fractures research group. Ann Intern Med. 1998;128(10):829–32.
22. Chang YS, Lee MD, Lee SK, Kim HM, Fitzpatrick LA. HMG CoA reductase inhibitors increase BMD in type 2 diabetes mellitus patients. J Clin Endocrinol Metab. 2000;85(3):1137–42.
23. Edwards CJ, Hart DJ, Spector TD. Oral statins and increased bone mineral density in postmenopausal women. Lancet. 2000;355(9222):2218–9.
24. Bauer DC, Mundy GR, Jamal SA, Black DM, Cauley JA, Harris F, et al. Statin use, bone mass and fracture: an analysis of two prospective studies. J Bone Miner Res. 1999;14 Suppl 1:S179.
25. Chan KA, Andrade DE, Boles M, Buist DS, Chase GA, Donahue JG, et al. Inhibitors of hydroxymethylglutaryl-coenzyme A reductase and risk of fracture among older women. Lancet. 2000;355(9222):2185–8.
26. Meier CR, Schlienger RG, Kraenzlin ME, Schlegel B, Jick H. HMG-CoA reductase inhibitors and the risk of fractures. JAMA. 2000;283(24):3205–10.
27. Wang PS, Solomon DH, Mogun H, Avorn J. HMG CoA reductase inhibitors and the risk of hip fractures in elderly patients. JAMA. 2000;283(24):3211–6.
28. Wang GJ, Chung KC, Shen WJ. Lipid clearing agents in steroid induced osteoporosis. J Formos Med Assoc. 2000;94(10):589–92.
29. Mundy G, Garret R, Harris S, Chan J, Chen D, Rossini G, et al. Stimulation of bone formation in vitro and in rodents by statins. Science. 1999;286(5446):1946–9.
30. Sirola J, Sirola J, Honkanen R, Kröger H, Jurvelin JS, Mäenpää P, Saarikoski S. Relation of statin use and bone loss: a prospective population-based cohort study in early postmenopausal women. Osteoporos Int. 2002;13(7):537–41.
31. LaCroix A, Cauley J, Pettinger M, Hsia J, Bauer DC, McGowan J, et al. Statin use, clinical fracture and bone mineral density in postmenopausal women: results from the women's health initiative observational study. Ann Intern Med. 2003;139(2):97–104.
32. Peña J, Aspberg S, MacFadyen J, Glynn RJ, Solomon DH, Ridker PM. Statin therapy and risk of fracture: results from the JUPITOR randomized clinical trial. JAMA Intern Med. 2015;175(2):171–7. doi:10.1001/jamainternmed.2014.6388.
33. Cockcroft JR, Pedersen ME. β-blockade: benefits beyond blood pressure reduction? J Clin Hypertens. 2012;14(2):112–20. doi:10.1111/j.1751-7176.2011.00553.x.
34. Sosa M, Saavedra P, Gómez de Tejada MJ, Mosquera J, Pérez-Cano R, Olmos JM, et al. β-blocker use is associated with fragility fractures in postmenopausal women with coronary heart disease. Aging Clin Exp Res. 2011;23(2):112–7. doi:10.3275/7041.
35. Ruths S, Bakken MS, Ranhoff AH, Hunskaar S, Engesaeter LB, Engeland A. Risk of hip fracture among older people using antihypertensive drugs: a nationwide cohort study. BMC Geriatr. 2015;15:1–10. doi:10.1186/s12877-015-0154-5.

36. Yang S, Nguyen ND, Eisman JA, Nguyen TV. Association between beta-blockers and fracture risk: a Bayesian meta-analysis. Bone. 2012;51(5):969–74. doi:10.1016/j.bone.2012.07.013.
37. Toulis KA, Hemming K, Stergianos S, Nirantharakumar K, Bilezikian JP. β -adrenergic receptor antagonists and fracture risk: a meta-analysis of selectivity, gender, and site-specific effects. Osteoporos Int. 2014;25(1):121–9. doi:10.1007/s00198-013-2498-z.
38. Rejnmark L, Vestergaard P, Mosekilde L. Treatment with beta blockers, ACE inhibitors, and calcium-channel blockers is associated with a reduced fracture risk: a nationwide case-control study. J Hypertens. 2006;24(3):581–9.
39. Shimizu H, Nakagami H, Osako MK, Hanayama R, Kunugiza Y, Kizawa T, et al. Angiotensin II accelerates osteoporosis by activating osteoclasts. FASEB J. 2008;22(7):2465–75. doi:10.1096/fj.07-098954.
40. Garcia Delgado I, Gil-Fraguas L, Robles E, Martinez G, Hawkins F. Clinical factors associated with bone mass loss previous to cardiac transplantation. Med Clin (Barc). 2000;114(20):761–4.
41. Dolgos S, Hartmann A, Isaksen GA, Simonsen S, Bjortuft O, Boberg KM, et al. Osteoporosis is a prevalent finding in patients with solid organ failure awaiting transplantation - a population based study. Clin Transplant. 2010;24(5):E145–52.
42. Kulak CA, Borba VZ, Kulak Jr J, Custodio MR. Osteoporosis after transplantation. Curr Osteoporos Rep. 2012;10(1):48–55.
43. Oz MC, Argenziano M, Catanese KA, Gardocki MT, Goldstein DJ, Ashton RC, et al. Bridge experience with long-term implantable left ventricular assist devices. Are they an alternative to transplantation? Circulation. 1997;95(7):1844–52.
44. Liang B, Feng Y. The association of low bone mineral density with clinically stable COPD. Endocrine. 2012;42(1):190–5.
45. Sheikh S, Gemma S, Patel A. Factors associated with low one mineral density in patients with cystic fibrosis. J Bone Miner Metab. 2015;33(2):180–5. doi:10.1007/s00774-014-0572-z.
46. Cystic Fibrosis Foundation, What is cystic fibrosis/about cystic fibrosis, https://www.cff.org/What-is-CF/About-Cystic-Fibrosis. Accessed 3 Feb 2016.
47. Lehouck A, Boonen S, Decramer M, Janssens W. COPD, bone metabolism, and osteoporosis. Chest. 2011;139(3):648–57. doi:10.1378/chest.10-1427.
48. Graat-Verboom L, Wouters EF, Smeenk FW, van den Borne BE, Lunde R, Spruit MA. Current status of research on osteoporosis in COPD: a systemic review. Eur Respir J. 2009;34(1):209–18.
49. Heron M. Deaths: leading causes for 2012. Nat Vital Stat Rep. 2015;64(10):1–93.
50. Qaseem A, Snow V, Shekelle P, Hopkins R, Forciea MA, Owens DK. Screening for osteoporosis in men: a clinical practice guideline from the American College of Physicians. Ann Intern Med. 2008;148(9):680–4.
51. Førli L, Mellbye OJ, Halse J, Bjørtuft O, Vatn M, Boe J. Cytokines, bone turnover markers and weight change in candidates for lung transplantation. Pulm Pharmacol Ther. 2008;21(1):188–95.
52. Silva DR, Coelho AC, Dumke A, Valentini JD, de Nunes JN, Stefani CL, et al. Osteoporosis prevalence and associated factors in patients with COPD: a cross-sectional study. Respir Care. 2011;56(7):961–8. doi:10.4187/respcare.01056.
53. Graat-Verboom L, van der Borne BE, Smeenk FW, Spruit MA, Wouters EF. Osteoporosis in COPD outpatients based on bone mineral density and vertebral fractures. J Bone Miner Res. 2011;26(3):561–8.
54. Graat-Verboom L, Spruit MA, van den Borne BE, Smeenk FW, Lunde R, Wouters EF, et al. Correlates of osteoporosis in chronic obstructive pulmonary disease: an underestimated systemic component. Respir Med. 2009;103(8):1143–51. doi:10.1016/j.rmed.2009.02.014.
55. Ferguson GT, Calverley PM, Anderson JA, Jenkins CR, Jones PW, Wilits LR, et al. Prevalence and progression of osteoporosis in patients with COPD: results from the TOwards a Revolution in COPD Health study. Chest. 2009;136(6):1456–65. doi:10.1378/chest.08-3016.

56. Sin DD, Man JP, Man SF. The risk of osteoporosis in Caucasian men and women with obstructive airways disease. Am J Med. 2003;114(1):10–4.
57. Iqbal F, Michaelson J, Thaler L, Rubin J, Roman J, Nanes MS. Declining bone mass in men with chronic pulmonary disease: contribution of glucocorticoid treatment, body mass index, and gonadal function. Chest. 1999;116(6):1616–24.
58. Sabit R, Bolton CE, Edwards PH, Pettit RJ, Evans WD, McEniery CM, et al. Arterial stiffness and osteoporosis in chronic obstructive pulmonary disease. Am J Respir Crit Care Med. 2007;175(12):1259–65.
59. Bolton CE, Ionescu AA, Shiels KM, Pettit RJ, Edwards PH, Stone MD, et al. Associated loss of fat-free mass and bone mineral density in chronic obstructive pulmonary disease. Am J Respir Crit Care Med. 2004;170(12):1286–93.
60. Jørgensen NR, Schwarz P, Holme I, Henriksen BM, Petersen LG, Backer V. The prevalence of osteoporosis in patients with chronic obstructive pulmonary disease: a cross sectional study. Respir Med. 2007;101(1):177–85.
61. Nuti R, Siviero P, Maggi S, Guglielmi G, Caffarelli C, Crepaldi G, Gonnelli S. Vertebral fractures in patients with chronic obstructive pulmonary disease: the EOLO Study. Osteoporos Int. 2009;20(5):989–98. doi:10.1007/s00198-008-0770-4.
62. Papaioannou A, Parkinson W, Ferko N, Probyn L, Ioannidis G, Jurriaans E, et al. Prevalence of vertebral fractures among patients with chronic obstructive pulmonary disease in Canada. Osteoporos Int. 2003;14(11):913–7.
63. McEvoy CE, Ensrud KE, Bender E, Genant HK, Yu W, Griffith JM, et al. Association between corticosteroid use and vertebral fractures in older men with chronic obstructive pulmonary disease. Am J Respir Crit Care Med. 1998;157(3):704–9.
64. Rabe KF, Hurd S, Anzueto A, Barnes PJ, Buist SA, Calverley P, et al. Global strategy for the diagnosis, management, and prevention of chronic obstructive pulmonary disease: GOLD executive summary. Am J Respir Crit Care Med. 2007;176(6):532–5.
65. van Staa TP, Leufkens HG, Cooper C. The epidemiology of corticosteroid-induced osteoporosis. Osteoporos Int. 2002;13(10):777–87.
66. Drummond MB, Dasenbrook EC, Pitz MW, Murphy DJ, Fan E. Inhaled corticosteroids in patients with stable chronic obstructive pulmonary disease: a systematic review and meta-analysis. JAMA. 2008;300:2407–16.
67. Jaramillo JD, Wilson C, Stinson DS, Lynch DA, Bowler RP, Lutz S, et al. Reduced bone density and vertebral fractures in smokers. Ann Am Thorac Soc. 2015;12(5):648–56. doi:10.1513/AnnalsATS.201412-591OC.
68. Loke YK, Cavallazzi R, Singh S. Risk of fractures with inhaled corticosteroids in COPD: systemic review and meta-analysis of randomised controlled trials and observational studies. Thorax. 2011;66(8):699–708. doi:10.1136/thx.2011.160028.
69. Panday K, Gona A, Humphrey MB. Medication induced osteoporosis: screening and treatment strategies. Ther Adv Musculoskelet Dis. 2014;6(5):185–202. doi:10.1177/1759720X14546350.
70. Tantucci C. COPD and osteoporosis: something more than a comorbidity. Endocrine. 2012;42(1):5–6. doi:10.1007/s12020-012-9686-z.
71. Rossini M, Gatti D, Adami S. Involvement of WNT/β-catenin signaling in the treatment of osteoporosis. Calcif Tissue Int. 2013;93(2):121–32. doi:10.1007/s00223-013-9749-z.
72. Kondo T, Kitazawa R, Maeda S, Kitazawa S. 1α,25 dihydroxyvitamin D3 rapidly regulates the mouse osteoprotegerin gene through dual pathways. J Bone Miner Res. 2004;19(9):1411–9.
73. Halfon M, Phan O, Teta D. Vitamin D: a review on its effects on muscle strength and the risk of fall and frailty. Biomed Res Intl. 2015. Article ID 953241:1–11. http://dx.doi.org/10.1155/2015/953241.
74. Bischoff-Ferrari HA, Dawson-Hughes B, Willett WC, Staehelin HB, Bazemore MG, Zee RY, et al. Effect of vitamin D on falls: a meta-analysis. JAMA. 2004;291(16):1999–2006.
75. Broe KE, Chen TC, Weinberg J, Bischoff-Ferrari HA, Holick MF, Kiel DP. A higher dose of vitamin D reduces the risk of falls in nursing home residents: a randomized, multiple-dose study. J Am Geriatr Soc. 2007;55(2):234–9.

76. Kim HC, Mofarrahi M, Hussain SN. Skeletal muscle dysfunction in patients with chronic obstructive pulmonary disease. Int J Chron Obstruct Pulmon Dis. 2008;3(4):637–58.
77. Mineo TC, Ambrogi V, Mineo D, Fabbri A, Fabbrini E, Massoud R. Bone mineral density improvement after lung volume reduction surgery for severe emphysema. Chest. 2005;127(6):1960–6.
78. Corhay JL, Dang DN, Van Cauwenberge H, Louis R. Pulmonary rehabilitation and COPD: providing patients a good environment for optimizing therapy. Int J Chron Obstruct Pulmon Dis. 2014;9:27–39. doi:10.2147/COPD.S52012.
79. Susiwala S. A detailed description on breathing exercises. http://www.slideshare.net/sharminsusiwala22/a-detailed-description-on-breathing-exercises. Accessed 13 Mar 2016.
80. Garritan SL. Physical therapy interventions for persons with chronic obstructive pulmonary disease. In: Bach JR, editor. Pulmonary rehabilitation: the obstruction and paralytic conditions. Philadelphia: Hanley and Belfus; 1996. p. 85–98.
81. Janssens W, Lehouck A, Carremans C, Bouillon R, Mathieu C, Decramer M. Vitamin D beyond bones in chronic obstructive pulmonary disease: time to act. Am J Respir Crit Care Med. 2009;179(8):630–6. doi:10.1164/rccm.200810-1576PP.
82. Garrod R, Lasserson T. Role of physiotherapy in the management of chronic lung diseases: an overview of systematic reviews. Respir Med. 2007;101(12):2429–36.
83. Camp PG, Appleton J, Reid WD. Quality of life after pulmonary rehabilitation: assessing change using quantitative and qualitative methods. Phys Ther. 2000;80(10):986–95.
84. American Lung Association. Nutrition guidelines. 2016. http://www.lung.org/lung-health-and-diseases/lung-disease-lookup/copd/living-with-copd/. Accessed 13 Feb 2016.
85. Borg GA. Psychophysical bases of perceived exertion. Med Sci Sports Exerc. 1982;14(5):377–81.
86. Smith BJ, Laslett LL, Pile KD, Phillips P, Phillipov G, Evans SM, et al. Randomized controlled trial of alendronate in airway disease and low bone mineral density. Chron Respir Dis. 2004;1(3):131–7.
87. Compston J. US and UK guidelines for glucocorticoid-induced osteoporosis: similarities and differences. Curr Rheumatol Rep. 2004;6(1):66–9.
88. Grossman JM, Gordon R, Ranganath VK, Deal C, Caplan L, Chen W, et al. American College of Rheumatology 2010 recommendations for the prevention and treatment of glucocorticoid-induced osteoporosis. Arthritis Care Res (Hoboken). 2010;62(11):1515–26. doi:10.1002/acr.20295.
89. LiPuma JJ. The changing microbial epidemiology in cystic fibrosis. Clin Microbiol Rev. 2010;23(2):299–323.
90. American Lung Association. Lung health and diseases: learn about cystic fibrosis. 2016. http://www.lung.org/lung-health-and-diseases/lung-disease-lookup/cystic-fibrosis/learn-about-cystic-fibrosis.html. Accessed 4 Mar 2016.
91. Spoonhower KA, David PB. Epidemiology of cystic fibrosis. Clin Chest Med. 2016;37(1):1–8.
92. Cystic Fibrosis Foundation. Cystic fibrosis foundation patient registry: annual data report, 2014. Cystic Fibrous Foundation. Bethesda, MD. 2015, p 73. Accessed 4 Mar 2016.
93. Gore AP, Kwon SH, Stenbit AE. A roadmap to the brittle bones of cystic fibrosis. J Osteoporos. 2011; 926045. http://dx.doi.org/10.4061/2011/926045.
94. Mischler EH, Chesney PJ, Chesney RW, Mazess RB. Demineralization in cystic fibrosis detected by direct photon absorptiometry. Am J Dis Child. 1979;133(6):632–5.
95. Conway SP, Morton AM, Oldroyd B, Truscott JG, White H, Smith AH, et al. Osteoporosis and osteopenia in adults and adolescents with cystic fibrosis: prevalence and associated factors. Thorax. 2000;55(9):798–804.
96. Aris RM, Ontjes DA, Buell HE, Blackwood AD, Lark RK, Caminiti M, et al. Abnormal bone turnover in cystic fibrosis adults. Osteoporos Int. 2002;13(2):151–7.
97. Aris RM, Renner JB, Winders AD, Buell HE, Riggs DB, Lester GE, et al. Increased rate of fractures and severe kyphosis: sequelae of living into adulthood with cystic fibrosis. Ann Intern Med. 1998;128(3):186–93.

98. Paccou J, Zeboulon N, Combescure C, Gossec L, Cortet B. The prevalence of osteoporosis, osteopenia, and fractures among adults with cystic fibrosis: systematic literature review with meta-analysis. Calcif Tissue Int. 2010;86:1–7. doi:10.1007/s00223-009-9316-9.
99. Goalski JL, Aris RM. In: Bush A, Bilton D, Hobson M, editors. Hudson and Geddes' cystic fibrosis. 4th ed. Boca Raton: CRC Press; 2016. p. 365.
100. Putnam MS, Baker JF, Ulner A, Herlyn K, Lapey A, Sicilian L, et al. Trends in bone mineral density in young adults with cystic fibrosis over a 15 year period. J Cyst Fibro. 2015;14:526–32. doi:10.1016/jcf.2015.01.011.
101. Stalvey MS, Clines GA. Cystic fibrosis-related bone disease: insights into a growing problem. Curr Opin Endocrinol Diabetes Obes. 2013;20(6):547–52. doi:10.1097/01.med.0000436191.87727.ec.
102. Henderson RC, Madsen CD. Bone density in children and adolescents with cystic fibrosis. J Pediatr. 1996;128(1):28–34.
103. Javier RM, Jacquot J. Bone disease in cystic fibrosis: what's new? Joint Bone Spine. 2011;78(5):445–50. doi:10.1016/jbspin.2010.11.015.
104. Teramoto S. Mechanism of osteoporosis in patients with cystic fibrosis. Thorax. 2000;55(5):439. doi:10.1136/thorax.55.5.43.
105. Morrell MR, Pilewski JM. Lung transplantation for cystic fibrosis. Clin Chest Med. 2016;37(1):127–38. doi:10.1016/j.ccm.2015.11.008.
106. Aris RM, Neuringer IP, Weiner MA, Egan TM, Ontjes D. Severe osteoporosis before and after lung transplantation. Chest. 1996;109(5):1176–83.
107. Dif F, Marty C, Baudoin C, de Vernejoul MC, Levi G. Severe osteoporosis in CFTE-null mice. Bone. 2004;35(3):595–603.
108. King SJ, Topliss DJ, Kotsimbos T, Nyulasi IB, Bailey M, Ebeling PR, et al. Reduced bone density in cystic fibrosis: delta F508 mutation is an independent risk factor. Eur Respir J. 2005;25(1):54–61.
109. Pashuck TD, Franz SE, Altman MK, Wasserfall CH, Atkinson MA, Wronski TJ, et al. Murine model for cystic fibrosis bone disease demonstrates osteopenia and sex-related differences in bone formation. Pediatr Res. 2009;65(3):311–6. doi:10.1203/PDR.0b013e3181961e80.
110. Shead EF, Haworth CS, Condliffe AM, McKeon DJ, Scott MA, Compston JE. Cystic fibrosis transmembrane conductance regulator (CFTR) is expressed in human bones. Thorax. 2007;62(7):650–1.
111. Aris RM, Merkel PA, Bachrach LK, Borowitz DS, Boyle MP, Elkin SL, et al. Guide to bone health and disease in cystic fibrosis. J Clin Endocrinol Metab. 2005;90(3):1888–96.
112. Tangpricha V, Kelly A, Stephenson A, Maguiness K, Enders J, Robinson KA, et al. An update on the screening, diagnosis, management, and treatment of vitamin D deficiency in individuals with cystic fibrosis: evidence-based recommendation from the Cystic Fibrosis Foundation. J Clin Endocrinol Metab. 2012;94(4):1082–93. doi:10.1210/jc.2011-3050.
113. Nicolaidou P, Stavrinadis I, Loukou I, Papadopoulou A, Georgouli H, Douros K, et al. The effect of vitamin K supplementation on biochemical markers of bone formation in children and adolescents with cystic fibrosis. Eur J Pediatr. 2006;165(8):540–5.
114. Hind K, Truscott JG, Conway SP. Exercise during childhood and adolescence: a prophylaxis against cystic fibrosis-related low BMD? Exercise for bone health in children with cystic fibrosis. J Cyst Fibros. 2008;7(4):270–6. doi:10.1016/j/jcf.2008.02.001.
115. Conwell LS, Chang AB. Bisphosphonates for osteoporosis in people with cystic fibrosis. Cochrane Database Syst Rev. 2009;4(4):CD002010. doi:10.1002/14651858.CD002010.pub2.
116. Bianchi ML, Colombo C, Assael BM, Dubini A, Lombardo M, Quattrucci S, et al. Treatment of low bone density in young people with cystic fibrosis: a multicentre, prospective open-label observational study of calcium and calcifediol followed by a randomised placebo-controlled trial of alendronate. Lancet Respir Med. 2013;1(5):377–85.
117. Boyle MP. Update on maintaining bone health in cystic fibrosis. Curr Opin Pulm Med. 2006;12:453–8.

118. Thaker V, Haagensen, Carter B, Fedorowixcz Z, Houston BW. Recombinant growth hormone therapy for cystic fibrosis in children and young adults. Cochrane Database Syst Rev. 2013;6(5):CD008901. doi:10.1002/14651858.CF008901.pub3.
119. Cystic Fibrosis Foundation. CF Patient Registry. 2016. https://www.cff.org/Our-Research/CF-Patient-Registry.
120. Mogazel Jr LJ, Dunitz J, Marrow LC, Hazle LA. Improving chronic care delivery and outcomes: the impact of the cystic fibrosis care center network. BMJ Qual Saf. 2014;23 Suppl 1:13–8.
121. Hruska KA, Siefert M. Pathophysiology of chronic kidney disease mineral bone disorder (CKD-MBS). In: Rosen CJ, editor. Primer on the metabolic bone diseases and disorders of mineral netabolism. 8th ed. Ames: Wiley Blackwell; 2013. p. 632–9.
122. Isakova T, Wahl P, Vargas GS, Gutierrez OM, Scialla J, Xie H, et al. Fibroblast growth factor 23 is elevated before parathyroid hormone and phosphate in chronic kidney disease. Kidney Int. 2011;79(12):1370–8.
123. Rodríguez M, López I, Muñoz J, Aguilera-Tejero E, Yolanda Almaden Y. FGF 23 and mineral metabolism: implications for CKD-MBD. Nefrologia. 2012;32(3):275–8. doi:10.3265/Nefrologia.pre2012.Mar.11415.
124. Bellorin-Font E, Ambrosoni P, Carlini RG, Carvalho AB, Correa-Rotter R, Cueto-Manzano A, et al. Clinical practice guidelines for the prevention, diagnosis, evaluation, and treatment of mineral and bone disorders in chronic kidney disease (CKD-MBD) in adults. Nefrologia. 2013;33 Suppl 1:1–28.
125. Data obtained from Quest Diagnostics, Dept of Billing, Madison NJ 07940. Accessed 7 Aug 2015.
126. Langton CM, Palmer SB, Porter RW. The measurement of broadband ultrasonic attenuation in cancellous bone. Eng Med. 1984;13(2):89–91.
127. Taal MW, Mawsud T, Green D, Cassidy MJ. Risk factors for reduced bone density in haemodialysis patients. Nephrol Dial Transplant. 1999;14(8):1922–8.
128. Gordon PL, Frassetto LA. Management of osteoporosis in CKD stages 3 to 5. Am J Kidney Dis. 2010;55(5):941–56.
129. Stehman-Breen CO, Sherrard D, Walker A, Sadler R, Alem A, Lindberg J. Racial differences in bone mineral density and bone loss among end-stage renal disease patients. Am J Kidney Dis. 1999;33(5):941–6.
130. Alem AM, Sherrard DJ, Gillen DL, Weiss NS, Beresford SA, Heckbert SR, et al. Increased risk of hip fracture among patients with end-stage renal disease. Kidney Int. 2000;58(1):396–9.
131. Coco M, Rush H. Increased incidence of hip fractures in dialysis patients with low serum parathyroid hormone. Am J Kidney Dis. 2000;36(6):1115–21.
132. Stehman-Breen C. Bone mineral density measurements in dialysis patients. Semin Dial. 2001;14(3):228–9.
133. Mathew S, Tustison KS, Sugatani T, Chaudhary LR, Rifas L, Hruska KA. The mechanism of phosphorus as a cardiovascular risk tor in chronic kidney disease. J Am Soc Nephrol. 2008;19(6):1092–105.
134. Kasiske BL, Zeier MG, Chapman JR, Craig JC, Ekberg H, Garvey CA, et al. KDIGO clinical practice guideline for the diagnosis, evaluation, prevention, and treatment of chronic kidney disease-mineral and bone disorder (CKD-MBD). Kidney Int Suppl. 2009;113:S1–130. doi:10.1038/ki.2009.188.
135. Alshayeb HA, Quarles LD. Treatment of chronic kidney disease-metabolic bone disorder (CKD-MBD). In: Rosen CJ, editor. Primer on the metabolic bone diseases and mineral metabolism. 8th ed. Ames: Wiley; 2013. p. 640–50.
136. Messa P, Macario F, Yaqoob M, et al. The OPTIMA study: assessing a new cinacalcet (Sensipar/Mimpara) treatment algorithm for secondary hyperparathyroidism. Clin J Am Soc Nephrol. 2008;3(1):36–45.

137. Lafage MH, Combe C, Fournier A, Aparicio M. Ketodiet, physiological calcium intake and native vitamin D improve renal osteodystrophy. Kidney Int. 1992;42(5):1217–25.
138. Lafage-Proust M-H, Combe C, Barthe N, Aparicio M. Bone mass and dynamic parathyroid function according to bone histology in nondialyzed uremic patients after long-term protein and phosphorus restriction. U Clin Endocrinol Metab. 1999;84(2):512–9.
139. Lindberg JS. New vitamin D analogs. Semin Dial. 2001;14:229–30. doi:10.1046/j.1525-139X.2001.00057-3.x.
140. Slatopolsky E, Finch J, Ritter C, Denda M, Morrissey J, Brown A, et al. A new analog of calcitriol, 19-nor-1,25-(OH)2D2, suppresses parathyroid hormone secretion in uremic rats in the absence of hypercalcemia. Am J Kidney Dis. 1995;26(5):852–60.
141. Martin KJ, Gonzalez EA, Gellens M, Hamm LL, Abboud H, Lindberg J. 19-Nor-1-alpha-25--dihydroxyvitamin D2 (Paricalcitol) safely and effectively reduces the levels of intact parathyroid hormone in patients on hemodialysis. J Am Soc Nephrol. 1998;9(8):1427–32.
142. Coburn JW, Tan AU, Levine BS, Mazess RB, Kyllo DM, Knutson JC, et al. 1 alpha-hydroxy-vitamin D2: a new look at an 'old' compound. Nephrol Dial Transplant. 1996;11 Suppl 3:153–7.
143. Frazao JM, Chesney RW, Coburn JW. Intermittent oral 1-alpha-hydroxyvitamin D2 is effective and safe for the suppression of secondary hyperparathyroidism in hemodialysis patients. 1alphaD2 Study Group. Nephrol Dial Transplant. 1998;13 Suppl 3:68–72.
144. Tan AU, Levine BS, Mazess RB, Kyllo DM, Bishop CW, Knutson JC, et al. Effective suppression of parathyroid hormone by 1 alpha-hydroxy-vitamin D2 in hemodialysis patients with moderate to severe secondary hyperparathyroidism. Kidney Int. 1997;51(1):317–23.
145. Matuszkiewicz-Rowinska J, Skorzewska K, Radowicki S, Sokalski A, Przedlacki J, Niemczk S, et al. The benefits of hormone replacement therapy in pre-menopausal women with oestrogen deficiency on haemodialysis. Nephrol Dial Transplant. 1999;14(5):1238–43.
146. Hernandez E, Valera R, Alonzo E, et al. Effects of raloxifene on bone metabolism and serum lipids in postmenopausal women on chronic hemodialysis. Kidney Int. 2003;63(6):2269–74.
147. Weisinger JR, Heilberg-Pfeferman I, Hernandez E, Carlini R, Bellorin-Font E. Selective estrogen receptor modulators in chronic renal failure. Kidney Int Suppl. 2003;85:S62–5.
148. Morello KC, Wurz GT, DeGregorio MW. Pharmacokinetics of selective estrogen receptor modulators. Clin Pharmacokinet. 2003;42(4):361–72.
149. Cremers SCLM, Pillai GC, Papapoulos SE. Pharmacokinetics/ Pharmacodynamics of bisphosphonates: use for optimization of intermittent therapy for osteoporosis. Clin Pharmacokinet. 2005;44(6):551–70.
150. Perazella MA, Markowitz GS. Bisphosphonate nephrotoxicity. Kidney Int. 2008;74(11):1385–93.
151. Boonen S, Sellmeyer DE, Lippuner K, Orlov-Morozov A, Adams K, Messenbrink P. Renal safety of annual zoledronic acid infusions in osteoporotic postmenopausal women. Kidney Int. 2008;74(5):641–8.
152. Bergner R, Henrich D, Hoffmann M, Schmidt-Gayk H, Lenz T, Upperkamp M. Treatment of reduced bone density with ibandronate in dialysis patients. J Nephrol. 2008;21(4):510–6.
153. Jamal SA, Bauer DC, Ensrud KE, Cauley JA, Hochberg M, Ishani A, et al. Alendronate treatment in women with normal to severely impaired renal function: an analysis of the fracture intervention trial. J Bone Min Res. 2007;22(4):503–8.
154. Miller PD, Roux C, Boonen S, Barton IP, Dunlop LE, Burgio DE. Safety and efficacy of risedronate in patients with age-related reduced renal function as estimated by the Cockcroft and Gault method: a pooled analysis of nine clinical trials. J Bone Min Res. 2005;20(12):2105–15.
155. Department of Transplant Surgery, University of California, San Francisco. Cirrhosis and end-stage liver disease (ESLD). 2015. http://www.transplant.surgery.ucsf.edu/conditions-procedures/cirrhosis.aspx. Accessed 25 Feb 2015.
156. U.S. Department of Health and Human Services, Organ Procurement and Transplantation Network. Facts about transplantation in the United States. 2016. http://aasld.org/sties/default/files/Weekly%20Fact%20Sheet%2019FEB2016.pdf.

157. Krol CG, Dekkers OM, Kroon HM, Rabelink TJ, van Hoek B, Hamdy NA. No association between BMD and prevalent vertebral fractures in liver transplant recipients at time of screening before transplantation. J Clin Endocrinol Metab. 2014;99(10):3677–85.
158. Guanabens N, Monegal A, Muxi A, Martinez-Ferrer A, Reyes R, Caballeria J, et al. Patients with cirrhosis and ascites have false values of bone density.: implications for the diagnosis of osteoporosis. Osteoporos Int. 2012;23(4):1481–7.
159. Alcade-Vargas A, Pascasio Acevedo JM, Gutierrez-Domingo I, Garcia-Jimenez R, Sousa Martin JM, Ferrier Rios MT, et al. Prevalence and characteristics of bone disease in cirrhotic patients under evaluation for liver transplantation. Transp Proceed. 2012;44(6):1496–8.
160. Mahmoudi A, Sellier N, Reboul-Marty J, Chales G, Lalatonne Y, Bourcier V, et al. Bone mineral density assessed by dual-energy X-ray absorptiometry in patients with viral or alcoholic compensated cirrhosis: a prospective study. Clin Res Hepatol Gastroenterol. 2011;35(11):731–7.
161. Nair S. Vitamin D, deficiency and liver disease. Gastroenterol Hepatol. 2010;6(8):491–3.
162. Kalaitzakis E, Simren M, Olsson R, Henfridsson P, Hugosson I, Bengtsson M, et al. Gastrointestinal symptoms in patients with liver cirrhosis: associations with nutritional status and health-related quality of life. Scand J Gastroenterol. 2006;419(12):1464–72.
163. Wang X, Li W, Zhang Y, Yang Y, Qin G. Association between vitamin D and non-alcoholic fatty liver disease /non-alcoholic steatohepatitis: results from a meta-analysis. Int J Clin Exp Med. 2015;8(10):17221–34.
164. Nelson JE, Roth CL, Wilson LA, Yates KP, Aouizerat B, Morgan-Stevenson V, et al. Vitamin D deficiency is associated with increased risk of non-alcoholic steatohepatitis in adults with nonalcoholic fatty liver disease: possible role for MAPK and NF-kβ. Am J Gastroenterol. 2016;111(6):852–63. doi:10.1038/ajg.2016.51.
165. Venu M, Martin E, Saeian K, Gawrieh ES. High prevalence of vitamin A and D deficiency in patients evaluated for liver transplantation. Liver Transpl. 2014;19(6):627–33.
166. Bang CS, Shin IS, Lee SW, Kim JB, Balk GH, Suk KT, et al. Osteoporosis and bone fractures in alcoholic liver disease: a meta-analysis. World J Gastroenterol. 2015;21(13):4035–47.
167. Yadav A, Carey EJ. Osteoporosis in chronic liver disease. Nutr Clin Pract. 2013;28(1):52–64.
168. Karatoprak O, Camurdan K, Ozturk, Ganiyusufoglu K, Aydogan M, Hamzaoglu A. Multiple-level cement vertebroplasty in patients with vertebral compression fractures from osteodystrophy in chronic liver disease. Acta Orthop Belg. 2008;74(4):566–8.
169. U.S. Department of Health and Human Services, National Institute of Diabetes and Digestive and Kidney Diseases. Primary biliary cirrhosis. 2014. http://www.nidk.nih.gov/health-information/health-topics/liver-disease/primary-biliary-cirrhosis/Pages/facts.aspx,. Accessed 25 Feb 2015.
170. Raszeja-Wyszomirska J, Miazgowski T. Osteoporosis in primary biliary cirrhosis of the liver. Prz Gastroenterol. 2014;9(2):82–7.
171. Menon KVN, Angulo P, Boe GM, Lindor KD. Safety and efficacy of estrogen therapy in preventing bone loss in primary biliary cirrhosis. Am J Gastroenterol. 2003;98(4):889–92.
172. Ormarsdottir S, Mallmin H, Naessen T, Petren-Mallmin M, Broome U, Hultcrantz R, et al. An open, randomized, controlled study of transdermal hormone replacement therapy on the rate of bone loss in primary biliary cirrhosis. J Intern Med. 2004;256(1):63–9.
173. Musialik J, Petelenz M, Gonciarz Z. Effects of alendronate on bone mass in patients with primary biliary cirrhosis and osteoporosis: preliminary results after one year. Scand J Gastroenterol. 2005;40(7):873–4.
174. Zein CO, Jorgensen RA, Clarke B, Wenger D, Keach JC, Angulo P. Alendronate improves bone mineral density in primary biliary cirrhosis: a randomized placebo-controlled trial. Hepatology. 2005;42(4):762–71.
175. Guanabens N, Pares A, Ros I, Alvarez L, Pons F, Caballeria L, et al. Alendronate is more effective than etidronate for increasing bone mass in osteopenic patients with primary biliary cirrhosis. Am J Gastroenterol. 2003;98(10):2268–74.
176. Guanabens N, Monegal A, Cerda D, Muxi A, Gifra L, Perls P, et al. Randomized trial comparing monthly ibandronate and weekly alendronate for osteoporosis in patients with primary biliary cirrhosis. Hepatology. 2013;58(6):2070–8.

177. Angelo P. Strengthening the bones in primary biliary cirrhosis. Hepatology. 2013;58(6): 1871–3.
178. Treeprasertsuk S, Silveira MG, Petz JL, Lindor KD. Parenteral bisphosphonates for osteoporosis in patients with primary biliary cirrhosis. Am J Therap. 2011;18(5):375–81.
179. Levy C, Harnois DM, Angulo P, Jorgensen R, Lindor KD. Raloxifene improves bone mass in osteopenic women with primary biliary cirrhosis: results of a pilot study. Liver Int. 2005;25(1):117–21.
180. Camisasca M, Crosignani A, Baltezzati PM, Albisetti W, Grandinetti G, Pietrogrande L, et al. Parenteral calcitonin for metabolic bone disease associated with primary biliary cirrhosis. Hepatology. 1994;2(3):633–7.
181. Rudic JS, Giljaca V, Krstic MN, Bjelakovic G, Glud C. Bisphosphonates for osteoporosis in primary biliary cirrhosis. Cochrane Database Syst Rev. 2011;(12):CD009144. doi:10.1002/14651858. CD009144. pub 2.

Chapter 15
Osteoporosis as a Complication of Transplant Medicine

Christina V. Oleson and Amanda B. Morina

Solid organ transplantation is increasingly available in many westernized nations for end-stage cardiac, pulmonary, liver, and kidney disease. The number of overall organ transplants is increasing as is the number of transplant survivors, raising concerns about complications that develop in the posttransplant stage, notably osteoporosis and fractures. Bone loss after transplantation is a combined result of compromised bone density prior to transplantation, poor nutrition before and after receiving a new organ, hypogonadrotrophic hypogonadism developing before or after surgery, and medications prescribed to address chronic health conditions associated with organ failure, including loop diuretics and heparin-based products. Some of these factors, combined with the negative effects of immunosuppressive medications, put patients at a heightened risk for bone loss and new fractures. Increasing attention has been given to evaluating and optimizing bone density prior to organ transplant, but as the prior chapter noted, attention to this critical issue often comes too late, long after bone loss has begun. This chapter considers the epidemiology of osteoporosis following solid organ transplantation as well as nonpharmacologic and pharmacologic interventions administered at the time of and following transplant which are specifically aimed at preventing further bone loss while potentially increasing bone density.

General Mechanisms of Bone Loss After Organ Transplantation

Kulak et al. [1] divide the process of bone loss into two phases: the first six months after organ transplantation constitute the *early* phase, and the subsequent year (approximately 6–18 months following transplant) represents the *later* phase. Steroids (glucocorticoids) at their highest doses, administered immediately following receipt of a new organ, inhibit osteoblast function as evidenced by decreased

C.V. Oleson, *Osteoporosis Rehabilitation*, DOI 10.1007/978-3-319-45084-1_15

serum osteocalcin levels, while they simultaneously increase osteoclastogenesis, thereby creating an environment that favors bone breakdown over bone formation. Glucocorticoid doses, often 0.5 mg/kg/day for the first month and then 5 mg/day for 2–6 months following transplant, also disrupt the hypothalamic–pituitary adrenal axis in such a way as to decrease levels of sex hormones that assist in building bone [2]. Moreover, glucocorticoids inhibit intestinal calcium absorption as well as renal transport of calcium, both of which indirectly result in increased levels of PTH.

Immunosuppressive agents are central to survival of the transplanted organ in its new environment. Calcineurin inhibitors, specifically cyclosporine A and tacrolimus, are nephrotoxic. Detrimental to the bone in the same manner as glucocorticoid agents, they are often used in liver and cardiac transplant but are also administered after other types of transplants [3, 4]. Of the two agents, cyclosporine A has more commonly been associated with lower bone density and higher fracture rates than has tacrolimus [5]. These factors contributing to posttransplantation bone loss are influential in varying degrees, depending on the particular organ being transplanted. Four of the most frequent organ transplants—cardiac, lung, liver, and kidney—will be considered in this chapter.

Cardiac Transplant

While the number of transplants is increasing worldwide, organ availability, especially for those needing a heart transplant, remains scarce. An increasing number of patients opt to undergo an intermediate procedure by inserting a left ventricular assistive device (LVAD) [6]. The implantation of such a device is challenging, and many recipients have difficulties not only in achieving desired anticoagulation levels but also in dealing with such adverse effects as gastrointestinal bleeding, orthostatic hypotension, and physical debility that limits weight-bearing activities and general mobility. Patients who ultimately undergo heart transplantation after first receiving an LVAD have additional osteoporotic risk factors, including prolonged use of anticoagulants and high-dose proton pump inhibitors as well as nutritional compromise. Indeed, this group may have even more risk factors for osteoporosis than patients who receive a transplant directly, due to the use of the above medications for potentially an indefinite period of time.

Bone Loss and Osteoporosis (Posttranplant Immunosuppression)

Following cardiac transplant, patients experience increased rates of rapid bone loss in the spine and hip, particularly in the femoral neck. At the same time, osteoporosis may already exist prior to transplant: According to Shane et al., osteopenia or osteoporosis, as defined by the World Health Organization criteria, is present in approximately half of patients awaiting cardiac transplant, despite relatively normal mean

T- and *Z*-scores [7]. In the six months following cardiac transplant, the rate of bone loss in the lumbar spine for patients with or without preexisting osteoporosis ranges between 6 and 10 %. Bone density declines by 6–11 % in the femoral neck during the same time interval [8]. Some studies suggest no further decline in the lumbar spine occurs beyond six months, but losses in the hip persist up to the end of the first year; there is limited evidence that partial recovery of lumbar spine BMD may take place in later years [9]. In a population of 41 cardiac transplant patients, Chou et al. found that 49 % were osteopenic and 17 % were osteoporotic [10]. Comparing two locations of common bone loss after a minimum of two years follow-up, the authors reported that 66 % of patients had either osteopenia or osteoporosis of the femoral neck and 26 % had one of these conditions in the lumbar spine. Osteoporosis can also exist in survivors of adolescent cardiac transplant as a result of not only preexisting osteoporosis and immunosuppressive therapy but also renal insufficiency, secondary hyperparathyroidism, and increased bone turnover [11].

Reduction in osteocalcin, a marker of bone formation, is found immediately following transplantation and continues to rise for the first year. In addition, levels of urinary telopeptides that reflect bone resorption are elevated shortly after transplantation but start to normalize after six months [12].

Fractures

The risk of vertebral fractures ranges from 22 to 35 % in the first three years after cardiac transplantation [2], with the percentage and timing of the fractures varying depending on the trial. A prospective study by Shane et al. [13] found that despite calcium and vitamin D supplementation, 36 % (7 women and 10 men) of 47 subjects sustained a fracture following cardiac transplantation; 85 % of this number did so in the first six months, with the highest risk found among those with low hip BMD prior to transplant. Similar trends for fracture risk in transplant recipients with pretransplant BMD below the fracture threshold were identified by Lee et al. [14] and Chou et al. [10]. These findings were supported by a European investigation five years later [15] that showed a 27 % incidence of vertebral fractures in the first two years after transplant among a group of 105 patients. During the investigation's 7-year course, 33 % of subjects had vertebral fractures, and of those, two-thirds had multiple vertebral fractures. In an analysis of femoral neck fractures [13], only 4 % of patients experienced a fracture, all due to falls.

Treatment Options

Physical Therapy

Resistive exercises and other forms of weight-bearing exercise are helpful in maintaining overall mobility and bone density following LVAD implantation [16]. Physicians must take advantage of any therapy possible to keep the bones and muscles of these patients optimized should they require future medical treatments. Instituted in the early postoperative phase, a 2015 study of the effect of the exercise training phase in 12 patients with LVAD devices has demonstrated improved functional capacity, albeit in a small number of subjects [17]. The ability to walk on a treadmill continuously for six minutes was a key goal, followed by an increase in the treadmill's speed to improve aerobic capacity. Subjects were necessarily limited by the need to carry the 2–2.5 kg batteries and controller, emphasizing the importance of close monitoring. Nonetheless, the researchers believe that the ability to achieve this objective by the time of discharge augurs well for adaptation to the daily needs of the posttransplant patient.

With regard to those who have undergone a full cardiac transplant, resistive training has been shown to maintain and, in some instances, restore bone mineral density losses following surgery. Braith and colleagues compared the 6-month outcomes of eight patients who underwent standard postoperative care, including a walking program, with another eight who performed structured resistance exercises (lumbar extension, duo decline chest press, and various other core muscle strengthening regimens); each group began two months after transplant and concluded six months posttransplant [18]. At two months posttransplant, both control and exercise groups demonstrated significant loss of bone density in the lumbar spine and femoral neck, relative to their baseline measurements immediately after surgery. In the resistance training group, BMD of the lumbar spine returned to within 1.9 % of immediate posttransplant levels, while the femoral neck improved to within 3.6 % of the original baseline level. By contrast, the control group saw no improvement in BMD between the 2-month and 6-month postoperative DXA scans.

Medications Alone and with Activity-Based Therapies

Over the last decade, combination therapies involving resistance training and alendronate or calcitonin have been investigated. Braith and colleagues performed a variant on the study described above by combining calcitonin and resistance exercises [19]. Six months of calcitonin therapy, initiated 48 h after transplant, was were compared with six months calcitonin therapy combined with resistance exercises beginning two months after transplant, a time when more aggressive activity is considered safe after sternotomy [20]. Although both groups lost 10–11 % of BMD in the first two months, femoral BMD in the calcitonin-alone group declined by 3.3 % at eight months post surgery, but BMD was maintained in the combined therapy cohort at the pretransplant BMD level. For the lumbar spine (L2 and L3), BMD in the group with calcitonin alone declined by 16.9 % eight months after transplant but only by 5 % in the mechanical loading group. Because both groups lost BMD early after transplant, it is unclear if the resistance group would have returned to baseline had the study extended further; however, once resistance training was permitted in the combination therapy group, subjects showed steady improvement. Although this study was limited by a small number of participants, it showed early promise of the value of physical exercise after transplant.

Alendronate has been examined in a similar manner by Braith et al. in a 2003 study, again combining resistance training with pharmacologic agents aimed to reduce bone loss [21]. Twenty-five participants were divided into three groups: The first was administered 10 mg daily alendronate beginning two months after surgery and the second received the same alendronate protocol but also participated in resistance training exercises (1–2 days/week). The third group was given no pharmacologic intervention or resistance exercises but did receive standard-of-care activities, including a walking program. DXA scans were performed at baseline, two months posttransplant, and eight months posttransplant. Results found that all three groups lost significant amounts of total body skeletal mass two months posttransplant (before interventions began) and showed regional bone losses of 5–6 % in the femoral neck and 11.2–12.5 % in the lumbar spine. While the total body BMD declined between months two (by 5.1 %) and eight (by 6.5 %) in the group receiving no pharmacologic intervention, the total body BMD loss of 5.3 % in the alendronate-only group at two months (prior to starting the drug) remained steady, neither improving nor declining by the end of the study. But when alendronate was combined with resistance training, the 5.6 % loss of BMD seen two months into the study had improved to a much smaller loss from baseline BMD of only 2.1 % by the end of the study, eight months following transplant.

In the lumbar spine, similar trends were found, except the decline at two months after transplant was in a significantly greater range of 12 %. Treatment with alendronate alone, given between months 2 and 8, only brought the BMD value up to a loss of 10.5 %. In contrast, patients receiving alendronate plus physical training involving lumbar extension exercises regained the majority of the lost bone, coming to within 3.4 % of the pretransplant BMD value.

Trials involving only bisphosphonates in the treatment of osteoporosis posttransplant have also been performed, with results measured over a longer time period. Again the studies were small and involved primarily pamidronate. For example, Shane et al. [13] examined the effect of a single intravenous infusion of pamidronate (60 mg) within two weeks of transplant, followed by oral etidronate and oral calcitriol in 18 patients compared with 52 subjects receiving only calcium and vitamin D supplementation. At 12 months after transplant, the pamidronate-etidronate therapy group experienced virtually no lumbar spine bone loss (0.2 %) in contrast to a significant decline in those without bisphosphonate therapy (6.8 %). Femoral neck fell by only 2.7 % in the therapy patients in contrast to 10.6 % in the non-therapy group. Whereas the therapy subjects experienced only three vertebral fractures, 17 patients in the non-bisphosphonate therapy group had 30 vertebral fractures, one hip fracture, and three episodes of rib fractures. Another trial by Krieg et al. [22] focused on the impact of a 3-year treatment of quarterly injections of 6 mg pamidronate; at the end point, the increase in BMD in the lumbar spine reached 18.3 % (14.3 % compared with BMD at the time of surgery), while bone loss in the femoral neck, which declined in the first posttransplant year by 3.4 %, completely recovered.

In cases where heart transplant patients cannot tolerate bisphosphonate treatment due to impaired renal function, denosumab may represent a viable alternative. A study of denosumab therapy in 46 kidney, liver, and heart transplant patients over a mean duration of 1.25 years indicates a mean increase of 9.8 % in the lumbar spine

BMD in 97 % of patients and a mean increase of 8.0 % BMD in the hip in all patients [23]. However, these are very preliminary findings, and more extensive research focused solely on heart transplant patients is needed.

These various therapies appear to be valuable in preserving bone density in heart transplant patients. Yet, as with many other conditions, the emphasis is on preserving the overall health of the organ, limiting rejection episodes, and improving cardiac conditioning. Preventing bone fractures and excess rapid bone loss that could lead to hypercalcemia are essential components of an overall plan. In the early postoperative phase, coordination of care among physiatrists, rehabilitation therapists, cardiologists, and transplant surgeons remains essential to achieve optimal health of the patient in the months and years following cardiac transplant.

Lung Transplant

Osteoporosis Prior to Transplant

Although far fewer transplants occur in lung disease than in heart, liver, and kidney, osteoporosis is a prevalent complication, both before and after transplant. In a study of 48 patients awaiting lung transplant, Jastrzebski et al. determined that osteoporosis was present in half the study population, with osteopenia occurring in 40 % [24]. The greatest increase in bone loss was evident in COPD patients who are also affected by both pancreatic insufficiency and reduced vitamin D and calcium absorption [25]. Confirmed by other studies, preexisting osteoporosis has become a matter of increasing concern. Growing recognition of its importance should enable physicians to implement anti-osteoporotic strategies during the waiting period before transplantation, ensuring that patients are in the best possible health at the time of the procedure [26]. Evaluation of bone mineral density and counseling about the risk of fracture posttransplant are now routinely recommended for patients with low BMD or fracture pretransplant [27].

Osteoporosis and Fractures Post Lung Transplant

As in the case of other solid organ transplants, bone loss is accelerated in the early months following lung surgery, primarily as a result of high doses of immunosuppressive medications that induce increased bone turnover. However improvement is indicated in more recent trials.

Earlier studies pointed to a marked decrease in lumbar spine BMD of 3.5–24 % occurring in the first 3–6 months. In their 1996 analysis of bone loss post lung transplant, Aris et al. reported that 73 % of patients had BMDs of the spine and femur below a fracture level defined as two SDs beneath the age-matched mean. The fracture rate was approximately 225 fractures per 1000 person-years which is equal to or greater than that for women with postmenopausal osteoporosis who have already experienced fractures. Biochemical markers of bone resorption were also significantly higher [25]. Osteoporosis was attributed not only to the cumulative steroid dose but also to the degree of preexisting bone demineralization—a condition that was often not fully recognized.

Other studies confirmed bone loss and fracture occurrence in varying degrees. Spira et al. [28] reported that the prevalence of osteoporosis increased from 54% prior to lung transplant to 78% posttransplant. A lesser decrease in BMD of about 5 % at both lumbar spine and femoral neck, as well as a high incidence of fractures at 18 %, was recorded 6–12 months after transplant. On the basis of these findings, the authors postulated that the modest decrease in BMD was still sufficient to impel patients over the fracture threshold especially in those with preexisting low bone mass, again emphasizing the importance of earlier screening and treatment. Women with low pretransplantation BMD and a history of pretransplant glucocorticoid therapy are at greater risk of fracture in the first year following transplant [29].

In this context, it is interesting to note that more recent investigations have produced better outcomes. In a 2014 study of a cohort of 210 lung transplant patients [30], 17 subjects (8.0 %) experienced fractures after transplantation, with the median time to first fracture occurring at 12 months and the mean time for fracture incidence occurring at 18 months. Calcium and vitamin D supplementation as well as glucocorticoid use did not differ in the fracture and nonfracture groups. Of the 17 who fractured, eight had COPD. Comprehensive bone care, including DXA scans; vitamin D screening before and immediately after transplantation; early initiation of antiresorptive therapy, at both the pretransplant and immediate posttransplant phase; and improved clinician awareness could account for these improved results.

Treatment

Therapy for bone loss and fracture risk post lung transplant must necessarily involve both the nonpharmacological and pharmacological strategies customarily used for osteoporosis alone. Studies focusing specifically on lung transplant recipients are limited in number and size; however, they do demonstrate the greater efficacy of bisphosphonates, particularly intravenous pamidronate.

Nonpharmacologic Interventions

Calcium and Vitamin D Supplementation

Studies indicate that calcium and vitamin D supplementation in lung transplant recipients appears to have little impact on glucocorticoid-induced osteoporosis. In a comparison with the bisphosphonate pamidronate, Trombetti et al. [31] found that, at one year, patients receiving only calcium and vitamin D supplementation had a

Z-scores of −0.4+/−0.1 at lumbar spine and −0.04+/−0.1 at femoral neck, in contrast to comparable scores of +0.2+/0.1 at lumbar spine and +0.2+/−01at femoral neck for bisphosphonate patients.

Exercise and Physical Therapy

In terms of exercise, weight-bearing and strengthening regimens are employed to improve and maintain bone density, while spinal posture and movement patterns may be beneficial in cases of vertebral fractures [32]. At the same time, exercise limitations, present before transplant, can persist well after transplant, suggesting chronic muscle deconditioning after lengthy pretransplant debilitation [33]. Cardiopulmonary exercise testing (CPET), incorporating maximal oxygen uptake, has been used for over two decades to assess aerobic capacity posttransplant, but results are mixed. Overall, Dudley et al. have shown that the absolute VO_2 capacity after transplant appears to be fixed at 50 % of predicted VO_2, regardless of pretransplant capacity [34]. Factors affecting exercise capacity include abnormalities in peripheral circulation and in skeletal muscle oxidative capacity as well as the effect of immunosuppressive medications.

As Seoane et al. have observed [35], the 6-min walk test (6-MWT) has essentially replaced CPET in evaluating lung disease itself, but only recently has it been applied to posttransplant patients. In their study of 49 lung transplant patients, they describe a normal distribution for the 6-MWT distance at six months following transplant, with improved distances continuing for a year. Although 6-MWT does not predict survival, it may have an as-yet undetermined predictive value for morbidity. However, its limitations, specifically the inability to determine peak oxygen uptake which, in turn, hinders assessment of the relative factors contributing to exercise capability, have led the American Thoracic Society to recommend that the 6-MWT be regarded as complementary to, but not a substitute for, CPET [34, 36].

To what extent is exercise beneficial for lung transplant patients? In a 2010 review of seven studies applying different forms of aerobic and resistance exercise, Wickerson et al. [37] concluded that a period of structured exercise training can have a positive effect on maximal and functional exercise capacity, skeletal muscle strength, and lumbar spine BMD. Several of the studies covered in the review and one completed more recently are noted here. A 6-month program of lumbar extension exercise [38] aimed at reversing vertebral osteoporosis post lung transplant revealed that lumbar BMD in the exercise group increased significantly (+9.25) over the period, whereas a control group lost bone mass, decreasing to 19.5 % less than pretransplantation levels. The lumbar spine was singled out because nearly all lung transplant patients have reduced BMD at that site, with lumbar spine compression fracture being the most debilitating consequence of glucocorticoid therapy and resulting in continued BMD loss. Another trial involving lung patients more than six months posttransplant reported that a period of normal daily activities exerted no impact on exercise performance in contrast to six weeks of aerobic endurance training which significantly improved submaximal and peak exercise performance [39]. A 2012 trial not only confirmed the benefits of exercise training in lung transplant patients but also added important information relating to broader health outcomes, specifically the impact of exercise on cardiovascular morbidity [40]. In patients between 40 and 65 years of age with an uncomplicated postoperative condition, those who underwent a 3-month structured exercise program (walking, stair climbing, cycling, and resistance training) immediately after the transplant, realized three major benefits:

1. After one year, walking time averaged 85 min per day versus 54 min for a control group.
2. Quadriceps force, 6MWT distance, self-reported physical functioning, and quality of life were improved in the intervention group.
3. The average 24-hour diastolic and systolic blood pressure was significantly lower in the exercise group, with positive implications for cardiovascular health.

Although lung transplant patients may be unable to attain full exercise capacity or maximum skeletal muscle strength, the benefits of exercise are indisputable. Further studies of the safety and efficacy of more intensive training programs as well as of the impact of exercise on patients with a more complicated postoperative experience, possibly involving comorbidities, are anticipated [37].

Pharmacologic Treatment

Long regarded as a mainstay of osteoporosis treatment, bisphosphonates have not been extensively studied in the lung transplant population and have recently been the subject of several safety advisories from the FDA. In a highly cited trial involving posttransplant cystic fibrosis patients, Aris et al. [25] found that in contrast to controls, intravenous pamidronate combined with calcium and vitamin D supplementation produced an 8.8 % gain in BMD at the lumbar spine and an 8.2 % gain in femur BMD at the end of two years; however, there was no difference in fracture rates between the two groups. A pilot study directed at bone loss and osteoporotic fracture in lung transplant patients [41] demonstrated that aggressive therapy with pamidronate and supplements reduced incident symptomatic fracture in the first year, with only 4 % of the 45 patients evidencing fracture. Lumbar spine and hip bone density remained stable or improved in 65 % and 86 % of patients, respectively, but significant bone loss was still apparent in 42 % of patients in the year following transplant. It is unclear when or whether bone remodeling normalizes in this population, indicating that the need for therapy may persist indefinitely. For the present, however, bisphosphonate use for 12 months prior to and posttransplant is generally recommended.

Possible combination regimens have also been examined. An analysis of alendronate together with mechanical loading [42] has shown that the blended prophylaxis produced a significantly increased lumbar spine BMD, with values 10.8+/−2.3 % greater than that prior to transplant, thus demonstrating that an antiresorptive agent plus resistance exercise is more effective than the agent alone.

Other treatments have shown limited efficacy. Short-term therapy with calcitriol or cyclical etidronate may be partially effective in reducing bone loss after lung transplant, but their use requires monitoring of calcium levels [43]. The application of parathyroid hormone and denosumab requires further investigation as does the potential of immune tolerance, which may be particularly difficult to achieve in pulmonary transplant recipients, given such factors as lack of bronchial artery circulation posttransplant and an imperfect barrier against invading pathogens [44].

Liver Transplant

Statistics compiled by the US Department of Health and Human Services indicate that the number of patients actively awaiting liver transplant far exceeds those on the waiting list for heart and lung together and is surpassed only by the extremely large number, over 66,000, registered for a kidney transplant. Here again osteoporosis is apparent before surgery. As recently as 2012, Kaemmerer et al. reported that the number of patients evidencing osteoporosis before transplantation ranged from 12 to 55 % and those with bone fractures from 3 to 35 % [45]. Moreover, low BMD or bone fractures before transplantation increase the risk of BMD loss and particularly vertebral fractures after transplantation.

Post Liver Transplant Osteoporosis

As Eberling has observed [46], bone loss and fracture rates are highest in the first 6–12 months after transplant but at times can occur as early as the first three months. However, recent trials have shown conflicting results with regard to bone loss. A 2002 study by Ninkovic et al. demonstrated a significant absence of bone loss and reduced fracture occurrence of 8 %, although it still found significant bone loss at the femoral neck of 4 %, compared to baseline, during the first three months [47]. In the authors' view, the decrease in both bone loss and fracture occurrence were most likely linked to the lower doses and reduced duration of glucocorticoids now in use, better bone health, and possibly the decision to implement the transplant option earlier in the course of chronic liver disease.

By contrast, a subsequent Mayo Clinic trial involving 360 posttransplant patients over a 16-year period (1985–2001) [5] continued to show a cumulative fracture incidence of 30 % in the first 12 months with an occurrence of almost 46 % by eight years. The greatest risk factors were pretransplant fracturing, primary binary cirrhosis, and corticosteroids. The researchers maintained that although other studies may have demonstrated an increase in the bone mass of liver recipients with fewer fractures, as of 2007, 25% of patients in their trial still developed new fractures in the posttransplant period. Another study focusing on BMD reported that women with primary binary cirrhosis had decreased BMD at three months post liver transplant followed by a subsequent increase, so that by 12 months, their median BMD was similar to that in the pretransplant stage and by 24 months was higher by 5 % [48].

Treatment

Nonpharmacologic Interventions

As in the case of other transplants, bone disease after a liver transplant was formerly attributable to the high dose of corticosteroids used as immunosuppressive agents. With corticosteroid administration now reduced to a minimum in favor of lower dosages and other immunosuppressive drugs, improvements in bone density over time are now being realized [49]. In addition to a decrease in the dose and duration of corticosteroid treatment, other nonpharmacologic measures including improved nutrition, cessation of smoking, and reduction of alcohol intake may improve bone health.

Vitamin D Supplementation

As Stein et al. have shown, severe vitamin D deficiency at the level of 25OHD <25 nmol/L existed in 30 % of 23 liver transplant recipients examined, while vitamin D deficiency at the level of 25OHD <50 nmol/L was common in the remainder of the cohort [50]. Levels are particularly low in liver recipients who experience impaired hepatic 25-hydroxylation of vitamin D. At a time when bisphosphonates are increasingly used following transplant, physicians should be aware that these drugs are not optimally effective in cases of severe vitamin D deficiency and that IV bisphosphonates may actually precipitate hypercalcemia in a deficient state. Depending on individual vitamin D levels, liver recipients require supplementation (generally administered with 1000 mg/day calcium) in varying dosages that will enable them to achieve serum levels of vitamin D25 OH above 20 ng/mL.

The status of vitamin D levels at the time of transplantation is also a matter of concern. A 2015 trial involving 127 patients receiving a transplant between July 2010 and July 2011 found that 84 % had vitamin D deficiency at the time of transplant evaluation and 74 % remained deficient at the time of transplant [51]. While this study found no association between vitamin D deficiency pretransplant and decreased BMD or fracture risk posttransplant, further research is needed to determine what effect the restoration of serum levels of vitamin D25 OH pretransplant might have on such posttransplant outcomes as the level of immunosuppressive therapy needed.

Physical Activity

In the past 15 years, increasing attention has been focused on the role of exercise in treating osteoporosis post liver transplant, primarily with respect to its effect on health-related quality of life. In conducting some of the earliest studies on this interaction, Painter et al. [52] observed that posttransplant conditions such as pain, weakness, loss of range of motion, and osteoporosis, coupled with significant weight gain, contribute to physical inactivity and adversely affect levels of physical functioning. Just as exercise is important for the general population, it should not be ignored in transplant patients.

Limited data is available on the direct effect of exercise on osteoporosis in post liver transplant patients. Instead, generalized benefits of exercise following solid organ transplant are extrapolated, taking into account the specific limitations imposed by liver replacement surgery and its consequences. Initially, exercise in these patients must be limited and carefully monitored to prevent complications from both suture breakage and the fatigue that so often occur post liver transplant. Several analyses have been conducted on potential physical activity programs for this population, aimed primarily at improving exercise capacity, muscular strength, and cardiorespiratory fitness, but beneficial to bones as well. In one trial, the "exercise prescription" for home-based training included walking and cycling, with a frequency of at least three times per week for a duration increasing to 30 minutes per session [53]. Because subjects and their families fear damaging a new organ, noncompliance with exercise results, making professional guidance essential in developing and maintaining much-needed resistance and aerobic exercise programs [54]. Additional studies are needed to develop the optimal exercise intervention for osteoporosis in the post liver transplant period.

Pharmacologic Intervention

Bisphosphonates

Bisphosphonates are effective in treating post liver transplant bone loss, provided that vitamin D deficiency is also addressed. Thus far, investigations of the effect of bone-protective therapy in transplant patients have been hindered by their small size, short duration, and insufficient power to compare different medications and detect fractures. They do, however, demonstrate some benefits, particularly with regard to pamidronate, alendronate, zoledronic acid (ZA), and ibandronate. A randomized 12-month study of 30 mg of IV pamidronate, administered with supplemental calcium and vitamin D, resulted in a significant increase in lumbar spine BMD as compared to controls, as well as a decrease in bone turnover. In a 12-month follow-up, the efficacy of pamidronate appeared to be limited to trabecular bone, with no effect on femoral neck bone loss [55].

Studies involving alendronate have produced limited positive results. A placebo-controlled trial in patients with primary biliary cirrhosis showed that alendronate was able to increase BMD after one year, in comparison with placebo and independent of concomitant estrogen therapy [56]. A nonrandomized investigation also indicated that alendronate produced an increase in BMD within 24 months of transplant [57]; another trial revealed significant increases of BMD at the lumbar spine, femoral neck, and total femur at 12–24 months but did not appear to offer protection against fractures [58].

Examinations of the impact of ZA and ibandronate have shown somewhat greater efficacy but still inconsistent findings. Although Crawford et al. reported that zoledronic acid prevented bone loss by 3.8–4.7 % at the lumbar spine, femoral neck, and total hip within the first year of transplant. They also found that it induced temporary secondary hyperparathyroidism and hypocalcemia; the trial was insufficiently powered to assess fractures [59]. Similar results were reported in a subsequent, randomized controlled trial by Bodingbauer et al. who compared ZA, combined with calcium and vitamin D, to controls receiving only calcium and vitamin D. The end points of fracture and death occurred in 26 % of patients on ZA and 46 % in controls. In addition, 75 % event-free survival time was achieved for 360 days in the ZA group compared to 200 days in the control group [60].

Most recently, an examination of bone disease in liver transplantation involved both *pre- and posttransplant treatment* with ibandronate [45]. An oral monthly dose of ibandronate (150 mg), combined with calcium and vitamin D, was administered to patients awaiting transplant, with follow-ups at 3-, 6-, 12-, and 24-months post surgery. BMD of the lumbar spine was measured both before and after transplant: the percentage change from baseline to 3 months was 13.59, reaching 17.1 % at six months, 18.78 % at 12 months, and 24.26 % at 24 months. Femoral neck BMD increased by 3.1 % at 3 months and 5.1 % at 6 months in the same cohort. A secondary end point in this study, the prevalence of fracture occurrence, was 3.2 % posttransplant. The results of this study warrant further examination, but it appears that immediate postoperative bone loss after liver transplantation can be significantly reduced by pretreatment.

Although much research remains to be done, bisphosphonates, particularly the more potent ZA and ibandronate, have demonstrated the importance of early treatment, as well as the need for a spinal x-ray prior to transplant to identify the status of bone mass. Clinical risk factors should also be considered as an integral part of the transplantation process. Large multicenter, randomized clinical trials are needed to produce more definitive findings.

Renal Transplant

The kidney is the most commonly transplanted solid organ in the United States and throughout the world, resulting in bone disorders caused by posttransplant conditions as well as those persisting from the pretransplant phase. As Bia has observed, bone loss in kidney transplantation differs from that for the heart, lung, and liver because of several factors: the presence of renal osteodystrophy which leads to low

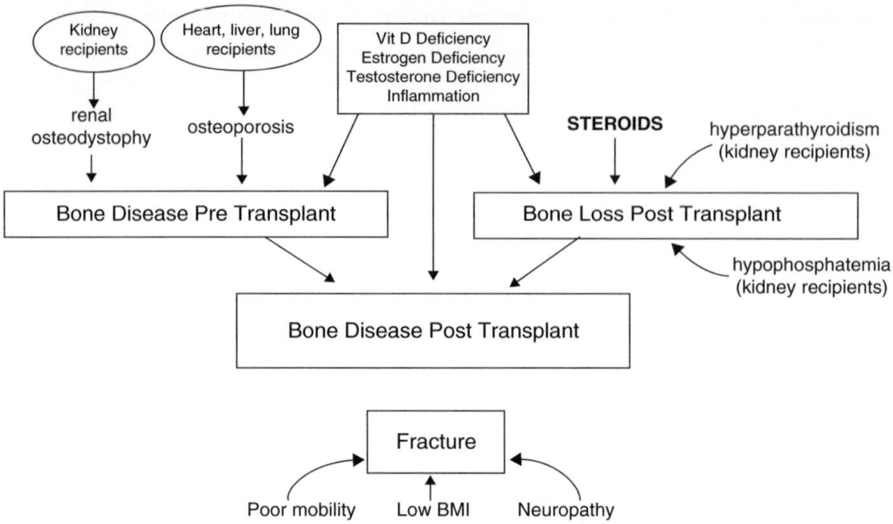

Fig. 1 Factors which contribute to posttransplant bone disease. Posttransplant steroid use plays a major role in bone loss, although other metabolic derangements, especially in kidney transplant patients, may also contribute (*Source*: Bia [61])

BMD; the location of fractures, which are more frequent in appendicular sites (lower limbs, feet, and hip) in kidney transplants than in axial sites (spine and ribs) as in other solid organ transplants; and the potential adverse effects of bisphosphonates that tend to cause "oversuppression" of bone turnover in kidney recipients (Fig. 1) [61].

Whereas patients with heart, lung, and liver disease tend to have preexisting osteoporosis, those with end-stage kidney diseases have what is termed renal osteodystrophy, which is an integral part of chronic kidney disease–metabolic bone syndrome (CKD–MBS) – also known as chronic kidney disease–mineral and bone disorder (CKD–MBD). This condition is marked by active vitamin D deficiency (low vitamin D-1.25-OH), hyperphosphatemia, secondary hyperparathyroidism, and excess aluminum levels—all of which may lead to reduced BMD and fractures but are distinct from osteoporosis as such [61]. While the magnitude of many of these metabolic abnormalities is lessened by kidney transplantation, some aspects of the CKD-MBS such as parathyroid hyperplasia are likely to remain [2]. Failure of enlarged parathyroid glands to involute means that PTH concentrations remain elevated after transplantation, a scenario true in 75 % of patients one year after renal transplant [62, 63]. In addition patients with end-stage kidney disease tend to be hypogonadal and thus could have already received treatment with immunosuppressive therapy (glucocorticoids or cyclosporine A) that will continue posttransplant [64]. Finally, transplant patients frequently still have chronic kidney disease with its attendant complications.

Posttransplant Osteoporosis, Bone Loss, and Fractures

In addition to the standard risk factors for osteoporosis including age and female gender, kidney transplant patients face other challenges, ranging from time since transplantation to the immunosuppressive regimen and graft dysfunction. Ahmadpoor et al. reported an incidence of osteoporosis at 26 % (20 of 77 patients who had undergone transplantation in the previous 6 months–2 years), with the most common sites being the hip and spine [65]. In a cohort of 44 patients followed up to 12 months posttransplant, Orzel et al. identified 43 % as osteopenic, 11 % as osteoporotic, and 46 % as normal, with younger age and high intact pretransplant parathyroid hormone levels as the principal risk factors [66].

As in the case of other transplants, improved results for BMD in kidney patients are evident in more recent studies. Whereas a 1991 investigation reported a BMD decline of 4–10 % in the first six months following transplant [67] due to the toxic effect of glucocorticoids, Bouquegneau et al. have pointed to newer trials that reveal a bone loss of only 0.1–5.7 % in the lumbar spine, reflecting reduced immunosuppressive therapy [68]. In 2014, a large trial ($n=326$) to assess long-term changes in BMD following kidney transplant used extensive DXA measurements to demonstrate that BMD typically improved or remained stable over a period of 8.2 years, with baseline values only slightly above average for age and sex. It should be noted, however, that baseline measurements did not begin until six months after transplantation, allowing for the well-established decline in BMD within the early posttransplant period. Over the long term, the single factor leading to a significant increase in mean BMD at all sites was osteoporosis treatment [69].

Similarly the results of later trials on fracture occurrence demonstrate improvement over earlier findings, mainly attributable to a reduction in the use of immunosuppressive agents; time after transplantation and the presence of diabetes are other contributing factors. Data from the US Renal Data System (USRDS) demonstrate that the demographic-adjusted incidence of hip fractures in kidney transplant recipients has declined significantly to the point where it is 45 % lower in patients transplanted in 2010 than in 1997 [70]. Explanations for this decline include not only changes in immunosuppressive regimens but also an altered lifestyle (smoking cessation, reduced alcohol consumption, enhanced physical activity) and increased bisphosphonate use, which, as noted later, remains a matter of concern in kidney transplant patients.

In one of the largest studies of fracture incidence in kidney transplant patients yet undertaken ($n=4821$) [71], Naylor et al. estimated the cumulative incidence of nonvertebral fractures at 3, 5, and 10 years in the period between 1994 and 2009 with the following results. The overall 3-year cumulative incidence of nonvertebral fractures was 1.6 %, with the number increasing over that time period; the hip fracture rate alone was 0.4 %. The overall 5- and 10-year cumulative incidence of nonvertebral fractures was 2.7 % and 5.5 %, respectively, with hip fractures alone at 1.7 % at the 10-year mark. The most common fracture site was the lower leg. These findings bear out the 2004 observation by Sprague et al. that "the more time since transplantation, the higher the reported fracture rate," but with fracture occurrence at a much lower level than the rates of 5–44 % cited in this earlier study [72]. To explain the lower fracture incidence now observed, Naylor et al. [71] cite the fact that earlier studies could not take into account patients transplanted after the year 2000 when decreased prednisone doses, as well as the use of bisphosphonates and vitamin D supplementation, came into play.

Another approach to reducing fracture risk in kidney transplant is early corticosteroid withdrawal. A study of 430 patients receiving transplants between 2000 and 2006 demonstrated that 31 % of patients discharged from the hospital without corticosteroids had a decreased risk of fracture compared with those discharged on a corticosteroid regimen – a finding that became significant at 24 months posttransplant [73]. Despite these encouraging signs, kidney recipients still have a nonvertebral fracture rate of 1.6 % compared with 0.5 % for the comparable healthy population; women aged 50 and over sustain the highest cumulative 3-year increase of 3.1 % [71].

Is there an association between low BMD and fractures in kidney transplant? In a study conducted over 20 years ago, Grotz et al. [74] showed that many transplant recipients did not experience fractures, concluding that low BMD values at the lumbar spine could, at best, only partially explain fracture occurrence. DXA measurements at the femoral neck indicated no relation to fractures. Findings that BMD assessment does not discriminate between patients with fractures and those without have led to increasing interest in measurements of *bone quality,* achieved with newer three-dimensional imaging techniques such as quantitative computed tomography. Recent evidence that lower femoral neck BMD may be linked with increased fracture risk in chronic kidney disease [75] calls for increased efforts to develop simplified, less invasive, and more cost-effective ways to conduct bone biopsies [76].

Diabetes compounds the fracture risk for patients with kidney transplants. Epidemiologic studies show that pretransplantation diabetes can more than double the risk for fracture after a kidney transplant [73]. Hypoinsulinemia, hyperglycemia, and other diabetic complications including peripheral neuropathy can all decrease bone strength. However, new research finds that a simultaneous pancreas–kidney transplant, as opposed to a kidney transplant alone, can result in lower fracture rates in kidney transplants, particularly in men [77]. Apparent within three months of transplantation, overall fracture incidence was 31 % lower in men over a 5-year period but was not significantly different in women. Higher levels of circulating estrogen in women under the age of 50, less severe bone loss at the lumbar spine and femoral neck, and prior medication aimed at fracture prevention may, in part, account for this difference. As the authors emphasize, further studies to determine the mechanisms underlying coincident type 1 diabetes and chronic kidney disease are required to serve as the basis for new fracture prevention strategies that can be used in men, concurrently with the combined transplantation, as well as to advance other therapies that will help to prevent fractures in women.

Treatment

Both nonpharmacologic and pharmacologic therapies have been employed to prevent bone loss posttransplant. In cases where the effect of these therapies have not been examined in kidney recipients directly, findings have been extrapolated from relevant trials involving other types of transplants, keeping in mind the special circumstances that define bone loss in the post-kidney transplant population. Given the sharp decline in bone loss that occurs in kidney as well as in other transplants immediately after surgery, therapeutic measures should be initiated at the earliest point.

Nonpharmacologic Regimens

Calcium and Vitamin D Supplementation

Hyperparathyroidism, abnormal vitamin D metabolism, and the use of prednisone all lead to reduced calcium absorption and further contribute to bone loss post kidney transplant. At the same time, calcium supplementation alone is ineffective in maintaining BMD or reducing fracture risk [78]. A Cochrane Database Review of 24 trials found that no *individual* intervention with either vitamin D, calcitonin, or bisphosphonates was associated with reduced fracture risk but that when the results of all trials were *combined*, *any* one of these treatments proved effective against fracture risk and all had a beneficial effect on BMD at the lumbar spine [79]. This study supports the concurrent use of vitamin D (with or without calcium) and bisphosphonates to reduce the deleterious effects of immunosuppressive therapy on bone density after transplant and indicates that any intervention to alter bone metabolism can reduce fracture risk in the year following surgery. With respect to calcium supplementation, Torres et al. report that intermittent-dose calcitriol during the first three months posttransplant, followed by oral calcium supplementation during the first year, decreased the rate of bone loss at the total hip compared with calcium supplementation alone, without any adverse effect on hypercalcemia levels [80].

The relation between vitamin D and hypercalciuria admits of mixed findings. A recent study reported that hypercalciuria occurred more frequently in a vitamin D supplementation group, leading to a reduction in the dosage or treatment discontinuation in 30 % of patients; calcium supplementation was also cited as a possible cause of hypercalciuria. It is clear that additional randomized controlled trials are required to determine the most effective dose and optimal duration of supplementation as well as to assess the specific impact on fracture risk [81]. Until then, the level of calcium and vitamin D supplementation is determined on an individual basis taking into account regular screening results to determine the extent of bone damage, as well as the severity of the disease and existing comorbidities such as diabetes.

Physical Activity

As in the case of dietary supplementation, exercise programs must be tailored to individual needs of the individual and, to the extent possible, should encompass mechanical loading, stretching, and strengthening regimens. Although the primary goal of exercise in the posttransplant phase is to reduce cardiovascular risk and improve graft function [81], the benefits of exercise extend to increasing BMD and preventing fractures by advancing motor fitness, improving balance, and decreasing fall risk. However, analyses of the efficacy and effectiveness of exercise post renal transplant are few in number, and the lack of evidence, in itself, represents one of the principal factors contributing to low exercise rates [82]. Gordon et al. point to several other reasons underlying reduced physical activity: (1) lack of motivation and interest, coupled with fear of injuring the graft, (2) limited knowledge of the benefits of exercise on the part of healthcare professionals faced with what they consider to be more immediate and compelling concerns, and (3) inadequate reimbursement for physical activity programs and counseling on the part of insurance carriers. Exercise may be particularly difficult to initiate in older renal transplant recipients with reduced physical performance prior to transplant, as well as in younger patients who have been shown to be less physically active pretransplant by a measure of 25 % in comparison with healthy subjects [83].

The guidelines adopted by Kidney Disease: Improving Global Outcomes (KDIGO) recommend that at least 30 min of moderate-intensity exercise (walking, cycling, slow jogging) be undertaken on most, preferably all, days of the weeks, as adapted to the needs and capacity of the individual [84]. In a highly cited randomized clinical trial, Painter et al. found that one year after transplant, an exercise intervention group increased its regular physical activity from 50 to 67 %, whereas the "usual care" group experienced a decline from 47 to 36 %; in addition the exercise group realized significantly greater gains in peak oxygen uptake (VO_2), muscle strength, and physical functioning [85]. Although guidelines and studies such as these have not directly addressed bone disease in renal transplant, they do raise awareness of the need to develop exercise regimens directed to individual needs as well as to conduct new empirical research on the safety and efficacy of specific exercise training programs with respect to the different outcomes of the transplant process including osteoporosis. Recent findings on the correlation between low physical activity and the risk of cardiovascular and all-cause mortality in renal transplant [86] may well stimulate further examinations of the impact of exercise on mineral and bone disorders as well as on fracture risk, leading to an improved quality of life.

Pharmacologic Measures

Bisphosphonates

As noted at the outset of this section, the value of bisphosphonates in kidney transplant is tempered by their potential to oversuppress bone metabolism. Given that concern, the general consensus is that bisphosphonates should not be used in kidney patients with low bone turnover that could be further exacerbated by these drugs, possibly increasing fracture risk. Studies of the effect of alendronate, pamidronate, and zoledronic acid have demonstrated benefits in terms of increased BMD.

In a 12-month analysis of kidney patients receiving 10 mg/day of alendronate plus calcitriol and calcium issued in 2001, BMD increased significantly by 5 % at the lumbar spine and 4 % at the femoral neck and bone turnover normalized; at the same time, bone continued to be lost due to prednisone treatment and persistent hyperparathyroidism [87]. Two intravenous doses of pamidronate given to male patients at the time of transplantation and one month later prevented early rapid bone loss, with no significant reduction at the lumbar vertebrae and femoral neck [88]. The regimen was well tolerated and easy to administer, with no detrimental effect on renal function and no discernible side effects. A subsequent study confirmed the efficacy of IV pamidronate in preserving bone mass but did observe an increased risk of low bone turnover [89].

A trial involving the third-generation bisphosphonate, zoledronic acid (ZA) reported that, at six months, two infusions of IV ZA increased trabecular calcium content significantly, with no change in BMD at the femoral neck. However, as Fratianni et al. have observed, the early bone-sparing effects of short-term ZA could not be sustained at three years after transplantation [90]. In addition, FDA warnings concerning the deterioration of renal function and renal failure resulting from ZA must also be taken into account, with dose reduction as recommended.

Still in their infancy, comparative analyses of these medications are impaired by the small sample sizes and the heterogeneous nature of the research, particularly with respect to time duration following transplant. Based solely on randomized controlled trials, a recent meta-analysis of bisphosphonates posttransplant [91] concluded that they were beneficial to BMD at the lumbar spine but not at the femoral neck. Although changes in vertebral and nonvertebral fractures or in adverse events were not associated with their use; bisphosphonates were not found to reduce fracture incidence. As a result of this study, the largest database on the use of bisphosphonates in patients undergoing renal transplantation is now in place and can serve as the basis for further analyses of their efficacy and safety as new information is obtained.

Other Medications

In general, bisphosphonates which are renally excreted are not recommended for kidney transplant patients with moderate to severe renal insufficiency. As an alternative, denosumab, the fully human monoclonal antibody against RANKL, has recently been investigated to determine its effect on BMD in renal transplant, with results indicating that it significantly increased areal BMD at vertebral and nonvertebral sites [92]. Unlike bisphosphonates it improved cortical volumetric BMD and thickness at the distal tibia and radius while decreasing levels of blood and urine biomarkers in bone turnover. Although associated with more frequent episodes of urinary tract infections, denosumab has the potential to improve bone health post-transplant and to sustain bone retention with long-term use. Synthetic parathyroid hormone (PTH) in the form of teriparatide does not improve BMD early after kidney transplantation, nor do histological analyses or bone markers provide evidence of improved bone turnover or mineralization [93].

The challenges of managing kidney recipients are many, emphasizing the importance of regular monitoring to determine the status of bone loss. Reduced doses of immunosuppressive therapy as well as early corticosteroid withdrawal, calcium and vitamin D supplementation as needed, increased physical activity, and the prudent use of bisphosphonates targeted at high-fracture risk recipients must be weighed carefully by an interdisciplinary team responsible for the care of transplant patients.

References

1. Kulak CAM, Barba VZC, Junior JK, Custodian MR. Bone disease after transplantation: osteoporosis and fracture risk. Arq Bras Endocrinol Metab. 2014;68(5):484–92.
2. Hawkins FG, Guadalix S, Sanchez R, Martinez. Post-transplantation bone disease. In: Dionyssiotis Y, editor. Osteoporosis. p. 299–322. ISBN: 978-953-51-0026-3. InTech, Available from: http://www.intechopen.com/books/osteoporosis/post-transplatation-bone-disease. Accessed 2 Mar 2016.
3. Giannini S, Nobile M, Cuiffreda M, Iemmolo RM, Dalle Carbonare L, Minicuci N. Long-term persistence of low bone density in orthotopic liver transplantation. Osteoporos Int. 2000;11(5):417–24.
4. Theibaud D, Krieg MA, Gillard-Berguer D, Jacquet AF, Goy JJ, Burckhardt P. Cyclosporine induces high bone turnover and may contribute to bone loss after heart transplantation. Eur J Clin Invest. 1996;26(7):549–55.
5. Guichelaar MM, Schmoll J, Malinchoc M, Hay JE. Fractures and avascular necrosis before and after orthotopic liver transplantation: long-term follow-up and predictive factors. Hepatology. 2007;46(4):1198–207.

6. Vanden Eynden F, Antoine M, El Oumeiri B, Chirade ML, Vachiery JL, Van Nooten GJ. How to cope with a temporarily aborted transplant program: solutions for a prolonged waiting period. Ann Transl Med. 2015;3(20):306. doi:10.3978/j.issn.2305-5839.2015.11.30.
7. Shane E, Mancini D, Aaronson K, Silverberg SJ, Seibel MJ, Addesso V, et al. Bone mass, vitamin D deficiency, and hyperparathyroidism in congestive heart failure. Am J Med. 1997;103(3):197–207.
8. Cohen A, Shane E. Osteoporosis after solid organ and bone marrow transplantation. Osteoporos Int. 2003;14(8):617–30.
9. Stein E, Eberling P, Shane E. Post-transplantation osteoporosis. Endocrinol Metab Clin. 2007;36(4):937–63.
10. Chou NK, Su IC, Kuo HL, Chen YH, Yang RS, Wang SS. Bone mineral density in long-term Chinese heart transplant recipients: a cross-sectional study. Transplant Proc. 2006;38(7):2141–4.
11. Cohen A, Addonizio LJ, Lamour JM, Addesso V, Staron RB, Gao P, et al. Osteoporosis in adult survivors of adolescent cardiac transplantation may be related to hyperthyroidism, mild renal insufficiency, and increased bone turnover. J Heart Lung Transplant. 2005;24(6):696–702.
12. Sambrook PN, Kelly PJ, Fontana D, Nguyen T, Keogh A, Macdonald P, et al. Mechanisms of rapid bone loss following cardiac transplantation. Osteoporos Int. 1994;4(5):273–8.
13. Shane E, Rodino MA, McMahon DJ, Addesso V, Staron RB, Seibel MJ, et al. Prevention of bone loss after heart transplantation with antiresorptive therapy: a pilot study. J Heart Long Transplant. 1998;17(11):1089–96.
14. Lee AH, Mull RL, Keenan GF, Callegari PE, Dalinka MK, Eisen HJ, et al. Osteoporosis and bone morbidity in cardiac transplant recipients. Am J Med. 1994;96(1):35–41.
15. Leidig-Bruckner G, Hosch S, Dodidou P, Ritschel D, Conradt C, Klose C, et al. Frequency and predictors of osteoporotic fractures after cardiac or liver transplantation: a follow-up study. Lancet. 2001;357(9253):342–7.
16. Oz M. Bridge experience with long term implantable left ventricular assist devices: are they an alternative to transplantation? Circulation. 1997;95(7):1844–52.
17. Blumberg Y, Kravits A, Dinkin D, Neimark A, Abu-Hatzira M, Shtein R, et al. Early physical rehabilitation after continuous flow left ventricular assist device implantation: suggested protocol and a pilot study. Int J Phys Med Rehabil. 2015;3(2):263–68. http://www/omicsonline.org/physical-medicine-rehabilitation.php. Accessed 10 Mar 2016.
18. Braith RW, Mills RM, Welsch MA, Keller JW, Pollock ML. Resistance exercise training restores bone mineral density in heart transplant recipients. J Am Coll Cardiol. 1996;28(6):1471–7.
19. Braith RW, Magyari PM, Fulton MN, Lisor CF, Vogel SE, Hill JA, et al. Comparison of calcitonin versus calcitonin +resistance exercise as prophylaxis for osteoporosis in heart transplant recipients. Transplantation. 2006;81(88):1191–5.
20. Braith RW, Welsch MA, Mills Jr RM, Keller JW, Pollock ML. Resistance exercise prevents glucocorticoid-induced myopathy in heart transplant recipients. Med Sci Sports Exerc. 1998;30(4):483–9.
21. Braith RW, Magyari MS, Fulton MW, Aranda J, Walker T, Hill JA. Resistance exercise training and alendronate reverse glucocorticoid-induced osteoporosis in heart transplant recipients. J Heart Lung Transplant. 2003;22(10):1082–90.
22. Krieg MA, Seydoux C, Sandino L, Goy JJ, Berguer DG, Thibeaux D, et al. Intravenous pamidronate as treatment for osteoporosis after heart transplantation: a prospective study. Osteoporos Int. 2001;12(2):112–6.
23. Brunova J, Kratochvilova S, Bruna J. Osteoporosis therapy with denosumab in patients after solid organ transplantation. Endocr Abs. 2016. doi:10.1530/endoabs.41.EP122.
24. Jastrzebski D, Lutogniewska W, Ochman M, Margas A, Kowalski K, Wyrwol J, et al. Osteoporosis in patients referred for lung transplantation. Eur J Med Res. 2010;15 Suppl 2:66–71.

25. Aris RM, Neuringer IP, Weiner MA, Egan TM, Ontjes D. Severe osteoporosis before and after lung transplantation. Chest. 1996;109(5):1176–83.
26. Shane E, Silverberg SJ, Donovan D, Papadopoulos A, Staron R, Addesso V. Osteoporosis in lung transplantation candidates with end-stage pulmonary disease. Am J Med. 1996;101(3):262–9.
27. Dodd VA, Staron RB, Papadopoulos A, Evans L, Schulman LL, Jorgensen B, et al. Bone densitometry should be included in the evaluation of candidates for lung transplantation. J Transpl Coord. 1999;9(2):119–23.
28. Spira A, Gutierrez C, Chaparro C, Hutcheon M, Chan CKN. Osteoporosis and lung transplantation: a prospective study. Chest. 2000;117(2):476–81.
29. Shane E, Papadopoulos A, Staron RB, Addesso V, Donovan D, McGregor C, et al. Bone loss and fracture after lung transplantation. Transplantation. 1999;68(12):220–7.
30. Hariman A, Alex C, Heroux A, Camacho P. Incidence of fracture after cardiac and lung transplantation: a single center experience. J Osteoporos. 2014. doi:10.1155/2014/573041.
31. Trombetti A, Gerbase MW, Spiliopoulos A, Slosman DO, Nicod LP, Rizzoli R. Bone mineral density in lung-transplant recipients before and after graft: prevention of lumbar spine post-transplantation-accelerated bone loss by pamidronate. J Heart Lung Transplant. 2000;19(8):736–43.
32. Scherer SA, Bookstein NA. Clinical perspective: framework and rationale for physical therapy management of lung transplant patients with osteoporosis. Cardiovasc Pulm Ther. 2001;12(3):75–82.
33. Williams TJ, Patterson A, Clean PA, Zamel N, Mauer JR. Maximal exercise testing in single and double lung transplant recipients. Am Rev Res Dis. 1992;145(1):101–5.
34. Dudley KA, El-Chemaly S. Cardiopulmonary exercise testing in lung transplantation: a review. Pulmon Med. 2012; Article ID 2337852. http://dx.doi.org/10.1155/2012/237852.
35. Seoane L, Alex S, Pirtie C, Gupta M, Taylor DE, Valentine VG, et al. Utility of the 6-minute walk test following lung transplantation. Ochsner J. 2010;10(4):227–30.
36. Crapo RO, Enright PL, Zeballos RJ. (Writing Committee Members) ATS Committee on Proficiency Standards for Clinical Pulmonary Function Laboratories. ATS statement: guidelines for the six-minute walk test. Am J Respir Crit Care Med. 2002;166(1):111–7.
37. Wickerson L, Mathur S, Brooks D. Exercise training after lung transplantation: a systematic review. J Heart Lung Transplant. 2010;29(5):497–503.
38. Mitchell MJ, Baz MA, Fulton MN, Lisor CR, Braith RW. Resistance training prevents vertebral osteoporosis in lung transplant recipients. Transplantation. 2003;76(3):557–62.
39. Stiebellehner L, Quittan M, End A, Wieselthaler G, Klepetko W, Haber P, et al. Aerobic endurance training program improves exercise performance in lung transplant recipients. Chest. 1998;113(4):906–12.
40. Langer D, Burtin C, Schepers L, Ivanoa A, Verleden G, Decramer M, et al. Exercise training after lung transplantation improves participation in daily activity: a randomized controlled trial. Am J Transplant. 2012;12(6):1584–92.
41. Cahill BC, O'Rourke MK, Parker S, Stringham JC, Karwande SV, Knecht TP. Prevention of bone loss and fracture after lung transplantation. Transplantation. 2001;72(7):1251–5.
42. Braith RW, Connor JA, Fulton MN, Lisor CF, Casey DP, Howe KS, et al. Comparison of alendronate vs alendronate plus mechanical loading as prophylaxis for osteoporosis in lung transplant recipients: a pilot study. J Heart Lung Transplant. 2007;26(2):132–7.
43. Henderson K, Eisman J, Keogh A, Macdonald P, Glanville A, Spratt P, et al. Protective effect of short-term calcitriol or cyclical etidronate on bone loss after cardiac or lung transplantation. J Bone Miner Res. 2001;16(3):565–71.
44. Jiang X, Nicholls MP. Working toward immune tolerance in lung transplantation. J Clin Invest. 2014;124(3):967–70.
45. Kaemmerer D, Schmidt B, Lehmann G, Wolf G, Settmacher U, Hommann M. Treatment of bone loss in patients with chronic liver disease awaiting liver transplantation. Transplant Res. 2012;1(1):7. doi:10.1186/2047-1440-1-7.

46. Eberling PR. Transplantation osteoporosis. In: Rosen CJ, editor. Primer on the metabolic bone diseases and disorders of mineral metabolism. 8th ed. Ames: Wiley; 2013. p. 495–507.
47. Ninkovic M, Love S, Tom BDM, Bearcroft PWP, Alexander GJM, Compston JE. Lack of effect of intravenous pamidronate on fracture incidence and bone mineral density after orthotopic liver transplantation. J Hepatol. 2002;37(1):93–100.
48. Eastell R, Dickson ER, Hodgson SF, Wiesner RH, Porayko MK, Wahner HW, et al. Rates of vertebral bone loss before and after liver transplantation in women with primary biliary cirrhosis. Hepatology. 1991;14(2):296–300.
49. Crippin JS. Bone disease after liver transplantation. Liver Transplant. 2001;7 Suppl 1:S27–35.
50. Stein EM, Cohen A, Freeby M, Rogers H, Kokolus S, Scott V, et al. Severe vitamin D deficiency among heart and liver transplant recipients. Clin Transplant. 2009;23(6):861–5.
51. Chaney A, Heckman MG, Diehl NN, Meek S, Keaveny AP. Effectiveness and outcomes of current practice in treating vitamin D deficiency in patients listed for liver transplantation. Endocr Pract. 2015;21(7):761–9.
52. Painter P, Krasnoff J, Paul SM, Ascher NL. Physical activity and health-related quality of life in liver transplant recipients. Liver Transplant. 2001;7(3):213–9.
53. Krasnoff JB, Vintro AQ, Ascher NL, Bass NM, Paul SM, Dodd MJ, et al. A randomized trial of exercise and dietary counseling after liver transplantation. Am J Transplant. 2006;6(89):1896–905.
54. Surgit O, Ersoz G, Gursel Y, Ersoz S. Effects of exercise training on specific immune parameters in transplant patients. Transplant Proc. 2001;33(7–8):3298.
55. Pennisi P, Trombetti A, Giostra E, Mentha G, Rizzoli R, Flore CE. Pamidronate and osteoporosis prevention in liver transplant recipients. Rheumatol Int. 2007;27(3):251–6.
56. Zein CO, Jorgensen RA, Clarke B, Wenger DS, Keach JC, Angulo P, et al. Alendronate improves bone mineral density in primary biliary cirrhosis: a randomized placebo-controlled trial. Hepatology. 2005;42(4):762–71.
57. Millonig G, Graziadei IW, Eichler D, Pfeiffer KP, Finkenstedt G, Muehllechner P, et al. Alendronate in combination with calcium and vitamin D prevents bone loss after orthotopic liver transplantation: a prospective single-center study. Liver Transplant. 2005;11(8):960–6.
58. Atamaz F, Hepguler S, Akyildiz M, Karase Z, Kilic M. Effects of alendronate on bone mineral density and bone metabolic markers in patients with liver transplantation. Osteoporos Int. 2006;17(6):942–9.
59. Crawford BA, Kam C, Pavlovic J, Byth K, Handelsman DJ, Angus PW, et al. Zoledronic acid prevents bone loss after liver transplantation: a randomized, double-blind, placebo-controlled trial. Ann Intern Med. 2006;144(4):239–48.
60. Bodingbauer M, Wekerle T, Paakrah B, Roschger P, Peck-Radpsavljevic M, Silberhumer G, et al. Prophylactic bisphosphonate treatment prevents bone fracture after a liver transplantation. Am J Transplant. 2007;7(7):1763–9.
61. Bia M. Evaluation and management of bone disease and fractures post-transplant. Transplant Rev. 2008;22(1):52–61.
62. Reinhardt W, Bartelworth H, Jockenhovel F, Schmidt-Gayk H, Witzke O, Wagner K, et al. Sequential changes of biochemical parameters after kidney transplantation. Nephrol Dial Transplant. 1998;13:436–42.
63. Parfitt AM. Hypercalcemic hyperparathyroidism following renal transplantation: differential diagnosis, management and implications for cell population control in the parathyroid gland. Miner Electrolyte Metab. 1982;8:92–112.
64. Rodino MA, Shane E. Osteoporosis after organ transplantation. Am J Med. 1998;104(5):459–69.
65. Ahmadpoor P, Reisi S, Ghafari MK, Sepehrvand N, Rahimi E. Osteoporosis and related risk factors in renal transplant recipients. Transplant Proc. 2009;4(7):2820–2.
66. Ozel L, Ata P, Ozel MS, Toros AB, Kara M, Unal E, et al. Risk factors for osteoporosis after renal transplantation and effect of vitamin D receptors Bsm I polymorphism. Transplant Proc. 2011;43(3):858–62.

67. Julian BA, Laskow DA, Dubovsky J, Dubovsky EV, Curtis JJ, Quarles LD. Rapid loss of vertebral mineral density after renal transplantation. N Engl J Med. 1991;325(8):544–50.
68. Bouquegneau A, Salam S, Delanaye P, Eastell R, Khwaja A. Bone disease after kidney transplantation. Clin J Am Soc Nephrol. 2016. doi:10.2215/CJN.11371015.
69. Naylor KL, Garg AX, Hodsman AB, Rush DN, Leslie WD. Long-term changes in bone mineral density in kidney transplant recipients. Transplantation. 2014;98(12):1279–85.
70. Sukumaran Nair S, Lenihan CR, Montez-Rath ME, Lowenberg DW, Chertow GM, Winkelmayer WC. Temporal trends in the incidence, treatment and outcomes of hip fracture after first kidney transplantation in the United States. Am J Transplant. 2014;14(4):943–51.
71. Naylor KL, Jamal SA, Zou G, McArthur E, Lam NN, Leslie WD, et al. Fracture incidence in adult kidney transplant recipients. Transplantation. 2016;100(1):167–75.
72. Sprague SM, Josephson MA. Bone disease after kidney transplantation. Sem Nephrol. 2004;24(1):82–90.
73. Nikkel LE, Mohana S, Zhang D, McMahon J, Boutroy G, Dube G, et al. Reduced fracture risk with early corticosteroid withdrawal after kidney transplant. Am J Transplant. 2012;12(3):649–59.
74. Grotz WH, Mundinger FA, Gugel B, Exner V, Girste G, Schollmeyer AJ. Bone fracture and osteodensitometry with dual energy x-ray absorptiometry in kidney transplant recipients. Transplantation. 1994;58(89):912–5.
75. Ketteler M, Elder GJ, Evenepoel P, Ix JH, Jamal SA, Lafage-Proust M-H, et al. Revisiting KDIGO clinical practice guideline on chronic kidney disease—mineral and bone disorder: a commentary from a kidney disease: improving global outcomes controversies conference. Kidney Int. 2015;87(3):502–28.
76. Wong J, Tan MZ-W, Chandran M. Fifty shades of gray: bone disease in renal transplantation. Proc Singap Healthc. 2015;24(4):225–32.
77. Nikkel LE, Iyer SP, Mohan S, Zhang A, MacMahon DJ, Tanriover B, et al. Pancreas-kidney transplantation is associated with reduced fracture risk compared to kidney alone transplantation in men with type 1 diabetes. Kidney Int. 2013;63(3):471–8.
78. Chadban S, Chan M, Fry K, Parwardhan A, Ryan C, Trevillian P, et al. Nutritional interventions for the prevention of bone disease in kidney transplant recipients. Nephrology. 2010;15 Suppl 1:S43–7.
79. Palmer SC, McGregor DO, Strippoli GF. Interventions for preventing bone disease in kidney transplant recipient. Cochrane Database Syst Rev. 2007;18(3):CD005015.
80. Torres A, Garcia S, Gomez A, Gonzalez A, Barrios Y, Concepcion MT, et al. Treatment with intermittent calcitriol and calcium reduces bone loss after renal transplantation. Kidney Int. 2004;65(2):705–12.
81. Romano G, Lorenzon E, Montanaro D. Effects of exercise in renal transplant recipients. World J Transplant. 2012;2(4):46–50.
82. Gordon EJ, Prohaska T, Skminoff LA, Minich PJ, Sehgal AR. Needed: tailored exercise regimens for kidney transplant recipient. Am J Kidney Dis. 2005;45(4):769–74.
83. Bellizzi V, Cupisti A, Capitanini A, Calella P, D'Alessandro C. Physical activity and renal transplantation. Kidney Blood Press Res. 2014;39(2–3):212–9.
84. Kidney Disease: Improving Global Outcomes Work Group. Management of progression and complications of CKD. In: KDIGO 2012 clinical practice guideline for the evaluation and management of chronic kidney disease. Kidney Int Suppl 2013;3(Suppl 1):73–90.
85. Painter PL, Hector L, Ray K, Lynes L, Dibble S, Paul SM, et al. A randomized trial of exercise training after renal transplantation. Transplantation. 2002;74(1):42–8.
86. Zelle DM, Corpeleijn E, Stolk RP, de Greef MHG, Gans ROB, van der Heide JJH, et al. Low physical activity and risk of cardiovascular and all-cause mortality in renal transplant recipients. Clin J Am Soc Nephrol. 2011;6(4):898–905.
87. Giannini S, D'Angelo A, Carraro G, Nobile M, Rigotti P, Bonfante L, et al. Alendronate prevents further bone loss in renal transplant patients. J Bone Miner Res. 2001;16(11):2111–7.

88. Fan SL-S, Almond MK, Ball E, Evans K, Cunningham KJ. Pamidronate therapy as prevention of bone loss following renal transplantation. Kidney Int. 2000;57(2):684–90.
89. Coco M, Glicklich D, Faugere MC, Burris L, Bogner I, Durkin P, et al. Prevention of bone loss in renal transplant recipients: a prospective, randomized trial of intravenous pamidronate. J Am Soc Nephrol. 2003;1(10):2669–76.
90. Fratianni CM. Osteoporosis in solid organ transplantation: overview of treatment 2013. http://emedicine.medscape.com/article/128108-overview. Accessed 2 Mar 2016.
91. Kan S-L, Ning G-Z, Chen L-X, Zhou Y, Feng S-Q. Efficacy and safety of bisphosphonates for low bone mineral density after kidney transplantation: a meta-analysis. Medicine. 2016;95(5):2679. doi:10.1097/MD.0000000000002679.
92. Bonani M, Frey D, Brockmann J, Fehr T, Meuller TF, Saleh L, et al. Effect of twice-yearly denosumab on prevention of bone mineral density loss in de novo kidney transplant recipients: a randomized controlled trial. Am J Transplant. 2016;16(6):1882–91.
93. Cejka D, Benesch T, Krestan C, Roschger P, Klauschofer K, Pietschmann P, et al. Effect of teriparatide on early bone loss after kidney transplantation. Am J Transplant. 2008;8(9):1864–70.

Chapter 16
Bone Disorders in Cancer

Christina V. Oleson

As life expectancy steadily increases, osteoporosis and cancer are becoming concurrent diseases in an aging population. Of the over 1.5 million new cancer cases diagnosed each year, some 80 % occur in people over 55 [1]. Osteoporosis most commonly affects individuals aged 50 and above, with the current number estimated at 54 million over the age of 50; the older a person gets, the greater the risk becomes [2]. In cancer, as in other diseases, patients and survivors are susceptible to *primary* osteoporosis caused by the aging process and other detrimental lifestyle factors. This chapter will focus on the *secondary* osteoporosis brought about by three types of cancer: hematologic malignancies (leukemias, lymphomas, myelomas), solid bone tumors that metastasize to bone (breast, prostate, lung, kidney), and primary bone tumors (osteosarcoma, chondrosarcoma, Ewing sarcoma). It will also consider prevailing cancer treatments ranging from medications including corticosteroids to radiation therapy which can be causal factors for osteoporosis. Tumors that metastasize to the spinal cord have a high risk of causing spinal cord injury and, consequently, have been addressed in the chapter on spinal cord disorders.

Hematologic Malignancies

Hematologic malignancies are a form of cancer that begins in the cells of blood-forming tissue such as bone marrow or in the cells of the immune system; they include leukemia, lymphoma, and myeloma. In all of these diseases, dysregulation of the normal bone-modeling process occurs, producing osteolytic, osteoblastic, and mixed osteolytic/osteoblastic lesions. Moreover, production of parathyroid hormone-related protein is stimulated by cancer cells, resulting in increased bone resorption and leading to hypercalcemia [3]. Diagnosis involves several tests including a physical examination and a complete blood count with a bone marrow biopsy used to confirm cancer findings.

C.V. Oleson, *Osteoporosis Rehabilitation*, DOI 10.1007/978-3-319-45084-1_16

Leukemia

Leukemia, which is present in blood and bone marrow, is caused by the rapid production of a high number of abnormal white blood cells which impair the ability of bone marrow to fight infection and to produce red blood cells and platelets [4]. Occurring in an acute and a chronic form, lymphoblastic leukemia involves the growth of cancerous white blood cells (lymphocytes) which affect the immune system; in contrast, myelogenous leukemia develops in marrow cells that become red blood cells, white blood cells other than lymphocytes, and platelets. About three out of four leukemias in children are acute lymphoblastic leukemia, also called acute lymphocytic leukemia (ALL); most of the rest are acute myelogenous leukemia (AML); chronic forms are rare in children.

Children with ALL evidence skeletal abnormalities at the time of diagnosis, following therapy, and even in the long-term, post therapy.

At Diagnosis: Well before therapy is initiated, reduced bone formation markers coupled with normal or reduced bone resorption markers evidence a low bone turnover rate with increased bone fragility [5]. Using a mouse model of AML, Frisch et al. [6] recently demonstrated that at a point when leukemia cells are barely discernible in the blood, they entrench themselves in the bone marrow and attack the production of healthy blood cells. Not only do leukemia stem cells trigger widespread severe loss of mineralized bone, but they also produce elevated levels of the protein, CCL3, which slows bone formation. By altering the balance between osteoblast and osteoclast activity, leukemia can result in a dysfunction in the bone marrow microenvironment; confirmation in human subjects is needed. Lower BMD at the time of diagnosis has also been found to indicate a high fracture risk; as Winkel et al. have shown, low values of bone mineral density of the lumbar spine at the time of diagnosis and during treatment, rather than the subsequent treatment-associated decline, result in an increased fracture risk of 17.8 % in ALL [7].

During Therapy: The fact that leukemia therapy is known to affect BMD in children with ALL underlies the need to incorporate the risk of osteoporosis as an integral part of disease management. During treatment with corticosteroids as well as with methotrexate and asparaginase, ALL patients experience reduced bone formation and increased resorption, leading to a decrease in total body BMD as well as greater incidence of fractures [8].

When does this damage begin? Recent research indicates that diminished bone density and skeletal fractures occur as early as the first month of treatment, much earlier than previously assumed, with important implications for treatment initiation [9]. Intervention measures include supplemental calcium and vitamin D and weight-bearing exercise. The safety and efficacy of bisphosphonates must be fully determined before they can be regarded as standard of care, although they are administered in severe cases [5].

The onset of childhood leukemia, coupled with poor nutrition and inactivity, is often concurrent with the development of peak bone mass, resulting in increased risk of bone deficits and fracture with greater severity in boys than in girls. Treatment-induced risk factors include chemotherapy components such as prolonged corticosteroid treatment and high-dose methotrexate; radiation which is used in cases of leukemia in the brain and testes; and hematopoietic stem cell transplantation (HSCT), now regarded as an established therapy for acute and chronic leukemia as well as for lymphoma and multiple myeloma [10].

Following Therapy: A number of studies of BMD and fracture risk in ALL survivors have been conducted, but their findings, particularly in the case of fractures, are compromised by their heterogeneous and cross-sectional nature and their limited sample size. For example, in leukemia survivors followed for a mean of 22 years after diagnosis, fracture prevalence was 42.2 % as compared with 46.6 % in siblings, a notable decrease despite chemotherapy and radiation exposure in the leukemia cohort (Table 1) [11]. As the age of survivors increases, further longitudinal studies will be needed to determine fracture rates in an aging childhood cancer population [11]. In terms of BMD, trials indicate that survivors treated with chemotherapy have normal BMD at the femoral neck and slight reduction in lumbar spine BMD [10], whereas those treated with radiation continue to experience significantly reduced total body and lumbar spine BMD [12]. Survivors of HSCT are reported to have a 2–10 % loss of BMD, with gonadal deficiency and lower femoral BMD [13]. These findings emphasize the importance of regular bone mass measurements in childhood leukemia survivors to monitor "late effects" including osteopenia and osteonecrosis and to determine the need for nonpharmacologic and pharmacologic interventions. Future research should be aimed at understanding changes in bone density and fracture risk over time to assess the impact of nutrition, mobility, exercise, and bisphosphonate therapy on the bone health of leukemia survivors.

Lymphoma

Unlike leukemia, lymphoma originates in the specific white blood cell line of lymphocytes, long established as critical components of the body's immune system. Lymphoma is divided into two broad types, based on the nature of the abnormal cells identified in a biopsy or on aspiration of the tumor tissue. The least common form, Hodgkin's disease or Hodgkin's lymphoma (HL), accounts for only 1 % of all cancers in the United States, and its occurrence is steadily declining; tumors occur in the lymph nodes and the chest area, with the disease progressing downward in an orderly manner from one contiguous lymph node to the next, seldom reaching a stage IV level. Comprised of more than 35 types, the most common form, non-Hodgkin's lymphoma (NHL), is characterized by tumors in the abdomen and a disorderly, unpredictable progression to any part of the body, with nearly 40 % of cases diagnosed at stage IV [14].

Hodgkin's Lymphoma

Bone mineral involvement, uncommon in HL and rarely encountered at diagnosis, signifies advanced stage disease and affects treatment and prognosis. As Ozdemirli et al. observe [15], the prognosis in stage IE (the earliest stage) is similar to that of a local nodal disease without osseous effect; by comparison, 5–15 % of stages III–IV

Table 1 The risk of fracture among survivors by childhood cancer diagnosis compared to siblings

	Males					Females				
	N	Fracture % ≧1	PR	95 % CI	*p*-value	*N*	Fracture ≧1 %	PR[a]	95 % CI	*p*-value
Leukemia	1229	42.2	0.91	(0.83–1.00)	0.045	1330	30.4	0.99	(0.88–1.12)	0.87
HL[b]	473	41.0	0.86	0.75–0.98	0.022	489	30.5	0.94	(0.80–1.10)	0.43
NHL[c]	376	46.3	0.98	0.86–1.12	0.75	176	30.7	0.98	(0.77–1.23)	0.84
CNS tumor[d]	469	30.7	0.66	0.56–0.76	<0.001	436	27.3	0.84	(0.71–1.00)	0.054

Source: Wilson et al. [11]

PR prevalence ratio, *CI* confidential interval

[a]Prevalence ratio adjusted for attained age and ethnicity

[b]Hodgkin lymphoma

[c]Non-Hodgkin lymphoma

[d]Central nervous system tumor

HL cases show evidence of diffuse bone involvement. The bone lesions that characterize HL generally respond to combined modality therapy consisting of chemotherapy and radiotherapy, but these interventions are likely to cause further bone deterioration, increasing the risk of vertebral and hip fractures. Whereas BMD deficits in ALL survivors are both serious and well documented, HL survivors examined at five years from therapy appear to have negligible deficits, possibly because of their older age at diagnosis [16]. At the same time, the proportion of HL survivors with BMD at 1.5–2.0 SD or lower is reported to be greater than anticipated, and males have a higher risk of a BMD lumbar *Z*-score of less than 1.5 % than females, emphasizing the need for subsequent screening as both genders age and encounter the risk of osteoporosis.

Non-Hodgkin's Lymphoma

Bone marrow involvement and low bone mineral density are more serious in non-Hodgkin's lymphoma (NHL). In contrast to the 5–14 % of HL patients who show evidence of lymphoma in the bone marrow at diagnosis, the percentage increases to 50–80 % for patients with low-grade (indolent) NHL and 25–40 % for those with high-grade (aggressive) NHL [17]. Moreover, bone marrow involvement is a critical factor in determining the staging of NHL and is generally associated with stage IV; it is treatable, as is the disease itself, with different combinations of chemotherapy, radiation, and bone marrow transplant depending on the nature and severity of the disease [18].

Although NHL therapy is associated with long-term sequelae including osteoporosis and the risk of vertebral and hip fractures, low BMD can also be present at the time of diagnosis. In patients age 50 and over, Westin et al. report that 54 % of men and 40 % of women had baseline osteopenia—a finding that was independent of disease stage or bone marrow involvement yet indicative of the observation that older men with lymphoma may be at higher risk of osteoporosis than those in the general population [19]. The Westin analysis of newly diagnosed patients with lymphoma determined that two doses of the third-generation bisphosphonate, zoledronic acid (ZA), together with calcium and vitamin D supplementation over a period of one year, prevented bone loss in this cohort. A subsequent 2014 study [20] of newly diagnosed adults with lymphoma receiving chemotherapy reported significant BMD loss at the lumbar spine (-2.7 ± 3.9) and total hip ($-2.6\,\% \pm 4.5\,\%$) as well as osteoporotic fractures after only one year of treatment, while an earlier study of 13,572 patients (age = ≥65) found increased risk of fracture and osteoporosis at up to 11 years of follow-up [21].

In studies of childhood survivors of lymphoma, estimates of osteoporosis risk is often conflicted due to varied degrees of disease severity, differing treatment strategies, small sample sizes, time from therapy completion, and study heterogeneity. For example, some researchers postulate that a decrease in BMD is time dependent, while others do not. An analysis of the long-term effects of treatment for BMD in both ALL and NHL, in which treatment protocols are similar [18], found that after five or more years of remission, more than one-third of patients treated with chemotherapy alone experienced a long-lasting BMD deficit. Those who received additional prophylactic irradiation had even lower BMD values, while others with bone marrow transplantation, combined with total body irradiation, had significantly reduced BMD at the total hip and femoral neck. The study further confirmed that male gender is a known risk factor for increased susceptibility to osteoporosis and fractures following chemotherapy, radiation, or bone marrow transplantation conditioned by total body irradiation. Yet, one of the few studies focused specifically on bone density in both types of lymphoma reported that childhood survivors evidenced no significant deficits in bone mass and maintained BMD within the normal range when examined 1–5 years following the end of therapy [22]. Because bone density loss is evident in lymphoma at baseline and can be exacerbated by standard treatment, some of the leading researchers in the field strongly advocate that routine screening should be part of the National Comprehensive Cancer Network guidelines, together with the use of prophylaxis in the form of calcium and vitamin D supplementation, zoledronic acid, and other bone-directed therapies [23].

Multiple Myeloma

Myeloma is a cancer that affects a type of white blood cells called plasma cells; as part of the immune system, they produce antibodies that protect the body from infection and disease. The disease is generally called "multiple myeloma" because malignant cells affect multiple areas of bone marrow. The incidence of myeloma increases with age (most people are diagnosed at age 65 or older), is almost twice as common in African-Americans than in Caucasians, and is relatively more prevalent in men than in women [24]. As the second most common hematologic malignancy accounting for about 15 % of these diseases, multiple myeloma has the highest occurrence of bone involvement—nearly 80 % of patients—among all malignant diseases [25].

Concentrated in the bone marrow and in the hard, outer parts of bone, myeloma cells collect in various bones, crowding out normal cells and creating multiple myelomas. As a result, "punched out" lytic lesions occur which weaken and damage bones, primarily the spine, pelvis, and rib cage. As bone density declines due to ongoing disease process, the relative risk for fracture increases [25]. See Fig. 1. Figure 2 shows diffuse myelomatous disease of the thoracolumbar spine in a patient with newly diagnosed multiple myeloma, demonstrating how quickly this disease can progress even in relatively young individuals. In terms of the mechanism [26], the receptor activator of nuclear factor kappa-B ligand (RANKL) is a potent inducer of osteoclast formation that binds to its receptor, RANK, located on osteoclasts. RANKL expression can also enhance the effects of other factors such as macrophage inflammatory protein 1 alpha (MIP-1α) and interleukin 6 (IL-6) in stimulating osteoclast formation and activity in the bone marrow microenvironment. The resulting bone resorption, in turn, leads to the release of growth factors that further increase myeloma cell production and can lead to hypercalcemia—an interaction known as the "vicious cycle of bone metastases" [3].

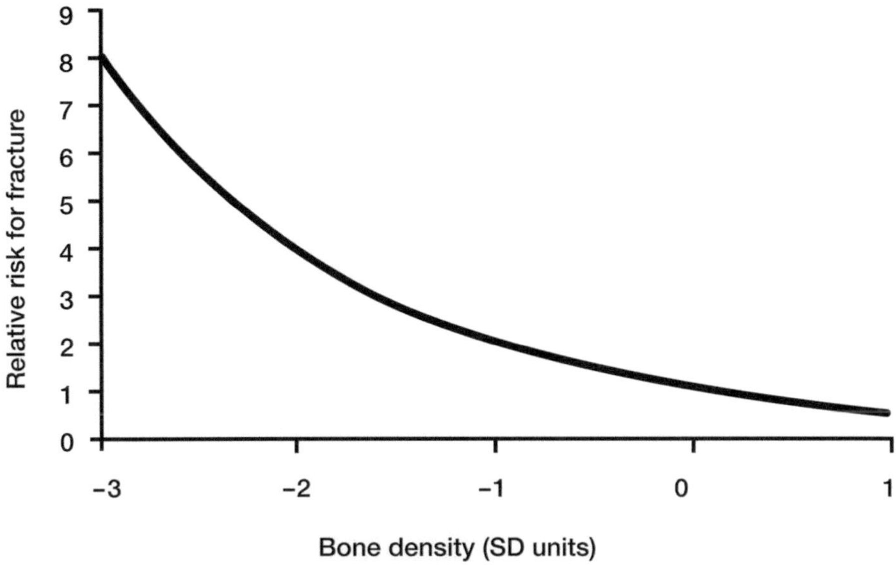

Fig. 1 Exponential relationship between bone density and fracture risk (*Source*: Adapted from Faulkner [25], with permission of the American Society for Bone and Mineral Research)

Precursor Diseases

In assessing the development of osteoporosis and fractures in multiple myeloma, attention must be given to its precursors: (1) monoclonal gammopathy of unknown significance (MGUS) which is generally regarded as asymptomatic but may progress to myeloma, and (2) "smoldering multiple myeloma," an early stage of multiple myeloma that is absent of bone lesions, hypercalcemia, and kidney damage [27]. Evidence now increasingly supports the theory that myeloma is a continuum of disease, from MGUS to smoldering myeloma to multiple myeloma.

Recent data indicate the presence of bone disease even in patients with these precursor conditions, precipitating a strong recommendation that routine DXA scans be employed to determine affected patients. A population-based retrospective cohort trial, involving 488 MGUS patients, reported a 6.3-fold increase in fracture risk at most axial, but not peripheral sites [28], while a subsequent study of 5326 MGUS patients revealed a 1.6-fold increased risk of *any fracture*, again with a higher degree of axial as opposed to distal fracture. Bisphosphonates, used in the clinical management of MAGUS and smoldering multiple myeloma, have a marked effect on BMD. A study by Pepe et al. involving alendronate in MGUS demonstrated a 6.1 increase in mean BMD of the lumbar spine and a 1.5 % increase in the total femur [29], while in a trial involving zoledronic acid, Berenson et al. reported a median increase in BMD of +15.0 % in lumbar spine and +6.0 % in total hip, with no new fractures [30]. However, neither alendronate, nor pamidronate, nor zoledronic acid are effective in halting the progression to active multiple myeloma [31].

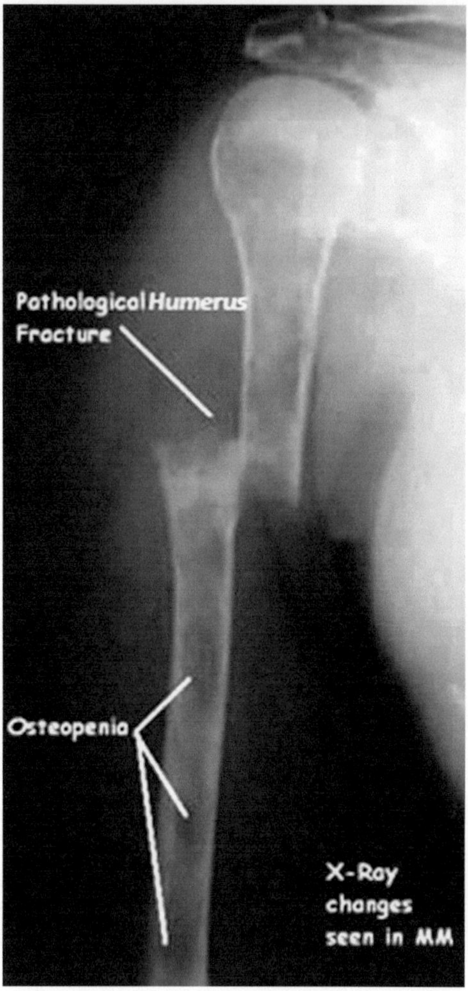

Fig. 2 Metastatic multiple myeloma of the thoracolumbar spine. Image demonstrates diffuse myelomatous disease of the thoracolumbar spine in a 30-year old female, with epidural soft tissue extension of the tumor at T-3. In addition, multiple compression deformities are seen along the thoracolumbar spine, the worst of which is at T-3 where there is vertebral plana (*Source*: Courtesy of Thomas Jefferson University Department of Radiology)

Active Multiple Myeloma

A number of interacting factors including increased osteoblastic activity and a heightened number of osteoclasts, decreased activity in the surrounding osteoblasts, increased markers of bone resorption with decreased markers of bone production, and persistent lytic lesions that inhibit bone repair all contribute to the severity of active multiple myeloma [32]. In newly diagnosed multiple myeloma patients, some 80 % have bone disease. Over 60 % of the cases of osteopenia, osteoporosis, and pathological fractures involve the spine as opposed to 90 % in metastatic prostate cancer and 75 % in metastatic breast cancer [33]. A study by Dhodapkar et al. found bone density to be significantly decreased at lumbar spine and femoral neck with duration of disease at >12 months as well as an independent association between female sex and lower BMD [34]. In another retrospective population-based cohort of 165 residents from Olmstead County, Minnesota, Melton et al. [35] reported that at the time of initial myeloma diagnosis, 16 times more fractures occurred than were expected and that subsequently a ninefold increase in fractures was observed. Although two-thirds were pathologic fractures of the vertebrae and the ribs, the risk of subsequent osteoporotic fracture was elevated twofold. Admittedly this increase coincides with a time of decreased survival probability.

Treatment

Bisphosphonates, which are used as therapy for osteoporosis, lytic bone lesions, and hypercalcemia, have become the standard of treatment in multiple myeloma. Administered intravenously, pamidronate and zoledronic acid (ZA) have proved particularly effective. For pamidronate, a dosage of 30 mg monthly has been recommended to protect against skeletal complications [36]. In comparison, 4 mg of ZA, administered every 3–4 weeks, has a more rapid infusion time and is more potent, reducing the overall risk of skeletal damage by an additional 16 % over pamidronate [37]. Moreover, despite the side effects including osteonecrosis of the jaw, ZA has been found to reduce bone loss and to independently improve overall survival, indicating a possible synergy with first-line myeloma therapies [38]. If myeloma should affect the spine resulting in a vertebral compression, both vertebroplasty and kyphoplasty (the injection of bone cement into the vertebrae) have been judged to be safe and effective [31].

Finally, daratumumab has recently become the first monoclonal antibody approved by the FDA for treatment of multiple myeloma cases that are refractory to proteasome inhibitors and immunomodulatory drugs. Given its favorable safety profile and its demonstrated efficacy, daratumumab is a much-needed targeted approach and a potentially transformative drug in the armamentarium of multiple myeloma [39, 40]. If this agent proves effective, future generations may not experience the lytic bone lesions and related disability that we now observe.

The incidence of osteoporosis and fractures in hematological malignancies is an active research area. In lymphoma and other childhood cancers affecting bone, further research on survivors should elucidate the impact on BMD of such risk factors as genetic predisposition, adverse treatment effects, poor nutritional status, restricted physical activity, and the natural aging process [41]. In myeloma, the marked improvement in 5-year survival rates from 12 % in 1960–1963 to 46.6 % in 2005–2011 [42, 43] with even significantly higher percentages at many institutions, underlines the need to ensure optimal use of bisphosphonates as well as to explore the treatment potential of newer agents such as recently FDA-approved monoclonal antibody, denosumab [31].

Solid Tumors

Whereas multiple myeloma affects the skeleton by means of bone lesions, solid tumors including breast, prostate, lung, and kidney metastasize to bone. Before examining the effect of solid tumors themselves as well as their treatments on bone, it might be helpful to consider the relation between solid tumor cancer, baseline BMD, and fracture risk, with particular reference to breast and prostate cancer. High rather than low bone mineral density is a known prognostic factor for both postmenopausal breast cancer in Caucasian women and prostate cancer. Zmuda et al. have shown that women 65 years and older with high BMD have a 2 to 2.5-fold increase in breast cancer risk [44], while a study by Zambetti and Tartter of postmenopausal women (median age = 57) with breast cancer confirmed the association between high BMD and high risk of breast cancer [45]. The authors speculate that elevated BMD in those with breast cancer may be related to estrogen levels, which are believed to increase the risk of breast cancer in some women but contribute favorably to bone mass accrual. While some early studies demonstrated a correlation between endogenous androgen levels and elevated BMD, findings were inconsistent based on limited hormonal assessment time points.

To address these discrepancies, Farhat et al. examined a cohort of older men with no history of prostate cancer [46]. Unexpectedly, they demonstrated that higher BMD of the total body was significantly related to lower risk for prostate cancer, supporting the findings of the NHANES I Epidemiology Follow-Up Survey. Although not significant statistically, NHANES data found a decline in prostate cancer risk was associated with higher quartiles of bone density [47]. Findings still remain difficult to interpret because total body BMD results in Farhat et al. were associated with lower prostate cancer in terms of high-grade tumors, yet no association with total hip or spine BMD or with low-grade tumors was observed. It remains uncertain if practitioners of rehabilitation patients can take comfort in higher BMD findings of a newly diagnosed patient with solid bone tumors. The above studies do not specifically address fracture risk. Moreover individuals undergoing active cancer treatment may be globally weak, predisposing them to falls that can lead to fracture.

Nonetheless, in patients with newly diagnosed breast and prostate cancer, low bone density and fracture risk resulting in osteopenia and osteoporosis do exist. In such cases, interventions should be taken to address the clinical risk of fracture. Both postmenopausal and premenopausal women with breast cancer may already have low BMD or develop this condition soon after diagnosis, leading to the American Society of Clinical Oncology's recommendation of routine DXA scans [48]. Moreover a study by Chen et al. demonstrates that both fracture and fall risks are significantly elevated after a diagnosis of breast cancer but not before [49].

In prostate cancer, low bone mineral density is again present at baseline. For example, Berruti et al. found that at baseline, 46 % of prostate cancer cases were osteopenic and 14 % were osteoporotic at lumbar spine, while 40 % were osteopenic and 4 % were osteoporotic at the hip [50].

Physiologic Basis of Bone Metastases

Bone metastasis is generally defined as the spread of cancer cells from their primary site through the blood stream or lymph system to a new organ where they can settle and grow [51]. Metastases are found primarily in bones in the center of the body, particularly the spine. Breast and prostate cancer account for 70–80 % of metastatic bone disease, while metastases occur in 40 % of advanced lung cancer patients [52]. In addition, multiple myeloma and thyroid and kidney cancers metastasize to bone [53].

Metastases manifest themselves in two ways: (1) by affecting osteoclasts and weakening bones without forming new bone, they result in the osteolytic or lytic lesions characteristic of breast cancer; (2) by affecting osteoblasts and promoting bone formation without destroying old bone, they produce abnormally hard bones (sclerosis) with the osteoblastic lesions evident in prostate cancer. As described in the discussion of multiple myeloma, bone metastases are the result of an interaction between tumor cells and the metastatic site characterized as a "vicious cycle": as tumor cells simulate bone cells to cause either bone destruction or bone formation, the bone microenvironment provides tumor cells with growth factors that stimulate the tumor cells to grow [26]. The resulting skeletal-related events (SREs), including severe bone pain, pathological fractures, spinal cord compression, hypercalcemia, impaired mobility, and the need for radiotherapy or surgery, are often exacerbated by the common risk factors for osteoporosis [54]. In a later section of this chapter, we will cover specific recommendations for fixation of metastatic bone lesions, precautions during physical therapy before and after fixation, and how to approach a patient with bone metastases that are not suitable for fixation.

Cancer Treatment-Induced Bone Loss

The challenges to bone health posed by cancer itself are further compounded by the drugs used to treat it, referred to as cancer treatment-induced bone loss (CTIBL). Although these drugs, specifically aromatase inhibitors in women (anastrozole, exemestane, letrozole) and androgen-deprivation therapy in men, have significantly increased the overall survival rates of cancer patients, they have exerted adverse effects on their bones, decreasing BMD and increasing the risk for osteopenia and osteoporosis. Moreover, these drugs have come into widespread use at the same time as age-related factors, contributing to bone degeneration, are exerting their effect across the cancer spectrum.

Patients under cancer treatment should not only adhere to the standard nonpharmaceutical therapies for osteoporosis, including calcium and vitamin D supplementation, weight-bearing exercise, and modification of such lifestyle factors as smoking and alcohol, but should also consider receiving bisphosphonate therapy with its established potency and known minimal effects [55]. The following section will consider the principal interventions used in treating breast and prostate cancer as well as strategies for maintaining bone health.

Breast Cancer

Early Menopause

Affecting 1 % of women under the age of 40 years [56], early menopause is precipitated by a number of factors ranging from genetics, smoking, and low body mass to autoimmune diseases, chromosome disease (Turner syndrome), and surgery (bilateral oophorectomy). In addition, chemotherapy used to treat breast cancer is likely to cause ovarian failure and loss of estrogen production, leading to sudden or premature menopause and increasing the risk of osteoporosis and fractures. Chemotherapy-induced ovarian failure (CIOF) occurs in more than 50 % of premenopausal women within the first year of treatment [57]. In a trial of 49 premenopausal women with stage I/II breast cancer receiving adjuvant chemotherapy, 39 experienced ovarian failure and, within that group, the median decrease in bone density was 7.7 % in lumbar spine and 4.6 % in femoral neck at 12 months [58]. Other studies have reported similar results confirming that early menopause leads to lower BMD and a higher risk of osteoporosis. The earlier menopause occurs, the greater the BMD loss later in life. In addition, tamoxifen, frequently used in premenopausal women with estrogen receptor-positive breast cancer, has been shown to produce an average annual decrease in lumbar BMD of 1.44 % over a 3-year period. (In comparison, tamoxifen prevents bone loss in postmenopausal women.) [59].

Given their superior efficacy and safety, aromatase inhibitors (AIs) such as anastrozole, letrozole, and exemestane are increasingly used to lower estrogen levels and impede tumor growth, but they too have a deleterious effect on bone. Although indicated for use only in postmenopausal women, recent studies have shown that AIs may have a positive effect in women with premature ovarian failure (POF) if they are combined with other medications. An examination of the effect of endocrine therapy together with zoledronic acid on such women [60] found that after a 3-year period, endocrine therapy alone resulted in a significant BMD loss of 11.3 % at lumbar spine and 7.3 % at trochanter. However, with the addition of zoledronic acid to the treatment regimen, BMD was stable at three years and increased at both lumbar spine and trochanter at five years.

Most recently, the results of two large clinical trials—the Tamoxifen and Exemestane Trial (TEXT) [61] and the Suppression of Ovarian Function Trial (SOFT) [62], indicated that the AI exemestane, combined with ovarian suppression to achieve low estrogen levels, was superior to both tamoxifen–ovarian suppression and tamoxifen alone. Although these results have been termed "practice changing," an increased use of exemestane, as opposed to the bone-conserving tamoxifen, will have adverse effects on bone.

An increased number of fractures are also evident in early menopause. In a Swedish study of 733 women with a follow-up at 11 years, those with early menopause had 50 % more fractures than those under the age of 70 who experienced a normal menopause [63]. The results of a 2004 Rotterdam population-based cohort study showed that early menopause compared with menopause at older than 50 years resulted in a significant increase in vertebral fractures at a relative risk of 2.4 but that, recognizing its adverse effects, estrogen use for more than three years was highly protective against fractures [64].

Postmenopausal Status

Whereas early menopause signifies that women will spend a longer time with weakened bone, postmenopausal women with breast cancer concurrently face issues posed not only by disease- and age-related bone loss but also by CTIBL. Osteoporosis may occur at any point in breast cancer progression: at the time of diagnosis as well as during cancer treatment and cancer-free survival, while hypogonadism induced by cancer therapy may further compound rapid loss of BMD [65]. Bone metastases and CTRBL require different interventions to prevent and stabilize BMD and fracture risk.

Cancer Treatment: Induced Bone Loss

Aromatase Inhibitors (AIs)

Favorable randomized trial results have led to the increasing use of AIs in breast cancer to the extent that they are now regarded as the first-line adjuvant therapy for postmenopausal women with hormone-responsive tumors. By lowering estradiol levels, both the nonsteroid reversible inhibitor, anastrozole, and the steroid irreversible inhibitor, exemestane, have been shown to reduce risk of breast cancer by at least 50 % [66, 67]. Although AIs have been demonstrated to have a positive effect on breast cancer risk, they have not been approved by the FDA for chemoprevention. Moreover, studies reveal that they exert damaging effects on bone.

With respect to bone loss and fracture risk, results of the Arimidex, Tamoxifen, Alone or in Combination (ATAC) trial indicate a significant loss in BMD of 6.08 % at the lumbar spine and 7.24 % at total hip after five years of anastrozole treatment; 43 % of women with normal BMD at treatment initiation developed osteopenia, compared with 9 % on tamoxifen. However, Eastell et al. have shown that anastrozole treatment-related bone loss does not continue into an off-treatment period: at six years after the ATAC trial, lumbar spine BMD increased by 2.35 % and at seven years by 4.02 %. Following two years of treatment with exemestane, loss of volumetric BMD at the distal radius and tibia was significantly greater than in a placebo group, while cortical thickness and area declined 7.9 % versus −1.1 % in the controls—a notable finding because 80 % of bone mass is cortical [68, 69]. At 24 months, patients on letrozole had a greater decrease in total hip BMD (3.6 %) and lumbar spine (5.35 %) than those on placebos [70]. All three AIs are associated with an increased risk of fractures conditions, and regular monitoring is recommended [71].

Chemotherapy and Radiation

Despite advances in cancer medications, chemotherapy and radiation therapy are still employed to achieve clearly defined objectives. Neoadjuvant (preoperative) chemotherapy is used to shrink or slow the growth of tumors, lowering the mastectomy rate, decreasing adverse events, and enabling researchers to assess tumor behavior in situ [72]. Patients treated with a high dose of radiation are at risk of rib fractures based on dosage: the lower the dosage (less than 50 Gy), the lower the fracture rate. Moreover, when radiation is combined with chemotherapy or surgery, the incidence of rib fractures increases compared to that in patients treated solely with a lower dose of radiation [65].

Selective Estrogen Reuptake Modulations

In terms of hormone therapies, studies indicate that the selective estrogen reuptake modulations (SERMs), tamoxifen and raloxifene, are efficacious and safe in breast cancer patients and do not appear to cause skeletal complications in postmenopausal women. Both agents are FDA approved for preventing breast cancer. As noted above, tamoxifen has different effects before and after menopause. Whereas tamoxifen is associated with bone loss in premenopausal women, it is linked to increased BMD following menopause, not only preserving and increasing BMD at the spine and hip but also reducing fracture risk [73]. A Canadian trial found that osteoporosis-related fracture risk decreased by 32 % and hip fracture risk by 53 % [74].

Originally FDA-approved for prevention and treatment of osteoporosis, raloxifene is now sanctioned for reduction of breast cancer risk in postmenopausal women with osteoporosis or those with elevated risk of breast cancer. As the STAR Breast Cancer Prevention trial revealed [75], raloxifene and tamoxifen are equally effective in reducing the risk of invasive breast cancer by about 50 %, with tamoxifen being somewhat more effective at preventing noninvasive disease. It should be noted, however, that tamoxifen has not gained widespread acceptance because it increases endometrial cancer and thromboembolic events including blood clots, whereas raloxifene leads to far less toxicity and retains its 38 % effectiveness over the long term.

Treatment of Bone Metastases

Several recent studies have elucidated the role of bisphosphonates in the treatment of skeletal-related events in postmenopausal breast cancer, comparing the most frequently used intravenous agent, ZA, with denosumab. A meta-analysis conducted by the Early Breast Cancer Trialists' Collaborative Group [76] determined that bisphosphonate therapy significantly reduced the development of bone metastasis and the rate of breast cancer recurrence, in addition to protecting bone health, particularly in women receiving aromatase inhibitors. The Zometa-Femara Adjuvant Synergy Trial (Z-FAST) focused on the timing of treatment with ZA in postmenopausal women with early-stage breast cancer receiving adjuvant letrozole therapy and found that upfront treatment with ZA, as opposed to delayed administration, significantly and progressively increased BMD, resulting in a mean difference in lumbar spine and total hip of 8.9 % and 6.7 %, respectively, at the 5-year mark [77]. Comparisons of ZA and denosumab tend to favor the latter, but individual circumstances must be taken into account in determining appropriate personalized treatment. In a randomized, double-blind study [78], denosumab demonstrated greater effectiveness in delaying or preventing SREs in women with breast cancer metastatic to bone; moreover, its benefits include the convenience of a subcutaneous injection and no requirement for renal monitoring. Overall survival, disease progression, and rate of adverse events were similar. Further, a 2012 trial [79] involving more than 2000 patients with advanced breast cancer, reported that fewer patients on denosumab compared with ZA had first SREs, multiple SREs, pathologic fractures, radiation therapy to bone, and hypercalcemia;

there was also a "clinically meaningful" improvement in health-related quality of life for those on denosumab. In addition to pamidronate and ZA denosumab was added to list of recommended treatments for bone metastases by the American Society of Clinical Oncologists in 2011 [80].

Treatment of CTIBL

The primary goal of managing CTIBL is to reduce fracture risk with a threefold approach; screening at age 60–65 for women with increased osteoporosis risk, lifestyle changes including calcium and vitamin D supplementation, weight-bearing exercises, and cessation of smoking, together with pharmacologic interventions, specifically bisphosphonates and, more recently, denosumab.

Although proven effective, first-generation oral bisphosphonates (clodronate) have largely given way to more potent second-generation intravenous compounds (pamidronate) and third-generation intravenous drugs (zoledronic acid-ZA) in treating CRIBL. As Blanchette et al. point out [81], oral bisphosphonates remain an affordable and "reasonable" treatment for breast cancer patients with limited bone disease; however, pamidronate, ZA, and denosumab have superior efficacy and are used in more advanced cancer and hypercalcemia. Denosumab is currently the only FDA-approved therapy for the treatment of AI-induced bone loss in women with early-stage breast cancer. Since FDA approval, a randomized, double-blind trial has further determined that denosumab, compared with placebo, has a significantly delayed time to first fracture in addition to an overall reduced number of fractures [82]. In 2015 a new trial showed that denosumab had an 18 % reduced risk of disease recurrence; together with its demonstrated 50 % reduction in fractures caused by adjuvant aromatase inhibitors [83].

Safety, compliance, and cost are also relevant factors in selecting treatment. Similar safety profiles exist for both ZA and denosumab; however, ZA is known to increase incidence of osteonecrosis of the jaw and renal toxicity, while denosumab poses a risk of severe hypocalcemia. Both denosumab, administered at 6-month intervals, and ZA, administered monthly for at least the first year, have greater compliance rates than oral bisphosphonates. Finally the advantages of denosumab must be balanced against its expense, particularly because ZA no longer has patent protection, potentially affecting its cost [84]. The cost of denosumab exceeds that of ZA and of oral bisphosphonates by a significant margin, raising potentially serious insurance issues. Cost-effectiveness studies, hindered by discrepant methodologies, end point variabilities, and changes in drug prices, are difficult to compare and await a more consistent, standardized approach [85].

Research to date clearly indicates that bone loss in breast cancer can be prevented and treated. What is needed is greater awareness of the incidence of concomitant bone loss and its consequences as well as more frequent screening. New findings on effective therapies are also emerging. For example, a recent phase III clinical trial established that following one year of monthly treatment with ZA, patients with metastatic breast cancer can scale back to an every 12-weeks maintenance dosing schedule with equal efficacy, reducing the risk of adverse side effects, patient inconvenience, and cost [86].

Prostate Cancer

Bone loss in breast and prostate cancer is similar in several respects, including time of occurrence, cause, and treatment. Like breast cancer, prostate cancer occurs primarily in the elderly and thus concurrently with osteoporosis. Bone is adversely affected by both the disease itself and by associated treatments, and bone loss responds to treatment with medications such as bisphosphonates and denosumab.

Just as aromatase inhibitors are used to lower estrogen levels in women, so androgen-deprivation therapy (ADT), involving bilateral orchiectomy or gonadotropin-releasing hormone (GnRH) analogues, is used to shrink prostate cancer cells or slow their growth by decreasing testosterone levels. Testosterone reduction, in turn, suppresses estrogen, now recognized as equally or potentially more important than testosterone in prostate cancer bone loss [87]. For many years, testosterone was regarded as the hormone primarily responsible for bone remodeling in men; now reduction in both circulating testosterone and estrogen is known to decrease osteoblasts and increase osteoclasts, leading to the erosion of trabecular bone by osteoclasts and the formation of structurally weak sclerotic-woven bone by osteoclasts [88]. Depending on the specific case, both the WHO Fracture Risk Assessment Tool (FRAX) and DXA testing are recommended to obtain baseline measurements.

Bone Metastases

In both breast and prostate cancer, bone metastases occur in up to 80–90 % of patients with advanced disease [89]. They lead to serious skeletal complications including pain, hypercalcemia, impaired mobility, spinal cord compression, and fractures, particularly in vertebral bones—conditions that are exacerbated in men by androgen-deprivation therapy (ADT), the principal treatment for metastatic prostate cancer [88]. However, it should be noted that only 7–16 % of fractures in prostate cancer are secondary to bone metastases. The others result from pretreatment low bone density, forms of cancer-induced treatment bone loss particularly due to AI or ADT, physical immobility, and nutrient deficiencies.

ADT encompasses (1) bilateral orchiectomy, (2) GnRH analogues, and (3) combined androgen blockade (CAB), which combines either GnRH analogues or orchiectomy with an antiandrogen such as bicalutamide [90]. Its objective is to prevent the production and use of androgens by the body, thereby impeding the growth and survival of cancer cells; however, it does not halt disease progression. Although most men with advanced prostate cancer initially respond well to ADT, the cancer can return, at which stage it is termed "castration resistant," signifying that ADT is no longer effective. A comparison of several cancer treatment modalities and their associated bone loss in the lumbar spine is presented in Fig. 3 [91].

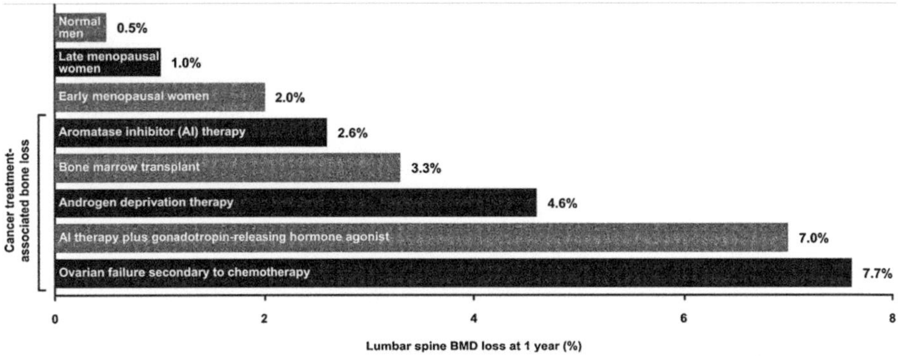

Fig. 3 Bone loss associated with various cancer therapies. Menopausal women lose bone at a rate of 1–2 % yearly. Cancer treatments, such as aromatase inhibitor therapy and chemotherapy, accelerate this process, leading to significant bone loss and subsequent skeletal complications (*Source*: Reproduced with permission from Guise [91])

Treatment of Bone Metastases

Bisphosphonates, particularly ZA and denosumab, have become the established therapies to slow or reverse bone loss caused by skeletal metastases. Although oral bisphosphonates cannot significantly reduce metastatic bone pain [92], intravenous forms, particularly ZA, have demonstrated positive results, with a potency of 100–1000 times that of pamidronate in vitro systems [92]. In 2002 the FDA approved ZA use for metastatic prostate cancer, citing a study by Saad et al. which found that fewer patients treated with 4 mg of ZA had SREs (33.2 %) compared with the placebo group (44.2 %); the median time to the first SRE was 488 days compared with 321 days for placebo [93]. As of 2016, several labeling changes have been instituted for Zometa including warnings about subtrochanteric and diaphyseal femoral fractures, acute phase reaction, and osteonecrosis of the jaw [94].

The steadily increasing role of denosumab in prostate cancer is supported by a number of clinical trials that demonstrate its efficacy not only in preventing or delaying fractures in men with metastases but also in slowing the spread of cancer to bone in men without metastases but with rising PSA levels [95]. In a path-breaking comparison of ZA with denosumab, involving 342 medical centers in 39 countries, Fizazi et al. [96] reported that the median time to the first SRE was significantly longer with denosumab (20.7 months) than with ZA (17.1 months); the former also resulted in a decreased rate of multiple SREs.

In cancer, both agents are used more frequently than they are for postmenopausal osteoporosis and studies indicate less frequent dosing with denosumab with respect to cancer patients. With both drugs approved for use, attention is now focused on dosing frequency and reduced dosages; if further randomized trials can confirm no significant difference between treatments every 6–12 months as opposed to every 3–4 weeks, the outcome would be lower costs for both patients and the healthcare system, as well as potentially decreased drug side effects [97]. Still, questions remain about the relative benefits of ZA and denosumab [98]: What is the cost-effectiveness of each treatment, particularly given the expiration of the ZA patent in 2013 and the probable extension of the patent for denosumab for some time in the future? Apart from clear recommendations of agents to treat osteoporosis in persons with impaired renal function, in which denosumab is an option but ZA is contraindicated, are there other reasons why some patients would benefit more from one agent than the other? Can denosumab be used to delay onset of metastasis? What is the effect of denosumab on bone pain and quality of life [99]?

Cancer Treatment-Induced Bone Loss

Whereas ADT was once used primarily in metastatic prostate cancer, it is increasingly administered in less serious stages of the disease. During ADT, circulating levels of testosterone decrease by >95 % and estrogen by >80 % [100] BMD begins to decrease within months of ADT initiation; at the end of the first year of therapy, it has declined by 2–8 % in the lumbar spine and from 1.8 to 6.5 % in the hip, continuing to diminish at a slower rate with long-term ADT [101]. Extended duration of ADT also markedly increases fracture risk, with an estimate of some 3000 excess fractures per year attributable to hormone agents; older age and more advanced stages of cancer may confound these results [102]. A 2015 study of risk fracture reported that patients receiving ADT experienced a 10.8 % fracture rate compared to 3.2 % for those not receiving ADT, results that are possibly confounded by pathologic fractures and spinal cord compression [103].

Two small randomized controlled trials with bisphosphonates have shown limited positive results in men without bone metastases. An investigation of the use of IV pamidronate in patients treated with the GnRH agonist, leuprolide, found pamidronate prevented bone loss in the hip and lumbar spine [104] while a subsequent study of 4 mg ZA as therapy for ADT in men with nonmetastatic prostate cancer demonstrated that, over a period of three months in one year, ZA actually significantly increased BMD in the lumbar spine by 5.6 % as opposed to placebo, with increases also observed in the BMD of the femoral neck, trochanter, and total hip. More recently, a once-yearly infusion of 4 mg ZA was shown to significantly increase the BMD at lumbar spine by 4.0 % in nonmetastatic prostate cancer, indicating that less-frequent dosing may be a more convenient but still effective strategy for preventing osteoporosis in men receiving GnRH [105].

Although these studies did not follow patients long enough to detect fracture risk, trials involving toremifene and denosumab have shown their efficacy in reducing fracture risk in high-risk prostate cancer patients receiving ADT. In a 2013 study comparing toremifene with placebo in such a population [106], the incidence of new vertebral fractures was 2.5 % in the toremifene group compared with 4.9 % in the placebo group—a significant relative risk reduction of 50 %. Toremifene also increased BMD at the lumbar spine, hip, and femoral neck and decreased markers of bone turnover. With regard to denosumab, the Hormone Ablation Bone Loss Trial (HALT-138) (NCT00089674) administered 60 mg of denosumab twice yearly to nonmetastatic patients at high risk for fractures; not only did BMD of the spine and hip increase significantly, but the incidence of new vertebral fractures decreased at 12, 24, and 36 months with a cumulative incidence of 1.5 % in the denosumab group versus 3.9 % in the placebo group at the end of three years—a 62 % reduction. These results were critical in gaining FDA approval for denosumab (Prolia) to increase bone mass and prevent fractures in men receiving ADT as well as in women taking AIs for breast cancer [107]. Routine bone scans every 1–2 years are recommended during treatment and relevant lifestyle modifications should be implemented [108].

Lung Cancer

Although research has concentrated on the impact of breast and prostate cancer on bone, a limited number of studies have examined the lung and, to a lesser extent, the kidney. After breast and prostate, the lung is the third most common site of origin for metastatic cancer deposits in bone, specifically the spine, pelvis, proximal long bones and, uniquely, the bones of the hands and feet. Lung cancer is divided into two categories based on cell size and tumor type (as determined by microscopic examination): non-small cell lung cancer (NSCLC) accounts for approximately 85 % of cases and small cell lung cancer (SCLC) comprises about 15 % [109]. However, SCLCs grow more rapidly and are more likely to metastasize, even to the point where metastasis can be evident at the time of diagnosis. The "vicious cycle of bone metastases," characteristic of other solid bone tumors, is evident in lung cancer as well.

In terms of the link between preexisting or concomitant osteoporosis and lung cancer, a study by McGlynn et al., one of the largest cancer follow-ups ever conducted among individuals hospitalized with osteoporosis, found that patients younger than 70 years with osteoporosis had an increased risk of NSCLC than those without osteoporosis [110]. A subsequent study confirmed these findings, reporting that a low BMD Z-score was strongly associated with a higher risk of NSCLC [111].

Bone Metastases

About 30–40 % of patients with lung cancer develop bone metastases, with a survival rate between 6–12 months [112]. In the first instance, most patients experience pain, followed by SREs including pathological fractures, spinal cord compression, the need for palliative radiotherapy or surgery to bone, and, less frequently, hypercalcemia. The development of these symptoms has led guideline agencies in the United States and Europe to recommend that bone scans, in the form of a combination of

18F-fluorodeoxyglucose (18F-FDG) positron emission tomography (PET) and computerized tomography (CT), be undertaken at the time of diagnosis [113].

Patients who develop SREs are 20–40 % more likely to die than those without SRE [114], with bone fractures being the most common SRE [112]. A recent Canadian study of 301 patients with metastatic NSCLC reported that 39 % had bone lesions, and 59 % had SREs, with two or more SREs related to smoking and a younger age; fractures accounted for 22 % of the SREs. The overall survival of patients with bone metastases is 5.5 months, compared with 9.9 months for those without bone lesions [115]. Although age, gender, and stage of NSCLC do not appear to influence the occurrence of SREs, a number of factors are associated with their development. Patients with a history of smoking have been found to be 6.7 times more likely to suffer SREs than those who never smoked; patients with poor performance status, less than ≥2, and those with multiple bone metastases were independently 3.3 times as likely to have SREs than those with a performance status of >2 or only a single bone metastasis [116, 117].

Treatment of Bone Metastases

For some time, platinum-based chemotherapies (cisplatin, the most common platinum-based chemotherapy drug, or carboplatin) have been regarded as the standard of care for NSCLC [112]. They are often used in combination with other drugs including third-generation chemotherapy agents (paclitaxel and docetaxel) and tyrosine kinase inhibitors (TKIs) (e.g., gefitinib). However, because the platinum-based components of these combined doses is associated with nephrotoxicity, third-generation agents or TKIs, alone or in combination, are also used, while recognizing that these regimens have lower response rates and are not known to prolong survival rates [116]. Single-agent chemotherapy is preferred in older patients.

As Brodowicz et al. have pointed out [118], unlike the bone loss associated with chemotherapy in breast and prostate cancer, the components of NSCLC therapy may have a beneficial effect on bone resorption. Not only does gefitinib inhibit bone resorption, but clinical trials have shown that a combination regimen of cisplatin, mitomycin C, and vinblastine decreases bone resorption, with patients experiencing less frequent bone metastases [119]. Research to identify less toxic and more effective platinum drugs is ongoing. A study by Park et al. identified phenanthriplatin as 4–40 times more powerful than cisplatin in destroying cancer cells across a range of cancer types and better able to evade cancer cell resistance [120].

Bone-Targeted Agents

In comparison with bone and prostate cancer, data on the use of bone-targeted agents in lung cancer is scarce. In a placebo-controlled, phase III trial of 773 patients with NSCLC, Rosen et al. were among the first to demonstrate the superior efficacy of ZA [121]. They reported that ZA was the first bisphosphonate to reduce SREs in lung cancer: patients taking a 4 mg dose of ZA had a 31 % risk of developing at least one SRE as opposed to 46 % with placebo; moreover, they also experienced a significantly delayed onset of complications as well as a significantly reduced annual incidence of SREs. Not only is ZA effective and safe but its short infusion time makes it more convenient for patient use.

Recent trials have further indicated that ZA may have anticancer effects on lung cancer. As Mahtani et al. have observed, preclinical and clinical studies provide limited evidence about the potential of ZA to exert positive effects on disease progression outside the bone, generally in combination with chemotherapy. But larger, prospective trials are needed to clarify the benefits of ZA therapy and to answer questions such as optimal dosing, initiation, duration of treatment, and the benefits of combination therapy [122].

Within the last decade, a therapy strategy directly targeting RANKL has emerged in the form of denosumab, now approved for the prevention of SREs in patients with solid tumor and bone metastases. The key study in gaining FDA approval was a phase III trial comparing denosumab with ZA in the treatment of advanced cancers and multiple myeloma, excluding breast and prostate cancer [123]. Focusing on a subset of lung cancer patients (both NSCLC and SCLC, $n=81$) from that analysis, Scagliotti et al. [124] found that denosumab was associated with significantly improved overall median survival of 8.9 months compared with 7.7 months for ZA, in addition to a statistically significant improvement in SREs and a delayed time to the first SRE of 20.6 months versus 16.3 months for ZA. Moreover, acute-phase reactions and nephrotoxicity occurred less often in the subcutaneous administration of denosumab than with ZA, indicating that despite its high incidence of hypocalcemia, denosumab may be more suitable for combination with platinum-based therapy in NSCLC [116].

Yet to be determined are the mechanisms underlying the action of denosumab and the relative cost-effectiveness of denosumab versus ZA; however, for patients with little time to live, increased survival time is a compelling factor in their decision process. The radioisotope, radium 223; the tyrosine kinase inhibitor, cabozantinib; and the c-Src (saracatinib) tyrosine kinase are novel bone-targeted agents, now showing promise in breast and prostate cancer and currently under investigation for their applicability in lung cancer [125]. The potential efficacy of these agents in *preventing* bone metastases is the subject of emerging research, holding the promise of a longer survival for patients with advanced lung cancer [126].

Renal Cell Carcinoma

Renal cell carcinoma (RCC) is the most common form of kidney cancer, occurring in nine out of ten cases, with clear cell carcinoma as the most common subcategory. The prognosis is better than for lung cancer but worse than for breast and prostate cancer, generally because RCC responds poorly to radiation and chemotherapy [127].

Bone Metastases

Approximately one-third of patients with newly diagnosed RCC have bone metastatic renal cell carcinoma (mRCC), together with SREs. Whereas the development of new therapies holds the promise of longer life spans in RCC, it is possible that bone will become, what Wood et al. term, a "sanctuary site" with increasingly frequent bone metastases [128]. As Woodward et al. have determined, the mean number of SREs in a cohort of 254 RCC patients with bone metastases was 2.4 % over the course of the disease, with only 37 patients experiencing no SRE [129]. Together with anticipated hypercalcemia, an unexpected incidence of spinal cord/nerve root compression occurred in 27 % of patients overall, increasing to 30 % in patients with bone metastases at time of diagnosis. As the authors emphasize, spinal cord compression requires emergency treatment and can result in paralysis, pointing up the importance of baseline and regular screening. A potentially "revolutionary" treatment for spinal metastases has emerged in the form of cement augmentation which stabilizes the vertebral body, providing pain relief and anterior column support and enabling patients to remain ambulant, continent, and pain free [130].

Treatment for Bone Metastases

Treatment for bone metastases has passed through a number of stages. With surgical resection now confined largely to localized RCC or a solitary metastasis and chemotherapy no longer accepted as a standard of care, cytokines became the mainstay of treatments in the period from the late 1980s to the mid-2000s. However, the cytokine agents, specifically interferon alpha (IFNα) and interleukin-2 (IL-2) have a low overall response rate with only modest improvements in survival (median overall survival of 12 months) and significant toxic consequences, which limit their widespread use [131].

Today, with advanced understanding of the pathogenesis of RCC, treatment has moved beyond the cytokine era to the era of targeted therapies. Molecular research has shown that in the process of metastasis, malignant tumors must necessarily produce growth factors to stimulate the formation of new blood vessels—a process known as angiogenesis. These growth factors include vascular endothelial growth factor (VEGF) and its receptor, platelet-derived growth factor receptor (PDGF-R), as well as the mammalian target of rapamycin (mTOR) [132–134]. By activating tyrosine kinases critical to the development of new blood vessels, the growth factors enable tumors to grow and metastasize. In 2005–2006, the FDA approved the first new treatment option for kidney cancer in over a decade: the tyrosine kinase inhibitors, sorafenib and sunitinib, followed in succeeding years by bevacizumab, a monoclonal antibody targeting VEGF, and other tyrosine kinase (pazopanib, axitinib) and mTOR inhibitors (everolimus, temsirolimus). By targeting both the tumor and the tumor blood vessel structure (the signaling pathways), these drugs interfere with the reproduction of cancer cells and slow their rate of growth. As single agents or in combination with INFα, they have become the new standard of care for most patients with metastatic RCC, as recommended by the 2016 National Comprehensive Cancer Network Guidelines [135].

Most of the studies on these treatment options have been conducted in patients with clear cell carcinoma, which is particularly responsive to targeted therapy and immunotherapy. Citing a number of phase III clinical trials of targeted therapies, Pickering [136] points to an improvement in overall survival from a baseline of 12–15 months to more than 30 months as well as higher response rates—substantially better results than were realized with cytokines. The typical paradigm for systematic therapy begins with VEGF-targeted therapy in a first-line setting; following relapse, the VEGF receptor (VEGFR), the TKI axitinib, or the mTOR inhibitor, everolimus, may be a used as a secondary line of treatment. New targeted treatments continue to emerge; the FDA approved nivolumab, an immune checkpoint inhibitor, in 2015 and the tyrosine kinase inhibitor, cabozantinib, in 2016. Compared with everolimus, nivolumab showed improved median overall survival and lower incidence of adverse effects [137], while cabozantinib demonstrated increased progression-free survival in comparison with everolimus [138].

However, the use of targeted therapies is not without drawbacks. A number of adverse side effects exist, ranging from rash, fatigue, and diarrhea to high blood pressure, hyperglycemia, and peripheral edema, depending on the agent. Sequencing of therapy to determine the order in which it should proceed and dosing and duration of treatment have yet to be determined [139]. The above adverse effects take their toll on the endurance, functional mobility, and psychological outlook of the cancer patient, which means the patient may not eat as well or participate in functional exercise, let alone structured physical and occupational therapy that could facilitate preservation of bone density. Future randomized trials are needed to determine the comparative advantage of one treatment over another as well as the effect of combination therapy on survival outcome and morbidity. Not uncommonly, the treatment of the cancer can have more adverse effects on the patient's physical condition than the cancer itself.

In this era of targeted agents, surgery and radiotherapy still have a role to play, albeit constrained and related primarily to pain control. As Wood et al. [128] have observed, surgery provides much-needed palliation and may be employed to reduce impending fracture risk, treat pathological fractures, and restore spinal integrity. Radiotherapy can be effective in reducing bone pain, strengthening destabilized bone, and treating spinal cord compression. In a study by Kijima et al. [140], radiotherapy combined with ZA resulted in a higher objective response rate and prolonged SRE-free survival compared with radiotherapy alone. However, further research is warranted to determine if this strategy should be pursued in the context of other treatment options.

Bone-Targeted Therapies

What, then, is the role of bisphosphonates or denosumab in metastatic RCC? How do they affect such skeletal complications as pain, pathologic fracture, and spinal cord compression? Of the available bisphosphonates, ZA demonstrated the greatest efficacy in terms of managing patients with metastatic RCC. In a subset of 74 RCC patients drawn from a large study of ZA in patients with solid tumors, a substantial portion of the results showed a reduction in the proportion of patients with an SRE of 37 % versus 74 % for placebo, as well as a decrease in the mean skeletal morbidity rate, extended time to the first SRE, longer time to progression of bone lesions, and a 61 % reduction in the risk of developing an SRE compared with placebo [141].

Several studies have also indicated that ZA has the potential to improve the outcome of systematic treatment including targeted therapies [142]. In a small Belgium study conducted by Beuselinck et al. [143], the concomitant use of bisphosphonates with sunitinib/sorafenib improved progression-free survival by a median of 16.3 months versus 3.4 months in patients without bisphosphonates. A subsequent study by Keizman et al. [144] indicated that bisphosphonates combined with sunitinib may improve response rate, progression-free survival, and overall survival; the authors propose that by inhibiting osteoblasts, bisphosphonates may be "additive or synergistic" with VEGF inhibition therapy. In both cases, however, these benefits must be weighed against the risk of osteonecrosis of the jaw, which is more frequent in the combined therapy than with bisphosphonates alone. Patient follow-up and monitoring is critical. Denosumab may also be used as an adjunct to targeted therapies. Larger prospective randomized will further elucidate the value and risks of combined therapies [145].

Physiatric Interventions for Cancer Patients

Precautions During Physical Therapy for Metastatic Long Bone Lesions

As patients begin to mobilize, impending pathological fractures are a significant concern for the physical therapist and physiatrist. Often lesions go unnoticed until a patient attempts to use a given limb for weight-bearing activities. While it is ideal for long bone series imaging to be performed prior to admission to rehabilitation, this step does not always occur, and, in cases of aggressive tumors, new lesions can form subsequent to prior imaging. Physiatrists and the related team members assisting the patient throughout rehabilitation (physical and occupational therapy, nursing, and psychologists) need to be aware of precautions during mobility to minimize pain and prevent future fractures. Factors to consider include the origin of the primary bone tumor, the site of involvement of the lesion, the degree of pain, and whether the lesion is blastic or lytic. Metastatic lesions that result in functional pain when a patient contracts muscles around a limb is a particularly ominous predictor of an impending fracture and should be brought to the attention of the cancer or orthopedic team associated with the patient's care [146]. Harrington et al. [147] has recommended that when 50 % of the cortex is destroyed, prophylactic internal fixation with rods, pins, or similar devices should be undertaken. In addition, if patients have humeral lesions greater than 3 cm in diameter or persistent pain following radiation therapy of the involved region, the bone should be stabilized surgically [53]. For metastatic lesions of the femur that are lytic in nature, have a diameter above 2.5 cm, or are causing pain with weight-bearing activity, even after radiation, prevention of impending fracture can be accomplished through elective internal fixation, before that lesion grows larger [148]. Some metastases are large enough that fixation is preferred to awaiting effects of radiation which can take longer to detect. Figure 4 is one example of such a case in which the metastatic lesion encompasses both the lateral and medial cortices. Figure 5 demonstrates successful intramedullary nailing of the impending fracture described in the above patient.

From the perspective of rehabilitation and overall mobility of the patient, metastasis in long bones that consume either 50 % of the bone diameter or 50 % of the cortical surfaces should be made non-weight-bearing until the area has been evaluated by the patient's cancer team, and orthopedic input has determined whether surgical stabilization is needed. A lesion of the above size within a long bone represents an impending bone fracture, regardless of the grade of the tumor or the type of primary cell.

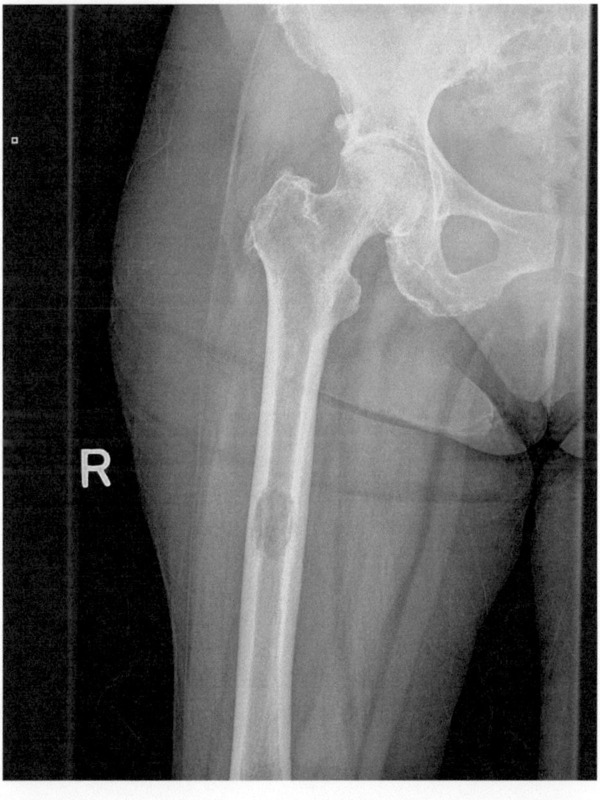

Fig. 4 Metastatic lesion encompassing lateral and medial cortices of the right femur. A 53-year-old female with metastatic cancer and large lytic lesion through mid-femoral shaft, encompassing both medial and lateral cortices (*Source*: Courtesy of Thomas Jefferson University Department of Radiology)

This recommendation holds true for metastatic lesions, whether from a hematologic malignancy to bone, such as multiple myeloma, or from one of several solid tumors that spread to long bones. Such patients should be issued offloading devices, such as a wheelchair or, alternatively, a walker for short-distance ambulation of a few feet maintaining single-leg stance until a decision has been made. If the decision is to defer surgery and off-load the limb, these adaptive strategies will continue for a period of weeks to months. While restrictions may be relaxed after consultation with bone specialists, such initial steps are essential to ensure patient safety.

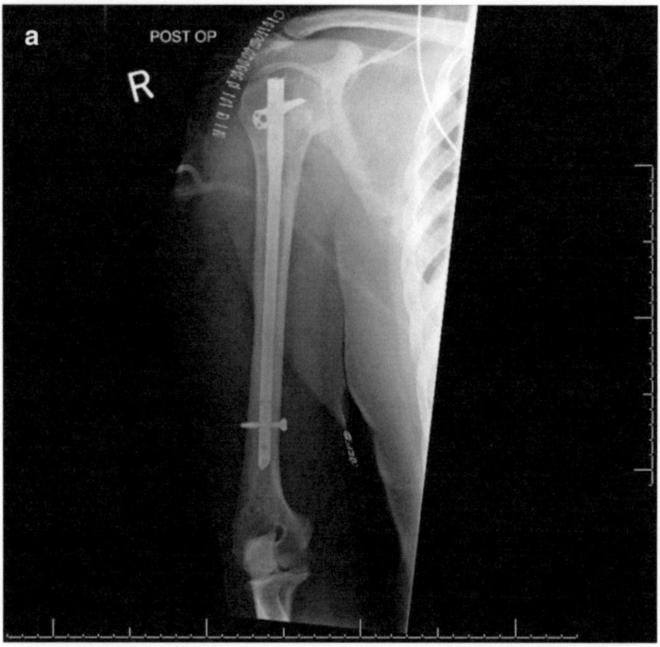

Fig. 5 (**a**) Intramedullary rod and screw fixation of the right humerus. Blastic metastases from metastatic prostate cancer are demonstrated at the elbow. (*Source*: Courtesy of Thomas Jefferson University, Philadelphia, PA)

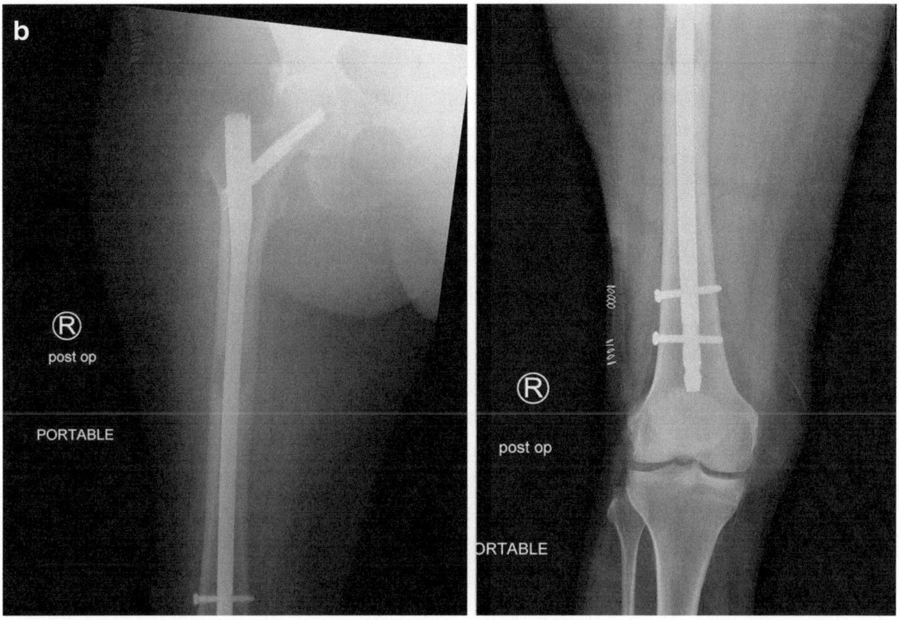

Fig. 5 (continued) (**b**) Intramedullary nailing of the right femur. Operative stabilization with intramedullary nailing required to stabilize impending fracture in patient with metastatic breast cancer. Right hip and knee joints maintain normal alignment even after procedure. (*Source*: Courtesy of Thomas Jefferson University Department of Radiology, Philadelphia PA)

Table 2 Weighted scoring system for metastatic lesions based on location, size, and cellular composition of the lesion (lytic or blastic)

	Score		
Variable	1	2	3
Site	Upper Limb	Lower limb	Peritrochanter
Pain	Mild	Moderate	Functional
Lesion	Blastic	Mixed	Lytic
Size	<1/3	1/3–2/3	>2/3

Composite score from each of the four variables is used to determine a total. Scores 9 and higher indicate increased risk of fracture from a metastatic lesion
Source: Mirels [148] Reproduced with permission

While the 50% cortical width rule of thumb is easy to apply, a more systematic approach is often followed based on a weighted scoring system developed by Mirels [148], involving relative risks of metastatic lesions by location, degree of pain, size, and cellular composition of the lesion (blastic or lytic) (Table 2). Each of the four variables is graded from 1 to 3 with a maximum score of 12. Based on Mirels' model, any patient with a score of nine or greater would be at sufficiently high risk of fracture that prophylactic internal fixation should be undertaken. However, some therapists feel that extremely aggressive tumors in patients with scores under 9 should mandate surgical intervention due to the rate at which certain tumors grow [146].

The Approach for Patients without Stabilization Surgery

Patients whose lesions do not meet the requirement for stabilization surgery yet are experiencing pain may nevertheless benefit from offloading devices such as a walker or cane. Assistive devices that enable full or partial weight-bearing can maintain mobility and prevent falls. In cases of partial or non-weight-bearing status, concerns do exist that the opposite limb may assume greater than 50 % weight-bearing, especially when a limb must remain off the ground and a patient is required to "hop" while using a walker. The additional weight borne in single-leg stance is effectively double the usual amount, and if bone density in the weight-bearing limb is poor, it too may ironically be at risk for fracture from the bone giving way. Essential knowledge of additional bone removed in stabilization of lytic or blastic metastases, types of hardware used to strengthen and repair the bone, any nerves or muscles damaged from the tumor not previously appreciated, and any muscles detached and subsequently reattached during surgery should be obtained from the operative report or through direct communication with the surgical team [149].

Throughout the continuum of cancer care, patients should receive ongoing education on measures of energy conservation; generalized conditioning; formal strengthening to the extent tolerated by their bones and muscles (under supervision of a physical therapist familiar with cancer rehabilitation); core strengthening with postural correction, unless spinal metastases are present; balance training; and essential skills in fall prevention [149]. For patients with mild or moderate strength deficits, educating patients and family on alternative ways to perform daily activities, reduce environmental hazards that can cause inadvertent falls, conserve energy, and provide formal education in adaptive equipment including alternative means of locomotion become the focus of rehabilitation. Patients with more significant impairments, be they temporary or permanent, will need to master wheelchair mobility and the use of transfer boards; in some cases, families will need to learn about weight shifts in wheelchairs and the use of a Hoyer lift. Prevention of contractures and pressure ulcers and management of orthostatic hypotension are additional areas of focus in those with moderate to severe impairments.

Continuing to be vigilant regarding areas of new pain, increased fatigue, and change in mental status is an ongoing responsibility and concern of physical and occupational therapists. Patients' endurance levels are important indicators of how they are coping physically and emotionally with their disease or, alternatively, with aggressive treatment in the form of radiation or chemotherapy. Depression, fear, and anxiety are common in both modalities of treatment [150, 151]. During radiation therapy, the skin can become red and blistered, and these regions undergoing desquamation should receive minimal hands-on treatment from a therapist. Physical therapy sessions are limited to active range of motion or active assistive range of motion. Because bones undergoing radiation treatment are weakened by the process and therefore are at higher risk of fracture during the acute phase of therapy, patients may need to be placed on limited weight-bearing status, necessitating the use of a cane or walker. In addition, resistive exercises are relatively contraindicated during this time of compromised bone integrity [149].

The Importance of a Multidisciplinary Approach

Given the significant advances made in the treatment in a number of solid tumor conditions over the last two decades, particularly renal cell carcinoma, attention is now being focused on achieving what Bex et al. [152] term "a continuum of care," with its potential to produce optimal use of treatment options. As in many instances of osteoporosis therapy cited in this book, the wide range and complexity of the various modalities points up the need for a multidisciplinary approach to adequately assess the costs and benefits of these approaches. Although a detailed analysis of each of these treatments is beyond the scope of this book, the need for a multidisciplinary team to determine therapy selection, dosing, administration, and management of related adverse side effects for the individual patient is apparent from the data presented here [153]. Beyond continued examination of the efficacy of existing and emerging drugs, factors that admit of future investigation include the use of sequential therapy and related resistance mechanisms; the positive and negative indications of surgery, particularly cytoreductive surgery followed by immunotherapy; the safety and tolerability of selected agents; and the potential for identifying prognostic biomarkers for disease occurrence, progression, and survival in patients with advanced metastases [152]. Understanding, integrating, and applying these elements, together with increasing knowledge of osteoporosis pathobiology, require input from varied specialties to achieve successful individualized treatment.

Primary Bone Cancer

At the most basic level, primary bone cancer should be distinguished from bone metastatic cancer, both of which can adversely affect the skeleton. Accounting for less than 0.2 % of all cancers, bone cancer is extremely rare, with estimates indicating that some 3,300 cases would occur in 2016 [1]. Originating within the bone itself, malignant bone tumors, known as sarcomas, may develop anywhere in the body but generally occur in the long bones and joints in the arms and legs. There are three basic types of sarcomas [154, 155]:

1. The most common type of primary bone disease, *osteosarcoma*, can occur at any age; however, its incidence is essentially bimodal: the first peak develops between the ages of 15–19 years and the second from 75 to 79 years, with a middle-level plateau from 25 to 49 years [156]. Arising from osteoid tissue, the tumors occur most often in bones of the arms, legs, and pelvis and are more common in males than in females.

2. *Chondrosarcoma*, the second most common type, originates in cartilage cells, primarily in the pelvis, leg, and arm bone. It is rare in children and adolescents; the risk increases from age 40 to 75 and occurs equally in women and men.
3. Generally occurring in childhood and rarely after the age of 30, the third most common type, *Ewing tumor or Ewing sarcoma*, affects the pelvis, chest wall, and long bones of the arms and legs and affects males more than females. It can originate in bone or in soft tissue.

Osteosarcoma can also be metastatic to the spine as shown in Fig. 6.

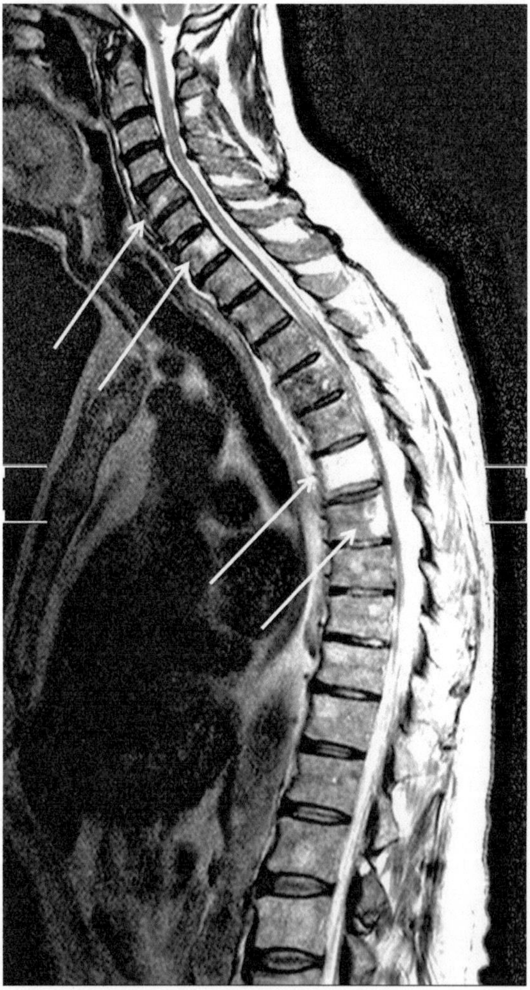

Fig. 6 Metastatic Osteosarcoma. Multiple metastatic lesions are seen throughout the lower cervical spine as well as the upper, middle, and particularly the lower thoracic spine. The patient's primary lesion was in the right hip (*Source*: Courtesy of Thomas Jefferson University Department of Radiology)

Treatment of Sarcoma

As cancer cells in bone grow out of control, they form a malignant tumor that results in pain and swelling at the tumor site, swelling in joints associated with the tumor, and a tendency to suffer bone fractures. Diagnosed through biopsies as well as imaging and bone tests and depending on the stage identified, several types of treatment are considered [155]. Limb-sparing surgery to remove the tumor and surrounding tissue from the bone is most common, but if unsuccessful, amputation is necessary. Used before or after surgery in osteosarcoma and Ewing sarcoma, chemotherapy exerts an adverse effect on bone by causing early menopause in premenopausal women as well as low blood counts and suppressed bone turnover rates. Radiation therapy can be both ineffective and damaging. Not only are renal cancer cells largely resistant to radiotherapy, but the high dosage required to be effective may destroy healthy tissue adjacent to the tumor. It should be noted, however, that a recent trial indicates that resulting pathologic fractures may not be due solely to radiation therapy. Dhakal et al. [157] have shown that radiotherapy did not uniformly decrease bone density, thus indicating that the risk of fractures is likely multifactorial, including possible alterations in bone remodeling.

Targeted therapies in the form of poly(ADP-ribose) polymerase (PARP) inhibitors combined with chemotherapy are now being investigated in cases of Ewing sarcoma. By interfering with the DNA repair mechanism (EWS-FLI1) needed to sustain and grow cancerous tumors, poly(ADP-ribose) polymerase (PARP) inhibitors have caused Ewing sarcoma to disappear in mice, with no relapse in 70 % of the population for over four months [158]. Further trials must be undertaken to confirm these promising results [159].

Bone-Targeted Agents

As in the case of solid tumors, not only does cancer itself weaken bone, but its treatment options lead to adverse effects on BMD and fracture risk. Several studies have been conducted on sarcoma and bone damage, but they are limited by their small size and by the failure to take into account other factors that damage bone. In adolescent sarcoma patients, the disease often occurs concurrently with the time of bone mass accrual. In a population of 95 osteosarcoma and Ewing sarcoma patients undergoing antitumoral treatment, Ruza et al. found BMD deficits in both the lumbar spine and femoral neck in about one-third of the cohort, with a corresponding risk of pathologic bone fractures [160]. More recently a small trial dealing with the impact of methotrexate-based chemotherapy on children with osteosarcoma reported that 78 % of femoral neck BMD and 44 % of lumbar spine BMD decreased in the course of treatment, while 11 % of the

Table 3 Summary of grades and stages of osteosarcoma

Stage		Tumor	Metastases	Grade
I	IA	≤8 cm	No	Low
	IB	>8 cm	No	Low
II	IIA	≤8 cm	No	High
	IIB	>8 cm	No	High
III		"Skipped" bone	To other sites in the same bone	High
IV	IVA	Any size	Only to the lung	Any
	IVB	Any size	To other distant sites	Any

Skipped bone means the tumor has migrated to other sites in the same bone, considered a regional metastasis but with poor prognosis. (*Source*: Tao et al. [156])

subjects experienced a fracture within five months following chemotherapy [161]. Reduced physical activity, extended immobilization if surgery is involved, and vitamin D deficiency also contribute to bone loss. The more aggressive tumors are often those of greatest concern for treatment. A summary of grades and stages of osteosarcoma is given in Table 3 [162].

Moreover, the long-term effects of sarcoma treatment may not become clinically significant until patients become older, indicating a need for physicians to anticipate these late events. In an analysis of Ewing sarcoma and osteosarcoma 7–8 years after diagnosis, Pirker-Fruhauf et al. [162] maintain that bone loss after chemotherapy may be underestimated in patients with sarcoma. Findings indicate that 21 % of their patients had osteoporosis and 37 % had osteopenia, with BMD reduction present in 58 % of patients and nontraumatic and nontumor-associated fractures in 16 %. A severe vitamin D deficiency was also identified in 88 % of patients. A study of long-term survivors of Ewing sarcoma produced a comparable reduction, with 31 of 56 patients experiencing low BMD and seven diagnosed with osteoporosis [163]. Interestingly, a 2016 investigation of chondrosarcoma survivors [164] who generally do not receive conventional adjuvant treatment also found a pathologic BMD as well as cases of osteopenia and osteoporosis, suggesting that factors other than chemotherapy, perhaps limited mobility, reduced physical activity, limited acquisition of bone mass, and nutritional deficiencies may be at work. Specific contributing factors are yet to be determined in all types of sarcoma.

These pilot studies will be followed by other, larger and more heterogeneous investigations, but they already indicate that regular evaluation of BMD is increasingly important as survival rates for sarcoma increase. Moderate weight-bearing exercise, supplemental calcium and vitamin D, and avoidance of smoking and alcohol should be implemented, and the potential positive effect of bisphosphonates and denosumab should be investigated [165]. In a mice model, ZA has proved effective in exerting an antitumor effect on osteosarcoma cells in vitro [166]. A 2016 study of the use of pamidronate in pediatric osteosarcoma revealed that it is both safe and effective in increasing BMD and relieving bone pain, although a reduction in fracture risk could not be ascertained [167]. The key is to provide early intervention for patients at risk of BMD deficits and fractures.

References

1. American Cancer Society. Cancer Facts and Figures 2016. Atlanta: American Cancer Society. http:www.cancer.org/rsearch/cancerfactsfigures. 2016. Accessed 3 Mar 2016.
2. Wright NC, Looker AC, Saag KG, Curtis JR, Delzell ES, Randall S, et al. The recent prevalence of osteoporosis and low bone mass in the United States based on bone mineral density at the femoral neck and lumbar spine. J Bone Miner Res. 2014;229(11):2520–6.
3. Silberman R, Rood GD. Hematologic malignancies and bone. In: Rosen CJ, editor. Primer on the metabolic bone diseases and disorders of mineral metabolism. Ames: Wiley; 2013. p. 694.
4. American Cancer Society. Learn about cancer: leukemia. http://www.cancer.org/cancer/leukemia. Accessed 5 Mar 2016.
5. Mostoufi-Moab S, Halton J. Bone morbidity in childhood leukemia: epidemiology, mechanisms, diagnosis, and treatment. Curr Osteoporos Rep. 2014;12(3):300–12.
6. Frisch BJ, Ashton JM, Xing L, Becker MW, Jordan CT, Calvi LM. Functional inhibition of osteoblastic cells in an in vivo mouse model of myeloid leukemia. Blood. 2012;119(2):540–50.
7. Winkel ML, Pieters R, Hop WC, Roos JC, Bokkerink JPM, Leeuw JA, et al. Bone mineral density at diagnosis determines fracture rate in children with acute lymphoblastic leukemia treated according to the DCOG-ALL9 protocol. Bone. 2014;59:223–6.
8. Tucci F, Arico M. Treatment of pediatric acute lymphoblastic leukemia. Haematologica. 2008;93(8):1124–8.
9. Orgel E, Mueske NM, Wren TA, Gilsanz V, Butturini AM, Freyer DR, et al. Early injury to cortical and cancellous bone from induction chemotherapy for adolescents and young adults treated for acute lymphoblastic leukemia. Bone. 2016;85:131–7.
10. Le Meignen M, Auquier P, Barlogis V, Sirvent N, Contet A, Simeoni MC, et al. Bone mineral density in adult survivors of childhood acute leukemia: impact of hematopoietic stem cell transplantation and other treatment modalities. Blood. 2011;118(6):1481–9.
11. Wilson CL, Dilley K, Ness KK, Leisenring WL, Sklar CA, Kaste SC. Fractures among long–term survivors of childhood cancer: a report from the childhood cancer survivor study. Cancer. 2012;118(23):5920–8.
12. Kaste SC, Jones-Wallace D, Rose SR, Boyett JM, Lustig RH, Rivera GK, et al. Bone mineral decrements in survivors of childhood acute lymphoblastic leukemia: frequency of occurrence and risk factors for their development. Leukemia. 2001;15(5):728–34.
13. Kang MJ, Lim JS. Bone mineral density deficits in childhood cancer survivors: pathophysiology, prevalence, screening, and management. Korean J Pediatr. 2013;56(2):60–7.
14. Dana Farber Cancer Institute. What is the difference between Hodgkin Lymphoma and Non-Hodgkin Lymphoma? 2015. http://dana-farber.org/insight/2015/07/what-is-the-difference-between-hodgkin-lymphoma-and-non-hodgkinlymphoma. Accessed 22 Mar 2016.
15. Ozdemirli M, Mankin HJ, Aisenberg AC, Harris NL. Hodgkin's lymphoma presenting as a solitary bone tumor: a report of four cases and review of the literature. Cancer. 1996;77(1):79–88.
16. Kaste SC, Metzger ML, Minhas A, Xiong Z, Rai SN, Ness K, et al. Pediatric Hodgkin lymphoma survivors at negligible risk for significant bone mineral density deficits. Pediatr Blood Cancer. 2009;52(4):516–21.
17. Carr R, Barrington SF, Madam B, O'Doherty MJ, Saunders CAB, van der Welk J, et al. Detection of lymphoma in bone marrow by whole-body positron emission tomography. Blood. 1998;91(9):3340–6.
18. Benmiloud S, Steffens M, Beauloye V, de Wandeleer A, Devogelaei J-P, Brichard B, et al. Long-term effects of bone mineral density of different therapeutic schemes for acute lymphoblastic leukemia or non-Hodgkin lymphoma during childhood. Horm Res Paediatr. 2010;74(4):241–50.
19. Westin JR, Thompson MA, Cataldo VC, Fayed LE, Fowler N, Fenale MA, Neelapu S, et al. Zoledronic acid for prevention of bone loss in patients receiving primary therapy for lymphomas, a prospective randomized controlled Phase III trial. Clin Lymphoma Myeloma Leuk. 2013;13(2):99–105. doi:10.1016/j.ciml2012.11.002.

20. Paccou J, Merlusca L, Henry-Desally I, Parcelier A, Gruson B, Royer B, et al. Alterations in bone mineral density and bone turnover markers in newly diagnosed adults with lymphoma receiving chemotherapy: a 1-year prospective pilot study. Adv Med Sci. 2014;59(2):200–5.
21. Cabanillas ME, Lu H, Fang S, Du XL. Elderly patients with non-Hodgkin lymphoma who receive chemotherapy are at higher risk of osteoporosis and fracture. Leuk Lymph. 2007;48(8):1514–21.
22. Muszynska-Roslan K, Latoch E, Konstantynowicz J, Panasiuk A, Stewart A, Krawczuk-Rybak M. Bone mineral density in pediatric survivors of Hodgkin and non-Hodgkin lymphomas. Adv Med Sci. 2014;59(2):200–5. http://dx. doi.org/10.1016 /jadvms.2014.02.004.
23. Thompson MA, Westin JR, Hagemeister FB. Bone mineral density screening should be routine in lymphoma patients. Ann Oncol. 2014;25(4):913–4. doi:10.1093/annonc/mdu044.
24. Johns Hopkins Medicine. Multiple myeloma. http://www.hopkinsmedicine.org/kimmel_cancer_center/types_cancer/multiple_myeloma.html. Accessed 28 Mar 2015.
25. Faulkner KG. Bone matters: are density increases necessary to reduce fracture risk? American Society for Bone and Mineral Research. J Bone Miner Res. 2000;15:183–7.
26. Guise TA. The vicious cycle of bone metastases. J Musculoskel Neuron Interact. 2002;2(6):570–2.
27. Shinohara E, Kuhn EN. Multiple myeloma: an overview. OncoLink: Abramason Cancer Center, University of Pennsylvania. 2013. http://www.oncolink.org/types.article.cfm?c=13&id=9552. Accessed 30 Mar 2016.
28. Melton III LJ, Rajkumar SV, Khosla S, Achenbach SJ, Oberg AL, Kyle RA. Fracture risk in monoclonal gammopathy of undetermined significance. J Bone Min Res. 2004;19(1): 25–30.
29. Pepe J, Petrucci MT, Mascia ML, Piemonte S, Fassino V, Romagnoli E, et al. The effects of alendronate treatment in osteoporotic patients affected by monoclonal gammopathy of undetermined significance. Calcif Tissue Int. 2008;2(6):418–26.
30. Berenson JR, Yellin O, Boccia, Flam W, Wong SF, Batuman O, et al. Zoledronic acid markedly improves bone mineral density for patients with monoclonal gammopathy of underdetermined significance and bone loss. Clin Cancer Res. 2008;14(19):6289–95.
31. Kristinsson SY, Minter AR, Korde N, Tan E, Landgren O. Bone disease in multiple myeloma and precursor disease: novel diagnostic approaches and implications in clinical management. Expert Rev Mol Diagn. 2011;11(6):593–603.
32. Minter AR, Simpson H, Weiss BM, Landgren O. Bone disease from monoclonal gammopathy of undetermined significance to multiple myeloma: pathogenesis, interventions, and future opportunities. Semin Hematol. 2011;48(1):55–65.
33. Tosi P. Diagnosis and treatment of bone disease in multiple myeloma: spotlight on spinal involvement. Scientifica. 2013;2013:104546. doi:10.1155/2013/104546.
34. Dhodapkar MV, Weinstein R, Tricot G, Jagannath S, Parfitt AM, Manolagas S, et al. Biologic and therapeutic determinants of bone mineral density in multiple myeloma. Leuk Lymphoma. 1998;32(1–2):1227.
35. Melton LJ, Kyle R, Achenbach SJ, Oberg AL, Rajkimar SV. Fracture risk with multiple myeloma: a population-based study. J Bone Min Res. 2005;20(3):487–93.
36. Berenson JR, Lichtenstein A, Porter L, Demopoulos MA, Bordoni R, Sebastian G, et al. Efficacy of pamidronate in reducing skeletal events in patients with advanced multiple myeloma. N Engl J Med. 1996;334(8):488–93.
37. Rosen LS, Gordon D, Kaminski M, Howell A, Beich A, Mackey J, et al. Long-term efficacy and safety of zoledronic acid compared with pamidronate disodium in the treatment of skeletal complications, in patients with advanced multiple myeloma or breast carcinoma: a randomized, double-blind, multicenter, comparative trial. Cancer. 2003;98(8): 1735–44.
38. Morgan GJ, Davies FE, Gregory WM, Cocks K, Bell SE, Szibert AJ, et al. First-line treatment with zoledronic acid as compared with clodronic acid in multiple myeloma (MRC Myeloma IX): a randomized controlled trial. Lancet. 2010;376(9759):744–51.

39. Lonial S, Weiss BM, Usmani SZ, Singhal S, Chari A, Bahlis A, et al. Daratumumab monotherapy in patients with treatment-refractory multiple myeloma (SIRIUS): an open-label, randomized, phase 2 trial. Lancet. 2016;387(10027):1551–60. doi:10.1016/S0140-6736(15)01120-4.
40. Rajkumar SV. Daratumumab in multiple myeloma (Comment). Lancet. 2016;387(10027):1490–2. doi:10.1016/S0140-6736(15)01226-X.
41. Kaste SC, Chesney RW, Hudson MM, Lustig RG, Rose SR, Carbone LD. Bone mineral status during and after therapy of childhood cancer: an increasing population with multiple risk factors for impaired bone health. J Bone Min Res. 1999;14(12):2010–4.
42. Leukemia and Lymphoma Society. Facts and Statistics. http://www.lls.org/nttp%3A/llsorg.prod.acquia-sties.com/facts-and-statistics/acts-and-statistics-overivew.facts-and-statistics. Accessed 4 Apr 2016.
43. National Cancer Institute; Surveillance, Epidemiology, and End Results Program. SEER stat fact sheets: myeloma. http://seer.cancer.gov/statfacts/html/mulmy.html. Accessed 4 Apr 2016.
44. Zmuda JM, Cauley JA, Ljung B-M, Bauer DC, Cummings SR, Kuller LH, et al. Bone mass and breast cancer risk in older women: difference by stage of diagnosis. J Nat Cancer Inst. 2001;93(12):930–6.
45. Zambetti A, Tartter P. Bone mineral density is a prognostic factor for postmenopausal Caucasian women with breast cancer. Breast J. 2013;19(2):168–72. doi:10.1111/tbj.12072.
46. Farhat GN, Taioli E, Cauley JA, Zmuda JN, Orwoll E, Bauer DC, et al. The association of bone mineral density with prostate cancer risk in the Osteoporotic Fracture in Men (Mros) study. Cancer Epidemiol Biomarkers Prev. 2009;18(1):148–54.
47. Nelson RL, Turyk M, Kim J, Pensky V. Bone mineral density and the subsequent risk of cancer in the NHANES I follow-up cohort. BMC Cancer. 2002;2(22):1–9.
48. Hadji P, Ziller M, Albert US, Kalder M. Assessment of fracture risk in women with breast cancer using current vs emerging guidelines. Br J Cancer. 2010;102(4):645–50.
49. Chen Z, Maricic M, Aragaki AK, Mouton C, Arendell L, Lopez AM, et al. Fracture risk increases after diagnosis of breast or other cancers in postmenopausal women—results from the Women's Health Initiative. Osteoporos Int. 2009;20(4):527–36.
50. Berruti A, Dogliotti L, Terrone C, Cerutti S, Isaia G, Tarabuzzi R, et al. Changes in bone mineral density, lean body mass and fat content as measured by dual energy X-ray absorptiometry in patients with prostate cancer without apparent bone metastases given androgen deprivation therapy. J Urol. 2002;167(6):2361–7.
51. American Cancer Society Bone metastasis. http://www.cancer.org/treatment/understandingyourdiagnosis/bonemetastasis/bone-metastasis-detailed-guide. Accessed 4 Apr 2016.
52. Coleman RE. Clinical features of metastatic bone disease and risk of skeletal morbidity. Clin Cancer Res. 2006;12 Suppl 20:6243s–9.
53. Sim FH, Pritchard DJ. Metastatic disease in the upper extremity. Clin Orthop Relat Res. 1982;169:83–94.
54. Coleman R, Body JJ, Aapro M, Hadji P, Herrstedt J. Bone health in cancer patients: ESMO clinical practice guidelines. Ann Oncol. 2014;25 Suppl 3:124–37.
55. Maxwell C, Viale PH. Cancer treatment-induced bone loss in patients with breast or prostate cancer. Oncol Nurs Forum. 2005;32(3):589–601.
56. Okeke TC, Anyaehie UB, Ezenyeaki CC. Premature menopause. Ann Med Health Sci Res. 2013;3(1):90–5.
57. Michaud LB, Goodin S. Cancer-treatment-induced bone loss, part 1. Am J Health Syst Pharm. 2006;63(5):419–30.
58. Shapiro CL, Manola J, Lenoff M. Ovarian failure after adjuvant chemotherapy is associated with bone loss in women with early-stage breast cancer. J Clin Oncol. 2001;19(140):3306–11.
59. Powles TJ, Hickish T, Kanis JA, Tidy A, Ashley S. Effect of tamoxifen on bone mineral density measured by dual-energy x-ray absorptiometry in healthy premenopausal and postmenopausal women. J Clin Oncol. 1996;14(1):78–84.

60. Gnant M, Mineritsch BB, Luschin-Ebengreuth G, Kainberger F, Kassmann H, Pioswanger-Solkner JC, et al. Adjuvant endocrine therapy plus zoledronic acid in premenopausal women with early stage breast cancer: 5 year follow-up of ABCSG-12 bone-mineral density sub-study. Lancet Oncol. 2008;9(9):840–9.
61. Pagani O, Regan MM, Walley BA, Fleming GF, Colleoni M, Lang I, et al. Adjuvant exemestane with ovarian suppression in premenopausal breast cancer (TEXT study). N Engl J Med. 2014;37(2):107–18.
62. Francis PA, Regan MM, Fleming GF, Lang I, Ciruelos E, Bellet M, et al. Adjuvant ovarian suppression in premenopausal breast cancer. N Engl J Med. 2015;372(5):436–46.
63. Gardsell P, Johnell O, Nilsson BE. The predictive value of bone loss for fragility fractures in women: a longitudinal study over 15 years. Calcif Tissue Int. 1991;49(2):90–4.
64. van der Klift M, de Laet CE, McCloskey EV, Johnell O, Kanis JA, Hofman A, et al. Risk factors for incident vertebral fractures in men and women: the Rotterdam Study. J Bone Min Res. 2004;19(7):1172–80.
65. Choksi P, Williams M, Clark PM, van Poznak C. Skeletal manifestations of treatment of breast cancer. Curr Osteoporos Rep. 2013;11(4):319–28. doi:10.1007/s11914-013-0179-7.
66. Goss PE, Ingle JN, Ales-Martinez JE, Cheung AM, Chiebowski RT, Wactawski-Wende J, et al. Exemestane for breast-cancer prevention in postmenopausal women. N Engl J Med. 2011;364(24):2381–91.
67. Cuzick J, Sestak K, Forbes JF, Dowsett M, Knox J, Cawthorn S, et al. Anastrozole for prevention of breast cancer in high-risk postmenopausal women (IBIS-II): an international, double-blind, randomized placebo-controlled trial. Lancet. 2014;383(9922):1041–8.
68. Cheung AM, Tile L, Cardew S, Pruthi S, Robbins J, Tomlinson G, et al. Bone density and structure in healthy postmenopausal women treated with exemestane for the primary prevention of breast cancer: a nested substudy of the MAP 3 randomized controlled trial. Lancet Oncol. 2012;13(3):275–84.
69. Cauley J. Bone loss associated with prevention of breast cancer. Lancet. 2012;13(3):221–2.
70. Perez EA, Josse RG, Pritchard KI, Ingle JN, Martino S, Findlay BP, et al. Effect of letrozole versus placebo on bone mineral density in women with primary breast cancer completing 5 or more years of adjuvant tamoxifen: a companion study to NCIC CTG MA,17. J Clin Oncol. 2006;24(22):3629–35.
71. Mincey BA, Duh MS, Thomas SK, Moyneur E, Marynchencko M, Boyce SP, et al. Risk of cancer treatment-associated bone loss and fractures among women with breast cancer receiving aromatase inhibitors. Clin Breast Cancer. 2006;7(2):127–32.
72. Mieog JS, van der Hage JA, van der Velde CJ. Neoadjuvant chemotherapy for operable breast cancer. Br J Surg. 2007;94(10):1189–200.
73. Love RR, Mazess RB, Barden HS, Epstein S, Newcomb PA, Jordan VC. Effects of tamoxifen on bone mineral density in postmenopausal women with breast cancer. N Engl J Med. 1992;326(3):852–6.
74. Cooke AL, Metge C, Lix L, Prior HJ, Leslie WD. Tamoxifen use and osteoporotic risk fracture: a population-based analysis. J Clin Oncol. 2008;26(32):5227–32.
75. Vogel VG, Costantino JP, Wickerman DL, Cronin WM, Cecchini RS, Atkins JN, et al. Update of the national surgical adjuvant breast and bowel project study of tamoxifen and raloxifene (STAR) P-2 trial: preventing breast cancer. Cancer Prev Res. 2010;3(6):696–706.
76. Coleman R, Gray R, Powles T, Paterson A, for the Early Breast Cancer Trialists' Collaborative Group. Adjuvant bisphosphonate treatment in early breast cancer: meta-analysis of individual patient's data from randomized trials. Lancet. 2015;386(10001):1353–61.
77. Brufsky AM, Harker WG, Beck JT, Bosserman L, Vogel C, Seidler C, et al. Final 5-year results of Z-FAST trial: adjuvant zoledronic acid maintains bone mass in postmenopausal breast banker patients receiving letrozole. Cancer. 2012;118(5):1192–201.
78. Stopeck AT, Lipton A, Body JJ, Steger GG, Tonkin K, de Boer RH, et al. Denosumab compared with zoledronic acid for the treatment of bone metastases in patients with advanced breast cancer: a randomized, double-blind study. J Clin Oncol. 2010;28(35):5132–9.

79. Martin M, Bell R, Bourgeois H, Brufsky A, Diel I, Enia A, et al. Bone-related complications and quality of life in advanced breast cancer: results from a randomized phase III trial of denosumab versus zoledronic acid. Clin Cancer Res. 2012;18(17):4841–9.
80. Van Poznik CH, Von Roenn JH, Temin S. American Society of Clinical Oncology clinical practice guideline update: recommendations on the role of bone-modifying agents in metastatic breast cancer. J Oncol Pract. 2011;7(2):117–21.
81. Blanchette PS, Pritchard KI. The role of bisphosphonates in early-and advanced-stage breast cancer: have we finally optimized care? http://www.cancernetwork.com/oncology-journal/role-bisphosphonates-early-and-advancedstage-have-we-finally-optimized care. Accessed 18 Apr 2016.
82. Gnant M, Pfeiler G, Dubsky PC, Hubalek M, Greil R, Jakesz R, et al. Adjuvant denosumab in breast cancer (ABCSG-18: a multicentre, randomized, double-blind, placebo-controlled trial. Lancet. 2015;386(9992):433–43.
83. Gnant M, Pfeiler G, Dubsky PC, Hubalek M, Greil R, Jackesz R, et al. The impact of adjuvant denosumab on disease-free survival: results from 3,425 postmenopausal patients of the ABCSG-18 trial. Presented at 2015 Breast Cancer Symposium, San Antonio, TX; 2015; Abstract S2-02.
84. Johnson GL. Denosumab (Prolia) for treatment of postmenopausal osteoporosis. Am Fam Physician. 2012;84(4):334–6.
85. Koo K, Law K, Mittmann N, Konski A, Dennis K, Zeng L, et al. Comparing cost-effectiveness analyses of denosumab versus zoledronic acid for the treatment of bone metastases. Support Care Cancer. 2013;21(6):1785–91. doi:10.1007/s00520-013-1790-y.
86. Himelstein AL, Qin R, Novotny PJ, Seisler DK, Khatcheressian JK, Robert JD, et al. CALGB 70604 (Alliance): a randomized phase III study of standard dosing vs longer interval dosing of zoledronic acid in metastatic cancer. J Clin Oncol. 2015;33 (suppl; abst 9501).
87. Munch KJ. Reinventing bone loss and fracture in cancer patients. OncoLog. 2010;55(3). http://www2.mdanderson.org/depts/oncolog/articles/pdf/10/3-mar/3-10-2.pf.html.
88. Saylor PJ, Smith MR. Bone health and prostate cancer. Prostate Cancer Prostatic Dis. 2010;13(1):20–7.
89. Body JJ. Treatment and prevention of bone metastases and myeloma bone disease. In: Rosen CR, editor. Primer on the metabolic bone diseases and disorders of mineral metabolism. Ames: Wiley; 2013. p. 741.
90. Brown SA, Guise TA. Cancer-associated bone disease. Curr Osteoporos Rep. 2007;5(3):120–7.
91. Guise TA. Bone loss and fracture risk associated with cancer therapy. Oncologist. 2006;11(10):1121–31.
92. Coleman RE. Metastatic bone disease: clinical features, pathophysiology and treatment strategies. Cancer Treat Rev. 2001;27(3):165–76.
93. Saad F, Gleason DM, Murray R, Tchekmedyian S, Venner P, Lacombe L, et al. Long-term efficacy of zoledronic acid for the prevention of skeletal complications in patients with metastatic hormone-refractory prostate cancer. J Natl Cancer Inst. 2004;96(11):879–82.
94. U.S. Food and Drug Administration. Zometa (zoledronic acid) for injection. http://www.fda.gov/safety/medwatch/safetyinformation/ucm244411.htm. Accessed 17 Apr 2016.
95. American Cancer Society. Preventing and treating prostate cancer spread to bones. 2016. http://www.cancer.org/cancer/prostate-cancer-treating-treating-pain. Accessed 10 May 2016.
96. Fizazi K, Carducci M, Smith M, Damiao R, Brown J, Karsh L, et al. Denosumab versus zoledronic acid for treatment of bone metastases in men with castration-resistant prostate cancer: a randomized, double-blind study. Lancet. 2011;377(9768):813–22. doi:10.1016/S0140-6736(10)62344-6.
97. Hong BY, Ibrahim MFK, Fernandez R, Mazzarello S, Hutton B, Shirr R, et al. De-escalation of bone-targeted agents for metastatic prostate cancer. Curr Oncol. 2016;23(1):e77–8. doi:10.3747/co.23.2913.
98. Aragon-Ching JB. Unravelling the role of denosumab in prostate cancer. Lancet. 2011;377(9768):785–6.

99. Gomez-Veiga F, Ponce-Reixa J, Martinez-Breijo S, Planas J, Morote J. Advances in prevention and treatment of bone metastases in prostate cancer. Role of RANK/RANKL inhibition. Actas Urol Esp (English Edition). 2013;37(5):292–304.
100. Smith MR. Bisphosphonates to prevent osteoporosis in men receiving androgen deprivation therapy for prostate cancer. Drugs Aging. 2003;20(3):175–83.
101. Diamond TH, Higano CS, Smith MR, Guise TA, Singer FR. Osteoporosis in men with prostate carcinoma receiving androgen-deprivation therapy: recommendations for diagnosis and therapies. Cancer. 2004;100(5):892–9.
102. Shahinian VS, Kuo YF, Freeman JL, Goodwin JS. Risk of fracture after androgen deprivation for prostate cancer. N Engl J Med. 2005;352(2):154–64.
103. Wang A, Obertova Z, Brown C, Karunasinghe N, Bishop K, Ferguson L, et al. Risk of fracture in men with prostate cancer on androgen deprivation therapy: a population-based cohort study in New Zealand. BMC Cancer. 2015;15:837. doi:10.11867/s12885-015-1843-3.
104. Smith MR, McGovern FJ, Zietman AL, Fallon MA, Hayden DL, Schoenfeld DA, et al. Pamidronate to prevent bone loss during androgen-deprivation therapy for prostate cancer. N Engl J Med. 2001;345(13):948–55.
105. Michaelson MD, Kaufman DS, Lee H, McGovern FJ, Kantoff PW, Fallon MA, et al. Randomized controlled trial of annual zoledronic acid to gonadotropin-releasing hormone agonist-induced bone loss in men with prostate cancer. J Clin Oncol. 2007;25(9):1038–42.
106. Smith MR, Morton RA, Barnette KG, Sieber PR, Malkowicz SB, Rodriguez D, et al. Toremifene to reduce fracture risk in men receiving androgen deprivation therapy for prostate cancer. J Urol. 2013;189 Suppl 1:S45–50. doi:10.1016/j.juro.2012.11.016.
107. Smith MR, Egerdie B, Hernandez N, Feldman R, Tammela TLJ, Saad F, et al. Denosumab in men receiving androgen-deprivation therapy for prostate cancer. N Eng J Med. 2009;361(8):745–55. doi:10.1056/NEJMoa0809003.
108. Body JJ. Prevention and treatment of side-effects of systematic treatment: bone loss. Ann Oncol. 2010;21 Suppl 7:180–5.
109. Hansell DM. Classification of diffuse lung disease: why and how. RSNA Radiol. 2013;268(3):628–40. http://dx.doi.org/10.1148/radiol.13120908.
110. McGlynn KA, Gridley G, Mellemkjaer L, Anderson KC, Caporaso NE, et al. Risks of cancer among a cohort of 23,935 men and women with osteoporosis. Int J Cancer. 2008;122(8):1879–84.
111. Hatlin P, Langhammer A, Forsmo S, Carlsen SM, Amundsen T. Bone mineral density, fracture history, self-reported osteoporosis as proxy variables for estrogen and the risk of non-small-cell lung cancer—a population based cohort study, the HUNT study: are proxy variables friends of faults? Lung Cancer. 2013;81(1):39–46.
112. D'Antonio, Passaro A, Gori B, Del Signore E, Migliorino MR, Ricciardi S. Bone and brain metastasis in lung cancer: recent advances in therapeutic strategies. Ther Adv Med Oncol. 2014;6(3):101–4.
113. Song J, Oh Y, Shim T, Kim W, Ryu J, Choi C. Efficacy comparison between 18 F-FDG PET/TC and bone scintigraphy in detecting bone metastases of non-small lung cancer. Lung Cancer. 2009;65(3):333–8.
114. Saad F, Lipton A, Cook R, Chen Y, Smith M, Coleman R. Pathologic fractures correlate with reduced survival in patients with malignant bone disease. Cancer. 2007;110:1860–7.
115. Azvolinsky, A. Bone metastases in lung cancer patients linked with poorer prognosis. http://www.physicianspractice.com/bone-metastases/bone-metastases-lung-cancer-patients--linked-poorer-prognosis. Accessed 12 Mar 2016.
116. Kuchuk M, Kuchuk I, Sabri E, Hutton B, Clemons M, Wheatley-Price P. The incidence and clinical impact of bone metastases in non-small cell lung cancer. Lung Cancer. 2015;89(2):197–202. doi:10.1016/j.lungcan.2015.04.007.
117. Da Silva GT, Bergmann A, Thuler LC. Skeletal related events in patients with bone metastasis arising from non-small cell lung cancer. Support Care Cancer. 2016;24(2):731–6.
118. Brodowicz T, O'Byrne K, Manegold C. Bone matters in lung cancer. Ann Oncol. 2012;23(9):2215–22.

119. Kolaczkowska M, Junik K, Rzymkowska M, Ramer L. The effect of chemotherapy on bone metabolism in patients with non-small cell lung cancer. Pneumonol Alergol Pol. 1998;66(5–6):283–9.
120. Park GY, Wilson JJ, Song Y, Lippard SJ. Phenanthriplatin, a monofunctional DNA-binding platinum anticancer drug candidates with unusual potency and cellular activity profiles. Proc Natl Acad Sci U S A. 2012;109(30):11987–92. doi:10.1073/pnas.1207670109.
121. Rosen LS, Gordon D, Tchekmedyian NS, Yanagihara R, Hirsh V, Krzakowski M, et al. Long-term efficacy and safety of zoledronic acid in the treatment of skeletal metastases in patients with nonsmall cell lung carcinoma and other solid tumors: a randomized, phase III, double-blind, placebo-controlled trial. Cancer. 2004;100(12):2613–21.
122. Mahtani R, Khan R, Jahanzeb M. The potential application of zoledronic acid as anticancer therapy in patients with non-small- cell lung cancer. Clin Lung Cancer. 2011;12(1):26–32.
123. Henry D, Costa L, Goldwasser F, Hirsh V, Hungria V, Prausova J, et al. Randomized, double-blind study of denosumab versus zoledronic acid in the treatment of bone metastases in patients with advanced cancer (excluding breast and prostate cancer) or multiple myeloma. J Clin Oncol. 2011;29(9):1125–32.
124. Scagliotti GV, Hirsh V, Siena S, Henry DH, Woll PJ, Manegold C, et al. Overall survival improvement in patients with lung cancer and bone metastases treated with denosumab versus zoledronic acid. J Thorac Oncol. 2012;7(12):1823–9.
125. Silva SC, Wilson C, Woll PJ. Bone-targeted agents in the treatment of lung cancer. Ther Adv Med Oncol. 2015;7(4):219–28. doi:10.1177/1758834015582178.
126. Hirsh V. Targeted treatments of bone metastases in patients with lung cancer. Front Oncol. 2014;4:146. doi:10.3389/fonc.2014.00146.
127. Fottner A, Szalantzy M, Wirthmann L, Stahler M, Baur-Melnyk A, Jannsson V, et al. Bone metastases from renal cell carcinoma: patients' survival after surgical treatment. BMC Musculoskelet Disord. 2010;11:145. doi:10.1186/1471-2474-11-145.
128. Wood SL, Brown JE. Skeletal metastasis in renal cell carcinoma: current and future management options. Cancer Treat Rev. 2012;38(4):284–91.
129. Woodward E, Jagdev S, McParland L, Clark K, Gregory W, Newsham A, et al. Skeletal complications and survival in renal cancer patients with bone metastases. Bone. 2011;48(1):160–6.
130. Langdon J, Way A, Heaton S, Bernard J, Molloy S. The management of spinal metastases from renal cell carcinoma. Ann R Coll Surg Engl. 2009;91(8):649–52. doi:10.1308/003588409X432482.
131. Li P, Wong YN, Armstrong K, Haaş N, Subedi P, Davis-Cerone M, et al. Survival among patients with advanced renal cell carcinoma in the pretargeted versus targeted therapy eras. Cancer Med. 2016;5(2):169–81. doi:10.1002/cam4.574.
132. Kidney Cancer Association. Therapies for advanced kidney cancer. 2016. http://www.kidneycancer.org/knowledge/learn/therapies-for-advanced-kidney-cancer. Accessed 5 May 2016.
133. Mathias J, Rini B. Angiogenesis inhibitor therapy in renal cell cancer. In: Lara Jr PN, Jonasch E, editors. Kidney cancer: principles and practice. New York: Springer; 2015. p. 282.
134. Motzer RJ. New perspectives on the treatment of metastatic renal cell carcinoma: an introduction and historical overview. Oncologist. 2011;16 Suppl 2:1–3. doi:10.1634/theoncologist.2011-S2-01.
135. National Comprehensive Cancer Network. NCCN clinical practice guidelines in oncology: kidney cancer. 2016. https://www.nccn.org/professionals/physician_gls/f_guidelines.asp. Accessed 5 May 2016.
136. Pickering LM. Advances in systematic therapy for renal cell carcinoma. Genitourinary Cancers Symposium. 2016. http://gucasym.org/daily-news/advances-systematic-therapy-renalcell-carcinoma. Accessed 5 May 2016.
137. Motzer RJ, Excudier B, McDermott DF, George S, Hammers HJ, Srinivas SS, et al. Nivolumab versus everolimus in advanced renal-cell carcinoma. N Engl J Med. 2015;373(19):1803–13.

138. Choueiri TK, Escudier B, Powles T, Mainwaring PN, Rini BI, Donskov F, et al. Cabozantinib versus everolimus in advanced renal-cell carcinoma. N Engl J Med. 2015;373(19):1814–23. doi:10.1056/NEJMoa1510016.
139. Logan JE, Rampersaud EN, Sonn GA, Chamie K, Belidegrun AS, Pantuck AJ, et al. Systematic therapy for metastatic renal cell carcinoma: a review and update. Rev Urol. 2012;14(304):65–78.
140. Kijima T, Fuji Y, Usama T, Okubo Y, Yamamoto S, Masuda H, et al. Radiotherapy to bone metastases from renal cell carcinoma with or without zolendronate. BJU Int. 2009;103(5):620–4. doi:10.1111/j.1464-410X.2008.08124.x.
141. Lipton A, Zheng M, Seaman J. Zoledronic acid delays the onset of skeletal-related effects and the progression of skeletal disease in patients with advanced renal cell carcinoma. Cancer. 2003;98(5):962–7.
142. Vrdoljak E, Rini B, Schmidinger M, Omrcen T, Torday L, Szczylik C. Bisphosphonates and vascular endothelial growth factor-targeted drugs in the treatment of patients with renal cell carcinoma metastatic to bone. Anticancer Drugs. 2013;25(5):431–40. doi:10.1097/CAD.0b013e328360335f.
143. Beuselinck B, Wolter P, Karadimou A, Elaidi R, Dumez H, Rogiers A, et al. Concomitant oral tyrosine kinase inhibitors and bisphosphonates in advanced renal cell carcinoma with bone metastases. Br J Cancer. 2012;107(10):1665–71. doi:10.1038/bjc.2012.385.
144. Keizman D, Ish-Shalom M, Pili R, Hammers H, Eisenberger MA, Sinbaldi V, et al. Bisphosphonates combined with sunitinib may improve the response rate, progression free survival and overall survival of patients with bone metastases from renal cell carcinoma. Eur J Cancer. 2012;48(7):1031–7.
145. Keizman D, Ish-Shalom M, Maimon N, Gottfried M. Are bisphosphonates an indispensable tool in the era of targeted therapy for renal cell carcinoma and bone metastases? World J Urol. 2014;32(1):39–45.
146. O'Toole GC, Boland PJ, Herklotz M. Bone metastasis. In: Stubblefield MD, O'Dell MW, editors. Cancer rehabilitation: principles and practice. New York: Demos; 2009. p. 773–82.
147. Harrington KD, Sim FH, Enis JE, Johnston JO, Diok HM, Gristina AG. Meethylmethacrylate as an adjunct in internal fixation of pathological fractures. Experience with three hundred and seventy-five cases. J Bone Joint Surg Am. 1976;58(8):1047–55.
148. Mirels H. Metastatic disease in long bones: a proposed scoring system for diagnosing impending pathologic fractures. Clin Orthop Relat Res. 2003;415(Suppl):S4–13.
149. Fitzpatrick TW. Principles of physical and occupational therapy in cancer. In: Stubblefield MD, O'Dell MW, editors. Cancer rehabilitation; principles and practice. New York: Demos; 2009. p. 785–96.
150. Liavaag AH, Dorum A, Fossa SD, Trope C, Dahl AA. Controlled study of fatigue, quality of life and somatic and mental morbidity in epithelial ovarian cancer survivors: how lucky are the lucky ones? J Clin Oncol. 2007;25(15):2049–56.
151. Liavaag AH, Dorum A, Fossa SD, Trope C, Dahl AA. Morbidity associated with "self-rated health" in epithelial ovarian cancer survivors. BMC Cancer. 2009;9(2):1–11.
152. Bex A, Gore M, Mulders P, Sternberg CN. Recent advances in the treatment of advanced renal cell carcinoma: towards multidisciplinary personalized care. BJU Int. 2012;110(9):1289–300. doi:10.1111/j.1464-410X.2012.11100.x.
153. Rini B. Renal cell carcinoma treatment regimens. 2016. http://www.cancertherapyadvisor.com/renal-cell-carcinoma-treatment-regimens/article/218161.
154. Bone Sarcoma and Subtypes. Sarcoma Alliance. 2016. http://sarcomaalliance.org/what-you-need-to-know. Accessed 2 May 2016.
155. Bone Cancer. American Cancer Society, Atlanta. 2016. http://www.cancer.org/acs/groups/cid/documents/webcontent/003086-pdf.pdf. Accessed 5 Feb 2016.
156. Tao J, Bae Y, Wang LL, Lee B. Osteogenic osteosarcoma. In: Rosen C, editor. Primer on the metabolic bone diseases and disorders of mineral metabolism. Ames: Wiley; 2013. p. 702–10.

157. Dhakal S, Chen J, McCance S, Rosier R, O'Keefe R, Constine LS. Bone density changes after radiation for extremity sarcomas: exploring the etiology of pathologic fractures. Int J Radiat Oncol Biol Phys. 2011;80(4):1158–63. doi:10.1016/j.ijrobp.2010.04.012.
158. Stewart E, Goshorn R, Bradley C, Griffiths LM, Benavente C, Twaarog NR, et al. Targeting the DNA repair pathway to Ewing Sarcoma. Cell Rep. 2014;9(3):829–41.
159. Ordonez JL, Amaral AT, Carcaboso AM, Herrero-Martin D, del Carmen Garcia-Macias M, Sevillano V, et al. The PARP inhibitor olaparib enhances the sensitivity of Ewing sarcoma to trabectedin. Oncotarget. 2015;6(22):18875–90.
160. Ruza E, Sierrasesumaga L, Azona C, Patino-Garcia A. Bone mineral density and bone metabolism in children treated for bone sarcoma. Pediatr Res. 2006;59(6):866–71.
161. Ahn JH, Cho WH, Lee JA, Seo JH, Lim JS. Bone mineral density change during adjuvant chemotherapy in pediatric osteosarcoma. Ann Pediatr Endocrinol Metab. 2015;20(3):150–4.
162. Pirker-Fruhauf UM, Friesenbichler J, Urban EC, Obermayer-Pietsch B, Leithner A. Osteoporosis in children and young adults: a late effect after chemotherapy for bone sarcoma. Clin Orthop Relat Res. 2012;470(10):2874–85.
163. Hobusch GM, Noebauer-Huhmann I, Krall C, Holzer. Do long-term survivors of Ewing family of tumors experience low bone mineral density and increased fracture risk? Clin Orthop Relat Res. 2014;472(11):3471–9.
164. Hobusch GM, Tiefenboeck TM, Patsch J, Krall C, Holzer G. Do patients after chondrosarcoma treatment have age-appropriate bone mineral density in the long term? Clin Orthop Relat Res. 2016;474(6):1508–15.
165. Wasilewski-Masker K, Kaste SC, Hudson MM, Esiashvili N, Mattano LA, Meacham LR. Bone mineral density deficits in survivors of childhood cancer: long-term follow-up guidelines and review of the literature. Pediatrics. 2008;121(3):e705–13.
166. Ory B, Heymann MF, Kamijo A, Goulin F, Heymann D, Redini F. Zoledronic acid suppresses lung metastases and prolongs overall survival of osteosarcoma-bearing mice. Cancer. 2005;104(11):2522–9.
167. Lim SW, Ahn JH, Choi A, Cho WH, Lee JA, Kim DH, et al. Efficacy of pamidronate in pediatric osteosarcoma patients with low bone mineral density. Ann Pediatr Endocrinol Metab. 2016;21(1):21–5.

Chapter 17
Primary Osteoporosis in Conditions of Pediatric Onset

Christina V. Oleson

In the past, osteoporosis has been regarded as a disease of elderly women or of adults with diseases that cause progressive bone loss and fragility fractures. More recently, physicians and researchers have become aware of conditions that lead to low bone mineral density (BMD) and fractures not only later in life but also in childhood and adolescence. Diseases and disorders originating in childhood but with implications for adulthood fall into two categories: primary bone diseases, particularly osteogenesis imperfecta and juvenile idiopathic arthritis, and secondary bone diseases resulting from an underlying medical disorder, including cerebral palsy and Duchenne muscular dystrophy, which will be considered in the next chapter. (Other childhood diseases—spina bifida and the eating disorders, amenorrhea, and osteoporosis that constitute the female athlete triad—are considered elsewhere in this volume.) What is common to all is the fact that they have their onset in childhood, leading to osteoporosis by or before young adulthood so that by their mid-20s and mid-30s, patients have the bones of a 70–80-year-old. Compromised bone health from infancy to age 19 carries a lifetime risk of osteoporosis.

Assessment of Bone Mass in Children

Techniques to measure bone mass in adults, particularly DXA measurements and *T*-scores, cannot simply be transferred to children without recognizing the implications of growth and development [1]. DXA is a two-dimensional measurement of a three-dimensional bone. It calculates BMD by using area, as reflected in the term areal bone mineral density (aBMD), but it cannot account for volumetric bone density (vBMD), the depth value which is critical in determining continually changing bone dimensions in children. Another diagnostic tool, quantitative computer tomography (QCT), can be used to complement DXA findings. Unaffected by body or skeletal size, the three-dimensional QCT is able to assess vBMD and can distinguish between cortical and trabecular bone—an important factor in understanding

C.V. Oleson, *Osteoporosis Rehabilitation*, DOI 10.1007/978-3-319-45084-1_17

the bone dynamics of children. Despite its drawbacks, including limited availability and high radiologic doses, QCT, particularly peripheral QCT with its lower radiation, is considered to be a safe screening method for children and is increasingly used in clinical practice.

In addition, the *T*-score used to interpret DXA findings in adults cannot be used in children. *T*-scores compare bone density to that of a healthy young adult of the relevant sex, indicating bone loss since early adulthood. On the other hand, *Z*-scores compare bone density to a sex/age matched reference group, adjusted for height, weight, pubertal status, and ethnicity. A *Z*-score of ≤ -2 constitutes low bone density in children and adolescents [2].

The recommended sites for DXA testing in children are the lumbar spine and the total bone less head (TBLH); measurement of the hip region is not reliable because of variability in skeletal development. DXA scans can also lead to serious misdiagnoses, particularly if administered and interpreted by technicians with limited training. A trial involving 34 children aged 14–17 years demonstrated how errors can occur. The most frequent error (69 %) stemmed from the use of a *T*-score to diagnose osteoporosis; other errors were caused by reference to a database that did not incorporate gender or ethnic differences (21), incorrect bone mapping (21), failure to account for short stature (15 %), and other statistical misinterpretations (12 %) [3, 4]. As Binkovitz and Henwood point out, the pediatric radiologist must be a "clinical pathologist" trained to monitor the DXA measurement in terms of quality control data and clinical images, a statistician knowledgeable about the concept of *Z*-scores and the limitations and uses of a numerical result, and a "bone specialist" capable of translating a numerical value into a clinically useful result [5].

The objectives of bone densitometry are to identify patients at greatest risk of fracture, to inform treatment decisions, and to monitor the effect of therapy. In a pediatric position paper issued in 2013 [6], the International Society for Clinical Densitometry stated that although DXA measurement should be part of a comprehensive skeletal analysis, a diagnosis of osteoporosis in children and adolescents should not be based on densitometric information alone. Other factors to be taken into account include:

1. The presence of one or more vertebral compression fractures in the absence of localized disease or high-energy trauma.
2. The presence of both a clinically significant fracture history and BMD *Z*–score of ≤ -2.0 in the absence of a vertebral compression fracture. A clinically significant fracture history is defined as one or more of the following: (a) two or more long bone fractures by age 10; (b) three or more long bone fractures at any age up to 19.

Other factors associated with low bone density in children include the presence and severity of primary and secondary bone diseases, medication exposure, family history and genetic inheritance, poor nutrition, lack of weight-bearing activity or prolonged immobilization, pubertal delay, and obesity.

A wide range of diseases and disorders, associated with osteoporosis, affect the acquisition of bone mass in children and adolescents and that number is increasing with the heightened use of densitometric diagnostic measurements. The rise in the survival rate of children and adolescents with these diseases has resulted in a growing number of patients with reduced bone density in this age group. These conditions are generally divided into two categories: primary bone diseases caused by a genetic bone abnormality and secondary bone diseases due to an underlying medical condition and/or its treatment.

Osteogenesis Imperfecta

Classification and Pathophysiology

Osteogenesis imperfecta (OI) is the most common form of what is often called "primary osteoporosis," also known as "brittle bone disease." It is characterized by bones that fracture easily, with little or no apparent trauma. OI is caused by a dominant genetic (allelic) defect that affects production of type 1 collagen, a "scaffolding" protein with a long, flexible fiber that gives strength to the bone, skin, and cartilage. Occurring in one in every 20,000 to possibly as many as 50,000 people, OI is currently divided into 11 types, differentiated by levels of severity; they include the most frequent (50–60 % of the OI population) and mildest form, type 1, and the most severe, type 2, which is generally lethal at, or shortly after, birth. Patients with type 1 OI generally have normal collagen but in reduced quantities, while those with more severe forms of the disease evidence abnormal collagen production; both contribute to fractures [7]. Whereas the majority of OI cases are inherited from a parent, 25 % of children have no family history of OI; in such cases, the genetic defect is caused by a spontaneous mutation. Regardless of the source, the genetic defect remains dominant, signifying that patients have a 50 % chance of passing on the disorder to their children [8]. OI is distinguished from a second type of primary bone disease, idiopathic juvenile osteoporosis (IJO), by the fact that it has a direct cause in the form of a genetic defect, whereas IOP has no known cause; appears shortly before the onset of puberty (8–12 years of age) rather than at birth; and is active primarily in growing children with most cases disappearing spontaneously and resulting in complete recovery of bone loss [9].

A person is born with osteogenesis imperfecta and, in varying degrees, is affected by it throughout a lifetime. Clinical features of type 1 OI include bones predisposed to fracture; thin, smooth skin; loose joints and muscle weakness; sclera (whites of the eyes) with a blue, gray, or purple tint; near-normal stature; triangular face; and possibly brittle teeth and hearing loss; more severe case of OI are marked by short stature, respiratory problems, bowed arms and legs, kyphosis, and scoliosis [10]. Angular deformities characteristic of OI are pictured in Fig. 1. Identification of these clinical features, together with obtaining a medical and family history, should be the first steps in identifying OI; laboratory tests including x-rays and ultrasound to locate bone abnormalities, a skin biopsy to determine if the quality and quantity

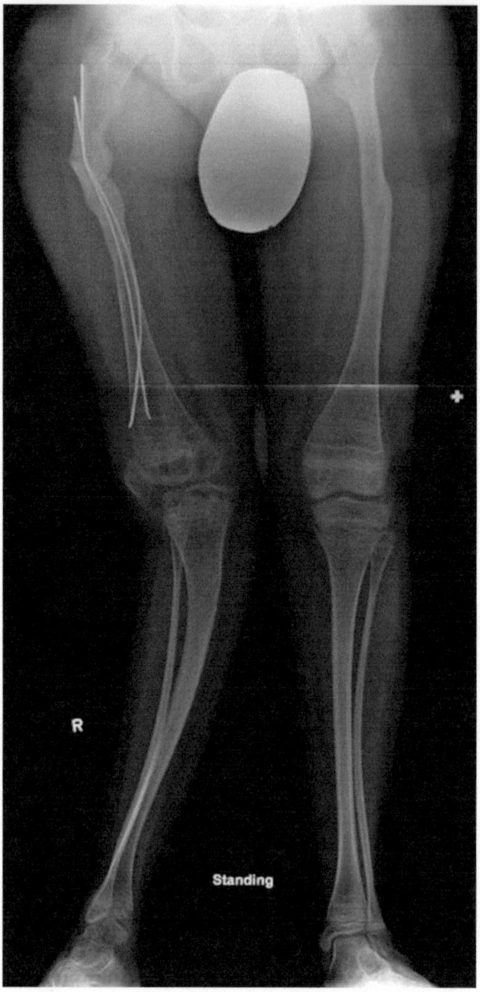

Fig. 1 Radiographic image of chronic bone changes and angular deformities in osteogenesis imperfecta. In this image, note healing fracture of the proximal shaft of the right femur, with two medullary pins. Both limbs demonstrate a degree of varus angulation. An age indeterminate partially remodeled fracture of the left femur is also evident, with a minor degree of residual deformity. Both legs are gracile in shape with bowing most marked of the right tibia, but seen in all bones (*Source*: http://radiopaedia.org/cases/osteogenesis-imperfecta-2. Accessed 27 Jan 2016)

of type 1 collagen are abnormal, and DNA sequencing from blood sample to identify a genetic mutation can help confirm a clinical OI diagnosis [11]. Clinical features of OI and initial diagnostic workup are illustrated in Table 1 [12].

One overriding concern for persons with OI is bone density. During their growth period, children are prone to bone loss, resulting in impaired bone development and the failure to reach peak bone mass at any age. Consequently, the National Institute of Arthritis and Musculoskeletal and Skin Diseases and related organizations continuously emphasize that osteoporosis is an almost universal consequence of OI. The goal of osteoporosis management in the context of OI is twofold: to increase bone density at every age and to minimize age-related bone loss [8]. Additional age-related osteoporosis is compounded by the preexisting effects of OI, and by middle age, fracture rates tend to increase.

Table 1 Classification of OI and key features

OI type	Relative morbidity/ mortality	Genetics	Collagen	Key features
1	Mildest form	Autosomal dominant	Normal quality	Bones fracture easily
			Insufficient quantity	Blue-gray discoloration of the sclera
			Defective type 1 collagen leads to discoloration of sclera	Poor muscle tone and loose joints
				Slight spinal curvature
				Slight protrusion of the eyes
				Early hearing loss in some children
2	Severe; often fatal within perinatal period	Autosomal dominant	Poor quality	Respiratory failure and other severe respiratory problems due to underdeveloped lungs
			Insufficient quantity	Intracerebral hemorrhage
				Severe bone deformity and small stature
3	Progressive; moderate in severity	Autosomal dominant	Poor quality	Considered progressive and deforming
			Sufficient quantity	Bones fracture easily
				Bone deformity (often severe)
				Triangular face
				Poor muscle tone and loose joints
				Blue-gray discoloration of the sclera
				Possible early hearing loss
				Short stature and spinal curvature
				Possible respiratory problems
4	Moderate in severity; variable	Autosomal dominant	Poor quality	Considered deforming
			Sufficient quantity	Bones fracture easily (prepuberty)
				Short stature and spinal curvature
				Barrel-shaped rib cage
				Mild to moderate bone deformities
				Early loss of hearing

(continued)

Table 1 (continued)

OI type	Relative morbidity/ mortality	Genetics	Collagen	Key features
5	Moderate in severity	Autosomal dominant	–	Clinically similar to type 4 Characteristic histologic findings (e.g., mesh-like bone) Calcification of interosseous membrane Hyperplasic callus at site of fractures Radial head dislocation Mixed hearing loss Long bone bowing
6	Moderate in severity	Autosomal recessive	–	Clinically similar to type 4 Characteristic histologic findings (e.g., fish-scale bone) Mineralization defect seen in bone Extremely rare
7	Lethal in all identified cases with a complete absence of the cartilage associated protein	Autosomal recessive	–	Some cases are clinically similar to type 4; other cases are clinically similar to type 2 Shortened long bones (e.g., humerus, femur) Short stature and coxa vara
8	Severe to lethal; associated with mutations in the LEPRE1 gene and leprecan protein	Autosomal recessive	–	Clinically similar to types 2 or 3 except that sclera remains white Severe growth deficiency Extremely under-mineralization of the skeleton

Source: Adapted from Facts about Osteogenesis Imperfecta, www.oif.org, [12]

Bone density measurements, including both dual-energy x-ray absorptiometry (DXA) and quantitative computer tomography (QCT) are essential in managing OI in both children and adults. For children, they are critical in assessing skeletal development and the likelihood of fracture occurrence while also providing a measure for studying the effects of different forms of therapy. They are also recommended for adults to establish a baseline for determining whether bone density changes over time or as a result of treatment. In individuals with OI, bone density measurements may be affected by such deformities as curvature of the spine or by the placement of metal rods.

Management of Type 1 OI and Osteoporosis in Children

Nonpharmacologic Treatment: Therapy and Surgical Intervention

Given the number of confounding conditions evident in OI, a multidisciplinary approach involving pediatricians, surgeons, physical therapists, nutritionists, and even parents and educators is the most effective way to manage the disease in children and adults [13]. Fracture management and protection are the mainstay of OI treatment. To prevent immobility-induced bone loss following a fracture, casting is recommended for only the short term, to be replaced by splints and braces that can be removed to permit appropriate physical therapy. The need to avoid twisting, jolting, and jarring movements is of paramount importance, underlying the value of water therapy and swimming which offer a gravity-free environment to reduce fracture risk. Coupled with water activities, hip extension and hip abduction exercises, walking, dancing, bicycling, and weight lifting, if permitted, can help promote maximum bone density and decrease muscle atrophy [14, 15].

In children with OI, physical activity and an appropriate diet are essential to prevent obesity, which results in less movement and places added stress on bones. Adequate amounts of calcium to help prevent bone loss, vitamin D to promote calcium absorption, and vitamin C to ensure healthy connective tissues are also recommended. Smoking and excess alcohol consumption that can result in falls and fractures should also be avoided although primarily relevant in older teenagers.

Surgical interventions are generally unnecessary in type 1 OI. However, if severe bone deformities or serious fractures are present, surgeons are able to insert metal rods into the long bones of the legs to reduce fracture risk. Using the Fassier-Duval Telescopic Intramedullary System designed for OI patients who are still growing, a rod is attached on the far end of each growth plate and telescopes as the bone grows, overcoming the fracture risk posed by older rods with a fixed length [16].

Pharmacologic Intervention

In recent years, research studies on the treatment of osteogenesis imperfecta and osteoporosis have focused increasingly on drug therapy and particularly on the role of bisphosphonates as antiresorptive medicines that reduce the rate at which osteoclasts remove the bone and thus prevent the loss of bone mass. Clinical trials on the effectiveness of bisphosphonates have focused on children with severe OI, but some have been expanded to encompass those who are mildly or moderately affected. Studies incorporating patients with type 1 OI indicate that although bisphosphonate use is not recommended for the group as a whole, it may have individualized benefits for patients with repeated fractures and low bone density findings. For example, in a study of intravenous pamidronate (the most commonly used bisphosphonates for OI), Zacharin and Kanumakaia reported improved bone quality, increased mobility, and reduced fracture occurrence in children with less severe OI [17].

Other trials involving a range of OI types and other bisphosphonates such as IV ZA and oral alendronate show promising results [18, 19]. Although no bisphosphonate is FDA approved as OI therapy for children, "off-label" bisphosphonates are increasingly becoming the standard of care in children with moderate to severe forms of OI, reflecting demonstrated positive effects ranging from increased BMD and enhanced vertebral height to pain relief and greater muscular strength and mobility [20]. However, concerns have been raised about both the efficacy of bisphosphonates in reducing fracture risk and the duration of their use in children. Citing the results of several recent studies [21–23], Brizola and Shapiro warn that despite positive results from individual studies, an overall analysis of numerous trials reveals no clear consensus on whether bisphosphonates consistently decrease the incidence of fractures in children or adults with OI, nor is there evidence to address the concern that continued long duration treatment may adversely affect bone [24].

Within the last few years, a series of new investigations have been published, further elucidating the effect of pharmacologic interventions in OI. In a systematic analysis of the clinical, biochemical, and radiological outcomes of ten studies involving only *children*, Rijks et al. found that six trials indicated a significant reduction in relative fracture risk as a result of bisphosphonate therapy, with the optimal duration of such therapy still unclear [25]. In an effort to assess long-term treatment outcomes with bisphosphonates (pamidronate/ZA), Palomo et al. reported that 37 children who began bisphosphonate therapy (pamidronate/ZA) before age five and were close to or at final height at the time of the study had increased *Z*-score for LS BMD and taller stature but still sustained frequent fractures of long bones and developed progressive scoliosis, underlining the role of bisphosphonates as an adjunct treatment [26].

Beyond bisphosphonates, the positive effects of other medications on OI, including combination therapies such as recombinant growth hormone plus bisphosphonates, have been examined. Moreover, the first prospective clinical trial of denosumab in OI children has demonstrated a mean relative change in LS BMD of +19 % and bone resorption suppression for a duration of 10–12 weeks, indicating that denosumab should be safe in a 1-year treatment regimen with calcium and vitamin D supplementation. The effect of denosumab on fracture occurrence and the optimal duration of treatment are yet to be assessed [27]. Greater understanding of the mechanisms underlying OI holds promise of developing novel molecular therapies through infusion of mesenchymal stem cells [28].

Management of Osteogenesis Imperfecta and Osteoporosis in Adults

Nonpharmacologic Treatment

Beginning in childhood, patients with OI should be taught to assume responsibility for themselves and to achieve as much independence as possible, given the severity level of the disease. Although generalized transition programs exist, they cannot encompass all the variable conditions associated with OI, underlying the need for approaches tailored to the medical condition and preferences of individual adults [29]. Critical to the transition is the continuity of medical care between pediatric and adult physicians and between physicians with limited knowledge of OI care and those with greater experience [30].

Clinicians must be aware of the confluence of conditions directly associated with OI and those affecting otherwise healthy aging adults, recognizing that, to a certain extent, the treatment for both may be the same. A decline in bone density can be related to immobilization from casts and lack of weight-bearing exercise as well as to age-related changes in the skeleton and hormonal system; however, symptoms of bone loss may appear at an earlier age than seen in people without OI. Periodic bone densitometry tests are recommended to identify osteoporosis, determine fracture risk, and monitor response to prescribed treatment. A healthy lifestyle, appropriate weight, adequate calcium and vitamin D through foods or supplements, smoking abstinence, limited alcohol use, and a safe exercise program, particularly aquatic therapy, will benefit patients with most types of OI. Those with type 1 may also be able to engage in noncontact sports that do not involve extensive twisting. Because they contribute significantly to bone loss, corticosteroids should be avoided [14].

Although fracture risk is known to decline following puberty, OI is a connective tissue disease, and adult patients with mild or moderate OI, particularly those with excessive joint flexibility, are likely to experience more soft tissue injuries as they age [30]. Impaired connective tissue can, in turn, lead to fractures as well as tendon, ligament, and muscle injuries and severe pain.

Pharmacologic Intervention

Bisphosphonate treatment has been studied in OI adults but to a more limited extent than in children and, thus far, with fewer positive results regarding fractures. Two studies of adult OI considered in a Cochrane review [21] revealed conflicting results. Although Adami et al. [31] reported a 14 % reduction in fracture incidence following treatment with IV pamidronate, further analysis of a subgroup of Adami's subjects who had incurred at least one fracture [21] demonstrated no difference in fractures between these patients and controls. In a study involving alendronate, Chevral et al. [32] indicated no difference in vertebral or peripheral fracture rates. Both trials showed a significant increase in bone density.

Since 2010, additional studies of bisphosphonate treatment of OI in adults by Pavon de Paz et al. [33], Shapiro et al. [34], and Bradbury et al. [35] all reported an increase in BMD, but the results for fracture rate reduction were inconclusive. Shapiro indicated that while bisphosphonates did not decrease fracture rate in type 1 OI, IV pamidronate did lead to fracture reduction in more severe forms of the disease; Bradbury's meta-analysis found no significant difference in fracture incidence in OI patients with oral bisphosphonates. At this point, insufficient evidence in support of the efficacy of bisphosphonates in reducing fracture rates does not justify a recommendation for general use, particularly over the long term when antiresorptive treatment has been associated with increased risk of atypical femoral fractures in OI patients [36]. Since there is such growing controversy in this area, expect to see more individualized approaches to treatment of patients with OI in terms of initiation of bisphosphonates.

The first trial examining the effect of the anabolic agent, teriparatide [37], on adult OI has produced positive results for type 1 in terms of increased hip and spine aBMD, vertebral vBMD, and markers of bone formation; efficacy was attenuated in more severe types 3 and 4. Larger trials are needed to evaluate teriparatide's ability to reduce bone fractures in OI as well as to compare its effectiveness with that of bisphosphonates and other anabolic agents and when used in combination with other antiresorptive treatments. Several new therapies requiring further investigations have the potential to benefit patients with OI; they include cell-based therapies including bone marrow transplantation and gene therapy that focus on silencing, decreasing, or replacing the allele carrying the causative variant, effectively transforming a severe type of OI into a milder form of the disease [38, 39].

As adults age, the effects of adult OI are likely to be compounded by age-related osteoporosis. For the present, patients with OI, particularly type 1 combined with osteoporosis, must rely on the most promising pharmacologic treatments as well as nonpharmacologic interventions including good nutrition, adequate amounts of calcium and vitamin D, physical therapy to strengthen muscles, and occupational therapy to address educational, work, and ADL needs.

Juvenile Idiopathic Arthritis

Once classified as juvenile rheumatoid arthritis in the United States and as juvenile chronic arthritis in Europe, the term "juvenile idiopathic arthritis" (JIA) has now been adopted as an international designation for a group of autoimmune diseases that result in chronic joint inflammation and stiffness, lasting more than six weeks in children aged 16 and younger. Some patients experience the disease only in childhood and adolescence; for others, JIA persists into adulthood.

Juvenile Idiopathic Arthritis in Children

Causes and Types

The underlying cause of JIA is thought to be both genetic and environmental. Research indicates that the genetic composition of a patient results in a tendency to develop the disease, which is then actually triggered by environmental factors such as early-age infections/viruses and possibly breastfeeding or maternal smoking [40]. A recent study of 153 children with JIA proposed another possible causal factor: exposure to antibiotics during childhood. Compared to children with no exposure to antibiotics, the ratio for developing JIA was 3:1 for those with one to two courses of antibiotics and 3:8 for those with three to five courses [41].

Divided into seven subgroups on the basis of the number of joints involved, the symptoms, and the presence of distinct antibodies in the blood, JIA will be separated into three broader categories for consideration in this chapter [42–44]:

1. *Oligoaricular (Pauciarticular) JIA*—Affecting half of JIA children with girls at greater risk than boys, it involves four or fewer joints in the 6-month onset period; if five or more joints become involved after the first six months, patients are said to have an "extended" form of the disease which develops in up to half of subjects and may persist into adulthood. Symptoms include large joint involvement of the lower extremities, particularly the knees, with little pain and little difficulty in functioning. About 70 % of patients are antinuclear antibody (ANA) positive, making them prone to eye diseases such as iritis and necessitating regular ophthalmologic examinations to prevent serious vision loss. This form of the diseases carries the best prognosis.
2. *Polyarticular JIA*—Occurring in 30 % of children with JIA, it affects five or more large and small joints, particularly those in the hands and feet, and is symmetrical, affecting the same joints on both sides of the body. Morning stiffness, joint swelling, and limited range of motion in the affected joints are among the symptoms. Complications include joint space narrowing, bone erosions, flexion contractures, and some growth disturbances. Because patients with this type of JIA generally have a positive blood test for proteins called rheumatoid factors, it may represent an earlier iteration of rheumatoid arthritis.
3. *Systemic JIA (Still's disease)*—Affecting the whole body and occurring in 10–15 % of those with JIA, it is characterized by two weeks of spiking fevers, a salmon-colored rash, and inflammation of internal organs; joint swelling in some patients may not appear until months later. Anemia, leukocytosis, thrombocytosis, and elevated liver enzymes are associated with systemic JIA as are such complications as osteoporosis, infection from immunosuppressive therapy, growth disturbances, and cardiac disease.

Diagnosis

No single test can diagnose JIA. The first step in the process is a thorough physical examination and a detailed medical history. Laboratory tests include a complete blood count to detect abnormalities in red blood cells, white blood cells, and platelets; liver function tests and ANA tests to detect autoimmunity and risk of eye disease; bone scans; and the erythrocyte sedimentation rate to measure how rapidly red blood cells settle to the bottom of a test tube, indicating inflammatory conditions within the body [45]. A differential diagnosis to rule out conditions with symptoms similar to those in JIA incorporates infections, malignancy, collagen vascular diseases, Lyme disease in oligoarticular JIA, and acute rheumatic fever in systematic JIA [44, 46]. Early diagnosis of JIA is imperative to prevent irretrievable damage to joints and organs, identify potential complications, reduce the risk of impaired vision and possible blindness and develop an effective treatment plan.

Treatment

Treatment of JIA involves a combination of medications, physical therapy, regular exercise, and nutrition.

Medications

Nonsteroidal anti-inflammatory drugs (NSAIDs) and corticosteroids, once the mainstay of JIA therapy, are now used largely as bridge or adjunctive therapies [47]. NSAIDs (aspirin, ibuprofen, naproxen, COX-2 inhibitors) reduce pain and inflammation, but their serious side effects including stomach, liver, kidney, and heart problems as well as high blood pressure and anemia outweigh their benefits, especially in comparison to biologic agents. Corticosteroids (hydrocortisone, prednisone) have been prescribed to treat serious symptoms such as inflammation of the lining of the heart, but adverse effects such as growth disturbances, weakened bones, osteoporosis, and increased susceptibility to infection inhibit their long-term use [45].

Disease-modifying antirheumatic drugs (DMARDs), particularly methotrexate, slow the progression of JIA and prevent the disorder from worsening but may take as much as 3–6 months to take effect. Administered in small doses, methotrexate does not incur dangerous side effects but can lead to anemia, immune suppression, low blood count, and kidney and liver problems, requiring regular physician monitoring. Nonetheless, as Stoll observes, its long track record of safety and efficacy justifies its standing as the "gold standard" therapy for children with JIA [47].

Genetically engineered biologic response modifiers, or biologics, are the newest class of medications in JIA therapy. They act by targeting specific proteins that cause inflammation in the body. The tumor necrosis factor inhibitor (TNFi), etanercept (Enbrel), inhibits the inflammatory protein, TNF, and, together with adalimumab

(Humira) and abatacept (Orencia), is FDA approved for treatment of polyarticular JIA in children older than two years of age. Other inflammatory proteins such as interleukin-1 and interleukin-6 in patients with systemic JIA have been effectively targeted with the biologics, anakinra and tocilizumab [48]. Biologics have proved to be both safe and effective in treating the more aggressive forms of JIA as well as uveitis, but long-term safety data has yet to be developed.

Concerns have been raised about the association of malignancy with prescribed medications in JIA. However, a trial based on data from 7,812 children found that although children with JIA had an increased rate of incident malignancy compared to those without JIA, the treatment including TNF inhibitors was not significantly associated with the development of malignancy [49].

Physical Therapy/Exercise/Nutrition

A physical therapy program based on the severity of the disease and appropriate regular exercise has long been regarded as an important element in the management of JIA. The principal goals are to control pain, alleviate stiffness, prevent or control joint damage, increase cardiovascular fitness, and maintain mobility. For example, one of the principal risk factors for osteopenia and osteoporosis is the avoidance of weight-bearing exercise in JIA [50]. In contrast to past trials indicating that exercise had a detrimental effect on JIA, newer studies show that exercise therapy has no detrimental effect nor does it exacerbate the symptoms of JIA [51]. Indeed, both RCAs and non-RCAs indicate some improvements with respect to the goals noted above, including, among others, a strong correlation between anaerobic physical fitness and functional ability [52]; decrease in the number of joints with swelling after aquatic training [53]; a relationship between physical activity and cardiorespiratory fitness [54]; weight-bearing exercises that increase muscular/bone strength, particularly in the legs; joint functionality to prevent osteoporosis [50, 55]; and stretching to maintain normal range of motion and to prevent joint contractures when a child has an acute inflammation [46, 50]. The new biologics may facilitate more aggressive therapy. Finally, children with JIA should be monitored for adequate calcium and vitamin D intake.

Osteoporosis in Children with JIA

Causes

Long recognized as a secondary consequence of all forms of JIA, osteoporosis in children and adolescents is caused by a number of interrelated factors: the disease process itself, the adverse effect of medications, poor nutrition, and restricted physical activity—all of which prevent the accrual of bone mass [56]. DXA evaluations indicate an association between decreased bone mineralization and low bone formation that is related to disease severity, with bone mass lower in polyarticular than in oligoarticular JIA; moreover, disease severity was highly correlated with decreases in markers of bone formation but not with those of bone formation [57]. Measurement with pQCT found that trabecular bone density was affected, particularly near inflamed joints [58].

The deleterious effects of high cumulative doses of corticosteroids, anticonvulsants, and immunosuppressive drugs negatively affect bone mass and induce growth retardation. Calcium and vitamin D deficiency and a decrease in the physical activity needed to strengthen bone, maintain bone mass, and improve balance and gait are also contributing factors [58]. The end result of these conditions is increased fracture susceptibility. In a population-based study of 1939 subjects (ages = 1–19), Burnham et al. reported a clinically significant increased fracture risk in children and adolescents, most pronounced in adolescent boys.

Treatment

Exercise and Nutrition

Before administering medications, appropriate exercise and optimized nutrition are regarded as the first course of action. As in the case of JIA without osteoporosis, a regular, structured program of weight-bearing activities, consistent with the severity of the disease, should be implemented to help increase bone density and promote bone growth as well as range of motion [56]. However, the optimal exercise program to promote bone mass accrual has yet to be determined and requires randomized controlled exercise trials with larger sample sizes [59]. High-impact sports including volleyball and gymnastics may be included in a physical activity program for JIA children with osteoporosis, depending on the patient's disease type and condition. For example, children with active polyarticular JIA are the most likely to have impaired anaerobic capacity and a much greater risk of injury from high-impact activities [60].

Routine supplementation of calcium and vitamin D is not recommended for this population, and its regular use in corticosteroid-induced osteoporosis is subject to conflicting interpretations, resulting in a general recommendation by the European Society for Paediatric Endocrinology to "assure adequate daily intake of calcium, vitamin D, and proteins" [61].

Medications

Bisphosphonates are a promising treatment for JIA children with osteoporosis, but, thus far, small-scale trials have produced limited results. A study involving ten patients indicated that intravenous pamidronate is a safe and useful therapy for corticosteroid-induced osteoporosis [62], while another trial with 13 patients demonstrated that treatment with disodium clodronate increased BMD by 8 %, while controls showed a BMD decrease of 7 % [63]. Further studies are needed to determine the safety and efficacy of bisphosphonates over the long term (beyond three years) and into adulthood; the optimal length of treatment and the gain in bone mass are likely to be achieved [64].

Management of JIA in Years of Transition to Adulthood

An informed and well-planned transition from pediatric to adult care for patients with JIA is critical. Many of the transition issues associated with other childhood diseases apply to JIA as well, notably the difficulty in transferring from a family-centered model with long-time providers to an unfamiliar, generally less supportive facility where patients must assume greater responsibility for their own care. In the case of JIA, it is particularly important to ensure coordination between the pediatric and the adult-care physicians as well as to identify a facility with physicians who are either trained in both pediatric and adult medicine or aware of the distinction between JIA and rheumatoid arthritis [65].

Juvenile Idiopathic Arthritis in Adults

Causes and Symptoms

Although a substantial number (estimated at 60 %) of children with JIA enter adulthood with no active functional limitations or synovitis (inflammation of the joint linings), between 30 and 56 % of adults continue to experience severe functional impairment, joint destruction, and synovitis [66]. Poly-onset JIA almost uniformly requires long-term therapy. In addition, some patients develop active flares of JIA after years of remission or after a period of effective disease control with disease-modifying antirheumatic drugs (DMARDs).

The persistence of active inflammation and the potential for joint injury are among the principal challenges in the management of JIA in adults. Differentiating inflammation from the pain and stiffness caused by joint injury is difficult. Morning stiffness is an uncertain guide to distinguishing between synovitis and mechanical joint pain; diagnostic tools such as an MRI and ultrasound may provide guidance [65]. Leg-length discrepancy stemming from childhood growth patterns results in pain, disfigurement, and complications, particularly if joint replacement is needed. Continued bone loss, joint contracture, and muscle wasting as well as pain and deformity that compromise function may dictate intervention in the form of total hip or knee replacement, recognizing that custom prostheses, generally requiring revision, may be required [67]. In a trial involving 123 JIA adults, over one-third affected with uveitis as children continued to experience symptoms as adults, with the greatest occurrence (20 %) in those with oligoarthritis [68]. In a 25-year follow-up study of 65 adults with active JIA, Zak et al. found that despite regular eye screening, 20 % of the cohort still experienced ophthalmic complications including partial vision, glaucoma, and cataracts [69]. Compromised vision may have a direct impact on frequency and severity of falls. Even near falls can put sudden increased forces on fragile joints, causing pain and adversely affecting gait. However, closer clinical surveillance, combined with access to immune-suppressing agents, is likely to result in improved outcomes of visual loss.

Treatment

In addition to surgical intervention for joint replacement, adults with JIA are treated with NSAIDs, DMARDs, and biologic drugs. In their study of 246 adult patients with long-standing JIA, Packham and Hall [66] found that 72.4 % of their cohort required NSAIDs and 30.1 % used simple analgesics such as ibuprofen and naproxen. However, the adverse effects of NSAIDs, particularly gastrointestinal disturbances, necessitated at least one incidence of withdrawal in 59 % of patients. In the same study, 74.4 % of the subjects had received DMARDs, most commonly methotrexate, to help control the disease by reducing inflammation and joint damage; 36.3 % of patients were still on the drug. Exposure to DMARDs in childhood does not decrease its effectiveness in adults.

Over the past two decades, biologics have produced positive results in both adults and children. By suppressing the immune system, they slow the progression of JIA, reducing pain, swelling, and stiffness. Thus far, the primary biologic used in adult JIA and the first to be FDA approved (1999) is the tumor necrosis factor (TNF), etanercept, used for "reducing signs and symptoms of moderate to severe polyarticular JIA in patients two years and older"; other biologics specially earmarked for polyarticular and systematic JIA have been approved more recently [70]. In a British study of the outcomes of biologic use in adults with JIA, McErlane et al. identified 225 patients who fulfilled the diagnostic criteria for JIA and initiated treatment as adults [71]. They reported that 42 % of their cohort remained on the primary biologic for five years, with 50 % of that group receiving more than one anti-TNF treatment. Although there is no consensus about the optimal management of JIA in adulthood and the factors influencing the choice of therapy, biologics have proven to be an important treatment option.

Osteoporosis in Adults with JIA

Causes and Risk Factors

An assessment of bone mineral density and an understanding of the factors underlying reduced bone mass are essential in diagnosing and treating osteoporosis in adult JIA. A trial examining disease activity in JIA patients 30 years after onset concluded that 41 % of the patients had active disease or were on medication and 28 % had a high symptom state [72]. In a study of BMD occurrence and predictors for low bone mineralization in 65 patients with a history of JIA [73], Zak et al. reported that for the hip, 46.6 % and 7.0 % of the cohort met the definition for osteopenia and osteoporosis, respectively, while 35.4 % and 7.7 % met the same criteria for the lumbar spine; they also reported an overall increased rate of bone turnover—bone formation and resorption—in their cohort. Other factors associated with low BMD included disease activity at the time of the study (a finding challenged by other researchers) [74], baseline erosions, polyarticular form of JIA, and a history of steroid treatment for more than one year; reduced physical activity and insufficient intake of calcium and vitamin D have also been implicated. It should be noted that in a trial differentiating between subjects with active disease and those in remission, Haugen et al. demonstrated that most young adults with JIA attain the same BMD as healthy subjects if the disease is in remission, but those with persistent JIA continue at an increased risk for osteopenia and osteoporosis [75].

Long-term corticosteroid therapy in adult JIA may be another causal factor for osteoporosis. Zak et al. and Haugen et al. noted an association between corticosteroid treatment and reduced bone mass in JIA [73, 75], although Haugen et al. observed that it is difficult to distinguish the impact of corticosteroid treatment from that of the disease itself, given the fact that corticosteroids are used primarily by those with high levels of disease activity. In addition, Thornton showed that JIA adults in recent trials received a stronger dose of corticosteroid and methotrexate than children currently being diagnosed with JIA and treated with less intense therapies, including etanercept rather than methotrexate [64]. In terms of fracture risk, a large, international study conducted by Kanis et al. [76] demonstrated that prior corticosteroid use by patients with chronic diseases is associated with a substantial increase in fracture risk—a risk that is independent of BMD or a prior fragility fracture. As Thornton et al. observe, further research is needed to better understand if *association* clearly denotes *causality* [64].

Treatment

JIA adults with osteoporosis should be guided by their physicians on the benefits of weight-bearing exercise and adequate calcium and vitamin D intake. Bone densitometry analysis should be conducted as part of routine clinical practice, particularly for those who are considering bisphosphonate treatment. The use of bisphosphonates in JIA has not been thoroughly examined; optimal dose, frequency of administration, and length of treatment periods have yet to be determined, and analyses of their effect in augmenting bone mass and reducing fracture risk in larger study sizes are still forthcoming [77]. In terms of other therapies, adult patients with closed linear growth may benefit from an intermittent administration of growth hormone therapy (PTH 1-34 or PTH 1-84) to restore previously lost bone structure [77]. Results indicating increased bone turnover in JIA adults with osteoporosis point to the possibility that inhibition of bone resorption may represent a new approach to preventing fractures in adult patients with active JIA or a history of the disease [73]. It is anticipated that future research will determine the predictors of low bone mass and fractures and the long-term effect of bisphosphonates in JIA adults with osteoporosis [64].

References

1. Laine C, Laine T. Diagnosis of osteoporosis in children and adolescents. Eur Endocrinol. 2013;9(2):141–4.
2. Langman CB, Trippe KA. Osteoporosis in children and adolescents. Osteoporosis clinical updates. Washington, DC: National Osteoporosis Foundation; 2010.
3. Gafni RI, Baron J. Overdiagnosis of osteoporosis in children due to misinterpretation of dual-energy x-ray absorptiometry (DEXA). J Pediatr. 2004;144(200):253–7.
4. Bachrach LK. Bone densitometry in children and adolescents. Pediatrics. 2011;127(1): 189–94.
5. Binkovitz LA, Henwood MJ. Pediatric DXA: technique and interpretation. Pediatr Radiol. 2007;37(1):21–31.
6. International Society for Clinical Densitometry. ICSD official position—pediatric—skeletal health assessment in children from infancy to adolescence. Middletown; 2013. http://www.iscd.org/official-positions/2013-iscd-official -positions-pediatric. Accessed 22 Dec 2015.
7. Marini JC. Osteogenesis imperfecta. In: Rosen CJ, editor. Primer on metabolic bone diseases and disorders of mineral metabolism. Ames: Wiley; 2013. p. 822–9.
8. National Institute of Arthritis and Musculoskeletal and Skin Diseases. What people with osteogenesis imperfecta need to know about osteoporosis. NIH Osteoporosis and Related Bone Diseases-National Resource Center; 2012. http://www.niams.nih.gov/Health_Info/Bone/Osteoporosis/Conditions_Behaviors/osteoporosis. Accessed 10 Aug 2015.
9. Bishop N, Glorieux FH. Juvenile osteoporosis. In: Rosen CJ, editor. Primer on the metabolic bone diseases and disorders of mineral metabolism. Ames: Wiley; 2013. p. 468–72.
10. Osteogenesis Imperfecta Foundation. OI issues: understanding type 1 OI. Gaithersburg; 2006. http://www.oif.org/sute/PageServer?pagename= Type 1. Accessed 9 Aug 2015.
11. National Institutes of Health. Guide to osteogenesis imperfecta for pediatricians and family physicians. Osteoporosis and Related Bone Diseases-National Resource Center, Bethesda. 2007. www.niams.nih.gov/Health_Info/Bone/default.asp. Accessed 10 Aug 2015.
12. National Osteoporosis Foundation. Facts about Osteogenesis Imperfecta. www.oif.org. Accessed 13 Feb 2016.
13. Osteogenesis Imperfecta Foundation. Linked clinical research centers. http://www.oi.org/site/PageServer?pagename=RS_lcrc. Accessed 15 Aug 2015.
14. National Institute of Arthritis and Musculoskeletal and Skin Diseases. OI issues: type I—understanding the mildest form of osteogenesis imperfecta. Bethesda; 2012. http://niams.nih.gov/Health_Info/Bone/Osteogenesis_Imperfecta/type_1/asp. Accessed 15 Aug 2015.
15. Rauch F, Glorieux FH. Osteogenesis imperfecta. Lancet. 2004;363(9418):1377–85.
16. Green DW. Osteogenesis imperfecta: a multidisciplinary approach to treatment in children. Hospital for Special Surgery; 2011. http://www.hss.edu/conditions_osteogenesis-imperfecta-approach-to-treatment.asp. Accessed 15 Aug 2015.
17. Zacharin M, Kanumakaia S. Pamidronate treatment of less severe forms of osteogenesis imperfecta in children. J Pediatr Endocrinol Metab. 2004;17(11):1511–8.
18. Brown JJ, Zacharin MR. Safety and efficacy of intravenous zoledronic acid in paediatric osteoporosis. J Pediatr Endocrinol Metab. 2009;22(1):225–7.
19. DiMeglio LA, Peacock M. Two-year clinical trial of oral alendronate versus intravenous pamidronate in children with osteogenesis imperfecta. J Bone Miner Res. 2006;21(12):132–40.

20. Ward LM, Petryk A, Gordon CM. Use of bisphosphonates in the treatment of pediatric osteoporosis. Int J Clin Rheumatol. 2009;4(6):657–72.
21. Dwan K, Phillipi CA, Steiner RD, Basel D. Bisphosphonate therapy for osteogenesis imperfecta. Cochrane Database Syst Rev. 2014;7. doi:10.1002/14651858.CD005088.
22. Hald JD, Evangelou E, Langdahl BL, Ralston SH. Bisphosphonates for the prevention of fractures in osteogenesis imperfecta: meta-analysis of placebo-controlled trials. J Bone Miner Res. 2015;30(5):929–33.
23. Marini JC. Bone: use of bisphosphonates in children—proceed with caution. Nat Rev Endocrinol. 2009;5:241–2. doi:10.1038/nrendo.2009.58.
24. Brizola E, Shapiro JR. Bisphosphonate treatment of children and adults with osteogenesis imperfecta: unanswered questions. Calcif Tissue Int. 2015;97(2):101–3. doi:10.1007/s00223-015-0021-6.
25. Rijks EBG, Bongers BC, Vlemmix MJL, Boot AM, van Dijk ATH, Sakkers RJB, et al. Efficacy and safety of bisphosphonate therapy in children with osteogenesis imperfecta: a systematic review. Horm Res Paediatr. 2015;84(1):26–42.
26. Palomo T, Fassier F, Ouellet J, Sato A, Montpetit K, Glorieux FH, et al. Intravenous bisphosphonate therapy of young children with osteogenesis imperfecta: skeletal findings during follow up throughout the growing years. J Bone Miner Res. 2015;30(12):2150–7.
27. Hoyer-Kuhn H, Franklin J, Allo G, Kron H, Netzer C, Eysel P, et al. Safety and efficacy of denosumab in children with osteogenesis imperfecta—a first prospective trial. J Musculoskelet Neuronal Interact. 2016;16(1):24–32.
28. Forlino A, Cabral WA, Barnes AM, Marini JC. New perspectives on osteogenesis imperfecta. Nat Rev Endocrinol. 2011;7(9):540–7.
29. Dogba MJ, Rauch F, Wong T, Ruck J, Glorieux FH, Bedos C. From pediatric to adult care: strategic evaluation of a transition program for patients with osteogenesis imperfecta. Biomed Central Health Serv Res. 2014;14:489. doi:10.1186/s12913-014-0489-1.
30. Shapiro JR, German-Lee EL. Osteogenesis imperfecta: effecting the transition from adolescent to adult medical care. J Musculoskelet Neuronal Interact. 2012;12(1):24–7.
31. Adami S, Gatti D, Colapiero F, Fracassi F, Braga V, Rossini M. Intravenous neridronate in adult with osteogenesis imperfecta. J Bone Miner Res. 2003;18(1):126–30.
32. Chevrel G, Schott AM, Fontanges E, Charrin JE, Lina-Granade G, Duboeuf F, et al. Effects of oral alendronate on BMD in adult patients with osteogenesis imperfecta: a 3-year randomized placebo-controlled trial. J Bone Miner Res. 2006;21(2):300–6.
33. Pavon de Paz I, Iglesias Bolanos P, Duran Martinez M, Olivar Roldan J, Guijarro De Armas G, Parra Garcia JI. Effects of zoledronic acid in adults with osteogenesis imperfecta. Endocrinol Nutr. 2010;57(6):245–50.
34. Shapiro JR, Thompson CB, Wu Y, Nunes M, Gillenj C. Bone mineral density and fracture rate in response to intravenous and oral bisphosphonates in adult osteogenesis imperfecta. Calcif Tissue Int. 2010;87(2):120–9.
35. Bradbury LA, Barlow S, Geoghegan F, Hannon RA, Stuckey SL, Wass JA, et al. Risedronate in adults with osteogenesis imperfecta type 1 results in increased bone mineral density and decreased bone turnover, but high fracture rate persists. Osteoporos Int. 2012;223(1):285–94.
36. Bishop NJ, Walsh JS. Osteogenesis imperfecta in adults. J Clin Invest. 2014;124(2):476–7.
37. Orwell ES, Shapiro J, Veith S, Wang Y, Lapidus J, Vanek C, et al. Evaluation of teriparatide treatment in adults with osteogenesis imperfecta. J Clin Invest. 2014;142(2):491–8.
38. Lindahl K, Lindahl B, Ljunggren O, Kindmark A. Treatment of osteogenesis imperfecta in adults. Eur J Endocrinol. 2014;171(2):R79–90. doi:10.1530/EJE-14-0017.
39. van Dijk FS, Cobben JM, Kariminejad A, Maugeri A, Nikkeles PGJ, van Rijn RR. Osteogenesis imperfecta: a review with clinical examples. Mol Syndromol. 2011;2(1):1–20. doi:10.1159/00033228.
40. Ellis JA, Munro JE, Ponsonby AL. Possible environmental determinants of juvenile idiopathic arthritis. Rheumatology. 2010;49(3):411–25.
41. Horton DB, Scott FY, Haynes K, Putt ME, Rose CD, Lewis JD, et al. Antibiotic exposure and juvenile idiopathic arthritis: a case-control study. Pediatrics. 2015;136(2):e333–43.

42. Rheumatology Network. Early identification of juvenile idiopathic arthritis. 2010. http://www.rheumatologynetwork.com/juvenile-arthritis/early-identification-juvenile-idiopathic-arthritis. Accessed 5 Sept 2015.
43. Weiss JE, Ilowite NT. Juvenile idiopathic arthritis. Rheum Dis Clin North Am. 2007;33(3):441–70. vi.
44. Espinosa M, Gottlieb BS. Juvenile idiopathic arthritis. Pediatr Rev. 2012;33(7):303–12.
45. National Institute of Arthritis and Musculoskeletal and Skin Diseases. Juvenile arthritis: questions and answers about juvenile arthritis. 2015. http://www.niams.nih.gov/Health_Info/Juv_Arthritis/#5. Accessed 28 Dec 2015.
46. Kim KH, Kim DS. Juvenile idiopathic arthritis: diagnosis and different diagnosis. Korean J Pediatr. 2010;53(1212):931–5.
47. Stoll MJ, Cron RQ. Treatment of juvenile idiopathic arthritis: a revolution in care. Pediatr Rheumatol Online J. 2014. doi:10.1186/1546-0096-12-13.
48. NHS England Clinical Reference Group for Paediatric Medicine. NHS England clinical commissioning policy statement: biologic therapies or the treatment of juvenile idiopathic arthritis. NHS England (e-format). 2015. https://www.england.nhs.uk/commissioning/wp-content/uploads/sites/12/2015/10/e03pd-bio-therapies-jia-oct15.pdf. Accessed 13 Dec 2015.
49. Beukelman T, Haynes K, Curtis JR, Xie F, Cen L, Bemrich-Stolz CJ, et al. Rates of malignancy associated with juvenile idiopathic arthritis and its treatment. Arthritis Rheum. 2012;64(4):1263–71.
50. Kim SC, Pope J. Juvenile idiopathic arthritis: stretching and strengthening exercises. Scand J Rheumatol. 2012;28(1):19–26.
51. Takken T, Van Brussel M, Engelbart RH, van der Net J, Kuis H, Helders PJM. Exercise therapy in juvenile idiopathic arthritis. Cochrane Database Syst Rev. 2008. doi:10.1002/144651858.CD005954.pub2.
52. Takken T, van der Net J, Helders PJM. Relationship between functionality and physical fitness in juvenile idiopathic arthritis patients. Scand J Rheumatol. 2003;32(3):174–8.
53. Epps H, Ginnelly L, Utley M, Southwood T, Gallivan S, Sculpher M, et al. Is hydrotherapy cost effective? A randomized controlled trial of combined hydrotherapy programmes compared with physiotherapy land techniques in children with juvenile idiopathic arthritis. Health Technol Assess. 2005;9(39):iii–iv. ix-x: 1–59.
54. Takken T, van der Net J, Heiders PJM. Physical activity and health related physical fitness in children with juvenile idiopathic arthritis. Ann Rheum Dis. 2003. doi:10.1136/ard.62.9.885.
55. Sandstedt E, Fasth A, Eek MN, Beckung E. Muscle strength, physical fitness and well-being in children and adolescents with juvenile idiopathic arthritis and the effect of an exercise programme: a randomized controlled trial. Pediatr Rheumatol. 2013;11(1):7. doi:10.1186/1546-0096-11-7.
56. McDonagh JE. Osteoporosis in juvenile idiopathic arthritis. Curr Opin Rheumatol. 2001;13:399–404.
57. Pepmueller PH, Cassidy JT, Allen SH, Hillman LS. Bone mineralization and bone mineral metabolism in children with juvenile rheumatoid arthritis. Arthritis Rheum. 1996;39(5):746–57.
58. Roth J, Bechtold S, Borte G, Dressler F, Girschick HJ, Borte M. Osteoporosis in juvenile idiopathic arthritis-a practical approach to diagnosis and therapy. Eur J Pediatr. 2007. doi:10.1007/s00431-007-0484-1.
59. Hind K, Burrows M. Weight-bearing exercise and bone mineral accrual in children and adolescents: a review of controlled trials. Bone. 2007;40(1):14–27.
60. Klepper S. Making the case for exercise in children with juvenile idiopathic arthritis: what we know and where do we go from here. Arthritis Care Res. 2007;57(6):887–90.
61. Hochberg Z, Bereket A, Davenport M, Delemarre-van de Waal HA, De Schepper J, Levine MA, et al. Consensus development for the supplementation of vitamin D in childhood and adolescence. Horm Res. 2002;58(1):39–51.

62. Noguera A, Ros JB, Pavia C, Alcover E, Valis C, Villaronga M, et al. Bisphosphonates, a new treatment for glucocorticoid-induced osteoporosis in children. J Pediatr Endocrinol Metab. 2003;16(4):529–36.
63. Lepore L, Pennesi M, Barbi E, Pozzi R. Treatment and prevention of osteoporosis in juvenile chronic arthritis with disodium clodronate. Clin Exp Rheumatol. 1991;9 Suppl 6:33–5.
64. Thornton J, Ashcroft D, O'Neill T, Elliott R, Adams J, Robert C, et al. A systematic review of the effectiveness of strategies for reducing fracture risk in children with juvenile idiopathic arthritis with additional data on long-term risk of fracture and cost of disease management. Health Technol Assess. 2008;12:41–7.
65. Nigrovic PA, White PH. Care of the adult with juvenile rheumatoid arthritis. Arthritis Rheum. 2006;55(2):2208–16.
66. Packham JC, Hall MA. Long-term follow-up of 246 adults with juvenile idiopathic arthritis: social function, relationships and sexual activity. Rheumatology (Oxford). 2002;41(12):1440–3.
67. Scott RD. Total hip and knee arthroplasty in juvenile rheumatoid arthritis. Clin Orthop Relat Res. 1990;259:83–91.
68. Kotaniemi K, Arkela-Kautiainen M, Haapasaari J, Leirisalo-Repo M. Uveitis in young adults with juvenile idiopathic arthritis: a clinical evaluation of 123 patients. Ann Rheum Dis. 2005. doi:10.1136/ard.2004.026955.
69. Zak M, Fledelius H, Karup F. Ocular complications and visual outcome in juvenile chronic arthritis: a 25-year follow-up study. Acta Ophthalmol Scand. 2003;81(3):211–5.
70. Food and Drug Administration. Biologics: new treatments for juvenile arthritis. Silver Spring: Food and Drug Administration; 2014. http://www.fda.gov/ForConsumers/ConsumerUpdates/ucm403578.htm. Accessed 27 Dec 2015.
71. McErlane F, Foster H, Davies R, Lunt M, Watson KD, Symmons DPM, et al. Biologic treatment response among adults with juvenile idiopathic arthritis: results from the British Society for Rheumatology Biologics Register. Rheumatology. 2013;52(120):1905–13.
72. Selvaag AM, Aulie HA, Lilleby V, Flate B. Disease progression into adulthood and predictors of long-term active disease in juvenile idiopathic arthritis. Ann Rheum Dis. 2014. doi:10.1136/annrheumdis-2014-206034.
73. Zak M, Hassager C, Lovell DJ, Nielson S, Henderson CJ, Pedersen FK. Assessment of bone mineral density in adults with a history of juvenile chronic arthritis. Arthritis Rheum. 1999;42(4):790–8.
74. French AR, Mason T, Nelson AM, Crowson CS, O'Fallon WM, Khosla S, et al. Osteopenia in adults with a history of juvenile rheumatoid arthritis. A population-based study. J Rheumatol. 2002;29(5):1065–70.
75. Haugen M, Lien G, Flato B, Kyammen J, Vinje, Sorskaar D, et al. Young adults with juvenile arthritis in remission attain normal peak bone mass at the lumbar spine and forearm. Arthritis Rheum. 2000;43(7):1504–10.
76. Kanis JA, Johansson H, Oden A, Johnell O, de Laet C, Melton III LJ. A meta-analysis of prior corticosteroid use and fracture risk. J Bone Min Res. 2004;19(6):893–9.
77. Maresova KB. Secondary osteoporosis in patients with juvenile idiopathic arthritis. J Osteoporos. 2011. doi:10.4061/2011/569417.

Chapter 18
Secondary Osteoporosis in Conditions of Pediatric Onset

Christina V. Oleson

Continuing the themes set forth in the prior chapter, secondary osteoporosis can result from disorders of the central nervous system or directly from the muscles. This chapter will discuss two of the most common pediatric disorders seen in pediatric units, transitional care clinics, and "young adult" programs in rehabilitation hospitals: cerebral palsy and Duchenne muscular dystrophy. Other forms of muscular dystrophy, such as Becker's muscular dystrophy, produce significantly less disability and are not considered here.

Cerebral Palsy in Children

The classic definition of cerebral palsy (CP), developed by Risenbaum et al., is a "group of permanent disorders of the development of movement and posture, causing activity limitations that are attributable to nonprogressive disturbances that occur in the developing fetal or infant brain" [1]. It is the most common motor disability in children and the childhood disease most associated with osteoporosis. CP is characterized as *congenital* when brain damage occurs before or during birth as it does in 85–90 % of CP cases or *acquired* when damage occurs more than 28 days after birth, generally associated with an infection or a head injury [2].

Types of Cerebral Palsy

Several different *classification systems* are currently in use for CP, sometimes leading to a confused diagnosis especially if different specialists are involved. Severity level, body control: spastic (increased muscle tone) or nonspastic (decreased or

C.V. Oleson, *Osteoporosis Rehabilitation*, DOI 10.1007/978-3-319-45084-1_18

Table 1 The four types of cerebral palsy and their features

	Predominance	Damaged area	Diagnostic groups
Spastic	70–80 %	Aspects of the brain which control movement	Divided into three groups, *hemiplegia*, *diplegia*, and *quadriplegia*, reflecting the parts of the body affected and the level of severity
Hemiplegia	Principal characteristics defined by exaggerated reflexes and stiff muscles. Specifically defined by unilateral stiffness which typically affects the upper extremity as opposed to the lower extremity; almost all children can walk		
Diplegia	Principal characteristics of exaggerated reflexes and stiff muscles. Specifically defined by stiffness which typically affects the lower extremities as opposed to the upper extremities, which are typically unaffected; three in four children can walk		
Quadriplegia	Principal characteristics of exaggerated reflexes and stiff muscles. Specifically defined by stiffness which typically affects all four extremities, the trunk, and face. Quadriplegia is identified as the most severe form of spasticity; generally includes other associated conditions (e.g., vision and hearing loss, seizures, and intellectual disabilities); one in four children can walk		
Dyskinetic	10–20 %	Basal ganglia	Two basic subcategories: *athetoid* and *dystonic*
Athetoid	Abnormal muscle contractions resulting in slow, involuntary writhing movements of the arms, hands, feet, and legs which may result in a disruption of the normal abilities to sit straight, hold or grasp objects; dysfunctional gait		
Dystonic	Abnormal muscle contractions resulting in a twisted position caused by trunk movements that are affected more than limb muscles; general uncontrollable muscle spasms		
Ataxic	5–10 %	Cerebellum	
	Ataxic muscles are generally floppy, which may result in coordination impairments, unsteady or shaky movements, hand tremors, and other balance problems; functional standing, walking, and depth perception are all typically impaired. Ataxia is identified as the least severe form of cerebral palsy		
Mixed	A combination of several of the impediments characteristic of the other three forms		

Sources: Fairhurst [3]
National Institute of Neurological Disorders and Stroke [4]
Center for Disease Control and Prevention [5]

flexible muscle tone), gross motor function (impairment level), and topographical distribution (body parts affected) are the four principal categories as applied to four different *types* of CP (Table 1) [3–5].

Causes and Symptoms

The causes of CP stem from problems occurring at three different stages [6, 7]:

1. *Prenatal*: genetic and environmental factors; damaged nerve cell fibers in the white matter of the brain, hemorrhage, and brain malfunction; and maternal infections such as rubella
2. *Perinatal*: problems in birthing process leading to ruptured blood vessels or oxygen deprivation to the brain and maternal infections
3. *Postnatal*: trauma (accidental injuries), infection (meningitis), and asphyxia that disrupt synapses between brain cells

Risk factors that may lead to an increased chance of a child being born with CP include birth conditions, medical conditions, and unforeseen trauma (Fig. 1) [6, 7]. In an Australian study of four risk factors for CP—asphyxiated birth events, inflammation or other signs of infection, birth defects, and poor fetal growth including low birth weight—McIntyre et al. [8] reported that birth defects and poor fetal growth, seen in almost half of the children studied, were the most common contributing factors. Babies with severe cerebral palsy show symptoms of the disease (notably a weak or shrill cry, problems sucking and swallowing, and seizures) at or shortly after birth. However, most children are diagnosed between the ages of six months and two years. The first sign is generally a delay in developmental milestones such as crawling, walking, rolling over, controlling head movements, sitting without support, and rocking with one hand.

The primary symptoms of CP [9, 10] and their influence on fracture risk are:

1. Poor muscle tone
2. Impaired muscle coordination and control
3. Persistence of primitive reflexes
4. Damaged gross and fine motor skills
5. Diminished oral motor functions
6. Compromised posture and balance

Descriptions of each of the six features listed above are given in Table 2 [9].

Secondary conditions associated with CP include epilepsy (up to 36 % of children with CP experience these seizures by 12 months), visual and cognitive impairment, joint contractures, foot deformities, hip dysplasia, incontinence, and constipation, among others [4].

Diagnosis and Prognosis

Because there is no single medical test that definitively confirms cerebral palsy, the diagnosis is necessarily complex and can extend over a period of time, on occasion as many as 2–5 years. The parental stress brought about by this lengthy process, a concern that doctors may be overly cautious in undertaking the necessary diagnostic procedures, and recognition of the importance of early detection and intervention have led the American Academy of Pediatrics to issue a 12-step program focused on developmental surveillance and screening of motor skills at ages 9, 18, and, 30 months [11]. In addition, diagnosis should include a parental interview with family history, physical examination, laboratory tests, and imaging studies. Physicians

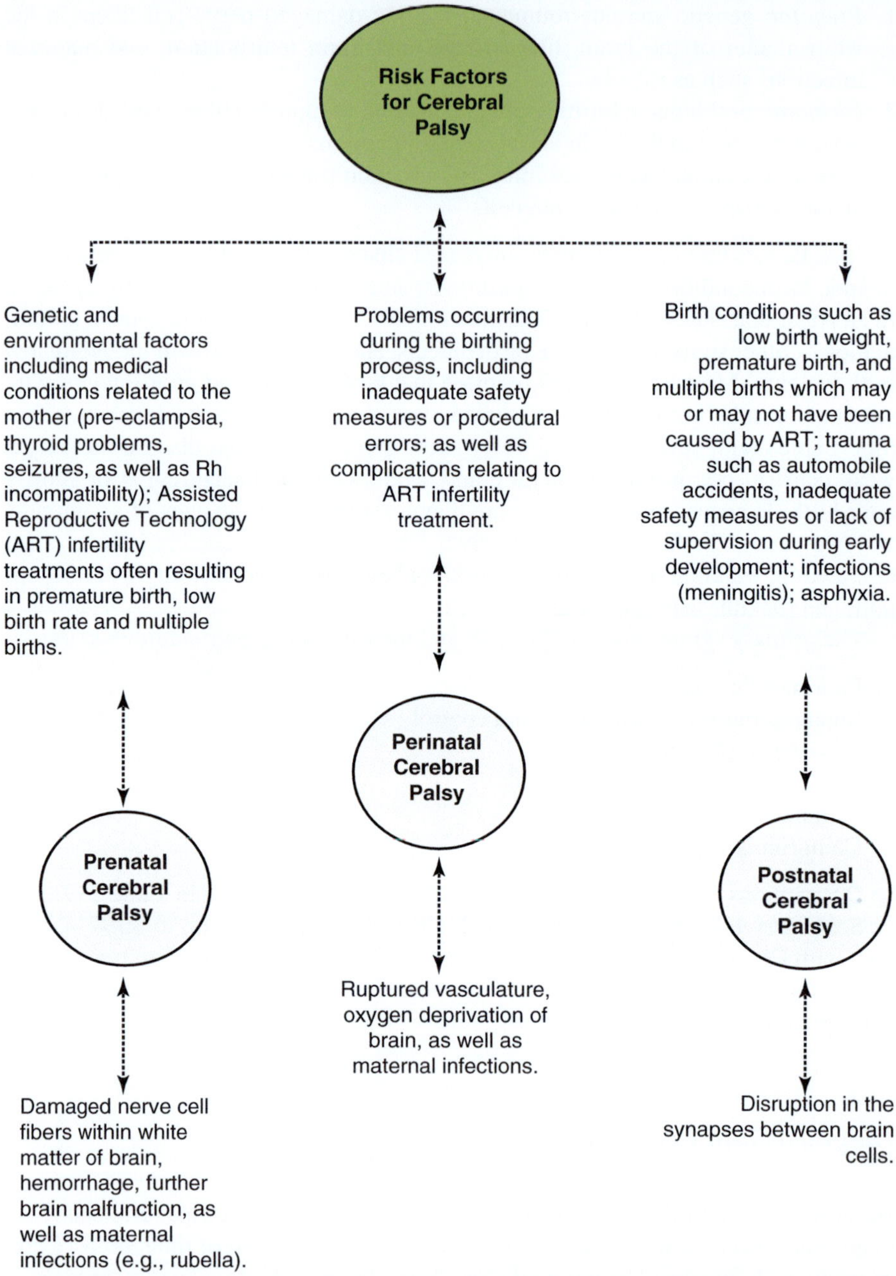

Fig. 1 Risk factors contributing to CP: Genetic, environmental factors and physiologic causes of CP, according to timing of onset (*Sources*: Nelson and Grether [6] and Reddihough and Collins [7])

Table 2 Primary symptoms associated with cerebral palsy

Primary symptom	Clinical description	Effect on bone
Poor muscle tone	The inability of muscles to work together with respect to both contracting and relaxing muscle fibers as needed is the most frequently observed symptom of CP. Exemplified by hypotonia: the floppy, rag doll appearance signifying decreased muscle resistance to passive movement or, more likely, by hypertonia, the stiffness or rigidity of muscles indicating increased resistance to passive movement	Compromised ability to reach peak bone density in the setting of weakened muscles limiting activities
Persistence of primitive reflexes	Reflexes such as sucking or grasping and holding an object persist beyond the typical and predictable time frame; in addition, a preference for use of the right or left hand is manifest before the normal age of 18 months	–
Damaged gross and fine motor skills	Abnormal muscle tone impairs crawling, standing, and walking; in addition it also affects the fine motor fibers necessary for precise movements such as picking up small objects and placing them in designated containers, turning book pages, or using a variety of writing and coloring instruments	–
Diminished oral motor functions	Difficulty conducting movement of the lips, jaw, and other facial muscles can result in feeding difficulties [117]. With respect to speech impediments, poor muscle control impedes air flow and posture; as well as negatively affecting the articulation of words and syllables [118]	Nutritional compromise may limit intake of calcium and other key vitamins and minerals
Compromised posture and balance	In contrast to the typical symmetrical posture, the asymmetrical posture characteristic of CP occurs because the right and left limbs do not mirror each other. Use of both hands for support in sitting, swaying when standing, and walking abnormally are all indications of balance abnormalities	Increase risk of fractures secondary to an increased fall risk

Sources: Jones et al. [9]
Reilly and Skuse [117]
Parkes et al. [118]

may use an assessment tool such as the Gross Motor Functional Classification System, an age-specific, five-level classification system, with five indicating total dependence [12]. Recently expanded to encompass a 12–18-year-old age group, it emphasizes functional abilities including movement and mobility, sitting, walking, and the need for assistive devices.

To establish an etiology and prognosis for children with CP, magnetic resonance imaging with its greater sensitivity is preferable to non-contrast computerized tomography (CT) as evidenced in studies showing that the yield of finding an abnormal MRI scan in a child is high (average of age 88 %) and greater than that reported using CT (77 %) [13].

Approaches to Management of CP in Children

Nonpharmacologic Management in Children

A multidisciplinary team of physicians, specialists, and therapists are needed to meet the complex needs of children with CP with a goal of increasing functional abilities, sustaining cognitive development, and achieving a sense of independence [3, 14, 15].

Physical therapy to improve muscle strength, balance, flexibility, and motor skills as well as to prevent contractures is one of the cornerstones of CP treatment. Resistance exercise has been shown to be effective in muscle strengthening, with no increase in spasticity [16]. Aqua exercises are also recommended. Braces, splints, casts, and ankle foot orthoses can help strengthen weak muscles and enhance joint motion, while gait function is improved with muscle strength training and orthoses. In a study of children with spastic diplegia, eight weeks of muscle strength training produced stronger muscles, higher GMFM scores, an increase in both stride length and hip extensor movement, and improved gait function [17]. Occupational therapy assists children in eating, grooming, dressing, attending school, and using a computer with a voice synthesizer; speech and language therapy enables them to gain greater control of jaw and mouth muscles, making their speech clearer and building their language skills.

Pharmacologic Management in Children

The most commonly prescribed medications for management of CP in children are oral and intrathecal baclofen (ITB), botulinum toxin (BT-A), diazepam, and tizanidine. Infused into the spinal canal with an inflatable pump, baclofen is a muscle relaxant that reduces muscle spasticity throughout the body. Administered by local injection, botulinum toxin is regarded as a standard treatment to reduce localized, segmental spasticity in the upper and lower extremities; it is most effective in children who have some control over their movements and when used in conjunction with a stretching program. Diazepam may be considered as a short-term treatment for generalized spasticity, while tizanidine has been found to be "possibly effective," recognizing that its impact on motor function has yet to be determined [18]. These medications may be important to improve the overall functional mobility of these patients, without which transfers and ambulation may be impossible. Maximizing mobility is an essential component of preventing osteoporosis.

Although surgery is rarely needed, it is recommended in some cases to reduce spasticity in legs, improve muscle development, lengthen or release tendons to increase mobility, and improve gait function. In addition, the insertion of spinal rods may be warranted to avoid the risk of musculoskeletal scoliosis [15].

Osteoporosis in Children with CP

Causes

In a frequently cited study, Houlihan and Stevenson observe that given their decreased bone density and bone mass, CP children suffer painful pathogenic fractures that are caused by poor bone mineralization. When inflicted with minimal trauma, such fractures result in compromised motor function and quality of life [19]. In the absence of mechanical loading by muscle force, the periosteal circumference of bone fails to expand; the long, narrow lever arms become weaker and more susceptible to fracture, and stiffness increases in the major joints, particularly in the hips and knees [20]. Other contributing causes of osteoporosis in CP are calcium and vitamin D deficiency, nutritional disorders associated with feeding and swallowing problems, anticonvulsant therapy, and delayed pubertal development that affects longitudinal bone growth and bone mineral accrual.

Diagnosis

As stipulated by the International Society for Clinical Densitometry (ISCD), DXA findings must be combined with evidence of a clinically significant fracture history to constitute a diagnosis of osteoporosis [21]. DXA scans in themselves pose special difficulties for children with CP [22]. Their smaller, thinner bones may lead to a false appearance of low BMD in these scans; abnormally shaped bones, prior surgeries, and surgical implants may also distort the results. Positioning the child in the scanner poses its own challenges. Excessive motion means that it is difficult to replicate positions from one scan to another, and these constantly changing positions can lead to a false BMD reading.

Adaptations in the use of conventional scanners are being made including supporting the extremities with splints and allowing the child to remain in a wheelchair, reducing or eliminating the need for sedation [23]. In addition, new, wider fan-beam scanners with their shorter span time minimize the effects of involuntary body movement [24]. Of particular significance, Henderson et al. have sought to counteract the effects of hip and knee contractures and scoliosis on the standard proximal femur testing site by developing an effective alternative: the measurement of BMD in the distal femur with the child in a lateral position [25].

Improved assessment tools are needed to increase understanding of the factors that promote bone quality in CP, including geometry and microarchitecture. Peripheral quantitative computed tomography (pQCT) is a more effective measure of the structural and material properties of bone, but it is not yet widely used in CP children, in part because of its lack of precision and high radiation doses [19]. It should be noted, however, that when used as a research tool, pQCT has demonstrated that bone strength in children with CP is due not to low cortical bone density but to the presence of smaller and thinner bone. Moreover, a recent assessment of the potential of high-resolution pQCT demonstrates what the authors term its "unprecedented ability" to measure bone microarchitecture in a clinical setting, providing much-needed insight into changes in bone quality as well as the impact of anti-osteoporosis treatment on bone quality. However, before it is generally accepted in routine clinical practice, researchers will need to demonstrate its utility for fracture prediction [26].

Treatment

In order of their increasing efficacy, the three basic categories of treatment for osteoporosis in children with CP are (1) weight-bearing interventions, (2) calcium and vitamin D supplementation, and (3) bisphosphonate medication [27]. Before treatment is initiated, consideration should be given to eliminating the risk factors for osteoporosis in CP children, specifically the anticonvulsant medications that reduce BMD and increase fracture risk.

Weight-Bearing Activities

Studies on the efficacy of weight-bearing interventions in improving BMD and preventing fractures have produced inconclusive, sometimes conflicting, results, which can be attributed to the small number of subjects involved, the short duration of the studies, their limited number, and the inadequate rigor of their research designs [28]. In an examination of 18 children (nine with cerebral palsy and nine controls), Chad et al. found that after eight months of physical activity, volumetric BMD increased 5.6 % in the cerebral palsy group compared with −6.3 % in controls, with femoral neck bone mineral content at 9.6 % in the cerebral palsy group and −5.8 % in controls [29]. However, interpreting the results may be problematic because the extent of the increase in BMD needed to affect fracture risk has yet to be determined for children with CP [19].

In a pilot trial to determine whether a 50 % longer standing time (with or without assistive devices) could increase BMD in nonambulatory children with CP, Caulton et al. found a significant 6 % mean increase in the vertebral trabecular BMD (vTBMD), but no change in the proximal tibial BMD (pTBMD) over a 9-month period. They conclude that while this result may reduce the risk of vertebral fractures, it is unlikely to reduce the risk of lower limb bone fractures: the most common site of trauma fracture in children with CP [30]. By contrast, in a 6-month trial involving short duration, low-magnitude, high-frequency mechanical stimuli, Ward et al. [31] demonstrated a 6.3 % mean increase in vTBMD in disabled children who stood on active devices as opposed to an 11.9 % decrease in those on placebo devices, representing a total net benefit of 17.7. On the basis of these findings, they conclude that low-magnitude mechanical loading may provide a surrogate for suppressed muscular activity in children with disabilities, representing a potential nonpharmacologic, noninvasive treatment. Although an analysis of the effect of stepping while standing revealed no added benefit to bone compared with passive standing [32], repetitive locomotor training with an electromechanical gait trainer led to improvements in 10 and 6-minutes walk tests, gait speed, and stride length [33]. Further research and stronger evidence are needed to justify an overall recommendation on weight training for osteoporosis treatment in cerebral palsy.

Nutrition

Children with limited exposure to sunlight and inadequate dietary intake, as in the case of those with cerebral palsy, are likely to experience vitamin D deficiency. The recommended daily requirement is 600 IU daily; however, a study by Kilpinen-Loisa et al. found that administration of 1,000 IU of vitamin D_3 daily five days a week for 10 weeks resulted in a significant increase in vitamin D concentration, without producing hypercalciuria or other adverse effects [34]. Calcium intake can be enhanced through diet or calcium supplementation, with diet as the preferred alternative, because it is more soluble and is associated with greater patient compliance [27]. Jekovec-Vrhovsek et al. conducted a study of 20 children ($n = 13$, 7 controls) with spastic quadriplegia and epilepsy, before and after vitamin D and calcium supplementation. Their results showed that in the treated group, BMD increased significantly, while the untreated group continued to experience bone loss [35].

Pharmacologic Intervention

Of the treatments currently in use, bisphosphonate therapy appears to be the most effective in increasing BMD and, to an extent, in reducing fragility fractures [27]. Despite concerns about long-term efficacy and safety in children, studies report generally favorable findings, specifically for the drug, intravenous pamidronate. In an evaluation of the effect of IV pamidronate on osteopenia in nonambulatory children with quadriplegic cerebral palsy [36], Henderson focused on six pairs of subjects with each pair matched by age, sex, and race. One subject in each group received a placebo; the other was administered with IV pamidronate for three consecutive days, repeated at 3-month intervals for one year, with continued evaluations for six months after the final treatment. The result was an $89\,\% \pm 21$ increase in BMD at the distal femur for the pamidronate group as opposed to a $9 \pm 6\,\%$ increase for the controls. Age-normalized *Z*-scores also increased for the pamidronate group, while controls showed no significant change.

Subsequent research on the effect of pamidronate has confirmed increases in BMD for femoral neck and lumbar spine, with increased *Z*-scores at both sites [37]. When used in combination with vitamin D, another bisphosphonate, risedronate, improved BMD in cerebral palsy patients for greater than one year [38]. Bisphosphonate intervention is generally recommended only after a child has sustained at least one fragility fracture and not as a preventative measure. Fehlings et al. further propose that treatments be initiated only if fractures continue after vitamin D and calcium have been optimized [27].

Another potential treatment for CP children with osteoporosis is growth hormone (GH) replacement therapy. In a study of 46 children (ages 3–11 years), Devesa et al. found that 70 % of the children had impaired GH secretion, making it the most common anterior pituitary abnormality in children with CP. Their analysis of other studies relating to GH (generally carried out in adults or rodents) emphasized that not only did GH increase the possibility of achieving normal height, but when combined with the insulin-like growth factor-1 (IGF-1), it also increased cell proliferation and survival in both the central and peripheral nervous system. Given these findings they propose that GH therapy be initiated as early as possible [39].

Cerebral Palsy in Adults

The number of adults living with cerebral palsy in the United States is estimated at about 400,000 and that number is expected to grow due to the heighted survival rate of low birth-weight infants as well as the increased longevity of the generalized adult population including those with CP. The initial challenge is the transition from pediatric to adult health care that offers more limited interdisciplinary care and rehabilitation services. Not only must a thorough and accurate medical history be provided to the adult facility, but provision should be made for initial overlap and continued communication, if needed, between pediatric care providers and adult health care professionals to ensure continuity of care. An interdisciplinary care center is the optimal adult facility given the needed to detect, monitor, and treat the multiple consequences of aging with cerebral palsy [40, 41].

Only within the last two decades have individuals with cerebral palsy lived long enough to encounter the effects of aging imposed upon their lifelong disability. Adults with CP experience early-onset aging in their 40s as developmental delays in childhood, continual spasms, and additional stress and strain result in deterioration of the cardiovascular and pulmonary systems as well as muscle groups. They may also have acute or chronic pain, generally situated in the hips, knees, ankles, and upper and lower back. Those with spastic cerebral palsy indicate pain at a greater number of sites and to a more intense degree than patients with other forms of CP [4]. In a study of 93 adults recruited from the University of Washington area, 67 % reported one or more areas of pain of a minimum of three months duration, most commonly in the lower extremities and back, with 56 % reporting pain on a daily basis [42]. In an analysis of the frequency and severity of several symptoms of cerebral palsy in 83 adults, Hirsh et al. [43] confirmed Schwartz et al.'s earlier findings that moderate-to-severe pain persisted in a cohort of 50 CP adults followed over a 2-year period.

Among the causes of pain in adult CP are osteoarthritis, contractures, spasticity, orthopedic deformity, fractures, poor nutrition, weakness, and fatigue [44]. The National Institute of Neurological Disorders and Stroke has reported that CP patients require three to five times the amount of energy to walk and move about than do normal persons [4].

An examination of 101 adults (aged 19–74) with cerebral palsy revealed that 76 % had multiple musculoskeletal problems; in 63 %, these occurred under the age of 50, suggesting that abnormal biomechanical forces and immobility led to excessive physical stress overuse syndromes and possibly early joint deterioration [45]. In a survey of 221 Swedish subjects (ages 25–58) [46], 35 % of the subjects reported decreased walking ability before age 35, with participants citing increased spasticity, balance problems, and musculoskeletal deterioration as the causes; researchers pointed to contractures in weight-bearing joints, immobility, knee pain, and the lack of physiotherapy as additional causal factors. One of the predictors of sustained walking is childhood experience: those better able to walk as a child persisted walking into adulthood for a longer period than those who used gait aids [47]. Other challenges facing adults with CP include communication, hearing and vision impairments, osteoarthritis, and depression which is three to four times greater in patients with such disabilities as CP, resulting primarily not from the disease itself but from the ability to cope with its consequences.

Medical Management and Symptom Control in Adult CP

The most critical need of patients with adult cerebral palsy is pain management. In a study of chronic pain in this population, Jensen et al. followed 50 patients (half women/half men) over the course of two years, finding that pain intensity did not change significantly over that period despite the use of several forms of treatment; although participants characterized a number of treatments as "moderately helpful," in their view, only three—whirlpool, ultrasound, and transcutaneous electrical nerve stimulation—were associated with decreased pain [48]. In a descriptive study of 64 adults (ages 18–76), Engel et al. reported that more than half of the participants used non-steroidal anti-inflammatory medications (i.e. acetaminophen, aspirin, ibuprofen) to treat pain, while one-third turned to anti-spasticity medications or opioids; all were reported to have limited success [49].

Intravenous botulinum toxin (BT-A) and intrathecal baclofen (ITB) have also been used in adults with limited success. Injected into muscles, BT-A is primarily directed at managing spasticity; its effect on pain is not fully understood and remains primarily anecdotal [44]. One of the most significant new advances in cerebral palsy, ITB, has been shown to be a safe and effective treatment for muscle spasticity in cerebral palsy, with demonstrated functional improvement and pain relief [50].

The positive effect of exercise in reducing pain has been examined in a number of disabilities including cerebral palsy. Patients themselves have indicated that physical therapy and strengthening exercises are beneficial. In an analysis of pain treatments in adults with CP [51], physical therapy, mobility/ROM exercises, and strengthening exercises were among the most common treatments, used with a rating of "moderately effective." However, more extensive studies are needed to demonstrate the effectiveness of various types of exercise and their direct relation to specific sites of pain and specific types of CP.

Beyond pain management, traditional physical therapy has long been one of the cornerstones of CP treatment and rehabilitation, with anticipated improvement in lung and heart efficiency, mobility, and bone strength as well as a reduction in the risk of complicating diseases such as osteoporosis. However, evidence on the actual effect of physical therapy remains limited. In a systematic review of 13 trials on the impact of physiotherapy on adults with CP, Jeglinsky et al. found that none met the criteria for high methodological quality and pointed up the need for new, well-designed studies [52].

At the same time, newer forms of exercise, notably strength training, have become prominent in both able-bodied and disabled individuals and have secured a place in the CP population. In previous decades, strength training was avoided because of the unfounded belief that it led to increased spasticity; even today, despite some evidence that it can improve strength and possibly improve motor function, strength training remains controversial, particularly in children and adolescents [53]. However, several studies of strength training in adults have shown promising results. In a study of the impact of a 10-week progressive strength training program focused on the lower extremities of a small group of adults with CP, Andersson et al. reported significantly improved muscle strength in hip extensors, resulting in improved walking ability, walking velocity, and gross motor function with no increase in spasticity [54]. A small study conducted at a community gymnasium demonstrated that during another 10-week intervention period, participants increased leg strength by 22.0% and arm strength by 17.2% [55]. Participating in a strength training program can have psychological and social benefits as well, even increasing adherence to the programs themselves. Participants in a trial involving adults aged 40+ cited enjoyment and social interaction as the principal benefits, leading to perceptions that their strength and ability to carry out everyday activities had improved [56]. Aquatic exercise, functional electrical stimulation, and whole body vibration in a community setting are other new techniques currently being studied for their efficacy in increasing muscle strength and motor performance, fostering social interaction without negatively affecting spasticity.

The adoption of new therapeutic approaches, coupled with a growing appreciation of the value of social involvement, is leading to a rethinking of how to assess physical interventions [57]. Instead of attempting to undertake and evaluate a multifaceted therapy program, researchers increasingly focus on assessing the value of a specific well-defined treatment. This is the goal of strength training evaluations. Other activity-based programs such as cycling and treadmill training aimed at increasing endurance and coordination require similar evaluations.

The extended life span of patients with CP and the fact that many lose their walking ability by the age of 35 have even led to questioning the value of the "symbolic" goal of independent walking for children and adolescents, resulting in significant implications for adults with the disease. As Bottos et al. emphasize [58], the need to plan for an entire life span, rather than focus on the childhood experience, has taken on a new importance. When walking is upheld as the ultimate achievement and is subsequently lost, frustration and disappointment are the inevitable result. In contrast, Damiano demonstrates that mobility, whether achieved independently or with motor devices, has positive effects in terms of the emotional and social development of the child and ultimately the adult. Children with increased motor ability are more likely to develop a "can do" attitude rather than retreat into a "help me" mode [57]. Independence achieved through the use of advanced assistive devices coupled with the benefits derived from social participation in the community should be among the altered and achievable goals of adults with CP who seek an improved quality of life [58]. Unfortunately, it must be noted that a number of "external" impediments impose limitations on access to exercise facilities. They range from the costs involved and the need for transportation to accessible fitness centers and for personal assistance at the centers themselves to the very existence of centers willing to accept adults with CP as well as lack of motivation on the part of some CP patients to engage in physical exercise [59].

Medications to Improve Functional Mobility

Botulinum toxin A (BoNT-A) is used to manage spasticity that interferes with motor control and function in CP adults, whereas ITB, injected in the spinal cord, has been reported to reduce dystonic and spastic tonal abnormalities, improve mobility and self-care, and increase stride length and walking speed [44].

Surgical Interventions

Orthopedic surgery is generally recommended to increase range of motion in CP patients with severe spasticity and stiffness [60]. Surgeons can lengthen or cut through muscles and tendons as well as attach a tendon to a different bone. Contracture release involving the cutting of an overly tight muscle is one of the most common procedures, often used to lengthen the Achilles tendon in an effort to correct contracture of the calf muscles. Foot deformities and hip displacement resulting in painful weight-bearing can also be corrected through a procedure called osteotomy, the selective removal of a small piece of bone which is then repositioned or reshaped. Hip arthrodeses, which fuse together bones that normally move independently, limit spastic muscles from pulling ankle and foot bones as well as hips out of position. Hip dislocation also responds to interposition arthroplasty which involves the use of muscles or tendons to separate inflamed bone surfaces in arthritic joints [44].

In terms of neurosurgery, selective dorsal rhizotomy (SDR), a procedure recommended only after more conservative treatments such as physical therapy and medications have been employed, involves cutting up to 50–70 % of the sensory nerve roots at the base of the spinal column to reduce muscle contractures and spasticity; the motor roots are left intact. It is most often used in cases of spastic diplegia to decrease chronic pain in the lower and upper extremities. In a trial involving 21 ambulatory adults with CP, Reynolds et al. reported that patients experienced significant improvements in lower extremity passive joint range of motion as well as decreased spasticity in all measured lower extremity muscles groups. Patients observed improvements in ambulatory ability, coordination, and overall quality of life, leading to the conclusion that SDR can be an effective treatment for adults with spastic diplegia [61].

Osteoporosis in Adults with Cerebral Palsy

By the time patients with CP reach adulthood, the bone and muscle impairment that adversely affected their earlier years has already been manifested in low bone mineral density (BMD), greater fracture risk, and increased number of fractures themselves, often occurring with minimal trauma. The neuromuscular impairments that affect the reliability of the standard DXA scans have been overcome, in large part, by the adaptation of the new lateral distal femur DXA scan to adults. Although administration of these scans requires special training and expertise, they promise to produce reliable, reproducible, and clinically relevant assessments of BMD in adults [62].

Several trials have documented low BMD in adults with cerebral palsy. In an examination of 48 premenopausal women and adults (age range: 25–46 years) [63], the mean BMD *Z*-scores were −1.40 for the lumbar spine, −1.36 for the total hip, and −1.02 for the femoral neck, with nonambulatory patients exhibiting significantly lower scores at all three sites. There was also a correlation between low BMD and low body mass index (BMI), reflecting the lower body fat generally observed in patients with cerebral palsy and confirming similar results for children and young adults reported by Henderson et al.

Causes

Among the principal causal factors for osteoporosis in adults are the degree of physical disability, prolonged immobilization or limited ambulatory status, nutritional deficits particularly in terms of calcium and vitamin D, and use of anticonvulsant drugs. A Japanese study of 123 institutionalized adults (51 men, aged 21–41, and 39 nonambulatory; 72 premenopausal women, aged 24–47, 54 nonambulatory) [64] examined the effect of mobility level, calcium status, and anticonvulsant drugs. Women who were nonambulatory had significantly lower BMD than those who were ambulatory; for nonambulatory men, BMD was also reduced, but it did not reach statistical significance. The use of anticonvulsant drugs (reported by 50 % of the patients) was significantly associated with lower BMD in both sexes. Anticonvulsants are known to be related to low levels of vitamin D as well as to hypocalcemia and higher serum alkaline phosphate levels. Twenty-nine percent of the patients in the study had abnormal calcium metabolism, while higher alkaline phosphate levels in the male participants were significantly associated with their low BMD. Patients in the study also evidenced shorter stature and lower weight than a comparable sample with normal height and weight values. Falls and resulting fractures are another risk factor for the development of osteoporosis. In a sample with a mean age of 44 years, one study found that 40 % of adults with CP fell monthly and that 75 % fell bimonthly [65, 66].

As in the normal population, osteoporosis may not be detected until a bone fracture actually occurs; in the case of cerebral palsy patients, the pain associated with fracture may not even be communicated by patients with cognitive or speech disabilities. Sheridan [67] observes that given the small number of studies on the prevalence and incidence of fractures in adults with CP, information must be extrapolated from pediatric studies to provide insight into the likelihood of fractures in adults. Specifically, he proposes that because adults have had a much longer exposure to bone deformities, joint surgeries, nutritional deficiencies, and the like, clinicians must assume a greater risk of fractures in adults than in children—a risk that will increase as the already compromised bone strength is compounded by the age-related decline in bone mass.

Nonpharmacologic Treatment

Physical Exercise

Osteoporotic patients are known to benefit from a regimen of physical activity that can increase bone mass through weight-bearing exercises and decrease fall risk by improving balance and coordination. However, the defining characteristics of adult cerebral palsy, including spasticity, degenerative arthritis, sarcopenia contractures, and pain, make such activity extremely difficult if not impossible in many cases. Assistive equipment including standers, standing frames, and standing on a vibrating platform are among the new approaches to osteoporosis treatment, but studies in adults are sparse. In several animal studies, low-magnitude, high-frequency whole body vibration (WBV) stimulation has produced an increase in trabecular bone mineral content and strength; investigations of the effect of WBV on postmenopausal women indicate an attenuation of the decline of BMD at the hip [68]. A recent trial involving older adults on vibration therapy demonstrated a significant improvement in all fall risk factors including a significant increase in the range of motion of ankle joints [69]. However, despite the beneficial effects shown in broader studies, little is known about the specific effect of WBV on CP patients faced with developing new motor skills and normal movement patterns. Moreover, WBV raises safety concerns about broken bones, musculoskeletal problems, and low back pain [70]—issues that may be especially problematic in adults with CP.

Nutrition

Bone quality in adults with CP, as in the broader population, is dependent on an adequate intake of calcium and vitamin D. In accordance with Institute of Medicine recommendations, the level for calcium is 1,000 mg/day for ages 19–50 and 1,200 mg/day for over age 50 up to a maximal limit of 2,500 mg/day. Because patients with CP are unlikely to be exposed to sunlight for a sufficient time period, vitamin D supplementation is needed in specified amounts for three different age categories: 200 IU/day for ages 50 and below; 400 IU/day for ages 50–70, and 600 IU/day for over age 70. Serum phosphate and parathyroid hormone (PTH) may also be recommended for patients with CP. Studies demonstrate that PTH, in its synthetic form, teriparatide, increases bone formation on all bone surfaces (trabecular, endosteal bone, and periosteal bone) and decreases the risk of vertebral and nonvertebral fractures [71].

Caloric intake for CP patients must be assessed on an individual basis. Muscular deformities, the inability to chew and swallow, gastroesophageal reflux disease, and malabsorption restrict caloric intake, while the specific form of paralysis can affect the energy needs of the CP individuals [67].

Pharmacologic Treatment

Estrogen replacement therapy and selective estrogen receptor modulators (SERMS) are known to increase BMD, but they are plagued with safety concerns and potentially harmful side effects including blood clots in the legs and lungs, particularly in patients who are inactive or immobile. Trials involving another option, growth hormone replacement therapy, indicate that after an initial 6–12 month period of bone resorption, GH results in both an improvement in balance and an increase in BMD that continues for 18–24 months after discontinuation of therapy. Moreover, concern persists as to whether long-term use of GH may promote tumor initiation or recurrence [72].

For the most part, the interventions outlined above have not been examined in adults with CP who face different and more complex challenges than those encountered by more able-bodied individuals with osteoporosis. In addition to further epidemiological research, trials focused on the impact of physical, nutritional, and pharmacologic therapies—both established and emerging—must be targeted *specifically* to these adults to better understand, possibly prevent, and more effectively treat osteoporosis in individuals with severely compromised bone strength and function [67].

Duchenne Muscular Dystrophy in Children

The most common form of muscular dystrophy, Duchenne muscular dystrophy (DMD), accounts for approximately half of muscular dystrophy cases and affects primarily young boys at an incidence of 1 in 3,500–6,000 male births in the United States [73].

Causes and Symptoms

Duchenne muscular dystrophy is caused by a mutation in the gene, dystrophin, which can be inherited in an X-linked recessive pattern; alternatively it can occur in individuals with no family history of the disease [74]. Dystrophin ensures muscle strength and health by maintaining the structure of muscle cells. Without it, profound muscle weakness and wasting caused by degenerating muscle fibers appear generally before the age of 6. The principal symptoms include frequent falls, a waddling gait, difficulty rising from a lying or sitting position, and enlarged calf muscles resulting from an accumulation of fat and connective tissue (pseudohypertrophy). As shown in Fig. 2, equinus of the feet and a hyperlordotic posture of the spine can compensate for balance loss temporarily, but a significant fall risk accompanies attempts to remain ambulatory using compensatory measures [75]. As the diseases progresses, the heart muscle weakens, scoliosis may develop, and the muscles associated with breathing and swallowing deteriorate to the point where ventilators must be used, initially at night but subsequently extending into the day. The thin, demineralized bone becomes osteoporotic and fractures occur easily. By early adolescence, children with DMD generally lose their ability to walk. Without the care of specialists from a number of disciplines and the use of advancing technologies and medication, these children die in their late teens or early 20s as a result of cardiac or respiratory failure; however, such interventions are now leading to survival rates in the 30s and even 40s [76, 77].

Diagnosis

Given the many complications of DMD, physicians may need to undertake a plethora of laboratory tests to confirm a diagnosis [78]. Among the most important are creatine kinase (CK) blood tests, genetic tests, and muscle biopsies. Following a thorough medical history and physical examination, one of the first tests to be conducted for DMD focuses on the identification of defective genes and neuromuscular disorders. Damaged muscles release the enzyme, CK, into the blood. Elevated CK levels including those found early in Duchenne indicate

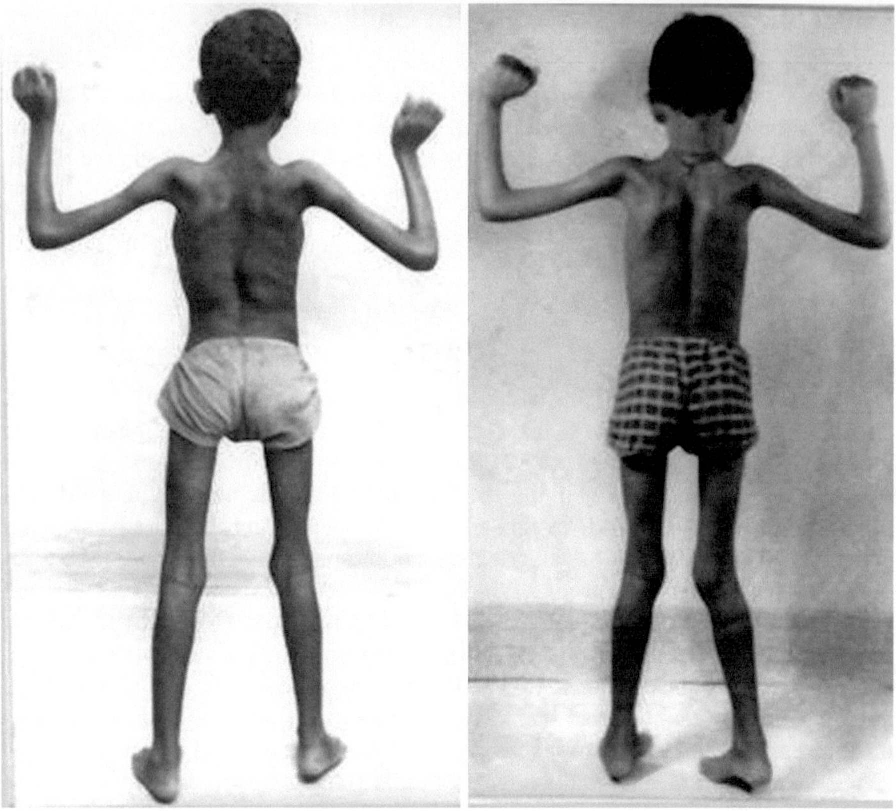

Fig. 2 Hyperlordotic posture and proximal muscle wasting of DMD. The photograph demonstrates muscle wasting in periscapular region, humerus, and thigh muscles but shows calf hypertrophy. In order to maintain balance, a hyperlordotic posture of spine can be adopted as a compensatory measure (*Source*: Wikipedia Public Domain (WPD) 1.0. Accessed 20 Dec 2015)

that muscles are being destroyed even before physical symptoms appear; however, the test may not indicate precisely what muscle disorder is involved.

Genetic testing, specifically single condition amplification/internal primer (SCAIP) sequencing [79], is increasingly recognized as the gold standard of diagnosis in inherited muscular dystrophy. Analysis of cell DNA can determine whether and where a mutation in the dystrophin gene has occurred and can identify women DMD carriers who are likely to pass the disease on to their sons and their carrier status on to their daughters. Knowledge of an individual's precise genetic mutation is essential not only for diagnosis but for the development of new therapies. Moreover, it provides the clinical information for genetic counseling that can identify whether mothers are carrying a mutated gene and thereby assist parents in planning for a family.

If these tests confirm a DMD diagnosis, no further testing is required. However, if the results show a high CK level and symptoms of DMD but no genetic mutation, a muscle biopsy is needed to determine whether dystrophin is present and, if so, in what amount and molecular size. The absence of dystrophin confirms a Duchenne diagnosis [78].

Treatment Approaches

Established forms of treatment for DMD encompass physical therapy and assistive devices, corrective surgery, medication, and dietary supplementation of calcium and vitamin D. Some newer approaches, as yet experimental but with implications for the severity of osteoporosis, are also in development.

Physical Therapy

Range-of-motion and stretching exercises, particularly those involving upper extremity muscles, are important for keeping muscles and joints as flexible and strong as possible; they may help patients maintain the ability to use a computer keyboard or control a wheelchair as well as delay contractures by preventing tendons from shortening prematurely. Passive stretching, carried out by a therapist and often used in conjunction with night splints, is also effective against contractures, whereas braces and standing frames enable DMD patients to stand for several hours a day, improving circulation and aiding bone strength. Therapy can help correct postural stance when a child is younger by strengthening those muscles with remaining function and using other modalities and supports to minimize lordosis (see Fig. 2). Aquatic exercises are examples of low-impact activities that use the buoyancy of the water to alleviate undue stress on muscles [80].

Surgical Intervention

Spinal fusion or the attachment of metal rods to the spine to correct posture and increase strength ease the adverse effects of scoliosis on sitting, sleeping, and even breathing. If severe contractures seriously impair movement, tendons or muscles can be lengthened to restore or improve range of motion. In terms of new surgical techniques, Forst et al. have reported that prophylactic surgery performed on the lower limbs and spine when patients are still ambulatory can delay the point at which they become wheelchair-bound by as much as two years; by enabling the patient to stand for a much longer period, it stimulates circulation and prevents or delays the onset of contractures, scoliosis, and osteoporosis. The long-term results may be a life expectancy of over 30 years and an improved quality of life [81]. End-stage dilated cardiomyopathy is recognized as an adverse outcome of DMD in patients who cannot tolerate cardiac transplantation. In such cases, a surgical technique involving the implantation of a ventricular assist device has been developed as a new therapeutic option [82].

Medications

The most widely used medications for DMD are corticosteroids, specifically prednisone (dose = 0.75 mg/kg) and deflazacort (dose = 0.9 mg/kg). Corticosteroids have been shown to attenuate muscle weakness, thereby prolonging ambulation and preserving cardiac and respiratory function. A 2008 Cochrane meta-analysis of four RCTs demonstrated that these drugs improved muscle strength and function in the short term—six months to two years [83]. However, this and subsequent studies have also shown that corticosteroids produce serious side effects ranging from rapid weight gain and myopathy to bone fragility and osteoporosis, with deflazacort having more bone-sparing qualities than prednisone [84].

In terms of new treatments, researchers using gene therapy are now developing strategies to replace the dystrophin gene or to bypass dystrophin mutations [85]. The skipping of sections of the genetic code called exons (exon skipping) is being investigated to determine if it would create partially functional dystrophin to lessen severe muscular weakness and atrophy [86]. If such treatment is successful and ambulation is extended for more years, the onset of osteoporosis would be proportionately delayed, potentially at a time when linear growth is occurring. Such measures would enable DMD patients to come closer to reaching peak bone density during puberty, an essential measure to limit future osteoporosis.

Osteoporosis in Children with DMD

Causes and Symptoms

The development of osteoporosis in DMD is generally attributed to decreased weight-bearing, progressive muscle weakness affecting bone loading, reduced mobility, and long-term use of corticosteroids. Side effects of corticosteroids include impaired osteoblast formation and mineralization, delayed puberty, and poor calcium absorption from the intestine [87]. Although long bone osteoporosis can occur in patients who are still ambulatory, vertebral bone osteoporosis, which is more susceptible to the effects of steroids, is generally not evident until boys are wheelchair-dependent [88].

Several studies have demonstrated the existence and effects of low BMD in this disease. An analysis of the interaction of bone density, mobility, and fracture in 41 DMD patients (31 nonambulatory) who had received no steroid treatment revealed that bone density in the lumbar spine and, to an even greater extent, in the proximal femur decreased, while the boys were still ambulatory. Moreover, 44 % of the boys sustained a fracture, with 66 % of the fractures involving the lower extremities; 44 % of nine boys who were walking with some support prior to the fracture never resumed walking [89]. In a subsequent study, a weakness in hip flexors as well as proximal femur and spine osteoporosis were apparent, despite continued ambulation [88].

When DMD patients are treated with corticosteroids, the incidence of both decreased BMD and fracture occurrence is even more pronounced. Bianchi et al. [90] evaluated bone mass and metabolism in 22 children on long-term prednisone therapy compared with 10 who had not been treated. Results indicated a correlation between corticosteroid dosage and decreased BMD at the spinal level as well as reduced BMD in the trunk and lower limbs, although the authors observed that the latter could be due to decreased weight-bearing on bone. Reduced intestinal calcium absorption was also observed. King et al. reported that not only did long bone fractures occur 2.6 times more frequently in steroid-treated DMD patients than in those untreated but also that 32 % of the steroid group experienced vertebral fractures compared with no fracture occurrence in the untreated group [91].

An analysis of the length of time between the initiation of corticosteroids and fracture occurrence indicated a latency period of 40 months before the first vertebral fracture appeared and predicted that 75 % of boys with DMD would experience a vertebral fracture following 100 months of steroid treatment [92]. In addition, a study of 408 steroid-treated patients reported that fracture prevalence, together with worsening motor function, progressively increases throughout the pediatric age span: 16.5 %, 37.45 %, and 83.3 % at ages 5, 10, and 15, respectively, with prevalence of vertebral fractures rising 4.4, 19.1, and 58.3 % for the same ages [93].

Diagnosis

The use of size-adjusted and subcranial analysis in DXA provides the most effective assessment of BMD in boys with DMD, indicating a deficit in total body BMD-for-age (*Z*-score of −1.2) that increases with age [94]. An international conference on corticosteroid treatment in DMD (2009) recommended that a baseline lumbar spine DXA be performed before such treatment is initiated and repeated at 12–24 month intervals while the patient continues on treatment [95]. Spinal screening for vertebral fractures in steroid-treated patients should also be performed to determine if fractures had occurred previously, an indication that bisphosphonates should be prescribed [87].

Treatment

Nutrition

With long-term corticosteroid treatment becoming the standard of care in DMD, the need for adequate calcium and vitamin D in this population assumes increasing importance. In a 2-year study of 33 DMD patients on corticosteroid therapy, first-line treatment with calcifediol (25-OH vitamin D_3), coupled with an adjustment in dietary calcium to the recommended dose, resulted in a significant increase in BMD in over 65 % of the patients, while bone resorption declined and bone mass increased in 78.8 % [96]. Bianchi et al. further recommend that when calcifediol levels are low, vitamin D metabolite, rather than vitamin D standard supplements, should be administered. Patients should adhere to at least the FDA recommended dose of calcium per age group in order to avoid hypocalcemia and an increase in bone turnover [90].

Exercise

The role of exercise in optimizing bone health is subject to conflicting reports. Light to moderate exercise appears to be beneficial in some forms of muscular dystrophy, but increased risk of muscle damage remains a serious concern. Some researchers point to the limited positive effect of standing programs and vibration therapy in cerebral palsy. However, the few studies focused specifically on muscular dystrophy demonstrate that although whole body vibration therapy (WBVT) was well tolerated and muscle damage did not occur, no improvements in bone density and muscle strength were observed [97, 98]. Further studies on larger cohorts are needed to evaluate the efficacy and safety of WBVT with attention to the duration and dose of exposure.

Medications

Thus far, the small number of trials involving bisphosphonate treatment and DMD patients on steroids has shown promising but limited results with respect to BMD and *Z*-scores. A study of boys (mean age = 10.2 years) using daily deflazacort [99] and treated with alendronate showed a positive effect on BMD, specifically maintenance of BMD *Z*-scores and the absence of symptomatic fractures, in contrast to the anticipated age-related decline in bone mass and increased fracture risk. During a 2-year follow-up period, the improvement in *Z*-scores was greatest in the youngest boys who received alendronate early in the course of the disease; the older boys were given a more conservative dose because of the prevailing concerns about a possible negative effect of bisphosphonates on longitudinal bone growth.

A more recent study indicated that *Z*-scores at the hip trended downward without alendronate and upward (stabilized) with alendronate, but the trends were not statistically significant [100]. In an analysis of the effect of intravenous bisphosphonates (pamidronate: 9 mg/kg/year or zoledronic acid: (0.1 mg/kg/year) on vertebral fractures caused by osteoporosis, back pain decreased or resolved completely and height ratios of previously fractured vertebrae stabilized or improved. However, such therapy did not completely prevent the development of new vertebral fractures [101]. Again, further research is needed to determine the long-term effects of bisphosphonate treatment, the most effective dose, frequency of treatment, optimal age to begin treatment, and relative efficacy of oral versus intravenous administration. Quinlivan et al. question the routine use of bisphosphonates to prevent fractures until these issues are addressed [95], while Hawker et al. indicate that they have been using daily deflazacort as a standard treatment [99]. Looking to the future, Buckner et al. recommended that the effect of such drugs as denosumab, recombinant parathyroid hormone (teriparatide), and melatonin on BMD and fracture risk be investigated [87].

Duchenne Muscular Dystrophy in Adults

Without intervention, progressive muscle degeneration, loss of ambulation, and other respiratory, cardiac, and orthopedic complications associated with DMD can lead to death at a mean age of 19 years [102]. However, significant advances in the management of DMD have now extended life expectancy into the late 20s and 30s [103]. Key to this improved prognosis has been the development of multidisciplinary teams incorporating physicians, therapists, psychologists, and other specialists to meet the complex challenges of DMD. The benefits of coordinated care underline the importance of an effective transition from childhood to adult facilities which can provide not only integrated medical therapy but also guidance about education, careers, living arrangements, social interaction, and, taken together, the demands of independent living [102].

Among the most critical issues in adult DMD are the complications caused by weakened breathing muscles or chest infections. At the onset of muscle weakness, lung function tests are conducted to monitor both muscle strength and oxygen levels in the blood. To counter breathing difficulties, "noninvasive ventilation," the use of a mask over the nose or mouth to deliver pressurized air, has emerged as a highly effective therapy, leading to higher survival rates. Initially used only overnight or from time to time, ventilation can be extended if muscle weakness progresses. In a study of the impact of nocturnal ventilation over the period 1967–2002, Eagle et al. demonstrated that the mean age of death in the 1960s was 14.4 compared with 25.3 years for patients ventilated since 1990. Although they acknowledged that the advent of more effective coordinated care has helped to advance life expectancy to 25 years (from 0 % in the 1960s to 4 % in the 1970s to 12 % in the 1980s), they emphasized that nocturnal ventilation improved the likelihood of survival to 53 % for those ventilated since 1990. These findings have been confirmed by subsequent trials [104, 105]; in addition, a later study, also led by Eagle, reported that ventilation combined with spinal surgery improved median survival to 30 years [106]. In the period since the original Eagle study, survival rates into the 30s with a few cases in the 40s and 50s have been reported [107]. Cough-assisted devices and manually assisted coughing may also be used in the early stages of breathing problems.

Whereas respiratory issues were the major cause of death in adult DMD until the 1980s–1990s, advances in respiratory treatments have focused attention on cardiac failure as an increasingly significant factor in morbidity and mortality. Caused by dilated cardiomyopathy (alone or in combination with infections and abdominal problems) and/or by cardiac arrhythmia [108], cardiac complications affect nearly all adults with DMD [103].

Diagnosis

The standard diagnostic tests to screen for cardiac abnormalities include electrocardiography (ECG), echocardiography, and cardiac magnetic resonance (CMR) imaging. ECGs are effective in determining cardiac arrhythmias such as atrial fibrillation but lack the sensitivity to assess structural cardiac disease. Echocardiography is used to assess left ventricular (LV) size, wall thickness, and valve function; it can be administered to patients in a wheelchair and offers cost and convenience benefits for DMD patients [103]. In addition to providing a more reliable assessment of LV size and function, CMR promises to provide insight into early cardiac involvement so that heart failure therapy may be initiated at a younger age, thereby delaying the onset and progression of left ventricular dysfunction [109]. However, its high cost and the blurred, ghostly images resulting from heart motion restrict greater use [103].

Medications

The most commonly used therapies for cardiac dysfunction in DMD are angiotensin-converting enzyme (ACE) inhibitors and beta (β) blockers. In some cases, evaluations of the efficacy of these drugs have been carried out in related disease populations, with applicable findings extended to those with DMD. For example, the effect of the ACE inhibitor, captopril, was analyzed in 2,231 patients (mean age = 59); they had no symptoms of heart failure but had experienced left ventricular dysfunction following myocardial infarction and had an ejection fraction (the amount of blood being pumped out of the left ventricle) of less than 40 %. The results showed not only an improvement in survival but also reduced morbidity and mortality resulting from major cardiovascular events [110]. In a more recent study, focused specifically on DMD, Duboc et al. reported that another ACE inhibitor, perindopril, administered between the ages of 9–13, delayed the onset of LV dysfunction and mortality, leading to their recommendation that ACE inhibitor treatment begin as early as nine years of age [111]. Now regarded as "first-line therapy," ACE inhibitors are customarily given to adult DMD patients who had never received this therapy, even if cardiac function is normal [103]. Studies supporting the use of β blockers point to their benefits in treating arrhythmia and improving LV ejection fraction when administered after the initiation of ACE inhibitor and in cases of symptomatic heart failure. A trial focusing on the effect of ACE inhibitors on cardiomyopathy in DMD, administered alone and in combination with β blockers, revealed no significant difference between the treatment groups [112].

Although corticosteroids are known to prolong ambulation in childhood, their continued use into adulthood remains controversial in terms of balancing the risks of long-term use against the potential benefits for cardiac and respiratory muscles. Whereas some trails in humans indicate improvement with steroid therapy, animal studies tend to indicate deleterious effects on myocardial function. These contradictory findings point up the need for further research on the impact of corticosteroid use in DMD [113].

Other Concerns and Challenges in Adult DMD

Given the limited motor abilities of adults with DMD, exercise must necessarily be restricted and studies of its efficacy are inconclusive. Stretching the upper extremity muscles, particularly finger flexors, may help minimize contractures and enable patients to use a computer keyboard or control a wheelchair joystick; stretching the lower extremity muscles, including hip and knee flexors, may relieve stiffness and pain [78]. Strenuous exercise is contraindicated in adult DMD because it can permanently damage already compromised muscle fibers and generate cardiac and respiratory problems. Hydrotherapy defined as moving in the water but not actually swimming may be beneficial. A recent systematic review of several trials on the effect of muscle exercise in DMD and other muscular dystrophies produced inconclusive results: given the absence of controls and the conflagration of different diseases in a single study, Gianola et al. could only conclude that "exercise might be useful, not useful, or even detrimental" while recommending that multicenter trials, focusing on muscle strength, fatigue, functional limitation, and pain, be undertaken as a next critical step [114].

Gastrointestinal problems in the form of constipation and gastroesophageal reflex are among other issues in adult DMD. Constipation responds to hydration, a balanced diet, stimulant laxatives, and stool softeners, whereas gastroesophageal reflex can be treated with proton pump inhibitors. With a multidisciplinary approach, dietitians can provide guidance on both undernutrition and obesity concerns, while swallowing/speech therapists deal with dysphagia and difficulties with oral expression and language comprehension [103].

Osteoporosis in Adult DMD

Maintenance of bone health is critical in patients with DMD, regardless of their age. Low bone mineral density in adults is attributed primarily to decreased weight-bearing, with the loss of ambulation occurring in the mid-teen years, and to the extended use of corticosteroids. At present, data on bone mineral density and fracture occurrence in this group are scarce. An analysis of one group of patients with neuromuscular disorders revealed fracture prevalence of 42 % with 72.5 % of the subjects experiencing a fall once a year [115]. Other causes of fractures, particularly in the lower limbs, include falls from wheelchairs resulting from tipping in transfers and sudden changes in wheelchair positions as well as accidents in the course of routine daily activities.

Although corticosteroids are effective in protecting cardiac and respiratory function and in delaying the onset of scoliosis in DMD, they lead to the development of vertebral compression fractures in what is known as "steroid-induced osteoporosis." Thus, annual DXA assessment is recommended to monitor bone density.

Treatment options for osteoporosis in adult DMD are much the same as those advocated in other childhood disorders, with necessary restrictions imposed by the progression of the disease. Because calcium and vitamin D deficiency contribute to bone resorption and osteoporosis, particularly in patients treated with corticosteroids, levels must be continually monitored with supplementation prescribed as needed. Whereas the impact of calcium alone is limited, research indicates that calcium in combination with vitamin D can improve bone mineral content and BMD. Bisphosphonates are known to increase BMD but their effect on vertebral fractures remains unclear [108].

For the first time, 60 % of patients with DMD are surviving into their third decade, dictating the need to further refine and develop national and international standards of care that will incorporate information on the transition to adult care and the challenges facing adults as the disease progresses. In addition to information relating to cardiac and respiratory issues as well as other complications noted above, guidelines on bone health in long-term steroid-treated adults as well as data on BMD in DMD adults and the effect of bisphosphonates should be incorporated in these standards [108]. Moreover, a recent assessment of the quality of life in men with DMD (mean age = 28 years) [116] reveals that DMD adults have an overriding concern not with their physical health but with their psychosocial needs ranging from intimacy and work capability to such measures as the "meaningfulness of life." Greater opportunities for social participation, education, and employment coupled with provision for transportation and assistance in undertaking leisure activities are a vital component of DMD therapy and should be addressed in the management guidelines for the disease.

References

1. Risenbaum P, Paneth N, Leviton A, Goldstein M, Bax M, Daniano D, et al. A report: the definition and classification of cerebral palsy. Dev Med Child Neurol Suppl. 2007;109:8–14.
2. National Center on Birth Defects and Developmental Disabilities, Centers for Disease Control and Prevention. Facts about cerebral palsy. http://www.cdc.gov/ncbdd/cp/facts/html. Accessed 25 Oct 2015.
3. Fairhurst C. Cerebral palsy: the whys and hows. Arch Dis Child Educ Pract Ed. 2012;97(4):122–31. doi:10.1136/edpract-2011-300593.
4. National Institute of Neurological Disorders and Stroke. Cerebral palsy: hope through research. National Institutes of Health; 2015. http://www.ninds.nih.gov/disordersofcerebralpalsy/detail_cerebral_palsy.htm. Accessed 9 Sept 2015.
5. Center for Disease Control and Prevention. Facts about cerebral palsy. http://ninds.nih.gov/ncbddd/cp/facts.html. Accessed 9 Sept 2015.
6. Nelson K, Grether J. Causes of cerebral palsy. Curr Opin Pediatr. 1999;11(6):487–91.
7. Reddihough DS, Collins KJ. The epidemiology and causes of cerebral palsy. Aust J Physiother. 2003;49(1):7–12.
8. McIntyre S, Blair E, Badawi N, Keogh J, Nelson KB. Antecedents of cerebral palsy and perinatal death in term and late preterm singletons. Obstet Gynecol. 2013;122(4):869–77.
9. Jones MW, Morgan E, Shelton JF, Thorogood C. Cerebral palsy: introduction and diagnosis (part 1). J Pediatr Health Care. 2007;21(3):146–52.
10. National Cerebral Palsy Foundation. Signs and symptoms of cerebral palsy. http://cerebralpalsy.org/about-cerebral-palsy/sign-and-symptoms/. Accessed 20 Sept 2015.

11. Noritz GH, Murphy NA, Neuromotor Screening Expert Panel. Motor delays: early identification and evaluation. Pediatrics. 2013;131(6):e2016–27. doi:10.1542/peds.2013-1056.
12. Palisano R, Rosenbaum P, Bartlett D, Livingston M. Content validity of the expanded and revised gross motor function classification system. Dev Med Child Neurol. 2008;50(10):744–50.
13. Ashwal S, Russman BB, Blasco PA, Miller G, Sandler A, Shevell M, et al. Practice parameter: diagnostic assessment of the child with cerebral palsy—report of the Quality Standards Subcommittee of the American Academy of Neurology and the Practice Committee of the Child Neurology Society. Neurology. 2004;62:851–63. doi:10.1212/01.WNL.0000117981.35364.1B.
14. Verma H, Srivastava V, Semwal BC. A review of cerebral palsy and its management. J Sci. 2012;2:54–62.
15. Krigger KW. Cerebral palsy: an overview. Am Fam Physician. 2006;73(1):91–100.
16. Fowler EG, Ho TW, Nwigwe AL, Dorey FJ. The effect of quadriceps femoris muscle strengthening exercises on spasticity in children with cerebral palsy. Phys Ther. 2001;81(6): 1215–23.
17. Eek MN, Tranberg R, Zugmer R, Alkema K, Beckrung E. Muscle strength training to improve gait function in children with cerebral palsy. Dev Med Child Neurol. 2008;50(10):759–64.
18. Delgardo MR, Hirtz D, Aisen M, Ashwal S, Fehlings DL, McLaughlin J, et al. Practice parameter: pharmacologic treatment of spasticity in children and adolescents with cerebral palsy (an evidence-based review): report of the Quality Standards Subcommittee of the American Academy of Neurology and the Practice Committee of the Child Neurology Society. Neurology. 2010;74(4):336–43.
19. Houlihan CM, Stevenson RD. Bone density in cerebral palsy. Phys Med Rehabil Clin N Am. 2009;20(3):493–508. doi:10.1016/j.pmr.2009.04.004.
20. Shaw NJ. Management of osteoporosis in children. Eur J Endocrinol. 2008;159:S33–9. doi:10.1530/EJE-08-0282.
21. International Society for Clinical Densitometry. ISCD official position-pediatric: skeletal health assessment in children from infancy to adolescence. International Society for ClinicalDensitometry;2013.http://www.iscd.org/official-positions/2013-iscd-official-positions-pediatric/.
22. Sheridan K. Assessing bone health in children: DXA scans play a vital role in management. Pediatr Perspect: Gillette Child Specialty Health Care. 2010;19(1):1–3.
23. Binkley T, Johnson J, Vogel L, Specker B. Bone measurements by peripheral quantitative computed tomography (pQCT) in children with cerebral palsy. J Pediatr. 2005;147(6): 7912–6.
24. Henderson RC, Kairella J, Abbas A, Stevenson RD. Predicting low bone density in children and young adults with quadriplegic cerebral palsy. Dev Med Child Neurol. 2004;46:416–9.
25. Henderson RC, Lark RK, Newman JE, Kecskemethy H, Fung EB, Renner JB, et al. Pediatric reference data for dual x-ray absorptiometric measures of normal bone density in the distal femur. AJR Am J Roentgenol. 2002;178(2):439–43. abs/10.2214/ajr.1780439.
26. Cheung AM, Adachi JD, Hanley DA, Kendler DL, Davison KS, Josse R, et al. High-resolution peripheral quantitative computed tomography for the assessment of bone strength and structure: a review by the Canadian Bone Strength Workshop. Curr Osteoporos Rep. 2013;11(2): 136–46.
27. Fehlings D, Switzer L, Agarwal P, Wong C, Sochett E, Stevenson R, et al. Informing evidence-based clinical practice guidelines for children with cerebral palsy at risk of osteoporosis: a systematicreview.DevMedChildNeurol.2012;54(2):106–16.doi:10.1111/j.1469-8749.2011.04091.x.
28. Pin TW. Effectiveness of static weight-bearing exercises in children with cerebral palsy. Pediatr Phys Ther. 2007;19(1):62–73. 10.1097/PEP.Ob013e318030211.
29. Chad KE, Bailey DA, McKay HA, Zello GA, Snyder RE. The effect of a weight-bearing physical activity program on bone mineral content and estimated volumetric density in children with spastic cerebral palsy. J Pediatr. 1999;135(1):115–7.
30. Caulton JM, Ward KA, Alsop CW, Dunn G, Adams JE, Mughal M. A randomised controlled trial of standing programmes on bone mineral density in non-ambulant children with cerebral palsy. Arch Dis Child. 2004;89(2):131–5. doi:10.1136/adc.2002.009316.

31. Ward K, Alsop C, Caulton J, Rubin C, Adams J, Mughal Z. Low magnitude mechanical loading is osteogenic in children with disabling conditions. J Bone Miner Res. 2004;19(3):360–9.
32. Eisenberg S, Zuk L, Carmelio E, Katz-Leurer M. Contribution of stepping while standing to function and secondary conditions among children with cerebral palsy. Pediatr Phys Ther. 2009;12(2):79–85.
33. Smania N, Bonetti P, Gandolfi M, Cosentino A, Waldner A, Hesse S, et al. Improved gait after repetitive locomotor training in children with cerebral palsy. Am J Phys Med Rehabil. 2011;90(2):137–49.
34. Kilpinen-Loisa P, Nenonen H, Pihko H, Makitie PO. High-dose vitamin D supplementation in children with cerebral palsy or neuromuscular disorder. Neuropediatrics. 2007;38(4):167–72.
35. Jekovec-Vrhovsek M, Kocijancic A, Prezeli J. Effect of vitamin D and calcium on bone mineral density in children with CP and epilepsy in full-time care. Dev Med Child Neurol. 2000;42(6):403–5.
36. Henderson RC, Lark RK, Kecshemethy HH, Miller F, Harcke HT, Bachrach SJ. Bisphosphonates to treat osteopenia in children with quadriplegic cerebral palsy: a randomized, placebo-controlled trial. J Pediatr. 2002;141(5):644–51.
37. Plotkin YH, Coughlin S, Kreikemeier R, Heidi K, Bruzoni M, Lerner G. Low doses of pamidronate to treat osteopenia in children with severe cerebral palsy: a pilot study. Dev Med Child Neurol. 2006;48(9):709–12.
38. Iwasaki T, Nonoda Y, Ishii M. Long-term outcomes of children and adolescents who had cerebral palsy with secondary osteoporosis. Curr Med Res Opin. 2012;28(5):737–47.
39. Devesa J, Casteleiro H, Roddicio C, Lopez N, Reimunde P. Growth hormone deficiency and cerebral palsy. Ther Clin Risk Manag. 2010;6:413–8.
40. Oskoui M. Growing up with cerebral palsy: contemporary challenges of health care transition. Can J Neurol Sci. 2012;39(1):23–5.
41. Viner R. Transition from paediatric to adult care: bridging the gaps or passing the buck? Arch Dis Child. 1999;81(3):271–5. doi:10.1136/adc.81.3.271.
42. Schwartz L, Engel JM, Jensen MP. Pain in persons with cerebral palsy. Arch Phys Med Rehabil. 1999;80(10):1243–6.
43. Hirsh AT, Gallegos JC, Gertz KJ, Engel JM, Jensen MP. Symptom burden in individuals with cerebral palsy. J Rehabil Res Dev. 2010;47(9):863–76. 10.1682/JRRD.2010.03.00224.
44. Tosi LL, Maher N, Moore DW, Goldstein M, Aisen ML. Adults with cerebral palsy: a workshop to define the challenges or treating and preventing secondary musculoskeletal and neuromuscular complications in this rapidly growing population. Dev Med Child Neurol. 2009;51 Suppl 4:2–11.
45. Murphy KP, Molnar GE, Lankasky K. Medical and functional status of adults with cerebral palsy. Dev Med Child Neurol. 1995;37(12):1075–84.
46. Andersson C, Mattsson E. Adults with cerebral palsy: a survey describing problems, needs and resources, with special emphasis on locomotion. Dev Med Child Neurol. 2001;43(2):76–82.
47. McGinley JL, Pogrebnoy D, Morgan P. Mobility in ambulant adults with cerebral palsy—challenges for the future. In: Svraka E, editor. Cerebral palsy—challenges for the future. InTech; 2014. http://dx.doi.org/10.5772/58344.
48. Jensen MP, Engel JM, Hoffman AJ, Schwartz L. Natural history of chronic pain and pain treatment in adults with cerebral palsy. Am J Phys Med Rehabil. 2004;83(6):439–45.
49. Engel JM, Kartin D, Jensen MP. Pain treatment in persons with cerebral palsy: frequency and helpfulness. Am J Phys Med Rehabil. 2002;81(4):291–6.
50. Van Schaeybroeck P, Nuttin B, Lagae L, Schrijvers E, Borghgraef C, Feys P. Intrathecal baclofen for intractable cerebral spasticity: a prospective placebo-controlled, double-blind study. Neurosurgery. 2000;46(3):603–12.
51. Hirsh AT, Kratz AL, Engbel JM, Jensen MP. Survey results of pain treatments in adults with cerebral palsy. Am J Phys Med Rehabil. 2011;90(3):207–16.

52. Jeglinsky I, Surakka J, Carlberg EB, Autti-Ramo I. Evidence on physiotherapeutic interventions for adults with cerebral palsy is sparse. A systematic review. Clin Rehabil. 2010;24(9):771–88.
53. Scianni A, Butler JMJ, Ada L, Teixeira-Salmela LF. Muscle strengthening is not effective in children and adolescents with cerebral palsy: a systematic review. Aust J Physiother. 2009;55(2):81–7.
54. Andersson C, Grooten W, Hellsten M, Kaping K, Mattsson E. Adults with cerebral palsy: walking ability after progressive strength training. Dev Med Child Neurol. 2003;45(4):220–8.
55. Taylor NF, Dodd KJ, Larkin H. Adults with cerebral palsy benefit from participating in a strength training programme at a community gymnasium. Disabil Rehabil. 2004;26(9):1128–34.
56. Allen J, Dodd KJ, Taylor NE, McBurney H, Larkin H. Strength training can be enjoyable and beneficial for adults with cerebral palsy. Disabil Rehabil. 2004;26(19):1121–7.
57. Damiano DL. Activity, activity, activity: rethinking our physical therapy approach to cerebral palsy. Phys Ther. 2006;86(11):1534–40.
58. Bottos M, Feliciangeli A, Sciuto L, Gericke C, Vianello A. Functional status of adults with cerebral palsy and implications for treatment of children. Dev Med Child Neurol. 2001;43(8):516–28.
59. Vogtle LK. Pain in adults with cerebral palsy: impact and solutions. Dev Med Child Neurol. 2009;51 Suppl 4:113–21. doi:10.1111/j.1469-8749.2009.03423.x.
60. Horstmann HM, Hosalkar H, Keenan MA. Orthopedic issues in the musculoskeletal care of adults with cerebral palsy. Dev Med Child Neurol. 1999;51 Suppl 4:99–105.
61. Reynolds MR, Ray WZ, Strom RG, Blackburn SL, Lee A, Park TS. Clinical outcomes after selective dorsal rhizotomy in an adult population. World Neurosurg. 2011;75(1):138–44. doi:10.1016/j.wneu.2010.09.010.
62. Henderson RC, Henderson BA, Kecshemethy HH, Hidalgo ST, Nikolava BA, Sheridan K. Adaptation of the lateral distal femur DXA technique to adults with disabilities. J Clin Densitom. 2015;18(1):102–8.
63. Fowler EG, Rao S, Nattiv A, Heberer K, Oppenheim WL. Bone density in premenopausal women and men under 50 years of age with cerebral palsy. Arch Phys Med Rehabil. 2015;96(7):1304–9. doi:10.1016/j.apmr.2015.03.012.
64. Nakano H, Aoyagi K, Ohgi S, Akiyama T. Factors influencing metacarpal bone mineral density in adults with cerebral palsy. J Bone Miner Metab. 2003;21(6):409–14.
65. Mosqueda L. Maintaining health and function. In: Kemp BJ, Mosqueda L, editors. Aging with a disability: what the clinician needs to know. Baltimore: Johns Hopkins University Press; 2004. p. 87–101.
66. Morgan P, McGinley J. Performance of adults with cerebral palsy related to falls, balance and function: a preliminary report. Dev Neurorehabil. 2013;16(2):113–20. doi:10.3109/17518423.2012.725107.
67. Sheridan KJ. Osteoporosis in adults with cerebral palsy. Dev Med Child Neurol. 2009;51 Suppl 4:38–51.
68. Totosy de Zepetnek JO, Giangregorio LM, Craven C. Whole-body vibration as potential intervention for people with low bone density and osteoporosis: a review. J Rehabil Res Dev. 2009;46(4):529–42.
69. Yang F, King GA, Dillon L, Su X. Controlled whole-body vibration training reduces risk of falls among community-dwelling older adults. J Biomech. 2015;48(12):3206–12.
70. Wysocki A, Butler M, Shamliyan T, Kane RL. Whole-body vibration therapy for osteoporosis: state of the science. Ann Intern Med. 2011;155(10):680–6.
71. Bukata SV. Systematic administration of pharmacological agents and bone repair: what can we expect. Injury. 2011;42(6):605–8.
72. Reed ML, Merrium GR, Kargi A. Adult growth hormone deficiency—benefits, side effects, and risks of growth hormone replacement. Front Endocrinol. 2013;4:64. doi:10.3389/fendo.2013.00064.

73. Bell JM, Blackwood D, Shields MD, Watters J, Hamilton A, Beringer T, et al. Interventions to prevent steroid-induced osteoporosis and osteoporotic fractures in Duchenne muscular dystrophy. Cochrane Database Syst Rev. 2014;(3):CD10899. doi:10.1002/14651858.CD010899.
74. National Human Genome Research Institute. Learning about Duchenne muscular dystrophy. http://www.genome.gov/19518854. Accessed 11 Oct 2015.
75. Oda T, Shimizu N, Yonenobu K, Ono K, Nabeshima T, Kyoh S. Longitudinal study of spinal deformity in Duchenne muscular dystrophy. J Pediatr Orthop. 1993;13(4):478–88.
76. Muscular Dystrophy Association. Duchenne muscular dystrophy: diagnosis. Bethesda: Muscular Dystrophy Association; 2015. https://www.mda.org/disease/duchenne-muscular-dystrophy/diagnosis. Accessed 12 Oct 2015.
77. National Institute of Neurological Disorders and Stroke. Muscular dystrophy: hope through research. Bethesda: National Institute of Neurological Disorders and Strokes; 2015. Accessed Oct 2015. http://www.ninds.nih.gov/disorders/md/detail_md.htm.
78. Bushby K, Finkel R, Birnkrant DJ, Case LE, Clemens PR, Cripe L. Diagnosis and management of Duchenne muscular dystrophy, part 1: diagnosis, and pharmacological and psychosocial management. Lancet Neurol. 2010;9:77–93.
79. Flanigan KM, von Niederhausern A, Dunn DM, Alder J, Mendell J, Weiss RB. Rapid direct sequence analysis of the dystrophin gene. Am J Hum Genet. 2003;72(4):931–9.
80. Lovering RM, Porter NC, Bloch RJ. The muscular dystrophies: from genes to therapies. Phys Ther. 2005;85(122):1372–88.
81. Forst J, Forst R. Surgical treatment of Duchenne muscular dystrophy patients in Germany: the present situation. Acta Myol. 2012;3(1):21–3.
82. Iodice F, Testa G, Averardi M, Brancaccio G, Amodeo A, Cogo P. Implantation of a left ventricular assist device as a destination therapy in Duchenne muscular dystrophy patients with end stage cardiac failure: management and lessons learned. Neuromuscul Disord. 2015;225(1):19–23. doi:10.1016/j.nmd.2014.08.008.
83. Manzur AY, Kuntzer T, Pike M, Swan A. Glucocorticoid corticosteroids for Duchenne muscular dystrophy. Cochrane Database Syst Rev. 2008;23(12), CD003725.
84. Angelini C, Tasca E. Drugs in development and dietary approach for Duchenne muscular dystrophy. Dove Press; 2015. http://dx.doi.org/10.2147/ODRR.S55677.
85. Rodino-Klapac LR, Chicoine LG, Kaspar BK. Gene therapy for Duchenne muscular dystrophy: expectations and challenges. Arch Neurol. 2007;64(9):1236–41.
86. Muscular Dystrophy Association. Duchenne muscular dystrophy: research. https://www.mda.org/disease/dhcuenne-muscular-dystrophy/research. Accessed 10 Dec 2015.
87. Buckner JL, Bowden SA, Mahan JD. Optimizing bone health in Duchenne muscular dystrophy. Int J Endocrinol. 2015;2015:1–9. (Article ID: 928385). 10.1155/2015/928385.
88. Aparicio LF, Jurkovic M, DeLullo J. Decreased bone density in ambulatory patients with Duchenne muscular dystrophy. J Pediatr Orthop. 2002;22(2):179–81.
89. Larson CMJ, Henderson RC. Bone mineral density on fractures in boys with Duchenne muscular dystrophy. J Pediatr Orthop. 2000;20(1):71–4.
90. Bianchi MJ, Mazzanti A, Galbiati E, Saraifoger S, Dubini A, Cornelio F, et al. Bone mineral density and bone metabolism in Duchenne muscular dystrophy. Osteoporos Int. 2003;14(9):761–7.
91. King WM, Ruttencutter R, Nagaraja HN, Matkovic V, Landell J, Hoyle C. Orthopedic outcomes of long-term daily corticosteroid treatment in Duchenne muscular dystrophy. Neurology. 2007;68(19):1607–13.
92. Bothwell JE, Gordon KE, Dooley JM, MacSween J, Cummings EA, Salisbury S. Vertebral fractures in boys with Duchenne muscular dystrophy. Clin Pediatr (Phila). 2003;42(4):353–6.
93. Tian C, Wong B, Hornung L, Khoury J, Miller L, Bange J, Tian C, Wong B, Hornung L, Khoury J, Miller L, Bange J, et al. Age-specific prevalence of osteoporosis and frequency of poor bone health indices to Duchenne muscular dystrophy (MON-0162). Neuromuscul Disord. 2014;24(9–10):857. doi.org/10.1016/j.nmd.2014.06.213.

94. King WM, Kissel JT, Visy D, Goel PK, Matkovic V. Skeletal health in Duchenne dystrophy: bone size and subcranial dual-energy x-ray absorptiometry analysis. Muscle Nerve. 2014;49(4):512–9.
95. Quinlivan R, Shaw N, Bushby K. 170th ENMC international workshop: bone protection for corticosteroid treated Duchenne muscular dystrophy. November 2009, Naarden, The Netherlands. Neuromuscul Disord. 2010;20(11):761–9. doi:10.1016/j.nmd.2010.07.272.
96. Bianchi ML, Morandi L, Andreucci E, Vai S, Frasunkiewicz J, Cottafava R. Low bone density and bone metabolism alterations in Duchenne muscular dystrophy: responses to calcium and vitamin D treatment. Osteoporos Int. 2011;22(2):529–39.
97. Myers KA, Ramage B, Khan A, Mah JK. Vibration therapy tolerated in children with Duchenne muscular dystrophy: a pilot study. Pediatr Neurol. 2014;51(1):126–9.
98. Soderpalm AC, Kroksmark AK, Magnusson P, Karlsson J, Tulinius M, Swolin-Eide D. Whole body vibration therapy in patients with Duchenne muscular dystrophy – a prospective observational study. J Musculoskelet Neuronal Interact. 2013;13(1):13–8.
99. Hawker GA, Rideout R, Harris VA, Chase CC, Fielding LJ, Rigger WD. Lendronate in the treatment of low bone mass in steroid-treated boys with Duchenne muscular dystrophy. Arch Phys Med Rehabil. 2005;86:284–8. doi:10.1016/j.apmr.2004.04.021.
100. Houston C, Mathews K, Shibli-Rahhai A. Bone density and alendronate effects in Duchenne muscular dystrophy patients. Muscle Nerve. 2014;49(4):506–11.
101. Shrocchi AM, Rauch F, Jacob P, McCormick A, McMillan HJ, Matzinger MA, et al. The use of intravenous bisphosphonate therapy to treat vertebral fractures due to osteoporosis among boys with Duchenne muscular dystrophy. Osteoporos Int. 2012;23(11):2703–11.
102. Rodger S, Steffensen BF, Lochmuller H. Transition from childhood to adulthood in Duchenne muscular dystrophy (DMD). Orphanet J Rare Dis. 2012;7 Suppl 2:A8. doi:10.1186/1750-1172-7-S2-A8.
103. Wagner KR, Lechzin N, Judge DP. Current treatment of Duchenne muscular dystrophy. Biochem Biophys Acta. 2007;1772(2):229–37.
104. Manzur AY, Kinali M, Muntoni F. Update on the management of Duchenne muscular dystrophy. Arch Dis Child. 2008;93(11):986–90.
105. Passamano L, Taglia A, Palladino A, Viggiano E, D'Ambrosio P, Sccutifero M, et al. Improvement of survival in Duchenne muscular dystrophy: a retrospective analysis of 835 patients. Acta Myol. 2012;31(2):121–5.
106. Eagle M, Bourke J, Bullock R, Gibson M, Mehta J, Giddings D, et al. Managing Duchenne muscular dystrophy—the additive effect of spinal surgery and home nocturnal ventilation in improving survival. Neuromuscul Disord. 2007;17(6):470–5.
107. LoMauro A, D'Angelo MG, Aliverti A. Assessment and management of respiratory function in patients with Duchenne muscular dystrophy: current and emerging options. Ther Clin Risk Manag. 2015;11:1475–88.
108. Rahbek J, Steffensen BF, Bushby K, de Groot IJM. 2006th ENMC international workshop: care for a novel group of patients—adults with Duchenne muscular dystrophy. Naarden, The Netherlands, 23–25 May 2014. Neuromuscul Disord. 2015;25:727–38.
109. Verhaert D, Richards K, Rafael-Fortney JA, Raman SV. Cardiac involvement in patients with muscular dystrophies: magnetic resonance imaging phenotype and genotypic considerations. Circ Cardiovasc Imaging. 2011;4(1):67–76.
110. Pfeffer MA, Braunwald E, Moye LA, Basta L, Brown Jr EJ, Cuddy TE, et al. Effect of captopril on mortality and morbidity in patients with left ventricular dysfunction after myocardial infarction trial. Results of the survival and ventricular enlargement (SAVE) trial. N Engl J Med. 1992;327(10):669–77.
111. Duboc D, Meune C, Lerebours G, Devaux JY, Vaksmann G, Becane HM. Effect of perindopril on the onset and progression of left ventricular dysfunction in Duchenne muscular dystrophy. J Am Coll Cardiol. 2005;45(6):855–7.
112. Viollet L, Thrush PT, Flanigan KM, Mendell JR, Allen HD. Effects of angiotensin-converting enzyme inhibitors and/or beta blockers on the cardiomyopathy in Duchenne muscular dystrophy. Am J Cardiol. 2012;110(1):98–102.

113. McNally EM, Kaitman JR, Benson DW, Canter CE, Cripe LH, Duan D, et al. Contemporary cardiac issues in Duchenne muscular dystrophy. Circulation. 2015;131(18):1590–8.
114. Gianola S, Pecoraro V, Lambiase S, Gatti R, Banfi G, Moja L. Efficacy of muscle exercise in patients with muscular dystrophy; a systematic review showing a missed opportunity to improve outcomes. PLoS One. 2013. doi:10.1371/journal.pone.0065414.
115. Quinlivan R, Roper H, Davie M, Shaw NJ, McDonagh J, Bushby K. Osteoporosis in Duchenne muscular dystrophy: its prevalence, treatment and prevention. Neuromuscul Disord. 2005;15(1):72–9.
116. Pangalila RF, van den Bos GA, Bartels B, Bergen MP, Kampelmacher MJ, Stam HJ, et al. Quality of life of adult men with Duchenne muscular dystrophy in the Netherlands: implications for care. J Rehabil Med. 2015;47:161–6.
117. Reilly S, Skuse D. Prevalence of feeding problems and oral motor dysfunction in children with cerebral palsy: a community survey. J Pediatr. 1996;129:877–82.
118. Parkes J, Hill N, Platt MJ, Donnelly C. Oromotor dysfunction and communication impairments in children with cerebral palsy: a register study. Dev Med Child Neurol. 2010;52:1113–9.

Chapter 19
Osteoporosis and the Female Athlete Triad

Christina V. Oleson and Tracy E. Ransom

Components of the Female Athlete Triad

Over the past four decades, an increase in the number of girls and women participating in sports has led to growing concerns about a series of three interrelated disorders observed by those involved in caring for the health of this cohort, namely, parents, coaches, athletic trainers, team physicians, and administrators at the high school and college level and, to a certain extent, at the level of professional sports. The American College of Sports Medicine (ACSM) was the first to identify the components of the female athlete triad in a "position stand," originally issued in 1992 and updated in 1997 and 2007 [1]. It identified the three components along a spectrum of dysfunction (Fig. 1).

Broadly defined, the components are:

1. Energy availability, from optimal energy availability to an end point of low energy availability with or without eating disorders
2. Menstrual function, from amenorrhea (normal menses) to an end point of amenorrhea (delayed menses or cessation for a period of three months)
3. Bone mineral density (BMD), from optimal bone density to an end point of osteoporosis

Although this book focuses on osteoporosis, it is important to understand that each of these components has implications for the next. Energy deficiency associated with eating disorders has a causal role in the development of menstrual irregularities; both energy deficiency and the hypoestrogenic environment linked to amenorrhea affect BMD. In addition, recent research suggests that this hypoestrogenic state could lead to endothelial dysfunction, resulting in cardiovascular disease. As Temme and Hoch have observed, this association could turn the triad into a tetrad [2].

C.V. Oleson, *Osteoporosis Rehabilitation*, DOI 10.1007/978-3-319-45084-1_19

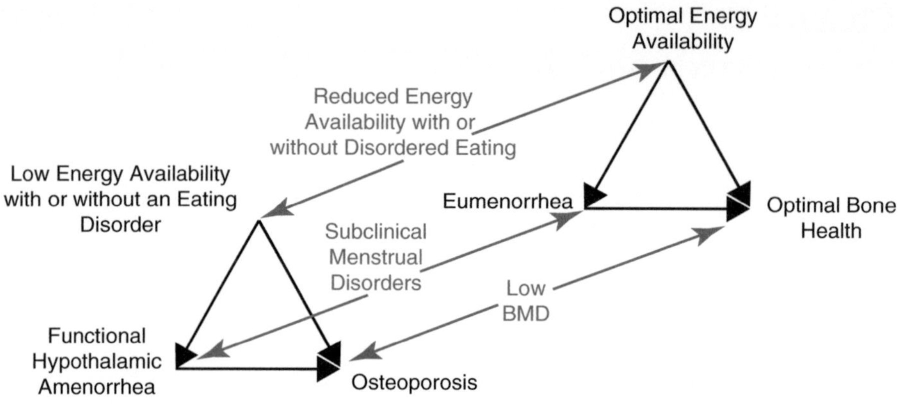

Fig. 1 Female athlete triad. The spectrum of energy availability, menstrual function, and bone mineral density (*Source*: Nattiv et al. [1]. Reproduced with permission)

Table 1 Sports most affected by the female athlete triad

Categorization of sports	Examples
Sports in which performance is subjectively scored	Dance, figure skating, diving, gymnastics, aerobics
Endurance sports emphasizing a low body weight	Distance running, cycling, cross-country skiing
Sports requiring body-contour-revealing clothing for competition	Volleyball, swimming, diving, cross-country running and skiing, track, speed skating, cheerleading
Sports using weight categories	Equestrian, some martial arts, wrestling, rowing
Sports emphasizing a prepubertal body for performance success	Figure skating, gymnastics, diving

Source: Otis et al. [3]

The ACSM 1997 Position Stand identifies several sports disciplines at high risk for promoting the development of one or more of the triad components (Table 1). It should be noted that triad components also occur in adolescent girls whose pursuit of thinness is influenced by role models in films, television, music, fashion, and other aspects of social media. According to a study by Ferguson et al., peer pressure may be even more significant than thin “idols” in promoting eating disorders [4].

Prevalence

Since the identification of the female athlete triad, numerous studies have been undertaken on the prevalence of this condition as a whole, for two or more components, and for individual components [2]. One of the most recent and comprehensive set of findings, developed by Gibbs et al., examines 65 studies ($n = 10{,}498$) of female high school students and premenopausal exercising women identified through an electronic search of the computerized databases PubMed and MEDLINE [5].

Findings from nine of these studies ($n = 991$) indicate that only a small percentage of athletes, 0–15.9 %, suffer from all three conditions presenting simultaneously. When two of the three components were considered, the prevalence ranged from 2.7 % to 27.0 % (seven studies, $n = 328$), but when only one component was taken into account, the prevalence increased markedly to a range of 16–60 % (six studies, $n = 537$). In another study, Thein-Nissenbaum and Carr used the self-report Eating Disorder Examination Questionnaire to determine that eating disorders and low energy availability (LEA) were present in 35.4 % of 331 female athletes [6]. A more recent analysis of professional ballet dancers by Hoch et al. found LEA in 77 %, eating disorders in 32 %, menstrual disorders in 36 %, low BMD in 23 %, and abnormal brachial artery flow-mediated dilitation (FMD)—the possible fourth component—in 64 % of the cohort [7].

Although significant advances have been made in determining the prevalence of the triad, comparisons among studies remain hindered by the use of different methodologies and varying definitions of the triad components as well as limitations in methods of assessment. In addition, there have been relatively few studies of the subclinical conditions along the spectrum of the triad. Although they may be less severe than the end point, these subclinical conditions remain linked with similar negative outcomes. Studies of subclinical conditions are needed to understand the full effect of the triad from a clinical perspective. Moreover, the highly personal nature of the triad research inevitably results in data often based on inaccurate self-reports, rather than on objective methods such as hormone analyses. If advances are to be made in the prevention and treatment of the triad, both subclinical and clinical outcomes must be measured in a research setting [5].

Causes and Consequences

Low Energy Availability and Eating Disorders

Low energy availability (LEA) is generally regarded as the amount of energy remaining for all physiological functions after it is expended for growth, exercise, and other daily activities. Ideal energy balance in the young occurs at an energy availability (EA) of about 45 kcal per kg of free fatty mass per day; bone formation and reproductive functions are diminished when the level falls to under 30 kcal [8]. The ACSM identifies EA, generally defined as energy intake minus energy expenditure, as the driving force in the triad [1]. The causes of LEA encompass a set of interrelated biological, social, cultural, and psychological factors. Young females at the greatest risk include those who:

- Intentionally or inadvertently restrict caloric intake
- Adhere to vegetarian diets
- Engage in prolonged periods of exercise, particularly in sports that favor lean physiques
- Begin their sport-specific training early
- Suddenly increase their training intensity

Quite apart from athletic participation, dieting has been identified as the principal factor in determining LEA in adolescents and young women. Patton et al. have shown that 8 % of 15-year-old girls dieted at a severe level and another 60 % dieted at a moderate level. Those who dieted at a severe level were 18 times more likely to develop an eating disorder within six months of initiating the diet; those who dieted at a moderate level were five times more likely to develop the disorder within the same time period [9]. Together and separately, comorbid psychological conditions including depression, anxiety, obsessive–compulsive disorder, low self-esteem, and hormonal factors, specifically decreased leptin and increased ghrelin, underlie the compulsion to diet. These influences can be encompassed under the term "psychiatric morbidity," as applied to competitive, determined women who are also perfectionists [16]. Athletes with high psychiatric morbidity can have a more than six times increased risk of developing an eating disorder.

In athletes, LEA may occur unintentionally if they fail to recognize that their caloric intact is insufficient to meet their training needs. Studies have shown that although dietary restriction increases hunger, energy deficiency caused by increased energy expenditure does not; thus, LEA can develop without clinical eating disorders [1]. More likely, however, it occurs deliberately when individuals engaged in excessive or highly competitive exercise knowingly reduce their caloric intake or increase their energy expenditure. In addition to the factors precipitating LEA in general, this behavior may be motivated by an athlete's internal pressure to be thin as well as by pressure from coaches, parents, and peers.

As noted earlier, LEA occurs across a spectrum, ranging from inadequate food intake to abnormal eating behaviors including skipping meals, fasting, diet pills, laxatives, diuretics, and vomiting to clinical disorders, specifically anorexia nervosa, bulimia nervosa, binge eating disorder (BED), and other feeding or eating disorders. The consequences of LEA are manifold and, in the case of severe anorexia nervosa, life threatening. The health of the individual is seriously affected when energy used for exercise is diverted from such physiological mechanisms as growth, reproduction, and cellular maintenance. For athletes, LEA can lead to decreased immunocompetence, which limits endurance and results in an increased chance of infection and declining performance levels. The greatest effect on performance is demonstrated by athletes in endurance sports, such as distance running and swimming as opposed to those with lower energy demands such as gymnastics and diving [10]. Moreover, in a study of long-distance runners, the ACSM reported that a tenfold increase in training intensity, <13 to >113 km week^{-1}, resulted in an increase in the prevalence of amenorrhea from 3 % to 60 % [1].

Anorexia nervosa (AN) is the most devastating type of eating disorder (ED), with the highest mortality rate of any psychiatric illness. Death rates are estimated as high as 17 % with 20 % of deaths attributable to suicide [11, 12]. It has been proposed that individuals with anorexia may be predisposed to suicide because they engage not only in dangerous eating behaviors to the point of starvation but also in self-harm behaviors: 25–45 % of individuals with ED engage in self-injury [13]. Of the patients who did not die from suicide, less than half recovered, one-third improved, and a fifth remained chronically ill [14].

Menstrual Disorders

Menstrual abnormalities include primary amenorrhea, secondary amenorrhea, and oligomenorrhea as defined below:

- Primary amenorrhea: the absence of menarche by the age of 15
- Secondary amenorrhea: loss of three or more periods after menarche has begun for a woman who is not pregnant
- Oligomenorrhea: the occurrence of cycles greater than 35 days apart

LEA, caused by insufficient dietary intake and/or excessive exercise, is the principal cause of what is termed "functional hypothalamic amenorrhea," characterized by suppression of the hypothalamic–pituitary–ovarian axis without an identifiable anatomic or organic cause.

In the absence of sufficient energy, the female body reacts by reducing the amount of energy used for growth and reproduction. With this condition, the pulsatile secretion of the gonadotropin-releasing hormone (GnRH) is disrupted, leading in turn to a disruption in the pulsatile secretion of the luteinizing hormone (LH) from the pituitary. Studies indicate that menstruation is impossible if levels of leptin, the "satiety hormone" that regulates the amount of fat stored in the body, fall below a critical level. Other metabolic hormones that contribute to menstrual dysfunction include ghrelin, the "hunger hormone" which signals hunger to the brain and has a role in regulating body weight, adiponectin which increases with prolonged fasting and weight reduction, as well as insulin, insulin-like growth factor-1, and cortisol [8].

The EA required to maintain normal menstruation is 30 kcal.kg^{-1} of lean body mass per day; LH pulsatility is disrupted when EA drops below that level. Neither intense athletic training nor low body weight can in themselves cause menstrual disorders, indicating that disrupted LH pulsatility is more directly attributable to low energy availability [15].

The consequences of menstrual dysfunction include infertility, decreased immune function, increased cardiovascular risks, and decreased BMD [10]. Unfortunately many young athletes and their coaches are unaware of these conditions or tend to ignore them; in fact, some women are actually relieved by the absence of their periods. However, there is now sufficient evidence to indicate that unless the situation is addressed, it will have long-term implications for the health of women in their training years and later in life.

Low Bone Density

In females, the greatest accretion of bone mass occurs between the ages of 11 and 14, with 25 % of bone mass accrual in the two years surrounding menarche. Healthy young women generally achieve 92 % or more of their total bone mineral content by age 18 and 99 % by age 26 [16]. Since bone mineral deposition occurs early in life, it is critical that a diagnosis be made in adolescence to detect high-risk females and avoid irreparable bone damage.

Evidence suggests that weight-bearing exercise at the pivotal times of bone deposition during puberty may result in improved BMD. Oleson and colleagues reported on a group of competitive figure skaters ages 14–20, all of whom were performing double and/or triple jumps. Those who had begun landing double jumps prior to menarche had statistically higher bone density as determined by quantitative ultrasound. Moreover, 10 of the 36 skaters evaluated had experienced fractures. This group on average mastered double jumps nearly two years later than the skaters without fractures, leading the authors to propose that an osteogenic stimulus contributes to the higher estimated BMD. Full advantage of this osteogenic stimulus appears to be possible only when present on or before menarche [17].

As in all aspects of the female athlete triad, bone density passes through a continuum from peak bone strength to osteopenia—BMD that is lower than peak but not as low as osteoporosis—to osteoporosis itself which is characterized by extremely low BMD, microarchitectural deterioration, and heightened risk of fractures. Decreased BMD is caused by reduced bone formation coupled with increased bone resorption. The causes of osteoporosis in postmenopausal females differ from the causes in younger women. Several decades ago, it was believed that osteoporosis in the young was caused by an estrogen deficiency, as is the case following menopause. Estrogen replacement therapy was used in an attempt to reverse the process but without significant benefit, even after years of such therapy. Estrogen has not been dismissed as a contributing factor in low BMD but more recent research reveals that the primary cause of osteoporosis in the young is lack of energy availability and low weight. When the body is malnourished, there is an inadequate intake of macronutrients including amino and fatty acids, as well as a lack of vitamins and minerals specifically calcium and vitamin D. Calcium is a critical factor in bone health and calcium deficiencies in young females can result in a 5–10 % difference in peak bone mass. When the body lacks sufficient energy, it can also experience hormonal changes, including high levels of cortisol and low levels of leptin and IGF-1, which contribute to further bone deterioration [18].

Female adolescents with anorexia nervosa are particularly predisposed to osteoporosis. Anorexia typically begins during the teenage years, at the same time that bones are growing and strengthening, thereby slowly or halting bone development. Moreover, if left untreated, anorexia can continue through the 20s and beyond, causing further bone loss. If females can recover from anorexia in their teens and 20s and bone loss is at a minimum, they may be able to recoup normal bone mass. However, a positive outcome will be affected by such factors as the amount of bone developed before the onset of anorexia, the amount lost during the period with anorexia, and the duration of the anorexia [19].

To a certain extent, low estrogen levels may also adversely affect the density and structure of bone mineral content. In patients affected by estrogen deficiency, osteoclasts live longer and more bone is resorbed. As this process continues, there is a loss in the density and structure of bone minerals, resulting in greater susceptibility to fractures in athletes, especially those whose bones are under increased mechanical stress [20]. A link between elevated fasting peptide (PYY) and decreased BMD has also been observed. Concentrations of PYY are negatively associated with bone turnover, indicating that PYY may contribute to detrimental bone pathology [21].

Endothelial Dysfunction

The "standard" components of the triad are long established, but, in the past two decades, researchers have identified another possible component of the triad, potentially transforming it into a tetrad. Endothelial dysfunction is a critical element in the pathogenesis of atherosclerosis and heart failure. The endothelium is the inner lining of blood vessels. When functioning normally, it controls the amount of fluid, electrolytes, and other materials that pass from the blood vessels into tissues; helps control blood clotting; forms new blood vessels; repairs damaged or diseased organs; and governs the dilation and constriction of blood vessels. Estrogen receptors on the endothelium of coronary and peripheral blood vessels regulate vascular function by stimulating the production of nitric oxide (NO) which, in turn, leads to the widening of blood vessels known as vasodilation. Nitric oxide is a strong vasodilator that helps to inhibit platelet aggregation, leukocyte adhesion, low-density lipoprotein, vascular smooth muscle proliferation and migration, and other atherosclerotic processes [22]. Dysfunction of the endothelium causes hypertension and thrombosis and can lead to impaired heart function, reduced blood flow to muscles, and the development of cardiovascular disease—the leading cause of female deaths in the United States [23].

Evidence shows that there may be a link between endothelial dysfunction, amenorrhea, and low estrogen bonds. Research by Hoch et al. demonstrates that female runners with athletic amenorrhea experience a significant reduction in endothelial-dependent arterial vasodilation [22]. Because amenorrheic females are known to have hormone profiles similar to those of postmenopausal women, Lancer et al. suggest that low estrogen levels will theoretically impair endothelial cell function and arterial dilation [24].

Screening and Diagnosis

According to the American College of Sports Medicine 2007 Position Stand, screening for the triad requires a thorough knowledge of the relationship among the individual components, the spectrum covered by each component, and rates of movement along the spectrum. Ideally, this screening should occur at the time of the preparticipation physical evaluation (PPE) and annual checkups. Athletes who experience one component of the triad should be examined for the others. Early detection of at-risk athletes is critical in preventing or delaying the progress of the triad [1].

Preparticipation physical evaluations (PPEs) cover a wide range of issues that may threaten the health and safety of athletes, ranging from heart and lung problems to cultural factors such as the expectations and behavior of athletes, parents, and coaches. The first step is generally a self-report questionnaire which now exists in several formats. In 2008, the Female Athlete Triad Coalition, consisting of member universities and organizations ranging from the ACSM and the International Olympic Committee to the American Academy of Orthopedic Surgeons and the American Academy of Pediatrics, drew up a questionnaire including eight questions on eating disorders, three on menstrual dysfunction, and one on bone health to be used as the primary screening for the triad (Table 2) [25]. Simple "yes"/"no" answers were requested [18].

Mencias et al. used these questions as a base measure in examining the PPEs used by 257 NCAA Division 1 universities. They found that 25 universities (9 %) included 9 of the 12 recommended items, whereas 127 universities (44 %) included only four or fewer items. Although all 257 universities required a PPE for incoming athletes, only 83 required PPEs for returning athletes [26].

Supported by six leading medical societies, the Fourth Edition PPE Evaluation Form (PPE-4, 2010) covers athletes from middle school through college and includes 8 of the 12 coalition-recommended questions. If widely adopted, it could improve the effectiveness of this tool by providing standardized criteria. However, in a 2015 study of PPE administrative policies in all 50 states and Washington,

Table 2 Female athlete triad screening questionnaire (2008)

Eating disorders	Do you worry about your weight or body composition?
	Do you limit or carefully control the food that you eat?
	Do you try to lose weight to meet weight or image appearance requirements in your sport?
	Does your weight affect the way you feel about yourself?
	Do you worry that you have lost control over how much you eat?
	Do you make yourself vomit or use diuretics or laxatives after you eat?
	Do you ever eat in secret?
Menstrual history	What age was your first menstrual period?
	Do you have monthly menstrual cycles?
	How many menstrual cycles have you had in the last year?
Bone health	Have you ever had a stress fracture?

Source: Adapted from Female Athlete Triad Coalition: An International Consortium [25]

D.C., Caswell et al. show that most states have been slow in adopting PPE-4 recommendations; they advocate adoption of a nationwide standardized PPE form and the use of an electronic PPE process to improve adherence and create a national database [27].

Low Energy Availability/Eating Disorders

Multiple factors including physical symptoms as well as psychological and behavioral characteristics must be taken into account in screening for energy availability. Physical symptoms encompass a wide range of cardiovascular, endocrine, gastrointestinal, and renal factors; psychological and behavioral issues include anxiety over weight gain, binging and purging behaviors, self-induced vomiting, use of laxatives and diet pills, extreme dieting, and excessive exercise. More than 50 % of the PPE forms examined in the Mencias study omitted questions relating to eating disorders.

Many physicians regard the Eating Disorder Examination (EDE) interview or Eating Disorder Examination Questionnaire (EDE-Q) as a more effective screening tool, but the interview is time consuming and requires training for those who administer it. The EDE-Q is a self-report with ratings for four subscales: restraint, eating concern, shape concern, and weight concern. Aardoom et al. demonstrate that it is highly accurate in discriminating between those with an ED and those without and find that it is a valid technique to assess a general level of ED psychopathology [28]. Often used in primary care settings, the SCOFF questionnaire, incorporating five questions concerning eating behavior, dieting, and a compulsion with food, is helpful in identifying anorexia nervosa and bulimia.

More recently, a new instrument, the Low Energy Availability in Female Questionnaire (LEAF-Q) has been developed to assess athletes at risk for the triad. Consisting of 25 questions about injuries, illness, dizziness, and gastronomical and reproductive functions, it was submitted by Melin et al. to 84 Swedish and Danish athletes aged 18–39 years who trained ≤5 times/week. Triad-associated disorders were common in this cohort, despite a normal BMI range. The results indicated that LEAF-Q is brief and easy to administer, has a specificity rate of 90 %, and may be successfully used to complement existing ED questionnaires [29].

In terms of diagnosing eating disorders, the *Diagnostic and Statistical Manual of Mental Disorders V* (DSM-V-2013) is regarded as the principal source book for clinicians. Anorexia nervosa (AN) is defined as a serious, potentially life-threatening psychiatric illness characterized by (1) persistent restriction of energy intake leading to significant low body weight in terms of what is minimally expected for age, sex, development, and physical health; (2) intense fear of gaining weight or persistent behavior that interferes with weight gain; and (3) distorted body image and lack of recognition of the seriousness of the low body weight [30]. Although not included in the DSM-V, the concept of anorexia athletica (sports anorexia) is often related to a triad diagnosis; in this condition, excessive exercise and the drive for thinness and high performance outweigh the body-image distortions seen with anorexia nervosa [31]. The DSM-V definition of bulimia nervosa incorporates (1) recurrent episodes of binge eating and (2) recurrent compensatory behaviors to prevent weight gain, including vomiting, diuretics, fasting, and excessive exercise. Both must occur, on average, at least once a week for three months. In DSM-V, binge eating disorder (BED) has been assigned a category unto itself. Occurring at least once a week over three months, it is marked by recurring episodes of eating large quantities of food, without purging; lack of control over eating; eating until uncomfortably full; and secretive eating.

Previously referred to as "Eating Disorders Not Otherwise Specified (EDNOS)," a fourth level, now titled "Feeding or Eating Disorders Not Elsewhere Classified (NEC)," is the most common eating disorder category, keeping in mind that eating disorder studies rely heavily on self-reports that may be inaccurate. NECs include less serious manifestations of the disorders specifically mentioned above, for example, atypical anorexia nervosa (all criteria for AN are met but weight is within or above normal range) and purging disorder (recurrent purging behavior in the absence of binge eating). It is anticipated that orthorexia, an obsession with healthy or rigorous eating, will be the next disorder added to this fourth category. Whereas the former EDNOS was highly diffuse, the NEC has been reorganized to achieve greater specificity, thereby providing new research opportunities as well as useful guidelines for clinical practice [32].

A physical exam, incorporating a PPE and the diagnostic guidelines set forth in DSM-V, is critical in identifying eating disorders. It should begin with basic height, weight, and vital signs and focus on specific physical factors specifically bradycardia and hypotension (cardiovascular); hair loss, lanugo hair, hand calluses or abrasions; dental enamel erosions (dermatological/dental); swollen parotid glands; constipation/diarrhea (gastrointestinal) and dehydration; electrolyte disturbances, edema (renal), as well as low body mass, significant weight loss, and frequent weight fluctuations. Laboratory tests should include a complete blood count, erythrocyte sedimentation rate, thyroid function tests, and urinalysis [18]. A psychologist should be consulted to examine contributing psychological and behavioral factors such as anxiety, obsessive–compulsive disorder, and perfectionism as well as low self-esteem and the need for self-control.

Menstrual Dysfunction

As in the case of eating disorders, a physical exam and thorough medical history are the essential first steps in identifying menstrual dysfunction. Females with functional hypothalamic amenorrhea may have a normal physical exam, but a pelvic exam may reveal signs of hypoestrogenism with vaginal atrophy. In general, their gonadotropins are low or normal, estradiol is low, and prolactin and thyroid-stimulating hormone are in normal range. In cases of primary/secondary amenorrhea, a pregnancy test should be administered, and endocrinopathies should be ruled out. Endocrinopathies include five primary areas of dysfunction, as described below [33]:

- Thyroid dysfunction
- Hyperprolactinemia
- Primary ovarian insufficiency
- Hypothalamic and pituitary disorder
- Hypoandrogenic conditions including polycystic ovary syndrome and virilizing ovarian insufficiency

Evaluation of menstrual dysfunction requires gonadotropin (follicle-stimulating hormone (FSH) and luteinizing hormone (LH) measurements to eliminate ovarian failure as a cause and to check for the increased FSH/LH ratios observed in polycystic ovary syndrome. In addition, workup should include a prolactin test to assess for a lactotropic-secreting tumor, and a thyroid-stimulating hormone test for thyroid disease. If the physical exam reveals evidence of androgen excess, further laboratory testing to diagnose polycystic ovary syndrome or congenital adrenal hyperplasia and a progesterone challenge test to assess the degree of hypoestrogen should be undertaken. Primary physicians may want to consult with endocrinologists in making this diagnosis [1].

Low Bone Mineral Density

Ultimately, low BMD is the result of a combination of low energy availability and menstrual dysfunction as well as genetics and hormonal functions. Initial studies of decreased BMD focused on the lumbar spine, but subsequent research indicates that the deficit occurs throughout the skeleton. A major consequence of this condition is the risk for fractures during an athlete's competitive years, leading to reduced performance and training time and resulting in chronic pain, delayed recovery, and disability, Moreover, fractures that occur in adolescence can predict fractures later in life [10]. Athletes with a high incidence of stress fractures, specifically endurance runners and dancers, generally exhibit high levels of dietary restraint and/or an extended history of anorexia or bulimia. Other studies show an association between fractures and amenorrhea [34]. In recent years, research has confirmed a relation between the components of the triad and musculoskeletal injuries in female high school athletes. Rauh et al. found that injured athletes had both higher EDE-Q scores and lower lumbar spine BMD, pointing to both menstrual dysfunction and low BMD as predictors of injury [35]. In the absence of more extensive research, it is difficult to assess the relative importance of one or the other triad components in determining the cause of injury. All three have a negative, long-term effect on bone.

A history of hypoestrogenism, eating disorders for 6 months or more, and stress fractures or fractures with minimal trauma warrant BMD assessment. Dual-energy x-ray absorptiometry (DXA) is regarded as the "gold standard" for evaluating BMD because of its speed, precision, safety, low cost, and widespread availability. It measures bone mass and areal BMD for the entire body as well for specific sites such as lumbar spine, hip, and distal radius [16]. Attention should be focused on the lumbar spine and forearm; they are rich in trabecular bone which is sensitive to changes in the hormonal environment and, thus, susceptible to poor bone quantity (mass) and bone quality (structure), leading to a risk of fracture [36]. In populations considered to be at risk for the triad, the prevalence of low BMD ranges from 1.4 % to 50 %.

The results of a DXA are reported as *T*-scores and *Z*-scores. The *T*-score, used for patients 20 years and older, is the number of standard deviations (SDs) by which a person's BMD differs from that of healthy adults of the same sex. The *Z*-score, reported for all ages, is the number of SDs by which a person's BMD differs from that of individuals of the same age and gender who have no fragility fractures. *Z*-scores are used to assess bone density in adolescent or premenopausal women because adolescents are still growing and have not achieved the BMD of women outside their age group [16]. Guidelines issued by the International Society for Clinical Densitometry stipulate a *Z*-score of −2.0 as "below the expected range for age," while a *Z*-score above −2.0 is "within the expected range of age." The diagnosis of osteoporosis is indicated by the presence of both a clinically significant fracture history and a *Z*-score of ≤ -2.0. The posterior–anterior spine and total body minus the head are the preferred sites for performing BMD measurements; the hip should be avoided due to variability in skeletal development. If symptoms persist, the DXA test should be repeated every 12 months, using the same equipment to ensure an accurate comparison [37].

Impaired bone microarchitecture should also be considered in assessing bone structure and fragility. Since DXA calculates BMD using an area measurement (DXA BMD is also known as areal bone mineral density), it cannot accurately measure volumetric BMD which incorporates a depth value. Other imaging technologies including axial quantitative computer tomography (QCT) and peripheral QCT (pQCT) are needed to measure bone mass and volumetric BMD as it occurs in both trabecular and cortical bone. DNA, QCT, and pQCT measure the inorganic element of the bone matrix; techniques to measure the organic component, primarily collagen, are yet to be perfected [38].

As Ducher et al. point out, diagnosing bone health in adolescents presents significant challenges given constant changes in bone mass, size, and shape. Bone growth can be compromised by childhood diseases as well as by LEA and hypoestrogenism, resulting in deficits in limb and spine dimensions as well as in volumetric BMD. Given these conditions, careful monitoring of young athletes is critical to ensure optimal skeletal development and peak bone mass. The distal forearm is a useful testing site for adolescents up to the age of 19 because it is a common site of fracture and is not loaded in activities such as running. Full recovery of bone strength may never be achieved because bone mineralization in young adults usually results in increased BMD, but not increased bone size [38].

Endothelial Dysfunction

The most common technique for evaluating endothelial function involves the use of a noninvasive, high-resolution ultrasound to examine the diameter of the brachial artery (a major blood vessel in the forearm) and to produce a brachial artery flow-mediated-dependent (FMD) vasodilation measurement. The diameter of the brachial artery and flow velocity are recorded at baseline and again following forearm occlusion with a blood pressure cuff. Deflating the cuff induces increased blood flow that stimulates an endothelium-dependent vasodilation of the brachial artery. The brachial artery FMD can be used successfully to study the early stages of atherosclerosis in children and young adults, thereby ensuring adequate time for prevention [39].

Using this technique, Hoch et al. tested the hypothesis that young female runners with athletic amenorrhea and oligomenorrhea show signs of early cardiovascular disease as manifested by decreased endothelium-dependent dilation of the brachial artery. Their results demonstrated that loss of FMD in conduit arteries compromises exercise-induced dilation of vessels and limits exercise capacity by restricting blood flow to muscles and that chronic impairment of endothelial function may accelerate the development of cardiovascular events [22].

Further studies show a positive relationship between brachial artery endothelial dysfunction and coronary artery endothelial dysfunction. For example, Schachinger et al. found that endothelial dysfunction in the brachial artery predicts atherosclerotic disease as well as cardiovascular events including heart attacks, strokes, and mortality [40]. Further research by Rickenlund et al. found a significantly decreased FMD in amenorrheic athletes as well as an unfavorable lipid profile with significantly higher total cholesterol and low-density lipoprotein [41]. A reasonable amount of exercise is cardioprotective, but the excessive exercise characteristic of amenorrhea can be counterproductive and instead increase the risk of cardiovascular events. Although the brachial artery FMD technique has been adopted widely, there remains significant variability regarding the protocols and methods of analysis used as well as the interpretation of results. Larger studies with improved and more consistent methodologies are needed to confirm the link between endothelial dysfunction and athletic amenorrhea and the possible extension of the female athlete into a tetrad.

General Approaches to Treatment

The first step in treating and preventing the female athlete triad is greater awareness of the syndrome on the part of healthcare professionals, trainers, physical therapists, coaches, and psychologists. The first "awareness" study on the triad, published in 2006, found that 48 % of physicians were able to identify all three components, but only 9 % were comfortable in treating them. The greatest recognition was among physical medicine and rehabilitation physicians at 69 % and orthopedic physicians at 63 % [42]. A 2013 study surveying 931 physicians at three academic medical centers identified only 37 % of the physicians as having heard about the triad, with the highest level of awareness among orthopedic surgeons (80.3 %) and the lowest level among psychiatrists (11.1 %) [43]. These findings underline the need for greater knowledge of the clinical guidelines for identifying the syndrome; they can be accessed at the website of the Female Athlete Coalition [44], an international advocacy group which serves as a clearing house for education and research about the triad.

There is a general consensus that only a multidisciplinary team ranging from primary care physicians and sports specialists including nutritionists, orthopedists, and psychotherapists to coaches, trainers, family, friends, and teammates can effectively treat the triad. Updated knowledge of both nonpharmacologic and pharmacologic therapy is essential, with pharmacologic treatment of secondary importance. The treatment goal is threefold: increase overall energy availability, restore normal menstrual cycle, and enhance BMD. Consideration should also be given to the role of endothelial dysfunction.

Behavioral Treatment

An understanding of psychological factors such as depression, anxiety, poor self-esteem, and poor self-image in addition to such personality traits as perfectionism and obsessiveness is critical in treating the consequences of the triad. The goals of behavioral treatment include restoring healthy eating habits, overcoming the compulsion to diet, ameliorating poor body image, and establishing greater control over thoughts and actions [1, 45]. There are a number of empirically based treatment options, described below, that can help reverse the effects of the triad.

Cognitive Behavioral Therapy (CBT)/Behavioral Contracting/ Treatment Plan Adherence

Backed by strong research support, the most widely used treatment for the triad is cognitive behavioral therapy or CBT. Based on the concept that emotions, behaviors, and thoughts are interconnected, this form of treatment consists of identifying distorted cognitions and views of the world along with maladaptive behaviors [46]. Treatment can provide those who suffer from the triad with information about how negative behaviors and attitudes are counterproductive to the goals of performance and how the development of appropriate strategies and skills can lead to increased self-esteem and self-worth. A key component of CBT is "behavioral contracting" which entails keeping a daily "diary" to document the athlete's negative thoughts and behavior patterns and to identify alternatives for better outcomes [1]. Treatment plan adherence focuses on personal methods of altering behavior and cognitions to reach performance goals, as well as on the individual's potential for nutritional education and counseling.

Cognitive Dissonance-Based Prevention (DBP)

The concept of cognitive dissonance centers on the mental distress that occurs when one or more feelings or behaviors contradict one or more thoughts (cognitions). In the triad, this would apply to athletes who restrict calories (behavior) yet recognize that energy availability is reduced for optimum performance (thoughts). In his seminal work, Festinger explains that human beings are driven to maintain internal consistency, meaning that thoughts, values, beliefs, and actions are in harmony [47]. Within a DBP program, female athletes are encouraged to utilize this framework when considering the thin ideal in terms of the dissonance related to performance and self-worth [48].

ATHENA Therapy and Athlete-Modified Health Weight Intervention (AM-HWI-Coach and Peer-Led Approaches)

ATHENA, an 8-week school-based and team-centered approach designed for middle and high school female athletes, has shown promising results. It focuses on identification and modification of disordered behaviors and uses cognitive restructuring to address risk factors for diet pill use. Depression, self-esteem, steroid-use, and societal and cultural pressures are key concerns. Participants engage in role-playing to practice "refusal skills"—saying "no" to dangerous situations—in cases of eating disorders and substance abuse. Peers and healthy athletes acting as mentors provide validation and encouragement, while the community component of the program offers an increased level of support for the athletes involved. ATHENA can also be a prevention program aimed at those who have not yet engaged in unhealthy behaviors [49]. In the Athlete-Modified Health Weight Intervention (AM-HWI) program, athletes are encouraged to make small, behavioral changes to address eating disorders. Often peer-led, it seeks to reduce thin-ideal internalization, body dissatisfaction, and the negativism that results from anorexic or bulimic behavior [48].

Mindfulness-Based Stress Reduction (MBSR)

Originating in Buddhist thought and practices, mindfulness training has received increasing attention as an intervention treatment for a variety of physiological and psychological problems, including eating disorders. One of the most popular and frequently cited examples of this approach is the mindfulness-based stress reduction (MBSR) program, developed by Jon Kabat-Zinn at the University of Massachusetts. Designed as an 8–10 week course in a group setting, it is based on teaching mindfulness by incorporating psychoeducation on stress reduction, coping, and pain control, together with instruction, discussion, and practice in mindfulness meditation skills and relaxation exercises [50].

"Seven attitudinal factors," espoused by Kabat-Zinn [51] are essential to mindfulness meditation (Table 3): (1) *non-judging*, (2) *patience*, (3) *beginner's mind*, (4)

Table 3 Seven attitudinal factors that are essential to mindfulness meditation

(1) Non-judging	Freeing your mind from judgmental thoughts and opinions
(2) Patience	Accepting the fact that events must occur in their own time and cannot be rushed
(3) Beginner's mind	A willingness to look at things with an open mind, always receptive to new possibilities
(4) Trust	Developing a better understanding of one's self, one's intuition, and one's actions, even if a mistake is made
(5) Non-striving	Seeking no other goal than to be yourself
(6) Acceptance	Understanding the world in the present moment and coming to terms with things as they actually are
(7) Letting go	Allowing experiences and thoughts to be what they are without disputing them

Source: F Kabat-Zinn [51]

trust, (5) *non-striving*, (6) *acceptance*, and (7) *letting go*. When considered as treatment for the triad, the MBSR clinic approach centers on (1) focusing attention on awareness and acceptance of the present moment and, in the case of the triad, on one's sport, (2) suspending judgment and developing an openness to new ideas, and (3) creating a sense of responsibility on the part of the individual for improved health and well-being [52].

How then does mindfulness work? It is proposed that stress and anxiety can be reduced through desensitization, self-exposure, and monitoring of thoughts; physiological impacts may also be involved as manifested by a change in the levels of neurotransmitters and cerebral blood flow, including an increase in dopamine during the meditative process [53]. However, physiological research on the mindfulness response to mind–body outcomes has not been studied extensively.

Mindfulness-Based Cognitive Therapy

Based on Kabat-Zinn MBSR program, mindfulness-based cognitive therapy (MBCT) is a manualized approach to "attentional" thought control that centers on accepting thoughts as what they are, simply thoughts. Focusing on anxiety and depression, it is designed to help prevent a relapse in major depression [54] by developing a detached view of one's thoughts, and, in a cognitive fashion, learning that thoughts are not facts and that they do not determine who a person is—a concept that is helpful for the treatment of the triad. Cognitive exercises such as hatha yoga, which are used in Kabat-Zinn's program, are emphasized and may be helpful for the treatment [55]. Through this approach, patients strengthen their relaxation responses, coping strategies, self-efficacy, insights, and self-determination. At the same time, it should be noted that CBT without mindfulness procedures is also effective in addressing anxiety and depression.

Dialectical Behavior Therapy (DBT)

Dialectical behavior therapy, a mindfulness approach developed by Marsha Linehan [56], encourages patients to change their behaviors and thought processes to build better lives. Participants are taught that the relationship between acceptance of one's situation and a motivation to change is the most profound dialectic. Mindfulness is a key component of DBT, because it allows the patient to observe and allow experiences to happen without suppressing or fighting them. Problem-solving approaches, such as explaining that the person's whole is greater than the sum of his or her parts, that parts are related, and that change involves incorporating all parts (emotions, behaviors, thoughts) in the process of change constitute the foundation of DBT [57].

Acceptance and Commitment Therapy

Developed by Steven Hayes at the University of Nevada, acceptance and commitment therapy (ACT, said as a word, not as an acronym) incorporates mindfulness techniques to assist patients in reducing their defensiveness so they may experience events as they really are. Instead of thought or emotional suppression, ACT's goal is to accept, experience, and deal with averse thoughts fully, to understand the actual words used to describe them, and then to defuse, rather than to avoid, them [58]. This approach suggests that much of psychopathology is due to maladaptive thoughts and that these thoughts, exacerbated by attempts to avoid then, result in movement away from goals—a common thought process for patients with the triad. ACT seeks to improve flexibility in six different psychological "realms": contact with the present moment, values, committed action, self as context, diffusion, and acceptance. Controlling these realms could enable triad patients to deal more effectively with their behavior [59].

Cognitive Behavioral Therapy and Mindfulness: Similarities and Differences

They are similar in that both help patients to recognize and change negative thought patterns and gain greater control over thoughts and feelings; both have been proved successful in treating depression and anxiety. They are different in that CBT focuses on actively pushing negative thoughts out of consciousness, whereas mindfulness advocates acceptance of thoughts without judgment, acknowledging their impermanence and letting them go [50, 60].

Family-Based and Coaching-Based Therapies

The above mentioned therapies center on individual or group treatment of the triad. It is important to note that influences from family and parents as well as coaches should not be overlooked. Family therapy can assist in identifying any external pressure or expectations from family members; in addition, coaching behavior and beliefs emphasizing the athlete's health rather than performance can often highly influence the approach to triad treatment.

Pharmacologic Treatment

Low Energy Availability and Eating Disorders

Increased energy availability is the key to reversing the female athlete triad: the longer the duration of low weight, the greater the risk of irreversible osteoporosis. For this component of the triad, few pharmacologic interventions have proved effective and those that demonstrate benefits are generally used in association with psychotherapy. However, antidepressant medications—including selective serotonin reuptake inhibitors (SSRIs, including the best known fluoxetine-Prozac), selective serotonin–norepinephrine reuptake inhibitors (SNRIs), and norepinephrine dopamine reuptake inhibitors (NDRIs)—may be helpful in treating LEA, secondary to chronic eating disorders, in athletes who experience concomitant depression, anxiety, and obsessive–compulsive behavior. These medications enable neurotransmitters to remain in neuron synapses for extended periods, thereby leading to a greater sense of well-being and a potential reduction in depressed mood. Moreover, they have few side effects and are well tolerated by most patients [61]. The American Psychiatric Association cites little evidence to warrant the use of medications in treating anorexia nervosa, but bulimia and binge eating have been found to respond to a combination of antidepressants and cognitive behavioral therapy [62]. Proper management and evaluation by a medical professional trained in administering these medications is essential, because frequent monitoring and feedback are needed to obtain the best results [33].

Menstrual Dysfunction

In 1989, the American Academy of Pediatrics recommended the use of oral contraceptive pills (OCPs) for young females with primary amenorrhea at age 15 or 16 and with secondary amenorrhea three months post menarche. However, studies of their efficacy are inconclusive, and some even demonstrate negative effects. For example, early investigations proposed that exogenous estrogen replacement could lead to premature growth plate closure in young athletes [18]. As Temme and Hoch point out, contraceptive therapy in the form of OCPs combining estrogen and progestin does not restore spontaneous menses, because it does not address the underlying metabolic changes that result in menstrual dysfunction [2]; specifically it does not normalize metabolic factors that impair bone formation and general health. Moreover, it does not address the fluctuations of such hormones as leptin, ghrelin, insulin-like growth factor-1 (IGF-1), follicle-stimulating hormone, and luteinizing hormone. Indeed, using OCPs to regulate menstrual cycles may produce a false sense of improvement when induced withdrawal bleeding occurs without a change in EA and can also deflect attention from proven efforts to restore EA through caloric intake [2]. A further disadvantage of OCP therapy is its suppression of the IGF-1, a major regulator of muscle mass and bone formation during development and a factor that is already at a low level in athletes with the triad.

Low Bone Mineral Density

Research on the efficacy of pharmacologic treatment in athletes with low BMD, stress fractures, and impaired bone accrual is also inconclusive as are studies that focus on whether such treatment prevents fracture or improves healing time and recovery from fractures already sustained. The 2014 Female Athlete Triad Coalition Consensus Statement states that the decision to use pharmacologic therapies should not depend solely on BMD Z-scores but should also take into account such risk factors as fracture history, genetic predisposition, triad conditions precipitating low BMD, bone stress injuries, and rate of bone loss with nonpharmacologic intervention [33]. OCP treatment does not increase BMD and may, in fact, further compromise bone health by lowering IGF-1.

However, it is recommended in the case of athletes who refuse to either follow dietary recommendations or reduce their exercise programs or who, despite nutrition or exercise counseling, fail to achieve restored menses after a 6-month period. OCP is not suggested for athletes under the age of 16 due to lack of research on this age group and concern for premature growth plate closure coupled with the knowledge that athletes oppose OCP because of a fear of weight gain [38]. Transdermal estradiol treatment with cyclic progesterone is being studied as an alternative to OCP therapy. Unlike OCP, it does not suppress IGF-1 and has been found to increase spine and hip BMD in young females with anorexia nervosa [63].

Bisphosphonates, which are commonly used to treat postmenopausal osteoporosis, are not generally recommended for young athletes. They act by inhibiting bone resorption and the difference in their effect in adults versus adolescents may relate to increased bone resorption in adults as compared with reduced bone resorption in adolescents. Because they remain active in the bone for as many as 10 years, bisphosphonates raise concerns about harm to the fetus during a subsequent pregnancy, specifically in the form of possible malformations and other defects in newborns. According to the Female Triad Coalition, they should be used only after consultation with an endocrinologist or a specialist in metabolic bone disease, with a decision made on a case-by-case basis [33].

Calcium and vitamin D supplements are recommended to improve bone health in athletes with the triad. According to the 2011 Institute of Medicine (IOM) guidelines, calcium intake for children ages 9–18 is 1,300 mg daily and for women 19–30, 1,000 mg; with 2,500 mg daily as the upper limit of safety, daily intake must be divided into multiple doses. As Ackerman and Misra point out, this recommended calcium intake is not sufficient to optimize bone density in athletes with amenorrhea

[64]. Some studies indicate that calcium supplementation may contribute to stress fracture prevention; further research is needed to make a definitive assessment but, in any case, calcium intake at the IOM level is safe.

Vitamin D is known to reduce the risk of stress fractures and impaired muscle function, yet vitamin D levels are often found to be low in the American population in general and particularly in adolescents. The IOM guidelines for adolescents and premenopausal women call for a daily intake of 600 IU, but a 2012 study proposes that patients receive 800–1,000 IU and perhaps as much as 2,000 IU daily of vitamin D3 because it is a safe treatment with a high therapeutic index [65].

With endothelial dysfunction now being considered as a possible fourth component of the triad, research on alleviating its effects is underway, producing some significant findings. Using a low-dose combined OCP in amenorrheic athletes with decreased FMD at baseline, Rickenlund et al. demonstrated a significant increase in FMD after nine months of treatment, indicating that OCP can improve endothelial function through estrogen's effect in increasing nitric acid's bioavailability. However, hormone replacement treatment in postmenopausal women reveals an increased risk of cardiovascular events and breast cancer, indicating a potential risk for younger women [24].

Given its known cardiovascular benefits, folic acid, which upgrades the production of nitric oxide, has recently been proposed as a treatment for decreased FMD. In studies of amenorrheic runners and ballet dancers, Hoch et al. found an increase in FMD following the administration of 10 mg of folic acid for four weeks; indeed the runners' vasodilator response rose from $3.0 \pm 2.3\,\%$ to $7.7 \pm 4.5\,\%$ [24]. Folic acid, a water-soluble vitamin regularly eliminated in urine, is well tolerated at a low dosage of 10 mg and appears to be a safe, effective treatment for the endothelial dysfunction that occurs in the triad.

Prevention and Early Intervention

Recognition of the components of the female athlete triad is the first step in preventing the serious consequences of the triad that cannot be alleviated through nonpharmacologic, pharmacologic, or a combination of both types of treatments. Ideally the multidisciplinary approach recommended for treatment should be in place to identify the symptoms of the triad and intervene before irreversible damage occurs, particularly with respect to bone density and the potential for osteoporosis. Barbara Drinkwater, one of the first researchers to coin the term "female athlete triad," was also among the first to study the effect of athletic amenorrhea on BMD. She found that following resumption of normal menses, amenorrheic athletes regained a small amount of bone density, but never returned to normal levels. Subsequent studies confirmed that the bone density of formerly amenorrheic athletes remained 15 % less than that of athletes who were never amenorrheic. These results underline the need for early intervention to avoid devastating consequences for younger athletes in the short and long term [66].

Lack of awareness coupled with the failure or unwillingness to admit that they are susceptible to the triad must also be overcome. A 2014 study of female collegiate cross-country runners at risk of osteoporosis illustrates this danger. Results showed that this group had minimal concern for osteoporosis; specifically, they did not perceive themselves as highly susceptible to the disease nor did they believe it was a serious disease even if they were afflicted with it [67].

The multidisciplinary team that is so critical in treating elements of the triad may be even more important in implementing prevention and intervention efforts. In the case of adolescents, parents who are knowledgeable about their children's general health and about the warning signs of the syndrome should intervene. More likely, it is team physicians or independent individual coaches who are in a position to observe destructive eating habits and irrational behavioral patterns. Simple recognition of the term "female athletic triad" is not sufficient; these individuals must be fully aware of the components and consequences of the syndrome if they are to address the perceptions and misunderstandings that surround it. A 2006 study of collegiate coaches reported that 64 % of the 91 respondents had heard of the triad but only 48 % thought they could identify its components; moreover, 24 % believed that irregular or absent menstruation was a "normal" consequence of intensive exercise. In contrast, knowledgeable coaches were in a position to welcome and even to coordinate a multidisciplinary assessment that could lead to informed judgments about effective treatment and prevention strategies and on when or whether athletes should "return to play." Perhaps most important, they were more interested in adopting strategies to educate the athletes themselves as well as instilling in them a personal sense of responsibility for actions that could have repercussions over a lifetime [68].

The question of whether preventative strategies and more informed judgments can overcome compulsive personality traits and the societal pressure to be thin admits of no easy answer. In-depth knowledge, increased awareness, and deliberate action on the part of a multidisciplinary team are all needed to meet the challenges of the female athlete triad and its devastating end point, osteoporosis.

References

1. Nattiv A, Loucks AB, Manore MM, Sanborn CF, Sundgot-Borgen J, Warren MP. American College of Sports Medicine position stand. The female athlete triad. Med Sci Sports Exerc. 2007;39(10):1867–82.
2. Temme KE, Hoch AZ. Recognition and rehabilitation of the female athlete triad/tetrad: a multidisciplinary approach. Curr Sports Med Rep. 2013;12(3):190–9. doi:10.1249/JSR.0b013e318296190b.
3. Otis CL, Drinkwater B, Johnson M, Loucks A, Wilmore J. American College of Sports Medicine position stand: the female athlete triad. Med Sci Sports Exerc. 1997;29(5):i–ix.
4. Ferguson CJ, Muñoz ME, Garza A, Galindo M. Concurrent and prospective analyses of peer, television, and social media influences of body dissatisfaction, eating disorder symptoms and life satisfaction in adolescent girls. J Youth Adolesc. 2014;43(1):1–4. doi:10.1007/s10964-012-9898-9.

5. Gibbs JC, Williams NI, De Souza MJ. Prevalence of individual and combined components of the female athlete triad. Med Sci Sports Exerc. 2013;45(5):985–96. doi:10.1249/MSS.0b013e31827e1bdc.
6. Thein-Nissenbaum JM, Carr KE. Female athlete triad symptoms in the high school athlete. Phys Ther Sport. 2011;12(3):108–16. doi:10.1016/j.ptsp.2011.04.002.
7. Hoch AZ, Papanek P, Szabo A, Widlansky ME, Schimke JE, Gutterman DD. Association between the female athlete triad and endothelial dysfunction in dancers. Clin J Sport Med. 2011;21(2):119–25. doi:10.1097/JSM.0b013e3182042a9a.
8. Marguez S, Molinero O. Energy availability, menstrual dysfunction and bone health in sports; an overview of the female athlete triad. Nutr Hosp. 2013;28(4):1010–7. doi:10.3305/nh.2013.28.4.6542.
9. Patton GC, Selzer R, Coffrey C, Carlin JB, Wolfe R. Onset of adolescent eating disorders: population passed cohort study over 3 years. BMJ. 1999;318(7186):765–8.
10. George CA, Leonard JP, Hutchinson MR. The female athlete triad: a current concepts review. S Afr J Sports Med. 2011;23(2):50–7.
11. Fedorowicz VJ, Falissard B, Foulon C, Dardennes R, Divac SM, Guelfi JD, et al. Factors associated with suicidal behaviors in a large French sample of inpatients with eating disorders. Int J Eat Disord. 2007;40(7):589–95.
12. Keel PK, Klump KL. Are eating disorders culture- bound syndromes? Implications for conceptualizing their etiology. Psychol Bull. 2003;129(5):747–69.
13. Siegfried N, Bartlett M. Anorexia and suicide. Eating for life alliance. www.eatingforlife.org, http://www.eating-disorders-research.com/. Accessed 25 Jan 2015.
14. Steinhausen HC. The outcome of anorexia nervosa in the 20th century. Am J Psychiatry. 2002;159(8):1284–93.
15. Loucks AB, Thuma JR. Luteinizing hormone pulsatility is disrupted at a threshold of energy availability in regularly menstruating women. J Clin Endocrinol Metab. 2003;88(1):297–311.
16. Nazem TG, Ackerman KE. The female athlete triad. Sports Health. 2012;4(4):302–11.
17. Oleson CV, Busconi BD, Baran DT. Bone density in competitive figure skaters. Arch Phys Med Rehabil. 2002;83(1):122–8.
18. Chu SM, Gustafson KE, Leiszler M. Female athlete triad: clinical evaluation and treatment. Am J Lifestyle Med. 2013;7(6):87–94.
19. Zanaker CL. Osteoporosis in eating disorders, March 2011. www.feast-ed.org.
20. Idris AI, van't Hof RJ, Greig IR, Ridge SA, Baker D, Ross RA, et al. Regulation of bone mass, bone loss and osteoclast activity by cannabinoid receptors. Nat Med. 2005;11(7):774–9.
21. Scheid JL, Toombs RJ, Ducher G, Gibbs JC, Williams NI, De Souza MJ. Estrogen and peptide YY are associated with bone mineral density in premenopausal exercising women. Bone. 2011;49(2):194–201. doi:10.1016/j.bone.2011.04.011.
22. Zeni Hoch A, Dempsey RL, Carrera GF, Wilson CR, Chen EH, Barnabei VM, et al. Is there an association between athletic amenorrhea and endothelial cell dysfunction? Med Sci Sports Exerc. 2003;35(3):377–83.
23. Reed J, editor. Eating disorders: an encyclopedia of causes, treatment and prevention. Santa Barbara: ABC-CLIO; 2012. Accessed 25 Jan 2015.
24. Lanser EM, Zach KN, Hoch AZ. The female athlete triad and endothelial dysfunction. PM&R. 2011;3(5):458–65. doi:10.1016/j.pmrj.2010.12.024.
25. Female Athlete Triad Coalition: An International Consortium. Introduction: female athlete triad pre participation evaluation. 2002. http://www.femaleathletetriad.org/~triad/wp-content/uploads/2008/11/ppe_for_website.pdf. Accessed 15 Apr 2015.
26. Mencias T, Noon M, Hoch AZ. Female athlete triad screening in national collegiate athletic association division 1 athletes: is the preparticipation evaluation form effective? Clin J Sport Med. 2012;22:122–5. doi:10.1097/JSM.0b013e3182425aee.
27. Caswell SV, Cortes N, Chabolla M, Ambegaonkar JP, Caswell AM, Brenner JS. State-specific differences in school sports preparticipation physical evaluation policies. Pediatrics. 2015;135(1):26–32. doi:10.1542/peds.2014-1451.

28. Aardoom JJ, Dingemans AE, Slop Op't Landt MC, Van Furth EF. Norms and discriminative validity of the Eating Disorder Examination Questionnaire (EDE-Q). Eat Behav. 2012;13(4):305–9. doi:10.1016/j.eatbeh.2012.09.002.
29. Melin A, Tornberg AB, Skouby S, Faber J, Ritz C, Sjödin A, et al. The LEAF questionnaire: a screening tool for the identification of female athletes at risk for the female athlete triad. Br J Sports Med. 2014;48(7):540–5. doi:10.1136/bjsports-2013-093240.
30. American Psychiatric Association. Feeding and eating disorders. DSM-V. 2013. http://www.dsm5.org/documents/eating%20disorders%20fact%20sheet.pdf. Accessed 15 Apr 2015.
31. National Eating Disorder Information Centre (NEDIC). 2014. http://medic.ca/know-facts/definitions. Accessed 13 Feb 2015.
32. Brown TA, Keel PK, Striegel RH. Feeding and eating conditions not elsewhere classified (NEC) in DSM-V. Psychiatr Ann. 2012;42(11):421–5.
33. De Souza MJ, Nattiv A, Joy E, Misra M, Williams NI, Mallinson RJ, et al. Female athlete triad coalition consensus statement on treatment and return to play of the female athlete triad: 1st International Conference San Francisco, California, May 2012 and 2nd International Conference held in Indianapolis, Indiana, May 2013. Br J Sports Med. 2014;48(4):289. doi:10.1136/bjsports-2013-093218.
34. Barrack MT, Ackerman KE, Gibbs JG. Update on the female athlete triad. Curr Rev Musculoskelet Med. 2013;6(2):195–204. doi:10.1007/s12178-013-9168-9.
35. Rauch MJ, Nichols JF, Barrack MT. Relationships among injury and disordered eating, menstrual dysfunction, and low bone mineral density in high school athletes: a prospective study. J Athl Train. 2010;45(3):243–52. doi:10.4085/1062-6050-45.3.243.
36. Mallinson RJ, DeSouza MJ. Current perspectives on the etiology and manifestation of the "silent" component of the female athlete triad. Int J Women's Health. 2014;6:451–67. doi:10.2147/IJWH.S38603.
37. Gordon CM, Leonard MB, Zemel BS. 2013 pediatric position development conference: executive summary and reflections. J Clin Densitom. 2014;17:219–24.
38. Ducher G, Turner AI, Kukuljan S, Pantano KJ, Carlson JL, Williams NI, et al. Obstacles in the optimization of bone health outcomes in the female athlete triad. Sports Med. 2011;41(7):587–607. doi:10.2165/11588770-000000000-00000.
39. Hoch AZ, Lal S, Jurva JW, Gutterman DD. The female athlete triad and cardiovascular dysfunction. Phys Med Rehabil Clin N Am. 2007;18(3):385–400. doi:10.1016/j.pmr.2007.05.001.
40. Schächinger V, Britten MB, Zehler AM. Prognostic impact of coronary vasodilator dysfunction on adverse long-term outcome of coronary heart disease. Circulation. 2000;101:1899–906.
41. Rickenlund A, Eriksson MJ, Schenck-Gustafson K, Hirschberg AL. Amenorrhea in female athletes is associated with endothelial dysfunction and unfavorable lip profile. J Clin Endocrinol Metab. 2005;90:1354–9.
42. Troy K, Hoch AZ, Stavikos JE. Awareness and comfort in treating the female athlete triad: are we failing our athletes? WMJ. 2006;105:21–4.
43. Curry EJ, Matzkin E. The female athlete triad: who falls under the umbrella? American Academy of Orthopaedic Surgeons, *AOOS Now*. 2013. http://www.aaos.org/new/aaosnow/nov13/clinical10.
44. Female Athlete Triad Coalition: an international consortium. 2002. http://www.femaleathletetriad.org/for-professionals/information-for-physicians/. Accessed 20 Feb 2015.
45. Nattiv A, Loucks AB, Manore MM, Sanborn CF, Sundgot-Borgen J, Warren MP. The female athlete triad: position stand. MSSE. 2007. doi:10.1249/mss.0b013e318149f111.
46. Beck JS. Cognitive behavior therapy: basics and beyond, vol. 2. New York: Guilford Press; 2011.
47. Festinger L. A theory of cognitive dissonance. Stanford: Stanford University Press; 1957.

48. Becker CB, McDaniel L, Bull S, Powell M, McIntyre K. Can we reduce eating disorder risk factors in female college athletes? A randomized exploratory investigation of two peer-lead interventions. Body Image. 2012;9:31–42.
49. Randy KW, Aiken LS, Mackinnon DP, Elliot DL, Moe EL, McGinnis W, et al. A mediation analysis of the ATHENA intervention for female athletes: prevention of athletic-enhancing substance use and unhealthy weight loss behaviors. J Pediatr Psychol. 2009;34:1069–83.
50. Baer RA. Mindfulness training as a clinical intervention: a conceptual and empirical review. Clin Psychol Sci Pract. 2003;10:125–43.
51. Kabat-Zinn J. Full catastrophe living: using the wisdom of your body and mind to face stress and pain. New York: Random House; 1990.
52. Kabat-Zinn J. Mindfulness-based interventions in context: past, present and future. Clin Psychol Sci Pract. 2003;10:144–56.
53. Marlette GA, Witkiewitz K, Dillworth TM, et al. Vipassana meditation as a treatment for alcohol and drug use. In: Hayes SC, Follette VM, Linehan MM, editors. Mindfulness and acceptance: expanding the cognitive-behavioral tradition. New York: Guilford Press; 2004. p. 261–87.
54. Segal Z, Teasdale JD, Williams JM. Mindfulness-based cognitive therapy: theoretical rational and empirical status. In: Hayes SC, Follette VM, Linehan MM, editors. Mindfulness and acceptance: expanding the cognitive-behavioral tradition. New York: Guilford Press; 2004. p. 46–65.
55. Teasdale JD, Segal Z, Williams JM. How does cognitive therapy prevent depressive relapse and why should attentional control (mindfulness) training help? Behav Res Ther. 1995;33:25–39.
56. Linehan MM. Cognitive-behavioral treatment of borderline personality disorder. 1st ed. New York: Guilford Press; 1993.
57. Robins CJ, Schmidt H, Linehan MM. Dialectical behavior therapy: synthesizing radical acceptance with skillful means. In: Hayes SC, Follette VM, Linehan MM, editors. Mindfulness and acceptance: expanding the cognitive-behavioral tradition. New York: Guilford Press; 2004. p. 30–44.
58. Blackledge JT, Hayes SC. Emotion regulation in acceptance and commitment therapy. J Clin Psychol. 2001;57:243–55.
59. Hayes SC. Acceptance and commitment therapy and the new behavior therapies: mindfulness, acceptance and relationship. In: Hayes SC, Follette VM, Linehan MM, editors. Mindfulness and acceptance: expanding the cognitive-behavioral tradition. New York: Guilford Press; 2004. p. 1–29.
60. Harley therapy, CCBT vs MBCT-what is the difference. *Harley therapy counselling blog*. http://www.harleytherapy.co.uk/counselling/cbt-mbct-differences.htm.
61. Marks H. How medication treats eating disorders, Everyday health. www.everydayhealth.com/eating-disorders/,medication-to-=treat-eatingdisorders.
62. Aigner M, Treasure J, Kaye W, Kasper S. WFSBP task force on eating disorders. World Federation of Societies of Biological Psychiatry (WFSBP) guidelines for the pharmacological treatment of eating disorders. World J Biol Psychiatry. 2011;12:400–43. doi:10.3109/15622975.2011.602720.
63. Misra M, Katzman D, Miller KK, Mendes N, Snelgrove D, Russell M, et al. Physiologic estrogen replacement increases bone density in adolescent girls with anorexia nervosa. J Bone Miner Res. 2011;26(10):2430–8. doi:10.1002/jbmr.447.
64. Ackerman KE, Misra M. Bone health and the female athlete triad in adolescent athletes. Phys Sportsmed. 2011;39(1):131–41. doi:10.3810/psm.2011.02.1871.
65. McCabe MP, Smyth MP, Richardson DR. Current concept review: vitamin D and stress fractures. Foot Ankle Int. 2012;33(6):526–33. doi:10.3113/FAI.2012.0526.

66. Quinn E. Amenorrhea in athletes. http://sportsmedicine.about.com/od/women/a/Amerorrhea.htm.
67. Nguyen VH, Wang Z, Okamura SM. Osteoporosis health beliefs in women with increased risk of the female athlete triad. J Osteoporos. 2014;2014:676304. doi:10.1155/2014/676304.
68. Pantano K. Current knowledge, perceptions and interventions used by collegiate coaches in the U.S. regarding the prevention and treatment of the female athlete triad. N Am J Sports Phys Ther. 2006;1(4):195–207.

Chapter 20
The Challenge of Osteoporosis: A Look to the Future

Christina V. Oleson

Osteoporosis is manifested not only in terms of personal physical, financial, and emotional costs but also in the costs imposed on the larger society, ranging from rising healthcare expenditures to lost productivity on the part of disabled workers and increased morbidity and mortality rates in the aging population. With growing life expectancy worldwide, osteoporosis has become an important public health priority, both in developed nations and in developing countries as they become increasingly westernized.

Studies cited throughout this book indicate the magnitude of the osteoporosis challenge. At the same time, some investigators have noted a trend, developing over the past two decades, toward a stabilized and subsequent declining rate of hip fractures in North America and Sweden (which have the highest incidences worldwide), together with a concomitant increased fracture risk in Asia and Latin America [1]. A study involving the entire population of Sweden over the age of 60 [2] speculated about several reasons for the decline, ranging from preventative measures to more effective treatment options and rising body weight. At this stage, however, causal factors remain a matter of conjecture. Moreover, this seemingly good news is tempered by the recognition that the lifetime risk of a hip fracture has not decreased given increased life expectancy and that survival after hip fracture has not improved. Ultimately the observed fracture reduction may be attributed not to a decline in the rate of osteoporosis but to changes in lifestyle. The question awaits further research as do many issues regarding the future of osteoporosis.

This book reviews the new approaches, strategies, and medications developed for the prevention and treatment of osteoporosis in itself and in the context of other diseases. Although it does not admit of a summary conclusion, it does offer the opportunity to review a number of broader concerns that must be addressed if we are to alleviate the burden of this disease.

C.V. Oleson, *Osteoporosis Rehabilitation*, DOI 10.1007/978-3-319-45084-1_20

Barriers to More Effective Osteoporosis Prevention and Treatment

In recent years, evidence-based guidelines for the diagnosis and treatment of osteoporosis have been issued in the United States, Canada, and countries around the world; in addition, important advances have been made in terms of diagnostic and therapy options [13] (Fig. 1). At the same time, studies continue to illustrate a disconnect between the presence of fracture risk, as well as actual fractures, and the implementation of preventative and treatment measures. In a study of 459 patients over the age of 60, chest radiography revealed that one in six (16 %) had clinically significant vertebral fractures of which only 60 % were recorded and only 25 % were diagnosed or treated for osteoporosis [3]. In a 2014 review of the "osteoporosis treatment gap," Kanis et al. reported that fewer than 20 % of subjects with fragility fractures received treatment to reduce fracture risk in the year following the incident, with an even greater gap for the elderly—as low as 10 % of elderly women with fractures—and for those in long-term care [4].

Obstacles to improving diagnosis and care stem from physician perspectives and practices, the policies of healthcare systems and insurance carriers, and the beliefs and actions of patients.

Physicians

In a leading-edge examination of physicians' knowledge of osteoporosis, Rizzoli et al. surveyed general practitioners/primary care physicians (GPs/PCPs) and specialists (rheumatologists, endocrinologists, gynecologists, orthopedists) in 13

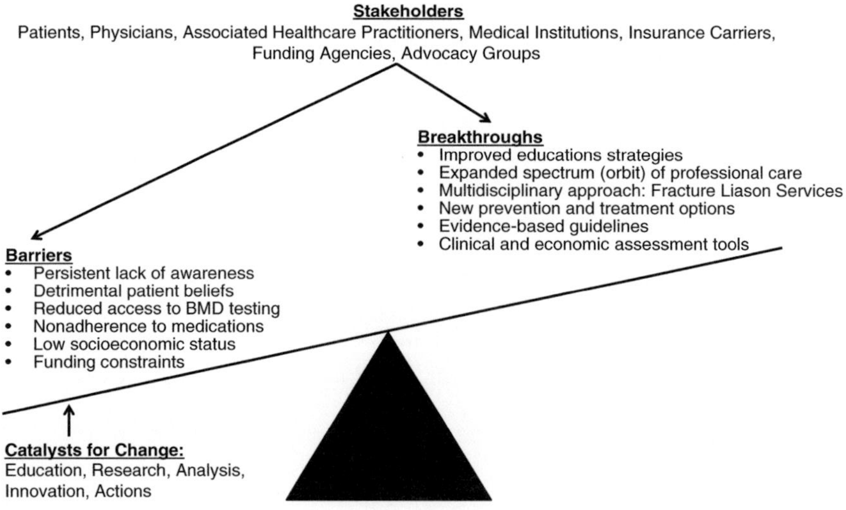

Fig. 1 Stakeholders are countering barriers with breakthroughs by utilizing catalysts for change

countries, finding that physicians did not fully recognize patient's concerns about the effect of osteoporosis on their quality of life [5]. Physicians underestimated the extent to which patients worry about (1) breaking a bone, (2) a potential decline in activity levels, (3) dependency on others, (4) inability to work as long as needed, and (5) compliance with prescribed treatments. For example, they believe that 71 % of patients forget to take medications, whereas patients put that figure at 20 %.

In terms of physician responsibility, osteoporosis remains, to a considerable extent, an "orphan" disease. The two groups most closely associated with osteoporosis care are orthopedic surgeons and GPs/PCPs. Because osteoporosis may remain undetected until a fracture actually occurs, the first point of contact for patients is likely to be an orthopedic surgeon. Although national and international organizations advocate greater involvement of orthopedic surgeons in osteoporosis management, a multinational survey of 3,422 orthopedic surgeons reported a failure or inability to assume this responsibility for reasons ranging from insufficient knowledge of fracture management to time constraints [6].

Much the same is true for primary care physicians who must deal with a number of preventative care issues in their limited time with patients. Without in-depth expertise in osteoporosis care, they are faced with conflicting information about the nature and availability of DXA testing, the adverse effects and long-term safety of osteoporosis medications, and potential complications in treating patients with comorbidities—all of which are exacerbated for doctors who have little or no contact with major hospital centers and for those practicing in rural areas [7]. Lack of clarity about where the responsibility lies in managing osteoporosis is, in itself, an impediment to effective care.

Healthcare Systems and Insurers

National healthcare systems and private insurers may have stated missions to improve osteoporosis care, but their actions often fail to live up to expectations. Inadequate support for osteoporosis testing, lack of incentives for preventative action, and limited opportunities for patient counseling and education are among the factors that hinder efforts to achieve optimal care and contribute to the rising financial burden of osteoporosis. Between \$3.1 billion and \$4.3 billion is spent annually on elderly osteoporosis patients with a bone fracture, and by 2025, the cost of osteoporotic-related fractures is expected to reach \$25.3 billion [8]. Medicare and Medicaid currently cover about 75 % of osteoporosis costs for women over age 45.

Early detection and preventative measures are crucial in controlling costs. Medicare reimbursement policies for osteoporosis DXA scans is an important case in point. The clinical benefits of DXA testing to diagnose osteoporosis, as well as to monitor response to drug therapy, have been clearly demonstrated. However, physician reimbursement for these scans, conducted in an office setting, has been reduced significantly from a high of about \$140 in 2006 to a low of approximately \$40 for both physicians' fees and technical costs, as of this writing—a 75 %

decrease. In a hospital setting, the rate is $110.28 for both the professional and technical component [9].

With physicians unable to recover the costs of administering the procedure, access to osteoporotic testing has been severely restricted. In 2002, 70 % of all DXA scans were performed in the offices of primary care doctors, rheumatologists, and endocrinologists or in small imaging centers; a decade and more later, many of these physicians can no longer afford to offer this protective service. From 2008 to 2011, the number of US physicians conducting office-based DXAs decreased by 12.9 %, with even larger declines, from 30 % to 60 %, in rural areas [10].

The implications of the shift to hospital-based DXAs and the detrimental impact on access to testing are both manifold and disquieting, potentially resulting in greater health and cost burdens in the long term. With scans increasingly undertaken by hospital radiology departments, lack of communication with referring physicians and failure to account for multiple chronic conditions may occur. Radiologists may not have full knowledge of the patients' preexisting conditions or medications, resulting in misdiagnosis and recommendations of inappropriate treatments. In making an osteoporosis diagnosis, all aspects of a patient's health must be considered, especially in the elderly who may well experience such comorbidities as heart disease, stroke, diabetes, hypertension, or kidney failure. Treatment of one condition may adversely affect treatment of another, or an emergency situation can overshadow the gradual, more "silent," development of osteoporosis. In a larger perspective, the societal cost of osteoporosis will inevitably rise as fracture prevention efforts diminish [11].

In the case of patients who have access to DXA testing, Medicare does provide coverage under one of several conditions [12]: (1) women determined by a physician to be estrogen deficient and at risk for osteoporosis; (2) persons whose x-rays show possible osteoporosis, osteopenia, and vertebral fractures; (3) individuals with vertebral abnormalities and primary hyperparathyroidism; and (4) those receiving steroid therapy or FDA-approved drugs that require regular monitoring. The likelihood of osteoporosis can be "discussed" as part of the no cost, one-time "Welcome to Medicare" preventative visit or once every two years at annual "Wellness" visits, but neither are the equivalent of a thorough physical examination and screening. Healthcare practitioners require more time, as well as the diagnostic tools, to assess risk factors for osteoporosis and determine prevention and treatment options.

Patients

Health Beliefs

Among the primary barriers to effective osteoporosis care are patients themselves, specifically their personal beliefs about osteoporosis and their failure to adhere to prescribed medications and other treatments. As defined in the *Health Belief Model*

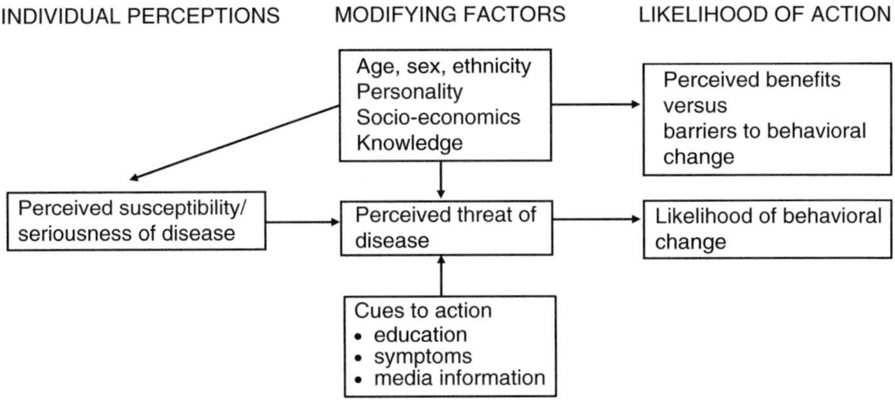

Fig. 2 Health belief model and its key components. How modifying factors, cues to action, and self-efficacy (#7 below) influence perceived susceptibility and seriousness, benefits and barriers, and ultimately likelihood of action. *Source*: Adapted from Champion and Skinner [55]

(HBM) [13] osteoporosis beliefs, originally confined to the categories of perceived benefits of exercise and calcium intake, have now been expanded to include:

1. Perceived susceptibility to osteoporosis
2. Perceived severity of the disease
3. Perceived benefits of action in terms of reducing risk and seriousness of the disease
4. Perceived barriers to action in terms of tangible and psychological costs (e.g. expense, negative side effects)
5. Modifying variables: age, gender, ethnicity, education, and socioeconomic level; past experiences
6. Internal and external cues to action—from pain and other symptoms to advice from family and physicians
7. Self-efficacy: confidence in one's ability to take action

The preceding figure outlines the interaction of these constructs (Fig. 2) [13]:

In a study of 1,268 women and men age 60 and over, Nayak et al. [14] identified the failure to recognize personal susceptibility to the disease as the strongest impediment to preventative and therapeutic action. Only 44.6 % of participants believed they were at risk for osteoporosis, and only 26.3 % thought they would develop it, despite the fact that age is the predominant factor in predicting osteoporosis. These findings are consistent with the results of earlier studies [15] and clearly demonstrate that to underestimate the health impact of osteoporosis is to create insurmountable obstacles to prevention and treatment.

Adherence

Another barrier is the failure to adhere to prescribed medications. Patients do not fill prescriptions, do not take the prescribed dose at the prescribed time, and do not follow instructions concerning restrictions on drug ingestion (medication preceding food intake by 30–60 min in the morning, upright positioning); moreover, they forget to take medications or discontinue their use altogether. Kothawala et al. demonstrated that one-third to one-half of patients fail to take their medications as directed and that nonadherence occurs shortly after treatment begins [16]. In terms of persistence, the Netherlands analysis of 8,626 patients treated with ten different oral osteoporosis drugs found a 12-month persistence rate of 43 % (in line with other findings of 30–52 % in the Netherlands); moreover, in an 18-month follow-up period, 78 % of patients who stopped treatment failed to restart. As indicated in other trials, persistence was lower for daily than for weekly bisphosphonate administration [17].

Simply forgetting to take medications is not the principal issue. As Donovan and Blake have demonstrated [18], lack of compliance is primarily the result of a conscious decision based on such circumstances as troubling side effects (nausea, heartburn), complexity of instructions for ingesting certain drugs (particularly in the case of oral bisphosphonates), doubts about the safety and efficacy of prescribed drugs, and apprehension about out-of-pocket costs. Some patients maintain that nonmedicinal interventions can alleviate the problem. In the absence of a fracture, patients are further deterred by the fact that they generally experience no symptoms and consequently lack the" pain relief syndrome" that can serve as a motivation [19].

Most recently, some striking figures have emerged relating to nonadherence, particularly with respect to bisphosphonates. In an analysis of FDA rulings and media reports relating to the safety of these drugs, specifically regarding osteonecrosis of the jaw, atrial fibrillation, and atypical femur fractures, Jha et al. [20] found that Internet searches for alendronate spiked markedly between 2006 and 2010 and that the use of oral bisphosphonates declined precipitously—by greater than 50 % between 2008 and 2012 after a period of increasing use for over a decade. A subsequent study demonstrated that among more than 22,000 patients with hip fractures, bisphosphonate use declined from an already low 15 % in 2004 to 3 % at the end of 2013 [21]. In an analysis of what they term "a crisis in the treatment of osteoporosis," Khosla and Shane emphasize that physicians must do more to educate patients about the benefits and costs of these treatments. In particular, they point to the tendency of patients to lose "all sense of proportion" about the relative versus the absolute risk of these medications, underlining the need to bring to bear the grave consequences of osteoporosis as opposed to the much most limited risks of bisphosphonates for those who must make an informed choice [22].

Thus far, efforts to improve compliance, ranging from extended dosing intervals and intravenous administration of some drugs to regular patient monitoring by physicians/nurses, have been implemented but with limited results. More effective steps, for example, a means of providing positive feedback to patients, are needed to advance adherence.

Strategies to Improve Osteoporosis Management

Collaboration and integration are the key to the most promising interventions designed to advance osteoporosis care. Healthcare professionals with knowledge vital to managing osteoporosis represent a wide range of expertise, from primary care physicians, rheumatologists, endocrinologists, and geriatricians, to nurses, pharmacists, nutritionists, physical and occupational therapists, and home health-care providers. To bring together the broad-based information they offer requires a multifaceted approach, combining education, counseling, and direct care.

Education-Based Approaches for Patients and Physicians

Information about all aspects of osteoporosis diagnosis and care abounds in a plethora of books, pamphlets, guidelines, brochures, articles, websites, and other sources. However, the sheer existence of these materials and their often-random dissemination, often termed "passive medical education," has had only a limited effect on the behavior of patients and physicians. Knowledge is an important first step in increasing awareness of osteoporosis, but it does not necessarily translate into changed beliefs or behaviors. Targeted, interactive educational interventions show greater promise of producing tangible results.

For Patients

Educational programs linked to the health belief model framework have produced mixed results. An analysis of several intervention programs based on these beliefs resulted in higher levels of knowledge, but no appreciable change in the health beliefs of the participants [23]. Applying the constructs of the health belief model, another approach, an osteoporosis prevention program for middle-aged women, incorporated visuals illustrating the adverse effects of osteoporosis, lectures by dieticians, physical activity programs, and a DXA test followed by a consultation to share the results with patients and to offer individualized advice [24]. Actual belief changes were not reported, but knowledge was enhanced through a highly interactive program.

However, more recent research has demonstrated promising results in terms of behavioral change. In an examination of postmenopausal women, Swaim et al. [25] showed that improving their self-efficacy was associated with improved calcium intake and engagement in exercise programs. A 2014 study of 240 females, based on a questionnaire employing HMD constructs [26], provided further insight into the factors influencing exercise behavior in osteoporosis. A subsequent trial involving women ages 30–50 [27] demonstrated that the use of the HBM over a 6-month period led to adoption of improved nutrition and walking behaviors as well as an increase in BMD. However, larger studies involving both men and women and accounting for educational backgrounds and socioeconomic factors are needed to determine the potential of interventions based on HBM.

In an examination of compliance with osteoporosis treatments, Warriner and Curtis [28] found that information garnered from an osteoporosis leaflet had the least effect, whereas provider–patient interaction produced a better result. Included in this exchange should be discussion of the results of DXA scans, changes in bone turnover markers, the benefits of osteoporosis medications, and feedback on treatment results. Direct involvement of patients in a dialogue about their experience with osteoporosis is critical in promoting effective therapy.

For Physicians

Whereas passive distribution of written information has been shown to have little effect on patients' behavior, physicians themselves seek up-to-date, easy-to-follow, evidence-based printed guidelines, applicable to their patient population and cognizant of their time limitations. These materials should focus on the clinical management of osteoporosis including bone densitometry screening and the safety and efficacy of available medications [29].

However, even for physicians, the educational strategies found to be most effective are both structured and interactive. For example, in a study focusing on recognition of vertebral fractures by general internists in a large teaching hospital, a two-phase intervention produced positive results [30]. In phase I, radiologists identified 34 % of patients with at least one vertebral fracture, independent investigators found 29 %, but internists detected only 22 %; following an internist education program that included lectures, discussions, and printed material (phase II), the detection rate among internists almost doubled to 43 %. Patients benefiting from this educational strategy increased from 11 % (phase I) to 40 % (phase II). Numerous continuing education programs to improve physicians' knowledge of osteoporosis exist, but the task of educating patients must still compete with other, often more pressing, demands placed on family physicians during their limited appointment times.

Additional Resources for Osteoporosis Education and Generalized Care

Given the fact that physicians cannot simultaneously serve as "educators" and "care providers," other resources, specifically support groups, nurse practitioners/physician assistants, pharmacists, nutritionists, and therapists can provide alternative means of informing and monitoring osteoporosis patients.

Support Groups

Both in person and online, support groups can serve as a resource for osteoporosis patients, family members, and caregivers by providing guidance and counsel about prevention, screening, treatment, and coping mechanisms as well as the opportunity to share experiences with others who encounter similar challenges on a daily basis. This interaction can also dispel myths about osteoporosis that persist despite the abundance of written and web-based educational materials. In a sympathetic yet inquisitive environment, group members can exchange information and perspectives to counter a wide range of misconceptions, i.e., only women have osteoporosis, osteoporosis is another form of arthritis, osteoporosis prevention takes too much effort, and instructions for treatment medications are too hard to follow [31].

Nurse Practitioners/Physician Assistants

As stated in the 2004 Surgeon General's report, expanding the role of nurse practitioners and physician assistants in the diagnosis and treatment of osteoporosis is one of the most promising ways to increase the efficacy of care. Nurses interact with patients in various settings—primary care, fracture clinics, long-term care facilities, and home care—as well as with the broader community through schools and outreach activities [32].

Through assessment, counseling, and education, on a one-to-one basis or in group sessions, nurses are in a unique position to advance patient understanding of the causes of osteoporosis, how it can be detected and controlled, the potential outcome of taking medications to reduce fracture risk, and the side effects of these drugs [33]. They can also offer psychosocial support aimed at ensuring compliance with medications and identifying and implementing coping mechanisms including pain management options [32]. In a randomized trial of 75 postmenopausal women taking reloxifene, Clowes et al. determined that monitoring by nurses increased adherence by 57 % compared with no monitoring and that bone marker monitoring provided no added improvement over nurse monitoring alone. They also cited a 25 % borderline significant increase in the monitored group's *persistence* with therapy compared with those under usual care, emphasizing the ability of healthcare professionals to bolster a positive patient response for a longer period [34].

However, to carry out this responsibility effectively, nurses require training in the assessment techniques, management skills, and evidence-based practices essential to the prevention and treatment of osteoporosis. Existing nursing-school curricula and osteoporosis-related continuing education should be enhanced to prepare nurses for this broader role.

Pharmacists

Pharmacists are another readily available source of information about osteoporosis and can potentially play a role in identifying patients at risk of the disease and improving adherence/persistence with therapy. In a Canadian study of patients [35] enrolled in a community pharmacy osteoporosis program, BMD screening more than doubled compared with controls—22 % versus 11 %—and calcium intake increased 30 % as against controls (19 %). Serving as a liaison between physicians and elderly patients with untreated atraumatic fractures, clinical pharmacists at Kaiser Permanente Colorado provided advice on calcium and vitamin D supplements, BMD testing, and pharmacotherapy options. As a result, 50 % of patients either initiated treatment or received a BMD test [36]. Other trials have demonstrated that pharmacists can improve patient compliance with nonpharmacological and pharmacological treatments [37] and identify patients who may be at risk of glucocorticoid-induced osteoporosis.

Project ImPACT: Osteoporosis, a program sponsored by the American Pharmacists Association Foundation, has added another component to the arsenal of community pharmacy interventions. In addition to considering the education, screening, and management services within the purview of pharmacists, it reported that patients as well as a third-party payer—United Healthcare of the Mid-Atlantic—were willing to compensate pharmacists for their assistance [38]. However, the risk of bias in these and other investigations necessitates further examination, as does the feasibility of implementing these interventions more broadly given such impediments as disruption of workflow, need for additional training, insufficient reimbursement, the absence of a collaborative relationship with area physicians, and the inability to access patient's medical records [39, 40].

Nonetheless, it is an opportune time to consider an expanded role for pharmacists in healthcare. As pharmacy technicians assume increased responsibility for drug dispensing tasks, pharmacists can enroll in specialized certification programs that offer training in osteoporosis screening and monitoring, prevention strategies, and drug therapy; such programs also incorporate business strategies for implementing pharmacist care, including the cost of portable BMD machines; contract arrangements with large employers, health clubs, and nursing homes; and collaboration with physicians to ensure reimbursement by Medicare and private insurers [41].

Nutritionists/Therapists

Nutritionists and dieticians can also provide information essential to osteoporosis prevention and treatment particularly given the fact that physicians' knowledge of nutrition is notably lacking. In a 2008–2009 survey of 105 targeted US medical schools, researchers found that only 27 % met the minimum 25 required hours of nutrition education set by the National Academy of Sciences, whereas in 2004, 38 % of 104 schools did [42]. In cooperation with nutritionists, physical and occupational therapists develop exercise programs aimed at regulating bone maintenance, stimulating bone formation, strengthening upper and lower body muscles, improving coordination and balance, preventing falls, and developing an increased sense of independence in undertaking daily activities.

Healthcare Delivery: Fraction Liaison Services

In osteoporosis as in many chronic diseases, the key to improving cost-effectiveness, increasing the efficacy of outcomes, and advancing medication compliance and persistence is a change in the healthcare delivery system. For osteoporosis patients who have experienced a fragility fracture, that change is represented by the introduction of Fracture Liaison Services (FLS)—a collaborative "systems" approach to identifying these patients and providing them with subsequent, integrated, multidisciplinary care. The key steps in the FLS pathway are identification, investigation, and intervention [43].

Central to the operation of a FLS are:

1. A physician "champion," usually an orthopedic surgeon, who makes the case for the program and determines funding options, contributes to the implementation of a system to identify fracture patients and to track outcomes and initiates the hiring of the FLS coordinator.
2. The FLS coordinator, generally a nurse practitioner or physician assistant knowledgeable about current osteoporosis guidelines and treatments, is responsible for screening eligible patients, recommending the necessary bone mineral density tests and FRAX reviews, initiating osteoporosis therapy, ensuring follow-up for treatment recommendations, and organizing educational programs. The coordinator must involve other specialists, such as physical and occupational therapists, nutritionists, and possibly psychologists, in the patient's care and inform the primary care provider of progress and impediments.
3. Nurse manager or "navigator," often the first point of contact with the program, ensures that all patients eligible for the program and wishing to participate are enrolled, facilitates communication within the care team including physicians and other specialists, and assists with osteoporosis education and medication administration [44, 45].

Analyses of the outcomes of Fracture Liaison Services demonstrate greatly improved quality of care as well as cost-effectiveness. As Miki et al. have observed [46], although hip fractures are directly associated with osteoporosis, the initiation of treatment following a fracture can be as low as 5–30 %. In their comparison of osteoporosis management by an orthopedic team as opposed to a primary care physician, the percentage of patients undergoing treatment at six months following fracture was significantly greater—58 %—when initiated by an orthopedic team at an osteoporosis clinic than when initiated by a PCP—29 %. Yates et al. are among a number of researchers confirming the efficacy of FLSs, adding that this form of osteoporosis intervention is not only welcomed by patients but also cost-effective [47]. Eighty-five of 90 questionnaire respondents reported that they were very satisfied or satisfied with their FLS. In terms of cost, the researchers estimated that when treatment is prescribed over five years, the cost would be $1,716 per patient with an incremental cost-effectiveness ratio of $31,749. In a recent Swedish study based on a hypothetical group of 1,000 fracture patients, 393 patients started treatment in a

FLS, resulting in the saving of 22 fractures, 19 quality-adjusted life years, and 40 added life years [48].

Among the two most prominent FLS models in the United States are the Kaiser Permanente "Healthy Bones" model and the Geisinger Health System osteoporosis disease management program. The National Bone Health Alliance, the American Society for Bone and Mineral Research, and the International Osteoporosis Foundation are among the organizations that strongly advocate implementation of the FLS model in the United States and around the world.

Analytical Tools in Assessing the Osteoporosis Burden

As noted above, the number of Americans with osteoporosis and low bone density, now estimated at 54 million, is expected to grow to 64.4 million by 2020 and to 71.2 million by 2030. Absolute numbers are one measure of the extent of the disease, but comparing the burden of osteoporosis with that of other chronic diseases provides a different, equally disturbing perspective on its severity and cost. In their comparative study of women 55 years and older, Singer et al. [49] reported than an estimated 50 % of women over 55 will experience an osteoporotic fracture (OF), whereas an estimated 13 % will be diagnosed with breast cancer over a lifetime. In terms of incidence of hospitalizations in the United States over the period 2000–2011, there were 4.9 million hospitalizations for OF, 2.9 million for myocardial infarction (MI), 3.0 million for stroke, and 0.7 million for breast cancer. The facility-related hospital costs were highest for OFs ($5.1 billion) compared with MI ($4.3 billion), stroke ($3.0 billion), and breast cancer ($0.5 billion.) Admittedly there are measures of disease burden other than hospitalization rates and costs, as well as treatment centers other than hospitals; however, these findings again underline the need for improving both primary and secondary fracture prevention efforts.

To an increasing extent, economic analysis is being employed to determine how limited financial resources can be most effectively allocated in terms of the osteoporosis challenge. Cost-effectiveness studies of available therapeutic options provide a basis for determining which interventions offer the greatest benefits [50]. As Tosteson illustrates, several studies focused on postmenopausal women have been critical in determining the amount of time required before treatment benefits can be realized—a finding that may exert a different influence on private insurers of women under 65 than on Medicare. Because the former typically have a 10-year time horizon, they may not regard testing and medication as being cost-effective, given the likelihood that a fracture will not occur during their coverage period, whereas Medicare could conclude that screening and interventions are cost-effective in terms of preventing fractures and their associated costs later in life.

Other analyses, often termed "burden-of-illness" studies, focus on time lost from work, leisure, or other unpaid activities, caretakers' expenses whether in a nursing home or at home, and, more broadly, the extent of the disease and its impact on national healthcare budgets and policies [51]. In contrast to cost-effectiveness analyses, they are generally used to increase understanding of the clinical and economic implications of osteoporosis as opposed to specific resource allocation. Employed on a global scale together with demographic projections, they are useful in assessing the extent and burden of osteoporosis in varying circumstances around the world.

The strategies outlined here—from education programs aimed at both physicians and patients and community support groups, both in person and on line to improved strategies for promoting adherence and persistence with medication and broader implementation of multidisciplinary, coordinated fracture liaison programs—are all critical elements in advancing knowledge about osteoporosis within the medical community, the broader public, and policy-makers. In addition, though a variety of multifaceted programs, national and international osteoporosis organizations work to increase public awareness; educate patients, physicians, and the wider public; establish guidelines for prevention and care; administer research programs; and advocate for increased funding to ensure that osteoporosis becomes a public health priority. In a position statement originally issued in 1993 and revised in 2014, the American Academy of Orthopedic Surgeons/American Association of Orthopedic Surgeons strongly stated the case for increased federal and private funding to evaluate current treatments, develop new therapeutic agents, institute effective educational programs, and expand team-oriented medical management [52].

The Case for Prevention and Early Treatment

Given the medical and societal consequences of osteoporosis, greater attention should be focused on developing effective prevention programs, both prior and subsequent to fracture occurrence. Taking a long-term perspective, osteoporosis prevention should ideally begin in childhood and adolescence with a healthy diet and a regular exercise program; unfortunately this is seldom the case. Because osteoporosis has few, if any, warning signs, healthcare practitioners must make every effort to initiate preventative measures, especially among the at-risk population. The US Preventive Services Task Force (USPSTF) identifies a twofold approach—advance screening and the reduction of controllable risk factors [53]:

1. DXA in combination with FRAX are the critical tools in the diagnosis of osteoporosis. Further research is needed on the cost, insurance coverage, and availability of DXA testing worldwide to determine how to increase access to what is regarded as "the gold standard" for measuring bone density.
2. The adoption of multifaceted approaches to educate physicians and patients must focus on information about the risk factors for osteoporosis and provide easily accessible guidelines for preventative action in the form of adequate calcium and vitamin D intake, a healthy diet, elimination of tobacco use, a regimen of weight-bearing exercises, the use of drugs as prescribed, and fall avoidance including increased balance and stability and elimination of environmental hazards in everyday activities.

To prevent secondary fractures following an initial incident, Fracture Liaison Services have proved to be one of the most significant new treatment programs to emerge in decades. Not only do they increase adherence to osteoporosis treatment, but they advance knowledge of the disease and increase patients' ability to oversee their own care in the context of an ongoing partnership with health professionals and their family/caretakers [54].

Ultimately, prevention and treatment of osteoporosis must be the responsibility of individual patients. They must fully understand and bear in mind the consequences of osteoporosis: pain, disability, restricted opportunities for work and leisure activities, loss of independence, and even possibly death. If patients schedule regular doctor visits, healthcare professionals can review symptoms, order screening tests, prescribe therapies, and adjust treatment plans to better conform to specific needs while repeatedly stressing the importance of calcium and vitamin D intake, exercise, and a healthy lifestyle. In the future, more effective ways to address prevailing—often devastating—health beliefs and to improve adherence to medications should lead to significant advances in osteoporosis care.

Osteoporosis is preventable, and its challenges can be met but only through the combined efforts of informed patients, knowledgeable physicians, coordinated care systems, dedicated researchers, determined impartial advocates for improved bone health, and increased funding for research, education, and innovations in healthcare delivery.

References

1. Cooper C, Cole ZA, Holroyd CR, Earl SC, Harvey NC, Dennison EM, et al. Secular trends in the incidence of hip and other osteoporotic fractures. Osteoporos Int. 2011;22(5):1277 88.
2. Karampampa K, Ahlborn A, Michaelsson K, Andersson T, Drefahl S, Modig K. Declining incidence trends for hip fracture have not been accompanied by improvements in lifetime risk of post-fracture survival—a nationwide study of the Swedish population 60 years and older. Bone. 2015;78:55–61. http://dx.doi.org/10/1016/j.bone.2015.04032.
3. Majumdar S, Kim N, Colman I, Chahal AM, Raymond G, Jen H, et al. Incidental vertebral fractures discovered with chest radiography in the emergency department: prevalence, recognition, and osteoporosis management in a cohort of elderly patients. Arch InternMed. 2005;165(8):905–9.
4. Kanis JA, Svedbom A, Harvey N, McCloskey EV. The osteoporosis treatment gap. J Bone Miner Res. 2014;29(9):1926–8.
5. Rizzoli R, Brandi ML, Dreinhofer K, Thomas T, Wahl DA, Cooper C. The gaps between patient and physician understanding of the emotional and physical impact of osteoporosis. Arch Osteoroporos. 2010;5:145–53.
6. Dreinhofer KE, Anderson M, Feron J-M, Herrera A, Hube R, Johnell O, et al. Multinational survey of osteoporotic fracture management. Osteoporos Int. 2005;16 Suppl 2:S44–53.
7. Saag, KG. Overcoming the barriers: strategies for improving osteoporosis management. Medscape Multispecialty. 2011. http://www.medscape.org/viewarticle/739558. Accessed 17 Jul 2015.
8. Ajayi A, Powell M, Obremskey WT, Jahangir A, Sethi MK. Osteoporosis: the orthopedic health policy perspective. AAOS News. 2012: http://www.aaos.org/news/aaosnow/jan12/advocacy6/.
9. Regulatory and 3rd party payer issues. International Society for Clinical Densitometry. 2015. http://www.iscd.org/publicpolicy/regulatory-payer-issues/. Accessed 12 Dec 2015.

10. King AB, Fiorentino DM. Medicare payment cuts for osteoporosis testing reduced use despite tests' benefit in reducing fractures. Health Aff (Millwood). 2011;30(12):2362–70. doi:10.1377/hlthaff.2011.0233.
11. Lewiechi EM, Laster AJ, Miller PD, Bilezikian JP. Viewpoint: more bone density testing is needed, not less. J Bone Miner Res. 2012;27(4):749–42.
12. Centers for Medicare and Medicaid . Services. Bone mass measurements (bone density). 2016. https://www.medicare.gov/coverage/bone-density.html. Accessed 16 Feb 2016.
13. Champion VL, Skinner CE. The health belief model. In: Glanz K, Rimer BK, Viswanath K, editors. Health behavior and health education: theory, research and practice. 4th edition Hoboken: Wiley; 2008. p. 47–50.
14. Nayak S, Roberts MS, Chang C-CH, Greenspan SL. Health beliefs about osteoporosis and osteoporosis screening in older women and men. Health Educ J. 2010;69(3):267–76.
15. Gerend MA, Erchull MJ, Aiken LS, Maner JK. Reasons and risk factors underlying women's perceptions of susceptibility to osteoporosis. Maturitis. 2006;55(3):227–37.
16. Kothawala P, Badamgarav E, Ryu S, Miller RM, Halbert RJ. Systematic review and meta-analysis of real-world adherence to drug therapy for osteoporosis. Mayo Clin Proc. 2007;82(12):1493–501.
17. Netelenbos JC, Geusens PP, Ypma G, Buijs SJE. Adherence and profile of non-persistence in patients treated for osteoporosis—a large-scale, long-term retrospective study in the Netherlands. Osteoporos Int. 2011;22(5):1537–46.
18. Donovan JL, Blake DR. Patient non-compliance: deviance or reasoned decision-making? Soc Sci Med. 1992;34(5):507–13.
19. Dontas IA, Yiannakopoulos CK. Risk factors and prevention of osteoporosis-related fractures. J Musculoskelet Neuronal Interact. 2007;7(3):268–72.
20. Jha S, Wang Z, Laucis N, Bhattacharyya T. Trends in media reports, oral bisphosphonate prescriptions, and hip fractures, 1996–2012: an ecological analysis. J Bone Miner Res. 2015;30(12):2179–87.
21. Kim SC, Kim DH, Mogun H, Eddings W, Polinski JM, Franklin JM, et al. Impact of the U.S. Food and Drug Administration's safety-related announcements on the use of bisphosphonates after hip fractures. J Bone Miner Res. 2016;31:1536. doi:10.1002/jbmr/2832.
22. Khosla S, Shane E. A crisis in the treatment of osteoporosis. J Bone Miner Res. 2016;31:1485. doi:10.1002/jbmr.2888.
23. Sedlak CA, Doheny MO, Jones SL. Osteoporosis education programs: changing knowledge and behaviors. Public Health Nurs. 2000;17(5):398–402.
24. Turner LW, Hunt SB, DiBrezzo R, Jones C. Design and implementation of an osteoporosis prevention program using the health belief model. Am J Health Stud. 2004;19(2):115–21.
25. Swaim RA, Barner JC, Brown CM. The relationship of calcium intake and exercise to osteoporosis health beliefs in postmenopausal women. Res Soc Admin Pharm. 2008;4(2):153–63.
26. Soleymanian A, Niknami S, Hajizadeh E, Shojacizadeh D, Montazeri A. Development and validation of a health-belief model based instrument for measuring factors influencing exercise behaviors to prevent osteoporosis in pre-menopausal women (HOPE). BMC Musculoskel Disord. 2014. doi:10.1186/1471-2474-15-61.
27. Jeihooni AK, Hidamai A, Kaveh MH, Hajizadeh E, Askan A. Effects of an osteoporosis prevention program based on health belief model among females. Nurs Midwifery Stud. 2015;4(3):e26731. doi:10.17795/nmsjournal26731.
28. Warriner AH, Curtis JR. Adherence to osteoporosis treatments: room for improvement. Curr Opin Rheumatol. 2009;21(4):356–62.
29. Jaglal SB, Carroll J, Hawker G, McIsaac WJ, Jaakkuimainen L, Cadarette SM, et al. How are family physicians managing osteoporosis? Qualitative study of their experiences and educational needs. Can Fam Physician. 2003;49:462–8.
30. Casez P, Uebelhart B, Gaspoz J-M, Ferrari S, Louis-Simonet M, Rizzoli R. Targeted education improves the very low recognition of vertebral fractures and osteoporosis management by general internists. Osteoporos Int. 2006;17(7):965–70.

31. McClung BL, Overdorf JH. Psychosocial aspects of osteoporosis. In: Rosen CW, editor. Osteoporosis: diagnostic and therapeutic principles. New York: Springer Science and Business Media; 1996. p. 73.
32. International Osteoporosis Foundation. The role of nurses in osteoporosis. 2006. http://www.iofbonehealth.org/role-nurses-osteoporosis. Accessed 24 July 2015.
33. Besser SJ, Anderson JE, Weinman J. How do osteoporosis patients perceive their illness and treatment? Implications for clinical practice. Arch Osteoporos. 2012;7:115–24.
34. Clowes JA, Peel NFA, Eastell RE. The impact of monitoring on adherence and persistence with antiresorptive treatment for postmenopausal osteoporosis: a randomized controlled trial. J Clin Endocrin Met. 2004;89(3):1117–23.
35. Yuksel N, Majumdar S, Biggs C, Tsuyuki R. Community pharmacist-initiated screening program for osteoporosis: randomized controlled trial. Osteoporos Int. 2010;21(3):391–8.
36. Nadrash TA, Plushner SL, Delate T. Clinical pharmacists' role in improving osteoporosis treatment rates among elderly patients with untreated atraumatic fractures. Ann Pharmacother. 2008;42(3):334–40.
37. Hall LN, Shrader SP, Ragucci KR. Evaluation of compliance with osteoporosis treatment guidelines after initiation of a pharmacist-run osteoporosis service at a family medicine clinic. Ann Pharmacother. 2009;43(11):1781–6.
38. Goode JV, Swiger K, Bluml BM. Regional osteoporosis screening, referral, and monitoring program in community pharmacies: findings from Project ImPACT: osteoporosis. J Am Pharm Assoc. 2004;44(2):152–60.
39. Elias MN, Burden AM, Cadarette SM. The impact of pharmacist interventions on osteoporosis management: a systematic review. Osteoporos Int. 2011;22(10):2587–96.
40. Phillips L, Ferguson R, Diduck K, Lamb D, Jorgenson D. Integrating a brief pharmacist intervention into practice: osteoporosis pharmacotherapy assessment. Can Pharm J. 2012;145(5):218–20.
41. Wynn P. Pharmacists boning up on osteoporosis care. Drug Top. 2004;148:18s. http://drugtopics.modernmedicine.com/drug-topics/content/pharmacists-boning-osteoporosis-care?page=ful.
42. Adams KM, Kohlmeier M, Zeisel SH. Nutrition education in U.S. medical schools: latest update of a national survey. Acad Med. 2010;85(9):1537–42.
43. Eisman JA, Bogoch ER, Dell R, Harrington JT, McKinney Jr RE, McLelllan A, et al. Making the first fracture the last fracture: ASBMR task force report on secondary fracture prevention. J Bone Min Res. 2012;27(10):2039–46.
44. Miller AN, Lake AE, Emory CL. Establishing a fracture liaison service: an orthopaedic approach. J Bone Joint Surg Am. 2015;97(8):675–81.
45. Curtis J, Silverman SL. Commentary: the five Ws of a fracture liaison service: why, who, what, where, and how? Osteoporosis: we reap what we sow. Curr Osteoporos Rep. 2013;11(4):365. doi:10.1007/s11914-013-0177-9.
46. Miki RA, Oetgen ME, Kirk J, Insogna KL, Lindskog DM. Orthopaedic management improves the rate of early osteoporosis treatment after hip fracture: a randomized clinical trial. J Bone Joint Surg Am. 2008;90(11):2346–53.
47. Yates CJ, Chauchard M-A, Liew D, Bucknill A, Wark JD. Bridging the osteoporosis treatment gap: performance and cost-effectiveness of a fracture liaison service. J Clin Densitom. 2015;18(2):150–6.
48. Jonsson E, Strom O, Borgstrom F. OC8: cost effectiveness evaluation of fracture liaison services for the management of osteoporosis in Sweden. Osteoporos Int. 2015;26(Suppl 1). doi:10.1007/s00198-015-3067-4.
49. Singer A, Exuzides A, Spangler L, O'Malley C, Colby C, Johnston K, et al. Burden of illness for osteoporotic fractures compared with other serious diseases among postmenopausal women in the United States. Mayo Clin Proc. 2015;90:53–62.
50. Tosteson A. "The Costs to Society" in the burden of disease, bone health, osteoporosis and related bone diseases: report of the surgeon general's workshop on osteoporosis and bone health. 12–13 Dec 2002. Washington, DC. http://www.ncbi.nlm.nih.gov/books/NBK44689.

51. Ben Sedrine W, Radican L, Reginster JY. On conducting burden of osteoporosis studies: a review of the core concepts and practical issues. A study carried out under the auspices of a WHO Collaborating Center. Rheumatology. 2001;40(1):7–14.
52. American Academy of Orthopedic Surgeons. Position Statement 1113: osteoporosis/bone health in adults as a national public health priority. 1993–1994. http://www.aaos.org/CustomTemplates/Content.aspx?id=5604.
53. US Preventive Services Task Force. Screening for osteoporosis: recommendations from the U.S. Preventive Services Task Force. Ann Intern Med. 2011;154:356–64. doi:10.7326/0003-4819-154-5-201103010-00307.
54. Rizzoli R, Chevalley T. Fracture liaison services and secondary fracture prevention. Medicographia. 2014;35:219–24.
55. Champion VL, Skinner CE. The health belief model. In: Glanz K, Rkimer BK, Viswanath K, editors. Health behaviors and health education: theory, research, and practice. 3rd ed. Hoboken: Wiley; 2002. p. 49.

Index

C.V. Oleson, *Osteoporosis Rehabilitation*, DOI 10.1007/978-3-319-45084-1

MIX
Papier aus verantwortungsvollen Quellen
Paper from responsible sources
FSC® C105338
FSC
www.fsc.org

If you have any concerns about our products,
you can contact us on
ProductSafety@springernature.com

In case Publisher is established outside the EU,
the EU authorized representative is:
Springer Nature Customer Service Center GmbH
Europaplatz 3, 69115 Heidelberg, Germany

Printed by Libri Plureos GmbH
in Hamburg, Germany